a LANGE medical book

Katzung & Trevor's
Pharmacology

Examination & Board Review

eighth edition

Anthony J. Trevor, PhD
Professor Emeritus of Pharmacology and Toxicology
Department of Cellular & Molecular Pharmacology
University of California, San Francisco

Bertram G. Katzung, MD, PhD
Professor Emeritus of Pharmacology
Department of Cellular & Molecular Pharmacology
University of California, San Francisco

Susan B. Masters, PhD
Professor & Academy Chair of Pharmacology Education
Department of Cellular & Molecular Pharmacology
University of California, San Francisco

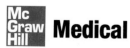 **Medical**

New York   Chicago   San Francisco   Lisbon   London
Madrid   Mexico City   Milan   New Delhi   San Juan
Seoul   Singapore   Sydney   Toronto

Katzung & Trevor's Pharmacology: Examination & Board Review, Eighth Edition

1 2 3 4 5 6 7 8 9 0   DOC/DOC   0 9 8 7

ISBN 978-0-07-148869-3
MHID 0-07-148869-3
ISSN 1063-8636

This book was set in Adobe Garamond by International Typesetting and Composition.
The editors were James Shanahan and Karen Davis.
The production supervisor was Sherri Souffrance.
Project management was provided by International Typesetting and Composition.
The text designer was Eve Siegel.
The cover designer was Pehrsson Design.
The cover photo shows a polarized light micrograph (PLM) of aspirin, also known as acetylsalicylic acid. Magnification: 4x.
Photo credit goes to Michael W. Davidson/Photo Researchers, Inc.
The index was prepared by Ken Hassman.
RR Donnelley was printer and binder.

This book is printed on acid-free paper.

Contents

Preface

This book is designed to help students review pharmacology and to prepare for both regular course examinations and board examinations. The eighth edition has been extensively revised to make such preparation as active and efficient as possible. As with earlier editions, rigorous standards of accuracy and currency have been maintained in keeping with the book's status as the companion to the textbook *Basic & Clinical Pharmacology*. The book divides pharmacology into the topics used in most courses and textbooks. Major introductory chapters (eg, autonomic pharmacology and CNS pharmacology) are included for integration with relevant physiology and biochemistry. The chapter-based approach facilitates use of this review book in conjunction with course notes or a larger text. We recommend several strategies to make reviewing more effective.

First, each chapter has a short discussion of the major concepts that underlie its basic principles or drug group, accompanied by explanatory figures and tables. Read the text thoroughly before you attempt to answer the study questions at the back of each chapter. If you find a concept difficult or confusing, consult a regular textbook, such as *Basic and Clinical Pharmacology*.

Second, each drug-oriented chapter (such as Chapter 7) opens with a "**Drug Tree**" that organizes the group of drugs visually. You should practice reproducing the Drug Tree diagram from memory.

Third, a list of **High-Yield Terms to Learn** and their definitions is near the front of each chapter. Make sure that you can define those terms.

Fourth, most chapters contain a "**Skill Keeper**" question ▶ that prompts you to review previous material and to see links between related topics. Try to answer the Skill Keeper questions on your own before checking the Skill Keeper answers that are provided at the end of the chapter.

Fifth, each drug-oriented chapter has a list of **Key Drugs** with drug names that you should recognize. For prototypes, you should be able to describe the mechanism of action and, if applicable, mechanisms of resistance to their action (eg, for antimicrobial and anticancer drugs). You should also know the pharmacokinetics and toxicity features that were emphasized in the chapter text. For each **Other Significant Agent** listed in the Key Drugs box, you should be able to identify its prototype and know the key way(s) in which it differs from the prototype.

Sixth, each chapter contains **sample questions** followed by a set of answers with explanations. For most effective learning, take each set of sample questions as if it were a real examination. After you have answered every question, work through the answers. When you are analyzing the answers, make sure that you understand why each choice is either correct or incorrect.

Seventh, each chapter ends with a **Checklist** of focused tasks that you should be able to do once you have finished with the chapter.

Eighth, when preparing for a comprehensive examination, you should review the list of drugs in Appendix I: Key Words for Key Drugs. Do this at the same time that you work your way through the chapters so that you can begin to recognize drugs out of the context of a chapter that discusses a restricted set of drugs.

Ninth, after you have worked your way through most or all of the chapters and have a good grasp of the Key Drugs, you should take the comprehensive examinations presented in Appendices II and III. These examinations are followed by a list of answers and the numbers of the chapters in which the answers are explained. Again, we recommend that you take an entire examination or a block of questions as if it were a real examination; commit to answers for the whole set before you check the answers. As you work though the answers, make sure you understand why each distracter is either correct or incorrect. If you need to, return to the relevant chapter(s) to review the text that covers key concepts and facts that form the basis of the question.

Tenth, you can use strategies in Appendix IV for improving your test performance. General advise for studying and approaching exams includes strategies for several types of questions that follow specific formats.

We recommend that this book be used with a regular text. *Basic & Clinical Pharmacology*, tenth edition (McGraw-Hill, 2007), follows the chapter sequence used here. However, this review book is designed to complement any standard medical pharmacology text. The student who completes and understands *Pharmacology: Examination & Board Review* will greatly improve his or her performance on examinations and will have an excellent command of pharmacology.

Because it was developed in parallel with the textbook *Basic & Clinical Pharmacology*, this review book represents the authors' interpretations of chapters written by contributors to that text. We are very grateful to these contributors, to our other faculty colleagues, and to our students—who have taught us most of what we know about teaching.

We very much appreciate the invaluable contributions to this text afforded by the editorial team of James Shanahan, Laura Libretti, Linda Conheady, Sherri Souffrance, and Karen Davis, and by Dr. S. Manikandan, Department of Pharmacology, Jawaharlal Institute of Postgraduate Medical Education and Research, Pondicherry, India.

Suggestions and criticisms regarding this study guide should be sent to us at the following address: Department of Cellular & Molecular Pharmacology, Box 0450, University of California School of Medicine, San Francisco, CA 94143-0450, USA.

Anthony J. Trevor, PhD
Bertram G. Katzung, MD, PhD
Susan B. Masters, PhD

PART I
Basic Principles

Introduction

Pharmacology is the body of knowledge concerned with the action of chemicals on biologic systems. **Medical pharmacology** is the area of pharmacology concerned with the use of chemicals in the prevention, diagnosis, and treatment of disease, especially in humans. **Toxicology** is the area of pharmacology concerned with the undesirable effects of chemicals on biologic systems. This chapter introduces basic principles that will be applied in subsequent chapters.

THE NATURE OF DRUGS

Drugs in common use include inorganic ions, nonpeptide organic molecules, small peptides and proteins, nucleic acids, lipids, and carbohydrates. Some are found in plants or animals, but many are partially or completely synthetic.

A. Size and Molecular Weight (MW)

Drugs vary in size from MW 7 (lithium) to over MW 50,000 (thrombolytic enzymes, other proteins). The majority of drugs, however, have molecular weights between 100 and 1000. Drugs smaller than MW 100 are rarely sufficiently selective, whereas drugs much larger than MW 1000 are often poorly absorbed and poorly distributed in the body.

B. Drug-Receptor Bonds

Drugs bind to receptors with a variety of chemical bonds. These include very strong covalent bonds (which usually result in irreversible action), somewhat weaker electrostatic bonds (eg, between a cation and an anion), and much weaker interactions (eg, hydrogen, van der Waals, and hydrophobic bonds).

THE MOVEMENT OF DRUGS IN THE BODY

In order to reach its receptors and bring about a biologic effect, a drug molecule (eg, a benzodiazepine sedative) must travel from the site of administration (eg, the gastrointestinal tract) to the site of action (eg, the brain).

A. Permeation

Permeation is the movement of drug molecules into and within the biologic environment. It involves several processes, the most important of which are discussed next.

1. Aqueous diffusion—Aqueous diffusion is the movement of molecules through the watery extracellular and intracellular spaces. The membranes of most capillaries have small water-filled pores that permit the aqueous diffusion of molecules up to the size of small proteins between the blood and the extravascular space. This is a passive process governed by Fick's law (see later discussion).

2. Lipid diffusion—Lipid diffusion is the movement of molecules through membranes and other lipid structures. Like aqueous diffusion, this is a passive process governed by Fick's law (see later discussion).

3. Transport by special carriers—Drugs that do not readily diffuse through membranes may be transported across barriers by mechanisms that carry similar endogenous substances. A very large number of such transporters have been identified, and many of these are important in the movement of drugs or as targets of drug action. Unlike aqueous and lipid diffusion, carrier transport is not governed by Fick's law and is capacity-limited.

HIGH-YIELD TERMS TO LEARN

Drugs	Substances that act on living systems at the chemical (molecular) level
Drug receptors	The molecular components of the body with which a drug interacts to bring about its effects
Distribution phase	The phase of drug movement from the site of administration into the tissues
Elimination phase	The phase of drug inactivation or removal from the body by metabolism or excretion
Endocytosis	Absorption of material across a cell membrane by enclosing it in cell membrane material and pulling it into the cell, where it can be released
First- and zero-order elimination	Mathematical descriptions of elimination processes that are proportional in rate to the concentration, or fixed and not dependent on concentration, respectively
Permeation	Movement of a molecule (eg, drug) though the biologic medium
Pharmacodynamics	The actions of a drug on the body, including receptor interactions, dose–response phenomena, and mechanisms of therapeutic and toxic action
Pharmacokinetics	The actions of the body on the drug, including absorption, distribution, metabolism, and elimination. Elimination of a drug may be achieved by metabolism or by excretion. *Biodisposition* is a term sometimes used to describe the processes of metabolism and excretion.
Transporter	A specialized molecule, usually a protein, in a membrane that carries a drug, transmitter, or other molecule across the membrane

Selective inhibitors for these carriers may have clinical value; for example, several antidepressants act by inhibiting the transport of amine neurotransmitters back into the nerve endings from which they have been released. Probenecid, which inhibits transport of uric acid, penicillin, and other weak acids in the nephron, is used to increase the excretion of uric acid in gout. The family of P-glycoprotein transport molecules, previously identified in malignant cells as one cause of cancer drug resistance, has been identified in the epithelium of the gastrointestinal tract and in the blood-brain barrier. After release, amine neurotransmitters (dopamine, norepinephrine, serotonin) and some other transmitters are recycled into nerve endings by transport molecules.

4. Endocytosis, pinocytosis—Endocytosis occurs through binding to specialized components (receptors) on cell membranes, with subsequent internalization by infolding of that area of the membrane. The contents of the resulting intracellular vesicle are subsequently released into the cytoplasm of the cell. Endocytosis permits very large or very lipid-insoluble chemicals to enter cells. For example, large molecules such as proteins may cross cell membranes by this mechanism. Smaller, polar substances such as vitamin B_{12} and iron combine with special proteins (B_{12} with intrinsic factor and iron with transferrin), and the complexes enter cells by this mechanism. Because the substance to be transported must combine with a membrane receptor, endocytotic transport can be quite selective. **Exocytosis** is the reverse process, ie, the expulsion of membrane-encapsulated material from cells.

B. FICK'S LAW OF DIFFUSION

Fick's law predicts the rate of movement of molecules across a barrier; the concentration gradient ($C_1 - C_2$) and permeability coefficient for the drug and the area and thickness of the barrier membrane are used to compute the rate, as follows:

$$\text{Rate} = (C_1 - C_2) \times \frac{\text{Permeability coefficient}}{\text{Thickness}} \times \text{Area} \quad \textbf{(1)}$$

This relationship quantifies the observation that drug absorption is faster from organs with large surface areas, such as the small intestine, than from organs with smaller absorbing areas (the stomach). Furthermore, drug absorption is faster from organs with thin membrane barriers (eg, the lung) than from those with thick barriers (eg, the skin).

C. WATER AND LIPID SOLUBILITY OF DRUGS

1. Aqueous diffusion—The aqueous solubility of a drug is often a function of the electrostatic charge (degree of ionization, polarity) of the molecule, because water molecules behave as dipoles and are attracted to charged drug molecules, forming an aqueous shell around them. Conversely, the lipid solubility of a molecule is inversely proportionate to its charge.

2. Lipid diffusion—Many drugs are weak bases or weak acids. For such molecules, the *pH of the medium* determines the fraction of molecules charged (ionized) versus uncharged (nonionized). If the pK_a of the drug and the pH of the medium are known, the fraction of molecules in the ionized state can be predicted by means of the Henderson-Hasselbalch equation:

$$\log\left(\frac{\text{Protonated form}}{\text{Unprotonated form}}\right) = pK_a - pH \qquad (2)$$

"Protonated" means *associated with a proton* (a hydrogen ion); this form of the equation applies to both acids and bases.

3. Ionization of weak acids and bases—Weak bases are ionized—and therefore more polar and more water-soluble—when they are protonated. Weak acids are not ionized—and so are less water-soluble—when they are protonated.

The following equations summarize these points:

$RNH_3^+ \rightleftharpoons \qquad RNH_2 \qquad + \qquad H^+$
protonated weak base (charged, more water-soluble) 　unprotonated weak base (uncharged, more lipid-soluble) 　proton

$\qquad\qquad\qquad\qquad\qquad\qquad\qquad (3)$

$RCOOH \rightleftharpoons \qquad RCOO^- \qquad + \qquad H^+$
protonated weak acid (uncharged, more lipid-soluble) 　unprotonated weak acid (uncharged, more water-soluble) 　proton

$\qquad\qquad\qquad\qquad\qquad\qquad\qquad (4)$

The Henderson-Hasselbalch relationship is clinically important when it is necessary to estimate or alter the partition of drugs between compartments of differing pH. For example, most drugs are freely filtered at the glomerulus, but lipid-soluble drugs can be rapidly reabsorbed from the tubular urine. If a patient takes an overdose of a weak acid drug, eg, aspirin, the excretion of this drug may be accelerated by alkalinizing the urine, eg, by giving bicarbonate. This is because a drug that is a weak acid dissociates to its charged, polar form in alkaline solution, and this form cannot readily diffuse from the renal tubule back into the blood. Conversely, excretion of a weak base (eg, pyrimethamine, amphetamine) may be accelerated by acidifying the urine, eg, by administering ammonium chloride (Figure 1–1).

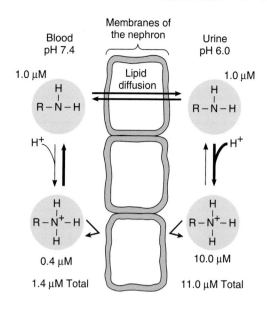

Figure 1–1. The Henderson-Hasselbalch principle applied to drug excretion in the urine. Because the nonionized form diffuses readily across the lipid barriers of the nephron, this form may reach equal concentrations in the blood and urine; in contrast, the ionized form does not diffuse as readily. Protonation will occur within the blood and the urine according to the Henderson-Hasselbalch equation. Pyrimethamine, a weak base of pK_a 7.0, is used in this example. At blood pH, only 0.4 μmol of the protonated species will be present for each 1.0 μmol of the unprotonated form. The total concentration in the blood will thus be 1.4 μmol/L if the concentration of the unprotonated form is 1.0 μmol/L. In the urine at pH 6.0, 10 μmol of the nondiffusible ionized form will be present for each 1.0 μmol of the unprotonated, diffusible, form. Therefore, the total urine concentration (11 μmol/L) may be almost 8 times higher than the blood concentration.

ABSORPTION OF DRUGS

A. ROUTES OF ADMINISTRATION

Drugs usually enter the body at sites remote from the target tissue or organ and thus require transport by the circulation to the intended site of action. To enter the bloodstream, a drug must be absorbed from its site of administration (unless the drug has been injected directly into the bloodstream). The rate and efficiency of absorption differ depending on a drug's route of administration. In fact, for some drugs, the amount absorbed may be only a small fraction of the dose administered when given by certain routes. The amount absorbed into the systemic circulation divided by the amount of drug administered constitutes its **bioavailability** by that route. Common routes of administration and some of their features include the following:

1. Oral (swallowed)—The oral route offers maximum convenience, but absorption may be slower and less complete than when parenteral routes are used. Ingested drugs are subject to the **first-pass effect,** in which a significant amount of the agent is metabolized in the gut wall, portal circulation, and liver before it reaches the systemic circulation. Thus, some drugs have low bioavailability when given orally.

2. Intravenous—The intravenous route offers instantaneous and complete absorption (by definition, bioavailability is 100%). This route is potentially more dangerous, however, because of the high blood levels reached if administration is too rapid.

3. Intramuscular—Absorption from an intramuscular injection site is often faster and more complete (higher bioavailability) than with oral administration. Large volumes (eg, >5 mL into each buttock) may be given if the drug is not too irritating. First-pass metabolism is avoided, but anticoagulants such as heparin cannot be given by this route because they may cause bleeding (hematomas) in the muscle.

4. Subcutaneous—The subcutaneous route offers slower absorption than the intramuscular route. Large-volume bolus doses are less feasible, but heparin does not cause hematomas when administered by this route. First-pass metabolism is avoided.

5. Buccal and sublingual—The sublingual route (under the tongue) permits direct absorption into the systemic venous circulation, bypassing the hepatic portal circuit and first-pass metabolism. This process may be fast or slow depending on the physical formulation of the product. The buccal route (in the pouch between the gums and cheek) offers the same features as the sublingual route.

6. Rectal (suppository)—The rectal route offers partial avoidance of the first-pass effect (though not as completely as the sublingual route). This is because suppositories tend to migrate upward in the rectum and absorption from this higher location is partially into the portal circulation. Larger amounts of drug and drugs with unpleasant tastes are better administered rectally than by the buccal or sublingual routes. Rectal administration is often used in patients who are vomiting. Some drugs administered rectally may cause significant irritation.

7. Inhalation—In the case of respiratory diseases, the inhalation route offers delivery closest to the target tissue. This route often results in rapid absorption because of the large and thin alveolar surface area available. Inhalation is particularly convenient for drugs that are gases at room temperature (eg, nitrous oxide, nitric oxide) or easily volatilized (many general anesthetics).

8. Topical—The topical route includes application to the skin or to the mucous membrane of the eye, ear, nose, throat, airway, or vagina for *local* effect. The rate of absorption varies with the area of application and the drug's formulation but is usually slower than any of the routes listed previously.

9. Transdermal—The transdermal route involves application to the skin for *systemic* effect. Absorption usually occurs very slowly (because of the thickness of the skin), but the first-pass effect is avoided.

B. Blood Flow

Blood flow influences absorption from intramuscular and subcutaneous sites and, in shock, from the gastrointestinal tract as well. High blood flow maintains a high drug depot-to-blood concentration gradient and thus facilitates absorption.

C. Concentration

The concentration of drug at the site of administration is important in determining the concentration gradient relative to the blood as noted previously. As indicated by Fick's law (Equation 1), the concentration gradient is a major determinant of the rate of absorption. Drug concentration in the vehicle is particularly important in the absorption of drugs applied topically for dermatologic conditions.

DISTRIBUTION OF DRUGS

A. Determinants of Distribution

The distribution of drugs to the tissues depends upon the following:

1. Size of the organ—The size of the organ determines the concentration gradient between blood and the organ. For example, skeletal muscle can take up a large amount of drug because the concentration in the muscle tissue remains low (and the blood–tissue gradient high) even after relatively large amounts of drug have been transferred; this occurs because skeletal muscle is a very large organ. In contrast, because the brain is smaller, distribution of a smaller amount of drug into it will raise the tissue concentration and reduce to zero the blood-tissue concentration gradient, preventing further uptake of drug.

2. Blood flow—Blood flow to the tissue is an important determinant of the *rate* of uptake, although blood flow may not affect the steady-state amount of drug in the tissue. As a result, well-perfused tissues (eg, brain, heart, kidneys, splanchnic organs) usually will achieve high tissue concentrations sooner than poorly perfused tissues (eg, fat, bone). If the drug is rapidly eliminated, the concentration in poorly perfused tissues may never rise significantly.

3. Solubility—The solubility of a drug in tissue influences the concentration of the drug in the extracellular fluid surrounding the blood vessels. If the drug is very soluble in the cells, the concentration in the perivascular extracellular space will be lower and diffusion from the vessel into the extravascular tissue space will be facilitated. For example, some organs (including the brain) have a high lipid content and thus dissolve a high concentration of lipid-soluble agents. As a result, a very lipid-soluble anesthetic will transfer out of the blood and into the brain tissue more rapidly and to a greater extent than a drug with low lipid solubility.

4. Binding—Binding of a drug to macromolecules in the blood or a tissue compartment will tend to increase the drug's concentration in that compartment. For example, warfarin is strongly bound to plasma albumin, which restricts warfarin's diffusion out of the vascular compartment. Conversely, chloroquine is strongly bound to extravascular tissue proteins, which results in a marked reduction in the plasma concentration of chloroquine.

B. APPARENT VOLUME OF DISTRIBUTION AND PHYSICAL VOLUMES

The apparent volume of distribution (V_d) is an important pharmacokinetic parameter that reflects the above determinants of the distribution of a drug in the body. V_d relates the amount of drug in the body to the concentration in the plasma (Chapter 3). In contrast, the physical volumes of various body compartments are less important in pharmacokinetics (Table 1–1).

METABOLISM OF DRUGS

Metabolism of a drug sometimes terminates its action, but other effects of drug metabolism are also important. Some drugs when given orally are metabolized before they enter the systemic circulation. This first-pass metabolism was referred to above as one cause of low bioavailability. Drug metabolism occurs primarily in the liver and is discussed in greater detail in Chapter 4.

A. DRUG METABOLISM AS A MECHANISM OF TERMINATION OF DRUG ACTION

The action of many drugs (eg, sympathomimetics, phenothiazines) is terminated before they are excreted because

Table 1–1. Average values for some physical volumes within the adult human body.

Compartment	Volume (L/kg body weight)
Plasma	0.04
Blood	0.08
Extracellular water	0.2
Total body water	0.6
Fat	0.2–0.35

they are metabolized to biologically inactive derivatives. Conversion to a metabolite is a form of **elimination.**

B. DRUG METABOLISM AS A MECHANISM OF DRUG ACTIVATION

Prodrugs (eg, levodopa, minoxidil) are inactive as administered and must be metabolized in the body to become active. Many drugs are active as administered and have active metabolites as well (eg, some benzodiazepines).

C. DRUG ELIMINATION WITHOUT METABOLISM

Some drugs (eg, lithium) are not modified by the body; they continue to act until they are excreted.

ELIMINATION OF DRUGS

Along with the dosage, the rate of elimination following the last dose (disappearance of the active molecules from the bloodstream or body) determines the duration of action for most drugs. Therefore, knowledge of the time course of concentration in plasma is important in predicting the intensity and duration of effect for most drugs. *Note:* Drug *elimination* is not the same as drug *excretion:* A drug may be eliminated by metabolism long before the modified molecules are excreted from the body. For most drugs and metabolites, excretion is primarily by way of the kidney. Anesthetic gases, a major exception, are excreted primarily by the lungs. For drugs with active metabolites (eg, diazepam), elimination of the parent molecule by metabolism is not synonymous with termination of action. For drugs that are not metabolized, excretion is the mode of elimination. A small number of drugs combine irreversibly with their receptors, so that disappearance from the bloodstream is not equivalent to cessation of drug action: These drugs may have a very prolonged action. For example, phenoxybenzamine, an irreversible inhibitor of α adrenoceptors, is eliminated from the bloodstream in less than 1 h after administration. The drug's action, however, lasts for 48 h.

A. FIRST-ORDER ELIMINATION

The term *first-order elimination* implies that the rate of elimination is proportionate to the concentration (ie, the higher the concentration, the greater the amount of drug eliminated per unit time). The result is that the drug's concentration in plasma decreases exponentially with time (Figure 1–2, left panel). Drugs with first-order elimination have a characteristic **half-life of elimination** that is constant regardless of the amount of drug in the body. The concentration of such a drug in the blood will decrease by 50% for every half-life. Most drugs in clinical use demonstrate first-order kinetics.

B. ZERO-ORDER ELIMINATION

The term *zero-order elimination* implies that the rate of elimination is constant regardless of concentration

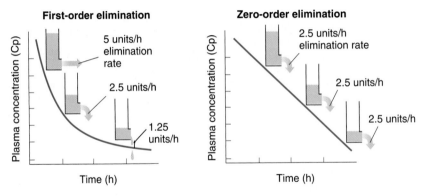

Figure 1–2. Comparison of first-order and zero-order elimination. For drugs with first-order kinetics (left panel), rate of elimination (units per hour) is proportionate to concentration; this is the more common process. In the case of zero-order elimination (right panel), the rate is constant and independent of concentration.

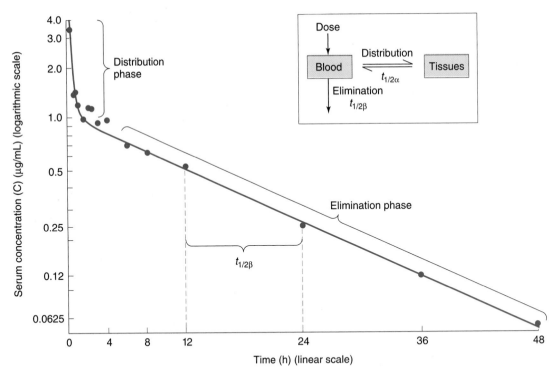

Figure 1–3. Serum concentration-time curve after administration of chlordiazepoxide as an intravenous bolus. The experimental data are plotted on a semilogarithmic scale as filled circles. This drug follows first-order kinetics and appears to occupy 2 compartments. The initial curvilinear portion of the data represents the distribution phase, with drug equilibrating between the blood compartment and the tissue compartment. The linear portion of the curve represents drug elimination. The elimination half-life ($t_{1/2\beta}$) can be extracted graphically as shown by measuring the time between any 2 plasma concentration points on the elimination phase that differ by twofold. (See Chapter 3 for additional details.) (Modified and reproduced, with permission, from Greenblatt DJ, Koch-Weser J: Drug therapy: Clinical pharmacokinetics. N Engl J Med 1975;293:702. Copyright © 1975 Massachusetts Medical Society. All rights reserved.)

(Figure 1–2, right panel). This occurs with drugs that saturate their elimination mechanisms at concentrations of clinical interest. As a result, the concentrations of these drugs in plasma decrease in a linear fashion over time. This is typical of ethanol (over most of its plasma concentration range) and of phenytoin and aspirin at high therapeutic or toxic concentrations.

PHARMACOKINETIC MODELS

A. MULTICOMPARTMENT DISTRIBUTION

After absorption into the circulation, many drugs undergo an early distribution phase followed by a slower elimination phase. Mathematically, this behavior can be simulated by means of a "2-compartment model" as shown in Figure 1–3. The 2 compartments consist of the blood and the extravascular tissues. (Note that each phase is associated with a characteristic half-life: $t_{1/2\alpha}$ for the first phase, $t_{1/2\beta}$ for the second phase. Note also that when concentration is plotted on a logarithmic axis, the elimination phase for a first-order drug is a straight line.)

B. OTHER DISTRIBUTION MODELS

A few drugs behave as if they are distributed to only 1 compartment (eg, if they are restricted to the vascular compartment). Others have more complex distributions that require more than 2 compartments for construction of accurate mathematical models.

QUESTIONS

1. A 3-year-old child is brought to the emergency department having just ingested a large overdose of promethazine, an antihistaminic drug. Promethazine is a weak base with a pK_a of 9.1. It is capable of entering most tissues, including the brain. On physical examination, the heart rate is 100/min, blood pressure 110/60 mm Hg, and respiratory rate 20/min. In this case of promethazine overdose,
   (A) Urinary excretion would be accelerated by administration of NH_4Cl, an acidifying agent
   (B) Urinary excretion would be accelerated by giving $NaHCO_3$, an alkalinizing agent
   (C) More of the drug would be ionized at blood pH than at stomach pH
   (D) Absorption of the drug would be faster from the stomach than from the small intestine
   (E) Hemodialysis is the only effective therapy

2. Which one of the following processes is best suited for permeation of very large protein molecules into cells?
   (A) Aqueous diffusion
   (B) Aqueous hydrolysis
   (C) Endocytosis
   (D) Lipid diffusion
   (E) Special carrier transport

3. A patient with a history of episodic attacks of coughing, wheezing, and shortness of breath is being evaluated in the asthma clinic. Several drug treatments with different routes of administration are under consideration. Which of the following statements about routes of administration is MOST correct?
   (A) Blood levels often rise more slowly after intramuscular injection than after oral dosing
   (B) The first-pass effect is the result of elimination of a drug after administration and before it enters the systemic circulation
   (C) Administration of antiasthmatic drugs by inhaled aerosol is usually associated with more adverse effects (eg, tachycardia, tremor) than is administration of these drugs by mouth
   (D) Bioavailability of most drugs is greater with rectal (suppository) administration than with sublingual administration
   (E) Administration of a drug by transdermal patch is often faster but is associated with more first-pass metabolism than oral administration

4. Aspirin is a weak organic acid with a pK_a of 3.5. What percentage of a given dose will be in the lipid-soluble form in the duodenum at a pH of 4.5?
   (A) About 1%
   (B) About 10%
   (C) About 50%
   (D) About 90%
   (E) About 99%

5. If the plasma concentration of a drug declines with "first-order kinetics," this means that
   (A) There is only 1 metabolic path for drug disposition
   (B) The half-life is the same regardless of the plasma concentration
   (C) The drug is largely metabolized in the liver after oral administration and has low bioavailability
   (D) The rate of elimination is proportionate to the rate of administration at all times
   (E) The drug is distributed to only 1 compartment outside the vascular system

6. Regarding termination of drug action,
   (A) Drugs must be excreted from the body to terminate their action
   (B) Metabolism of drugs always increases their water solubility
   (C) Metabolism of drugs always abolishes their pharmacologic activity
   (D) Hepatic metabolism and renal excretion are the 2 most important mechanisms involved
   (E) Distribution of a drug out of the bloodstream terminates the drug's effects

7. Distribution of drugs to specific tissues
   (A) Is independent of blood flow to the organ
   (B) Is independent of the solubility of the drug in that tissue
   (C) Depends on the unbound drug concentration gradient between blood and the tissue
   (D) Is increased for drugs that are strongly bound to plasma proteins
   (E) Has no effect on the half-life of the drug

8. Timolol is being considered for the treatment of glaucoma in a 58-year-old patient. Except for elevated intraocular pressure, the patient's history and physical examination are unremarkable. Timolol is a weak base of pK_a 9.2. Which of the following statements is MOST correct?
   (A) If given by the intravenous route, the concentration of timolol in the aqueous humor (pH 7.8) will be lower than the concentration in the duodenum (pH 5.5)
   (B) When administered as eyedrops, the rate of absorption into the eye will be slower if the drops are alkaline (pH 8.0) than if they are acidic (pH 5.0)
   (C) Excretion in the urine will be slower if urine pH is alkaline (pH 8.0) than if the urine pH is acidic (pH 5.8)
   (D) The proportion of timolol in the protonated form will be approximately 10% at pH 8.2
   (E) The proportion of timolol in the more lipid-soluble form will be approximately 10% at pH 10.2

9. A process by which a weak acid becomes less water soluble and more lipid soluble at low pH is
   (A) Distribution
   (B) Elimination
   (C) First-pass effect
   (D) Permeation
   (E) Protonation

10. The set of properties that characterize the effects of a drug on the body is called
    (A) Distribution
    (B) Permeation
    (C) Pharmacodynamics
    (D) Pharmacokinetics
    (E) Protonation

11. The set of properties that characterize the effects of the body on a drug is called
    (A) Absorption
    (B) Distribution
    (C) Elimination
    (D) First-order kinetics
    (E) Pharmacokinetics

12. The most general term for the process by which the amount of active drug in the body is reduced after absorption into the systemic circulation is
    (A) Distribution
    (B) Elimination
    (C) Excretion
    (D) First-order elimination
    (E) Metabolism

13. The process by which the amount of drug in the body is reduced after administration but before entering the systemic circulation is called
    (A) Excretion
    (B) First-order elimination
    (C) First-pass effect
    (D) Metabolism
    (E) Pharmacokinetics

14. The kinetics that are characteristic of the elimination of ethanol and high doses of phenytoin and aspirin are called
    (A) Distribution
    (B) Excretion
    (C) First-pass effect
    (D) First-order elimination
    (E) Zero-order elimination

ANSWERS

1. Questions that deal with acid-base (Henderson-Hasselbalch) manipulations are common on examinations. Since absorption involves permeation across lipid membranes, we can treat an overdose by decreasing absorption from the gut and reabsorption from the tubular urine by making the drug *less lipid soluble.* Ionization attracts water molecules and decreases lipid solubility. Promethazine is a weak base, which means that it will be more ionized (protonated) at acid pH than at basic pH. Choice **C** suggests that the drug would be more ionized at pH 7.4 than at pH 2.0: clearly wrong. Choice **D** says (in effect) that the more ionized form will be absorbed faster, which is incorrect. **A** and **B** are opposites because NH_4Cl is an acidifying salt and sodium bicarbonate an alkalinizing one. From the point of view of test strategy, opposites always deserve careful attention and, in this case, encourage us to exclude **E,** a distracter. Because an acid environment favors ionization of a weak base, we should give NH_4Cl. The answer is **A.** Note that similar questions may be designed around other compartments, eg, prostatic and vaginal fluids, and breast milk (more acidic than blood) and cerebrospinal fluid and aqueous humor (more alkaline).

2. Endocytosis is an important mechanism for transport of very large molecules across membranes. Aqueous diffusion is rarely used for transport across cell membranes. Lipid diffusion and special carrier transport are common for smaller molecules. Hydrolysis has nothing to do with the mechanisms of permeation; rather, hydrolysis is one mechanism of drug metabolism. The answer is **C**.

3. Blood levels usually rise more *rapidly* after intramuscular injection than after oral administration. Choice **C** is wrong: Delivering the drug directly to the target organ usually *reduces* adverse effects because the required total dose is smaller and the concentration reaching other organs is lower. Bioavailability is usually greater after sublingual than after rectal administration. Onset of effect is usually slower with transdermal administration than with any other route, but it does avoid the first-pass effect. The answer is **B**.

4. Aspirin is an acid, so it will be more ionized at alkaline pH and less ionized at acidic pH. The Henderson-Hasselbalch equation predicts that the ratio will change from 50/50 at the pH equal to the pK_a to 1/10 (protonated/unprotonated) at 1 pH unit more alkaline than the pK_a. For acids, the protonated form is the nonionized, more lipid-soluble form. The answer is **B**.

5. "First-order" means that the elimination rate is proportionate to the concentration perfusing the organ of elimination. The half-life is a constant. The rate of elimination is proportionate to the rate of administration only at steady state. The order of elimination is independent of the number of compartments into which a drug distributes. The answer is **B**.

6. Note the "trigger" words ("must," "always") in choices **A** and **B**. All drugs that affect tissues other than the blood or vascular endothelium act outside of the "bloodstream." The answer is **D**.

7. This is a straightforward question of distribution concepts. There are no trigger words to give the answer away, but it can be deduced without much trouble. From the list of determinants of drug distribution given previously, choice **C** is correct.

8. More Henderson-Hasselbalch concepts. Weak bases are more protonated in an acidic environment because more protons (hydrogen ions) are available. In the protonated state, weak bases are ionized, polar, and less lipid soluble. Therefore, less timolol is lipid soluble and able to diffuse back into the blood from the duodenum (pH 5.5) than is able to diffuse through the surface of the eye (pH 7.8). By the same reasoning, the drug diffuses faster if the eyedrops are alkaline than if they are acidic. Less drug diffuses back into the body from the urine if the urine pH is acidic than if it is alkaline, so excretion will be faster in acidic urine. The answer is **A**.

9. Protonation (combination with a proton, H^+) causes a weak acid to lose its negative electrical charge and become less polar and more lipid soluble. The answer is **E**.

10. More definitions. Pharmacodynamics is the term given to the properties of drug action on the body. The answer is **C**.

11. Pharmacokinetics is the general term that denotes all of the body's actions on the drug. The answer is **E**.

12. The amount of active drug is reduced by excretion and metabolism, processes that are included in the term "elimination." The answer is **B**.

13. "First-pass effect" is the term given to elimination of a drug before it enters the systemic circulation (ie, on its first pass through the portal circulation and liver). The answer is **C**.

14. The excretion of most drugs is determined by first-order kinetics. However, ethanol and, in higher doses, aspirin and phenytoin follow zero-order kinetics (ie, their elimination rates are constant regardless of blood concentration). The answer is **E**.

CHECKLIST

When you complete this chapter, you should be able to:

☐ Predict the relative ease of permeation of a weak acid or base from a knowledge of its pK_a, the pH of the medium, and the Henderson-Hasselbalch equation.

☐ List and discuss the common routes of drug administration and excretion.

☐ Draw graphs of the blood level versus time for drugs subject to zero-order elimination and for drugs subject to first-order elimination. Label the axes appropriately.

Pharmacodynamics

Pharmacodynamics deals with the effects of drugs on biologic systems, whereas pharmacokinetics (Chapter 3) deals with actions of the biologic system on the drug. The principles of pharmacodynamics apply to all biologic systems, from isolated receptors in the test tube to patients with specific diseases.

RECEPTORS

Receptors are the specific molecules in a biologic system with which drugs interact to produce changes in the function of the system. Receptors must be selective in their ligand-binding characteristics (so as to respond to the proper chemical signal and not to meaningless ones). Receptors must also be modifiable when they bind a drug molecule (so as to bring about the functional change). Many receptors have been identified, purified, chemically characterized, and cloned. The great majority are proteins; a few are other macromolecules such as DNA. The **receptor site** (also known as the **recognition site**) for a drug is the specific binding region of the receptor macromolecule and has a relatively high and selective affinity for the drug molecule. The interaction of a drug with its receptor is the fundamental event that initiates the action of the drug.

EFFECTORS

Effectors are molecules that translate the drug–receptor interaction into a change in cellular activity. The best examples of effectors are enzymes such as adenylyl cyclase. Some receptors are also effectors in that a single molecule may incorporate both the drug binding site and the effector mechanism. For example, a tyrosine kinase effector is part of the insulin receptor molecule, and a sodium-potassium channel is the effector part of the nicotinic acetylcholine receptor.

GRADED DOSE-RESPONSE RELATIONSHIPS

When the response of a particular receptor-effector system is measured against increasing concentrations of a drug, the graph of the response versus the drug concentration or dose is called a *graded dose-response curve* (Figure 2–1, panel A). Plotting the same data on a semilogarithmic concentration axis usually results in a sigmoid curve, which simplifies the mathematical manipulation of the dose-response data (Figure 2–1, panel B). The efficacy (E_{max}) and potency (EC_{50} or ED_{50}) parameters are derived from these data. The *smaller* the EC_{50} (or ED_{50}), the *greater* the potency of the drug.

GRADED DOSE-BINDING RELATIONSHIP & BINDING AFFINITY

It is possible to measure the fraction of receptors bound by a drug, and, by plotting this fraction against the log of the concentration of the drug, a graph similar to the dose-response curve is obtained (Figure 2–1, panel C). The concentration of drug required to bind 50% of the receptor sites is denoted the K_d and is a useful measure of the affinity of a drug molecule for its binding site on the receptor molecule. The smaller the K_d, the greater the affinity of the drug for its receptor. If the number of binding sites on each receptor molecule is known, it is possible to determine the total number of receptors in the system from the B_{max}.

QUANTAL DOSE-RESPONSE RELATIONSHIPS

When the minimum dose required to produce a specified response is determined in each member of a population, the quantal dose-response relationship is defined (Figure 2–2). For example, a blood pressure-lowering drug might be studied by measuring the dose required to lower the mean arterial pressure by 20 mm Hg in 100 patients. When plotted as the fraction of the population that shows this response at each dose versus the log of the dose administered, a cumulative quantal dose-response curve, usually sigmoid in shape, is obtained. The **median effective (ED_{50})**, **median toxic (TD_{50})**, and (in animals) **median lethal (LD_{50})** doses are derived from experiments carried out in this manner. Because the magnitude of the specified effect is arbitrarily determined, the ED_{50} determined by quantal dose-response measurements has no direct relationship to the

---

HIGH-YIELD TERMS TO LEARN

Receptor	A molecule to which a drug binds to bring about a change in function of the biologic system
Inert binding molecule or site	A molecule to which a drug may bind without changing any function
Receptor site	Specific region of the receptor molecule to which the drug binds
Spare receptor	Receptor that does not bind drug when the drug concentration is sufficient to produce maximal effect; present when $K_d > EC_{50}$
Effector	Component of a system that accomplishes the biologic effect after being activated by an agonist; often a channel or enzyme molecule
Agonist	A drug that activates its receptor upon binding
Pharmacologic antagonist	A drug that binds without activating its receptor and thereby prevents activation by an agonist
Competitive antagonist	A pharmacologic antagonist that can be overcome by increasing the concentration of agonist
Irreversible antagonist	A pharmacologic antagonist that cannot be overcome by increasing agonist concentration
Physiologic antagonist	A drug that counters the effects of another by binding to a different receptor and causing opposing effects
Chemical antagonist	A drug that counters the effects of another by binding the agonist drug (not the receptor)
Partial agonist	A drug that binds to its receptor but produces a smaller effect at full dosage than a full agonist
Graded dose-response curve	A graph of increasing response to increasing drug concentration or dose
Quantal dose-response curve	A graph of the fraction of a population that shows a specified response at progressively increasing doses
EC_{50}, ED_{50}, TD_{50}, etc	In graded dose-response curves, the concentration or dose that causes 50% of the maximum effect or toxicity. In quantal dose-response curves, the concentration or dose that causes a specified response in 50% of the population under study.
K_d	The concentration of drug that binds 50% of the receptors in the system
Efficacy, maximal efficacy	The maximum effect that can be achieved with a particular drug, regardless of dose

---

ED_{50} determined from graded dose-response curves. Unlike the graded dose-response determination, no attempt is made to determine the maximal effect of the drug.

EFFICACY

Efficacy—often called maximal efficacy—is the greatest effect (E_{max}) an agonist can produce if the dose is taken to very high levels. Efficacy is determined mainly by the nature of the drug and the receptor and its associated effector system. It can be measured with a graded dose-response curve (Figure 2–1) but not with a quantal dose-response curve. By definition, partial agonists have lower maximal efficacy than full agonists (see later discussion).

POTENCY

Potency denotes the amount of drug needed to produce a given effect. In graded dose-response measurements, the effect usually chosen is 50% of the maximal effect and the dose causing this effect is called the EC_{50} (Figure 2–1, panels A and B). Potency is determined mainly by the

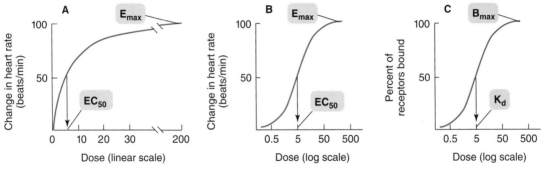

Figure 2–1. Graded dose-response and dose-binding graphs. (In isolated tissue preparations, *concentration (C)* is usually used as the measure of dose.) **A.** Relation between drug dose or concentration (abscissa) and drug effect (ordinate). When the dose axis is linear, a hyperbolic curve is commonly obtained. **B.** Same data, logarithmic dose axis. The dose or concentration at which effect is half-maximal is denoted EC_{50}, whereas the maximal effect is E_{max}. **C.** If the percentage of receptors that bind drug is plotted against drug concentration, a similar curve is obtained, and the concentration at which 50% of the receptors are bound is denoted K_d and the maximal number of receptors bound is termed B_{max}.

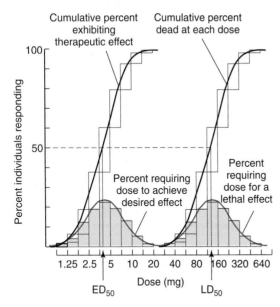

Figure 2–2. Quantal dose-response plots from a study of the therapeutic and lethal effects of a new drug in mice. Shaded boxes (and the accompanying curves) indicate the frequency distribution of doses of drug required to produce a specified effect, ie, the percentage of animals that required a particular dose to exhibit the effect. The open boxes (and corresponding curves) indicate the cumulative frequency distribution of responses, which are lognormally distributed. (Reproduced, with permission, from Katzung BG, editor: *Basic & Clinical Pharmacology*, 9th ed. McGraw-Hill, 2004.)

affinity of the receptor for the drug and the number of receptors available. In quantal dose-response measurements, ED_{50}, TD_{50}, and LD_{50} are also potency variables (median effective, toxic, and lethal doses, respectively, in 50% of the population studied). Thus, potency can be determined from either graded or quantal dose-response curves (eg, Figures 2–1 and 2–2), but the numbers obtained are not identical.

SPARE RECEPTORS

Spare receptors are said to exist if the maximal drug response (E_{max}) is obtained at less than maximal occupation of the receptors (B_{max}). In practice, the determination is usually made by comparing the concentration for 50% of maximal effect (EC_{50}) with the concentration for 50% of maximal binding (K_d). If the EC_{50} is less than the K_d, spare receptors are said to exist (Figure 2–3). This might result from 1 of 2 mechanisms. First, the duration of the *activation of the effector* may be much greater than the duration of the *drug–receptor interaction*. Second, the actual number of receptors may exceed the number of effector molecules available. The presence of spare receptors increases sensitivity to the agonist because the likelihood of a drug–receptor interaction increases in proportion to the number of receptors available. (For contrast, the system depicted in Figure 2–1, panels B and C, does not have spare receptors, since the EC_{50} and the K_d are equal.)

INERT BINDING SITES

Inert binding sites are components of endogenous molecules that bind a drug without initiating events leading to any of the drug's effects. In some compartments of the

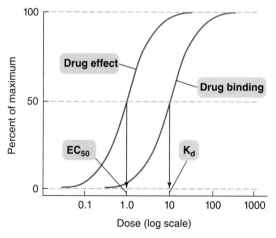

Figure 2–3. In a system with spare receptors, the EC_{50} is lower than the K_d, indicating that to achieve 50% of maximal effect, fewer than 50% of the receptors must be activated. Explanations for this phenomenon are discussed in the text.

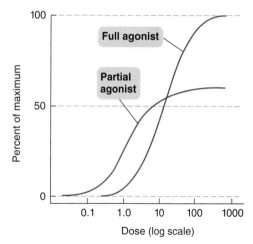

Figure 2–4. Comparison of dose-response curves for a full agonist and a partial agonist. The partial agonist acts on the same receptor system as the full agonist but cannot produce as large an effect (it has lower maximal efficacy), no matter how much the dose is increased. A partial agonist may be more potent (as in the figure), less potent, or equally potent; potency is an independent factor.

body (eg, the plasma), inert binding sites play an important role in buffering the concentration of a drug because bound drug does not contribute directly to the concentration gradient that drives diffusion. The 2 most important plasma proteins with significant drug-binding capacity are **albumin** and **orosomucoid** (α_1-acid glycoprotein).

AGONISTS & PARTIAL AGONISTS

An agonist is a drug capable of fully activating the effector system when it binds to the receptor. A partial agonist produces less than the full effect, even when it has saturated the receptors (Figure 2–4). In the presence of a full agonist, a partial agonist acts as an inhibitor.

ANTAGONISTS

A. COMPETITIVE AND IRREVERSIBLE PHARMACOLOGIC ANTAGONISTS

Competitive antagonists are drugs that bind to, or very close to, the receptor site in a reversible way without activating the effector system for that receptor. In the presence of a competitive antagonist, the log dose-response curve is shifted to higher doses (ie, horizontally to the right on the dose axis) but the same maximal effect is reached (Figure 2–5A). The agonist, if given in a high enough concentration, can displace the antagonist and fully activate the receptors. In contrast, an irreversible antagonist causes a downward shift of the maximum, with no shift of the curve on the dose axis

unless spare receptors are present (Figure 2–5B). Unlike the effects of a competitive antagonist, the effects of an irreversible antagonist cannot be overcome by adding more agonist. Competitive antagonists increase the ED_{50}; irreversible antagonists do not (unless spare receptors are present).

B. PHYSIOLOGIC ANTAGONISTS

A physiologic antagonist binds to a *different* receptor molecule, producing an effect opposite to that produced by the drug it antagonizes. Thus it differs from a pharmacologic antagonist, which interacts with the *same* receptor as the drug it is inhibiting. A familiar example is the antagonism of the bronchoconstrictor action of histamine (mediated at histamine receptors) by epinephrine's bronchodilator action (mediated at beta adrenoceptors).

C. CHEMICAL ANTAGONISTS

A chemical antagonist interacts directly with the drug being antagonized to remove it or to prevent it from reaching its target. A chemical antagonist does not depend on interaction with the agonist's receptor (although such interaction may occur). A common example of a chemical antagonist is dimercaprol, a chelator of lead and some other toxic metals. Pralidoxime, which combines avidly with the phosphorus in organophosphate cholinesterase inhibitors, is another type of chemical antagonist.

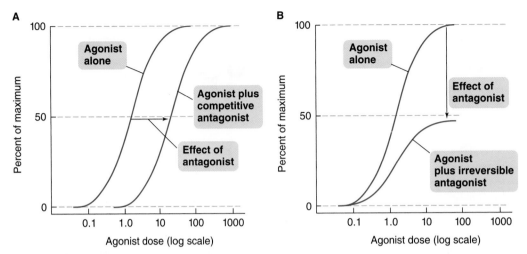

Figure 2–5. Agonist dose-response curves in the presence of competitive and irreversible antagonists. Note the use of a logarithmic scale for drug concentration. **A.** A competitive antagonist has an effect illustrated by the shift of the agonist curve to the right. **B.** A noncompetitive antagonist shifts the agonist curve downward.

THERAPEUTIC INDEX & THERAPEUTIC WINDOW

The therapeutic index is the ratio of the TD_{50} (or LD_{50}) to the ED_{50}, determined from quantal dose-response curves. The therapeutic index represents an estimate of the safety of a drug, because a very safe drug might be expected to have a very large toxic dose and a much smaller effective dose. For example, in Figure 2–2, the ED_{50} is approximately 3 mg and the LD_{50} is approximately 150 mg. The therapeutic index is therefore approximately 150/3, or 50. Obviously, a full range of toxic doses cannot be ethically studied in humans. Furthermore, factors such as the varying slopes of dose-response curves make this estimate a poor safety index even in animals.

The therapeutic window, a more clinically relevant index of safety, describes the *dosage range* between the minimum effective therapeutic concentration or dose, and the minimum toxic concentration or dose. For example, if the average minimum therapeutic plasma concentration of theophylline is 8 mg/L and toxic effects are observed at 18 mg/L, the therapeutic window is 8–18 mg/L. Both the therapeutic index and the therapeutic window depend on the specific toxic effect used in the determination.

SIGNALING MECHANISMS

Once an agonist drug has bound to its receptor, some effector mechanism is activated. For many drug–receptor interactions, the drug is present in the extracellular space

while the effector mechanism resides inside the cell and modifies some intracellular process. Thus, signaling across the membrane must occur. Five major types of transmembrane signaling mechanisms for receptor-effector systems have been defined (Figure 2–6).

A. RECEPTORS THAT ARE INTRACELLULAR

Some drugs, especially more lipid-soluble or diffusible agents (eg, steroid hormones, nitric oxide) may cross the membrane and combine with an intracellular receptor that affects an intracellular effector molecule. The receptor and effector may or may not be the same molecule, but no specialized transmembrane signaling device is required.

B. RECEPTORS LOCATED ON MEMBRANE-SPANNING ENZYMES

Drugs that affect membrane-spanning enzymes combine with a receptor site on the extracellular portion of the molecule and modify its intracellular activity. For example, insulin acts on a tyrosine kinase that is located in the membrane. The insulin receptor site faces the extracellular environment and the effector enzyme catalytic site is on the cytoplasmic side. When activated, such receptors dimerize and phosphorylate specific intracellular protein substrates.

C. RECEPTORS LOCATED ON MEMBRANE-SPANNING MOLECULES THAT BIND SEPARATE INTRACELLULAR TYROSINE KINASE MOLECULES

Like receptor tyrosine kinases, these receptors have extracellular and intracellular domains and form dimers.

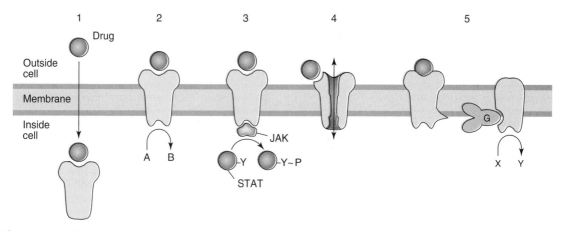

Figure 2–6. Signaling mechanisms for drug effects. Five major signaling mechanisms are recognized: (1) transmembrane diffusion of the drug to bind to an intracellular receptor; (2) transmembrane enzyme receptors, whose outer domain provides the receptor function and inner domain provides the effector mechanism converting A to B; (3) transmembrane receptors that, after activation by an appropriate ligand, activate separate cytoplasmic tyrosine kinase molecules (JAKs), which phosphorylate STAT molecules that regulate transcription (Y, tyrosine; P, phosphate); (4) transmembrane channels that are gated open or closed by the binding of a drug to the receptor site; and (5) G protein-coupled receptors, which utilize a coupling protein to activate a separate effector molecule. (Reproduced, with permission, from Katzung BG, editor: *Basic & Clinical Pharmacology,* 9th ed. McGraw-Hill, 2004.)

However, after receptor activation by an appropriate drug (often a cytokine) at the extracellular receptor site, associated but separate tyrosine kinase molecules (**Janus kinases; JAKs**) are activated, resulting in phosphorylation of **STAT** molecules (signal transducers and activators of transcription). STAT dimers (the effectors) then travel to the nucleus, where they regulate transcription.

D. RECEPTORS LOCATED ON MEMBRANE ION CHANNELS

Receptors that regulate membrane ion channels may directly cause the opening of the channel (eg, acetylcholine at the nicotinic receptor) or modify the ion channel's response to other agents (eg, benzodiazepines at the GABA-activated chloride channel). The channel molecule acts as both receptor and effector, and the result is a change in transmembrane electrical potential.

E. RECEPTORS LINKED TO EFFECTORS VIA G PROTEINS

A very large number of drugs bind to receptors that are linked by coupling proteins to intracellular or membrane-bound effectors. The best defined examples of this group are the sympathomimetic drugs, which activate or inhibit adenylyl cyclase (formerly called adenylate cyclase) by a multistep process: activation of the receptor (located in the membrane with the binding site facing the extracellular side) by the drug results in activation of separate G proteins (located in the intracellular face of the membrane) that either stimulate or inhibit the cyclase. Thus the receptor and effector are linked through the G coupling protein. Many types of G proteins have been identified; 3 of the most important are listed in Table 2–1. When G-coupled receptors bind agonist, the G protein is activated. This process involves replacement with GTP of

Table 2–1. Examples of receptors that are coupled to their effectors by G proteins.

Receptor Types	Coupling Protein	Effector	Effector Substrate	Second Messenger Response	Result
M_1, M_3, α_1	G_q	Phospholipase C	Membrane lipids	↑ IP_3, DAG	↑ Ca^{2+} and protein kinase activity
β, D_1	G_s	Adenylyl cyclase	ATP	↑ cAMP	↑ Ca^{2+} influx and enzyme activity
α_2, M_2	G_i	Adenylyl cyclase	ATP	↓ cAMP	↓ Ca^{2+} influx and enzyme activity; ↑ K^+ efflux

the GDP that is bound to the protein and subsequent dissociation of the trimeric G protein complex into a GTP-alpha moiety and a beta-gamma moiety. The GTP-alpha portion is the primary player in most interactions with effector molecules, but in some the beta-gamma moiety is the activator.

RECEPTOR REGULATION

Frequent or continuous exposure to agonists often results in a diminution of the receptor response, especially the responses of G protein-coupled receptors. Several mechanisms are responsible for this phenomenon. First, intracellular proteins may block access of the G protein to the activated receptor molecule. For example, the molecule β-arrestin has been shown to bind to an intracellular loop of the beta adrenoceptor, when the receptor is continuously activated. β-Arrestin prevents access of the G_s coupling protein and thus desensitizes the tissue to further beta agonist activation. Removal of the beta agonist results in removal of β-arrestin and restoration of the full response.

Second, agonist-bound receptors may be internalized by endocytosis, removing them from further exposure to extracellular molecules. The internalized receptor molecule may then be either reinserted into the membrane (eg, morphine receptors) or degraded (eg, beta adrenoceptors, epidermal growth factor receptors). In some cases, the internalization-reinsertion process may actually be necessary for normal functioning of the receptor-effector system.

QUESTIONS

1. A 55-year-old woman with heart failure is to be treated with a diuretic drug. Drugs X and Y have the same mechanism of diuretic action. Drug X in a dose of 5 mg produces the same magnitude of diuresis as 500 mg of drug Y. This suggests that
   (A) Drug Y is less efficacious than drug X
   (B) Drug X is about 100 times more potent than drug Y
   (C) Toxicity of drug X is less than that of drug Y
   (D) Drug X has a wider therapeutic window than drug Y
   (E) Drug X will have a shorter duration of action than drug Y because less of drug X is present for a given effect

2. Dose-response curves are used for drug evaluation in the animal laboratory and in the clinic. *Quantal* dose-response curves are
   (A) Used for determining the therapeutic index of a drug
   (B) Used for determining the maximal efficacy of a drug
   (C) More precisely quantitated than ordinary graded dose-response curves

   (D) Obtainable from the study of intact subjects but not from isolated tissue preparations
   (E) Used to determine the statistical variation (standard deviation) of the maximal response to the drug

3. The results shown in the graph below were obtained in a comparison of drugs that increase the force of cardiac contraction. Which of the following statements is correct?

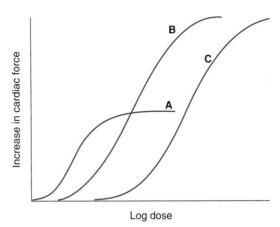

   (A) Drug A is most effective
   (B) Drug B is least potent
   (C) Drug C is most potent
   (D) Drug B is more potent than drug C and more effective than drug A
   (E) Drug A is more potent than drug B and more effective than drug C

4. In the absence of other drugs, pindolol causes an increase in heart rate by activating beta adrenoceptors. In the presence of highly effective beta stimulants, however, pindolol causes a dose-dependent, reversible decrease in heart rate. Therefore, pindolol should be classified as
   (A) A chemical antagonist
   (B) An irreversible antagonist
   (C) A partial agonist
   (D) A physiologic antagonist
   (E) A spare receptor agonist

5. Which of the following statements about spare receptors is MOST correct?
   (A) Spare receptors, in the absence of drug, are sequestered in the cytoplasm
   (B) Spare receptors may be detected by finding that the drug–receptor interaction lasts longer than the intracellular effect
   (C) Spare receptors influence the maximal efficacy of the drug–receptor system

(D) Spare receptors activate the effector machinery of the cell without the need for a drug

(E) Spare receptors may be detected by the finding that the EC_{50} is smaller than the K_d for the agonist

6. Two antihypertensive drugs, X and Y, were studied in a large group of patients and the percentages of the group showing a specific therapeutic effect (20 mm Hg decrease in systolic blood pressure) were determined. The results are shown in the table:

Drug Dose	Percent Responding to Drug X	Percent Responding to Drug Y
0.1 mg	1	10
0.3 mg	5	20
1.0 mg	10	50
3.0 mg	50	70
10.0 mg	70	90
30.0 mg	90	100

Which of the following statements about these results is correct?

(A) Drug X is safer than drug Y

(B) Drug Y is more effective than drug X

(C) The 2 drugs act on the same receptors

(D) Drug X is less potent than drug Y

(E) The therapeutic index of drug Y is 10

7. Leukotriene causes bronchoconstriction (mediated at leukotriene receptors) in a patient with asthma. When terbutaline (acting at adrenoceptors) is given to the patient during an asthmatic attack, bronchodilation usually results. In this situation, terbutaline is a

(A) Chemical antagonist

(B) Noncompetitive antagonist

(C) Partial agonist

(D) Pharmacologic antagonist

(E) Physiologic antagonist

8. Which of the following names best describes an antagonist that interacts directly with the agonist and not at all, or only incidentally, with the receptor?

(A) Chemical antagonist

(B) Noncompetitive antagonist

(C) Partial agonist

(D) Pharmacologic antagonist

(E) Physiologic antagonist

9. Which of the following terms best describes a drug that blocks the action of epinephrine at its receptors by occupying those receptors without activating them?

(A) Chemical antagonist

(B) Noncompetitive antagonist

(C) Partial agonist

(D) Pharmacologic antagonist

(E) Physiologic antagonist

10. Which of the following provides information about the variation in sensitivity to a drug within the population studied?

(A) Drug potency

(B) Graded dose-response curve

(C) Maximal efficacy

(D) Quantal dose-response curve

(E) Therapeutic index

11. Which of the following most accurately describes the transmembrane signaling process involved in steroid hormone action?

(A) Action on a membrane-spanning tyrosine kinase

(B) Activation of a G protein, which activates or inhibits adenylyl cyclase

(C) Diffusion across the membrane and binding to an intracellular receptor

(D) Diffusion of STAT molecules across the membrane

(E) Opening of transmembrane ion channels

12. Which of the following provides information about the largest response a drug can produce, regardless of dose?

(A) Drug potency

(B) Maximal efficacy

(C) Mechanism of receptor action

(D) Therapeutic index

(E) Therapeutic window

DIRECTIONS: 13–15. Each of the curves in the graph below may be considered a concentration-effect curve or a concentration-binding curve.

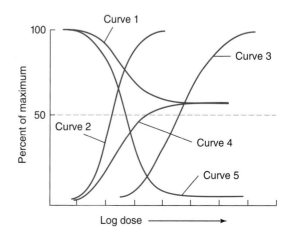

13. Which of the curves in the graph describes the percentage *binding* of a large dose of full agonist to its receptors as the concentration of a partial agonist is increased from low to very high levels?
    (A) Curve 1
    (B) Curve 2
    (C) Curve 3
    (D) Curve 4
    (E) Curve 5

14. Which of the curves in the graph describes the percentage *effect* observed when a large dose of full agonist is present throughout the experiment and the concentration of a partial agonist is increased from low to very high levels?
    (A) Curve 1
    (B) Curve 2
    (C) Curve 3
    (D) Curve 4
    (E) Curve 5

15. Which of the curves in the graph describes the percentage *binding* of the partial agonist whose *effect* is shown by curve 4 if the system has many spare receptors?
    (A) Curve 1
    (B) Curve 2
    (C) Curve 3
    (D) Curve 4
    (E) Curve 5

ANSWERS

1. No information is given regarding the magnitude of the maximum diuretic response to either drug. Similarly, no information about toxicity is provided. The fact that a given response is achieved with a smaller dose of drug X indicates that X is more potent than Y in the ratio of 500/5. The answer is **B**.

2. Graded (not quantal) dose-response curves must be used to determine maximum efficacy (maximum response). Quantal dose-response curves show only the frequency of occurrence of a specified response, which may be therapeutically effective (ED) or toxic (TD). Dividing the TD_{50} by the ED_{50} gives the therapeutic index. The answer is **A**.

3. Drug A produces 50% of its maximum effect at the lowest dose and thus is the most potent; drug C is the least. Drug A is less efficacious than drugs B and C. The answer is **D**.

4. Choices involving chemical or physiologic antagonism are incorrect because pindolol is said to act at beta receptors and to block beta stimulants. The drug effect is reversible, so choice **B** is incorrect. "Spare receptor agonist" is a nonsense distracter. The answer is **C**.

5. While some types of receptors appear to be sequestered in the cytoplasm under certain conditions, there is no difference between "spare" and other receptors. Spare receptors may be defined as those which are not needed for binding drug to achieve the maximum effect. Spare receptors influence the *sensitivity* of the system to an agonist because the statistical probability of a drug–receptor interaction increases with the total number of receptors. They do not alter the maximal efficacy. If they do not bind an agonist molecule, spare receptors do not activate an effector molecule. EC_{50} *less* than K_d is an indication of the presence of spare receptors. The answer is **E**.

6. No information is presented regarding the safety of these drugs. Similarly, no information on efficacy is presented. Although both drugs are said to be producing a therapeutic effect, no information on their receptor mechanisms is given. Since no data on toxicity are available, the therapeutic index cannot be determined. The answer is **D** because the ED_{50} of drug Y (1.0 mg) is less than that of drug X (3.0 mg).

7. Because terbutaline interacts with adrenoceptors and leukotriene with leukotriene receptors, terbutaline cannot be a pharmacologic antagonist of leukotriene. Because the results of adrenoceptor activation oppose the effects of leukotriene receptor activation, terbutaline must be a physiologic antagonist. The answer is **E**.

8. A chemical antagonist interacts directly (chemically) with the agonist drug and not with a receptor. The answer is **A**.

9. A pharmacologic antagonist occupies the receptors without activating them. The answer is **D**.

10. Quantal dose-response curves provide information about the statistical distribution of sensitivity to a drug. The answer is **D**.

11. Steroid hormones (eg, cortisol, sex hormones, and aldosterone) diffuse through the membrane of the cell into the cytoplasm and bind to an intracellular receptor. The hormone-receptor complex then modulates gene expression. The answer is **C**.

12. Maximal efficacy represents the largest response a drug can produce. The answer is **B**.

13. The binding of a full agonist will *decrease* as the concentration of a partial agonist is increased to very high levels. As the partial agonist displaces more and more of the full agonist, the percentage of receptors that bind the full agonist will drop to zero, ie, curve 5. The answer is **E**.

14. Curve 1 describes the *response* of the system when a full agonist is displaced by increasing concentrations

of partial agonist. This is because the increasing percentage of receptors binding the partial agonist will finally produce the maximum effect typical of the partial agonist. The answer is **A.**

15. Partial agonists, like full agonists, bind 100% of their receptors when present in a high enough concentration. Therefore, the binding curve (but not the effect curve) will go to 100%. If the effect curve is curve 4 and many spare receptors are present, the binding curve must be displaced to the right of curve 4 ($K_d > EC_{50}$). Therefore, curve 3 fits the description better than curve 2. The answer is **C.**

CHECKLIST

When you complete this chapter, you should be able to:

☐ Compare the efficacy and the potency of 2 drugs on the basis of their dose-response curves.

☐ Predict the effect of a partial agonist in a patient in the presence and in the absence of a full agonist.

☐ Describe the difference between receptor binding sites and inert binding sites and name 2 proteins in blood that have important inert drug binding sites.

☐ Name the types of antagonists used in pharmacology.

☐ Specify whether an antagonist is competitive or irreversible based on its effect on the dose-response curve of an agonist.

☐ Give examples of competitive and irreversible pharmacologic antagonists and of physiologic and chemical antagonists.

☐ Name the coupling and effector proteins usually activated by muscarinic receptors (M_1, M_2, M_3); α_1 and α_2 receptors; and β receptors.

☐ Name 5 transmembrane signaling methods by which drug–receptor interactions exert their effects.

☐ Describe 2 mechanisms of receptor regulation.

Pharmacokinetics

Pharmacokinetics denotes the effects of biologic systems on drugs. It deals with the processes of absorption, distribution, and elimination and makes possible the calculation of loading and maintenance doses.

EFFECTIVE DRUG CONCENTRATION

The effective drug concentration is the concentration of a drug *at the receptor site* (in contrast to drug concentrations that are more readily measured, eg, in blood). Except for topically applied agents, the concentration at the receptor site is usually proportionate to the drug's concentration in the plasma or whole blood at equilibrium. The plasma concentration is a function of the rate of input of the drug (by absorption) into the plasma, the rate of distribution to the peripheral tissues (including the target organ), and the rate of elimination, or loss, from the body. These are all functions of time; but if the rate of input is known, the remaining processes are well described by 2 primary parameters: **apparent volume of distribution** and **clearance.** These parameters are unique for a particular drug and may differ from patient to patient but have average values in large populations that can be used to predict drug concentrations.

VOLUME OF DISTRIBUTION (V$_d$)

The volume of distribution relates the amount of drug in the body to the plasma concentration (Figure 3–1) according to the following equation:

$$V_d = \frac{\text{Amount of drug in the body}}{\text{Plasma drug concentration}} \quad \text{(1)}$$

(Units = volume)

The calculated parameter for the volume of distribution has no direct physical equivalent; therefore, it is denoted the *apparent* V$_d$. If a drug is avidly bound in peripheral tissues, the drug's concentration in plasma may drop to very low values even though the total amount in the body is large. As a result, the volume of distribution may greatly exceed the total volume of the body. For example, 50,000 liters is the average V$_d$ for the drug quinacrine in persons whose average physical body volume is 70 liters. On the

other hand, a drug that is completely retained in the plasma compartment will have a volume of distribution equal to the plasma volume (about 4% of body weight). The volume of distribution of drugs that are normally bound to plasma proteins such as albumin can be altered by liver disease (through reduced protein synthesis) and kidney disease (through urinary protein loss).

CLEARANCE (CL)

Clearance relates the rate of elimination to the plasma concentration:

$$CL = \frac{\text{Rate of elimination of drug}}{\text{Plasma drug concentration}} \quad \text{(2)}$$

(Units = volume per unit time)

For a drug eliminated with first-order kinetics, clearance is a constant, ie, the ratio of rate of elimination to plasma concentration is the same regardless of plasma concentration (Figure 3–2). The magnitudes of clearance for different drugs range from a small fraction of the blood flow to a maximum of the total blood flow to the organs of elimination. Clearance depends on the drug and the condition of the organs of elimination in the patient. The clearance of a particular drug by an individual organ is equivalent to the extraction capability of that organ for that drug times the rate of delivery of drug to the organ. Thus, the clearance of a drug that is very effectively extracted by an organ (ie, the blood is completely cleared of the drug as it passes through the organ) is often *flow-limited*. For such a drug, the total clearance from the body is a function of blood flow through the eliminating organ and is

SKILL KEEPER 1: ZERO-ORDER ELIMINATION (SEE CHAPTER 1)

The great majority of drugs in clinical use obey the first-order kinetics "rule" described in the text. Can you name 3 important drugs that do not? The Skill Keeper Answer appears at the end of the chapter.

HIGH-YIELD TERMS TO LEARN	
Volume of distribution (apparent)	The ratio of the amount of drug in the body to the drug concentration in the plasma or blood
Clearance	The ratio of the rate of elimination of a drug to the concentration of the drug in the plasma or blood
Half-life	The time required for the amount of drug to fall to 50% of an earlier measurement. For drugs eliminated by first-order kinetics, this number is a constant regardless of the concentration.
Bioavailability	The fraction (or percentage) of the administered dose of drug that reaches the systemic circulation
Area under the curve (AUC)	The graphic area under a plot of drug concentration versus time after a single dose or during a single dosing interval
Peak and trough concentrations	The maximum and minimum drug concentrations achieved during repeated dosing cycles
Minimum effective concentration (MEC)	The plasma drug concentration below which a patient's response is too small for clinical benefit
First-pass effect, presystemic elimination	The elimination of drug that occurs after administration but before it enters the systemic circulation (eg, during passage through the gut wall, portal circulation, or liver for an orally administered drug)
Steady state	In pharmacokinetics, the condition in which the average total amount of drug in the body does not change over multiple dosing cycles (ie, the condition in which the rate of drug elimination equals the rate of administration)
Biodisposition	Often used as a synonym for pharmacokinetics; the processes of drug absorption, distribution, and elimination. Sometimes used more narrowly to describe elimination

limited by the blood flow to that organ. In this situation, other conditions—disease or other drugs that change blood flow—may have more dramatic effects on clearance than disease of the organ of elimination.

HALF-LIFE

Half-life ($t_{1/2}$) is a derived parameter, completely determined by volume of distribution and clearance. Half-life can be determined graphically from a plot of the blood level versus time (eg, Figure 1–3), or from the following relationship:

$$t_{1/2} = \frac{0.693 \times V_d}{CL} \qquad (3)$$

(Units = time)

One must know both primary variables (V_d and CL) to predict changes in half-life. Disease, age, and other variables usually alter the clearance of a drug much more than they alter its volume of distribution. The half-life of a drug may not change, however, despite a decreased

clearance if the volume of distribution decreases at the same time. This occurs, for example, when lidocaine is administered to patients with heart failure. The half-life determines the rate at which blood concentration rises during a constant infusion and falls after administration is stopped (Figure 3–3). The effect of a drug at 87–90% of its steady-state concentration is clinically indistinguishable from the steady-state effect; thus, 3–4 half-lives of dosing at a constant rate are considered adequate to produce the effect to be expected at steady state with chronic dosing at the dosage used.

BIOAVAILABILITY

The bioavailability of a drug is the fraction (F) of the administered dose that reaches the systemic circulation. Bioavailability is defined as unity (or 100%) in the case of intravenous administration. After administration by other routes, bioavailability is generally reduced by incomplete absorption (and in the intestine, expulsion of drug by intestinal transporters), first-pass metabolism, and any distribution into other tissues that occurs before the drug enters the systemic circulation. Even for drugs with equal

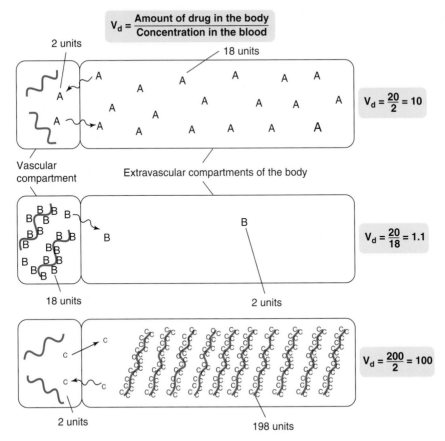

$$V_d = \frac{\text{Amount of drug in the body}}{\text{Concentration in the blood}}$$

2 units

18 units

$V_d = \frac{20}{2} = 10$

Vascular compartment

Extravascular compartments of the body

$V_d = \frac{20}{18} = 1.1$

18 units

2 units

$V_d = \frac{200}{2} = 100$

2 units

198 units

Figure 3–1. Effect of drug binding on volume of distribution. Drug A diffuses freely between the 2 compartments and does not bind to macromolecules (heavy wavy lines) in the vascular or the extravascular compartments of the hypothetical organism in the diagram. With 20 units of the drug in the body, the steady-state distribution leaves a blood concentration of 2 units. Drug B, on the other hand, binds avidly to proteins in the blood. At equilibrium, only 2 units of the total are present in the extravascular volume, leaving 18 units still in the blood. In each case the total amount of drug in the body is the same (20 units), but the apparent volumes of distribution are very different. Drug C is avidly bound to molecules in peripheral tissues, so that a larger total dose (200 units) is required to achieve measurable plasma concentrations. At equilibrium, 198 units are found in the peripheral tissues and only 2 in the plasma, so that the calculated volume of distribution is greater than the physical volume of the system.

bioavailabilities, entry into the systemic circulation occurs over varying periods of time depending on the drug formulation and other factors. To account for such factors, the concentration appearing in the plasma is integrated over time to obtain an integrated total **area under the plasma concentration curve** (**AUC,** Figure 3–4).

EXTRACTION

Removal of a drug by an organ can be specified as the extraction ratio, ie, the fraction of the drug removed from the perfusing blood during its passage through the organ (Figure 3–5). After steady-state concentration in plasma has been achieved, the extraction ratio is one measure of the elimination of the drug by that organ.

Drugs that have a high hepatic extraction ratio have a large first-pass effect; the bioavailability of these drugs after oral administration will be low.

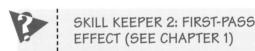

SKILL KEEPER 2: FIRST-PASS EFFECT (SEE CHAPTER 1)

What route of administration is most likely to have a large first-pass effect and therefore low bioavailability? The Skill Keeper Answer appears at the end of the chapter.

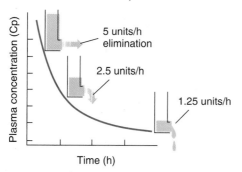

$$\text{Clearance, CL} = \frac{\text{Rate of elimination}}{\text{Plasma concentration (Cp)}}$$

Rate of elimination = CL x Cp

Figure 3–2. The clearance of most drugs is constant over a broad range of plasma concentrations. Since elimination rate is equal to clearance times plasma concentration, the elimination rate will be rapid at first and slow as the concentration decreases.

DOSAGE REGIMENS

A dosage regimen is a plan for drug administration over a period of time. An appropriate dosage regimen results in the achievement of therapeutic levels of the drug in the blood without exceeding the minimum toxic concentration. To maintain the plasma concentration within a specified range over long periods of therapy, a schedule of *maintenance doses* is used. If it is necessary to achieve the target plasma level rapidly, a *loading dose* is used to "load" the volume of distribution with the drug. Ideally, the dosing plan is based on knowledge of both the minimum therapeutic and minimum toxic concentrations for the drug, as well as its clearance and volume of distribution.

A. MAINTENANCE DOSAGE

Because the maintenance rate of drug administration is equal to the rate of elimination at steady state (this is the definition of steady state), the maintenance dosage is a function of clearance (from Equation 2).

$$\text{Dosing rate} = \frac{\text{Clearance} \times \text{Desired plasma concentration}}{\text{Bioavailability}} \quad (4)$$

Note that volume of distribution is not directly involved in the above calculation. The dosing rate computed for maintenance dosage is the average dose per unit time. When performing such calculations, make certain that the units are in agreement throughout. For example, if clearance is given in mL/min, the resulting dosing rate is a per-minute rate. Because convenience of administration is desirable for chronic therapy, doses should be given orally if possible and only once or a few times per day. The size of the daily dose (dose per minute × 60 min/h × 24 h/day) is a simple extension of the above information. The number of doses to be given per day is usually determined by the half-life of the drug and the difference between the minimum therapeutic and toxic concentrations (see Therapeutic Window, below).

If it is important to maintain a concentration above the minimum therapeutic level at all times, either a larger dose may be given at long intervals or smaller doses at more frequent intervals. If the difference between the toxic and therapeutic concentrations is small, then smaller and more frequent doses must be administered to avoid toxicity.

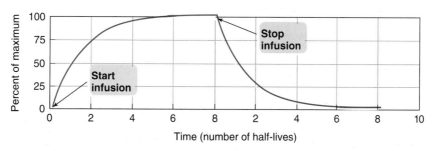

Figure 3–3. Plasma concentration (plotted as percent of maximum) of a drug given by constant intravenous infusion for 8 half-lives and then stopped. The concentration rises smoothly with time and always reaches 50% of steady state after 1 half-life, 75% after 2 half-lives, 87.5% after 3 half-lives, and so on. The decline in concentration after stopping drug administration follows the same type of curve: 50% is left after 1 half-life, 25% after 2 half-lives, etc. The asymptotic approach to steady state on both increasing and decreasing limbs of the curve is characteristic of drugs following first-order kinetics.

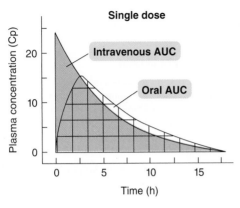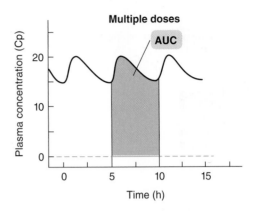

Figure 3–4. The area under the curve is used to calculate the bioavailability of a drug. The AUC can be derived from either single dose studies (left panel) or multiple dose measurements (right panel). Bioavailability is calculated from $AUC_{(route)}/AUC_{(IV)}$.

B. LOADING DOSAGE

If the therapeutic concentration must be achieved rapidly and the volume of distribution is large, a large loading dose may be needed at the onset of therapy. This can be calculated from the following equation:

$$\text{Loading dose} = \frac{\text{Volume of distribution} \times \text{Desired plasma concentration}}{\text{Bioavailability}} \quad (5)$$

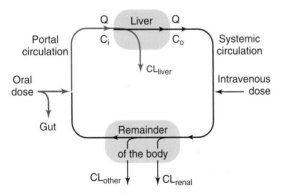

Figure 3–5. The principles of organ extraction and first-pass effect are illustrated. Part of the administered oral dose (color) is lost to metabolism in the gut and the liver before it enters the systemic circulation: this is the first-pass effect. The extraction of drug from the circulation by the liver is equal to blood flow times the difference between entering and leaving drug concentration, ie, $Q \times (C_i − C_o)$. (Reproduced, with permission, from Katzung BG, editor: *Basic & Clinical Pharmacology*, 8th ed. McGraw-Hill, 2001.)

Note that clearance does not enter into this computation. If the loading dose is very large (V_d much larger than blood volume), the dose should be given slowly to avoid excessively high plasma levels during the distribution phase.

THERAPEUTIC WINDOW

The therapeutic window is the safe range between the minimum therapeutic concentration and the minimum toxic concentration of a drug. The concept is used to determine the acceptable range of plasma levels when designing a dosing regimen. Thus, the minimum effective concentration will usually determine the desired **trough** levels of a drug given intermittently while the minimum toxic concentration determines the permissible **peak** plasma concentration. For example, the drug theophylline has a therapeutic concentration range of 8–15 mg/L but is toxic at concentrations of 16 mg/L and above. The therapeutic window for a given patient might thus be fixed in the range of 8–15 mg/L (Figure 3–6). Unfortunately, for some drugs the therapeutic and toxic concentrations vary so greatly among patients that it is impossible to predict the therapeutic window in a given patient. Such drugs must be titrated individually in each patient.

ADJUSTMENT OF DOSAGE WHEN ELIMINATION IS ALTERED BY DISEASE

Renal disease or reduced cardiac output often reduces the clearance of drugs that depend on renal function. Alteration of clearance by liver disease is less common but may occur. Impairment of hepatic clearance occurs (for high extraction drugs) when liver blood flow is reduced, as in heart failure. The dose in a patient with

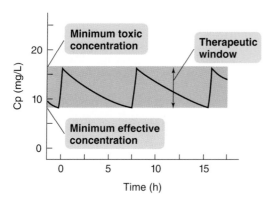

Figure 3–6. The therapeutic window for theophylline in a 13-year-old patient. The minimum effective concentration in this patient was found to be 8 mg/L; the minimum toxic concentration was found to be 16 mg/L. The therapeutic window is indicated by the colored area. To maintain the plasma concentration (Cp) within the window, this drug must be given at least once every half-life (7.5 h in this patient) because the minimum effective concentration is half the minimum toxic concentration and Cp will decay by 50% in 1 half-life. (**Note:** This concept applies to drugs given in the ordinary, prompt-release form. Slow-release formulations can often be given at longer intervals.)

renal impairment may be corrected by multiplying the average dose for a normal person times the ratio of the patient's altered creatinine clearance to normal creatinine clearance (approximately 100 mL/min, or 6 L/h).

$$\text{Corrected dose} = \text{Average dose} \times \frac{\text{Patient's creatinine clearance}}{100 \text{ mL/min}} \quad (6)$$

This simplified approach ignores nonrenal routes of clearance that may be significant. If a drug is cleared partly by the kidney and partly by other routes, the above equation should be applied to that part of the dose that is eliminated by the kidney. For example, if a drug is 50% cleared by the kidney and 50% by the liver and the normal dosage is 200 mg/d, the hepatic and renal clearances are each 100 mg/d. Therefore, the corrected dosage in a patient with a creatinine clearance of 20 mL/min will be

$$\text{Dose} = 100 \text{ mg/d} + 100 \text{ mg/d} \times \frac{20 \text{ mL/min}}{100 \text{ mL/min}}$$

$$\text{Dose} = 100 \text{ mg/d} + 20 \text{ mg/d} = 120 \text{ mg/d} \quad (7)$$

QUESTIONS

1–2. Mr Jones is admitted to the hospital with pneumonia due to gram-negative bacteria. The antibiotic tobramycin is ordered. The CL and V_d of tobramycin in Mr Jones are 80 mL/min and 40 L, respectively.

1. What maintenance dose should be administered intravenously every 6 h to eventually obtain average steady-state plasma concentrations of 4 mg/L?
   (**A**) 0.32 mg
   (**B**) 19.2 mg
   (**C**) 115 mg
   (**D**) 160 mg
   (**E**) 230 mg

2. If you wish to give Mr Jones an intravenous loading dose to achieve the therapeutic plasma concentration of 4 mg/L rapidly, how much should be given?
   (**A**) 0.1 mg
   (**B**) 10 mg
   (**C**) 115.2 mg
   (**D**) 160 mg
   (**E**) None of the above

3. Despite your careful adherence to basic pharmacokinetic principles, your patient on digoxin therapy has developed digitalis toxicity. The plasma digoxin level is now 4 ng/mL. Renal function is normal, and the plasma $t_{1/2}$ for digoxin in this patient is 1.6 days. How long should you withhold digoxin in order to reach a safer yet probably therapeutic level of 1 ng/mL?
   (**A**) 1.6 days
   (**B**) 2.4 days
   (**C**) 3.2 days
   (**D**) 4.8 days
   (**E**) 6.4 days

4. Verapamil and phenytoin are both eliminated from the body by metabolism in the liver. Verapamil has a clearance of 1.5 L/min, approximately equal to liver blood flow, whereas phenytoin has a clearance of 0.1 L/min. When these compounds are administered along with rifampin, a drug that markedly increases hepatic drug-metabolizing enzymes, which of the following is most likely?
   (**A**) The clearance of both verapamil and phenytoin will be markedly increased
   (**B**) The clearance of both verapamil and phenytoin will be markedly decreased
   (**C**) The clearance of verapamil will be unchanged, whereas the clearance of phenytoin will be increased
   (**D**) The clearance of phenytoin will be unchanged, whereas the clearance of verapamil will be increased
   (**E**) The clearance of both drugs will be unchanged

5. A 60-year-old man enters the hospital with a myocardial infarction and a severe ventricular arrhythmia. The antiarrhythmic drug chosen has a narrow therapeutic window: the minimum toxic plasma concentration is 1.5 times the minimum therapeutic plasma concentration. The half-life is 6 h. It is essential to maintain the plasma concentration above the minimum therapeutic level to prevent a possibly lethal arrhythmia. Of the following, the most appropriate dosing regimen would be
(A) Once a day
(B) Twice a day
(C) Three times a day
(D) Four times a day
(E) Constant intravenous infusion

6. A 50-year-old woman with metastatic breast cancer has elected to participate in the trial of a new chemotherapeutic agent. It is given by constant intravenous infusion of 8 mg/h. Plasma concentrations (Cp) are measured with the results shown in the following table.

Time After Start of Infusion (h)	Plasma Concentration (mg/L)
1	0.8
2	1.3
4	2.0
8	3.0
10	3.6
16	3.7
20	3.84
25	3.95
30	4.0
40	4.0

From these data, it may be concluded that
(A) Volume of distribution is 30 L
(B) Clearance is 2 L/h
(C) Elimination follows zero-order kinetics
(D) Half-life is 8 h
(E) Doubling the rate of infusion would result in a plasma concentration of 16 mg/L at 40 h

7. A city clinic is considering the substitution of generic drugs in order to save money. The clinical pharmacologist is asked to advise on the bioavailability of the generic products. She informs the head of the clinic that the bioavailability of drugs is
(A) Established by FDA regulation at 100% for preparations for intramuscular injection
(B) 100% for oral preparations that are not metabolized in the liver
(C) Calculated from the peak concentration of drug divided by the dose administered
(D) Important because bioavailability determines what fraction of the administered dose reaches the systemic circulation
(E) Equal to 1 (100%) only for drugs administered by a parenteral route

8. A 19-year-old woman is brought to the hospital with severe asthmatic wheezing. You decide to use intravenous theophylline for treatment. The pharmacokinetics of theophylline include the following average parameters: V_d 35 L; CL 48 mL/min; half-life 8 h. If an intravenous infusion of theophylline is started at a rate of 0.48 mg/min, how long will it take to reach 93.75% of the final steady-state concentration?
(A) Approximately 48 min
(B) Approximately 7.4 h
(C) Approximately 8 h
(D) Approximately 24 h
(E) Approximately 32 h

9–10. Your 74-year-old patient with a myocardial infarction has a severe cardiac arrhythmia. You decide to give lidocaine to correct the arrhythmia.

9. A continuous intravenous infusion of lidocaine, 1.92 mg/min, is started at 8 AM. The average pharmacokinetic parameters of lidocaine are: V_d 77 L; CL 640 mL/min; half-life 1.4 h. The expected steady-state plasma concentration is approximately
(A) 40 mg/L
(B) 3.0 mg/L
(C) 0.025 mg/L
(D) 7.2 mg/L
(E) 3.46 mg/L

10. Your patient has been receiving lidocaine for 8 h and the arrhythmia is suppressed. However, there are some signs of toxicity. You decide to obtain a plasma concentration measurement. When the results come back, the plasma level is exactly twice what you expected. The infusion rate should:
(A) Be changed to 0.48 mg/min
(B) Be changed to 0.96 mg/min

(C) Be halted for 1.4 h and then restarted at 0.96 mg/min
(D) Be halted for 1.4 h and then restarted at 1.92 mg/min
(E) Not be changed but the plasma level should be measured again

11. A patient requires an infusion of procainamide. Its half-life is 2 h. The infusion is begun at 9 AM. At 1 PM the same day, a blood sample is taken; the drug concentration is found to be 3 mg/L. What is the probable steady-state drug concentration, eg, after 12 or more hours of infusion?
(A) 3 mg/L
(B) 4 mg/L
(C) 6 mg/L
(D) 9.9 mg/L
(E) 15 mg/L

12. A young man is brought to the emergency room in a deep coma. His friends state that he self-administered a large dose of morphine 6 h earlier. An immediate blood analysis shows a morphine blood level of 0.25 mg/L. Assuming that the pharmacokinetics of morphine in this patient are V_d 200 L, and half-life 3 h, how much morphine did the patient inject 6 h earlier?
(A) 25 mg
(B) 50 mg
(C) 100 mg
(D) 200 mg
(E) Not enough data to predict

13. A normal volunteer will receive a new drug in a phase 1 clinical trial. The clearance and volume of distribution of the drug in this subject are 1.386 L/h and 80 L, respectively. The half-life of the drug in this subject will be approximately
(A) 83 h
(B) 77 h
(C) 58 h
(D) 40 h
(E) 0.02 h

14. Gentamicin is sometimes given in intermittent intravenous bolus doses of 100 mg 3 times a day to achieve target peak plasma concentrations of about 5 mg/L. Gentamicin's clearance (normally 5.4 L/h/70 kg) is almost entirely by glomerular filtration. Your patient, however, is found to have a creatinine clearance one third of normal. Your initial dosage regimen for this patient would probably be
(A) 20 mg 3 times/day
(B) 33 mg 3 times/day
(C) 72 mg 3 times/day
(D) 100 mg 2 times/day
(E) 150 mg 2 times/day

15–17. A new drug was studied in 20 healthy volunteers to determine basic pharmacokinetic parameters. A dose of 100 mg was administered as an intravenous bolus to each volunteer, and blood samples were analyzed at intervals as shown in the graph below. The average plasma concentrations at each time are shown by the solid circles at 10 and 30 min and at 1, 2, 3, 4, 6, and 8 h after administration.

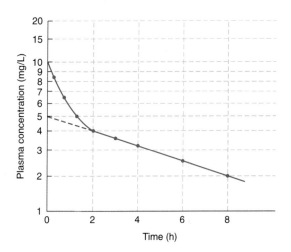

15. The elimination half-life of the new drug is approximately
(A) 1.5 h
(B) 2 h
(C) 4 h
(D) 6 h
(E) 8 h

16. The volume of distribution of the new drug is approximately
(A) 0.05 L
(B) 0.1 L
(C) 5 L
(D) 10 L
(E) 20 L

17. The clearance of the new drug is approximately
(A) 0.43 L/h
(B) 0.86 L/h
(C) 1.15 L/h
(D) 2.3 L/h
(E) Too few data to answer

ANSWERS

1. Maintenance dosage is a function of the target plasma level, bioavailability, and clearance only:

Rate in = Rate out at steady state

$$\text{Dosage} = \frac{\text{Plasma level}_{ss} \times \text{Clearance}}{\text{Bioavailability (F)}}$$

$$= \frac{4 \text{ mg/L} \times 0.08 \text{ L/min}}{1.0}$$

$$= 0.32 \text{ mg/min}$$

when given at 6-h intervals:

$$= 0.32 \text{ mg/min} \times 60 \text{ min/h} \times 6 \text{ h}$$

$$= 115.2 \text{ mg/dose every 6 h}$$

The answer is **C.**

2. Loading dose is a function of volume of distribution and target plasma concentration:

$$\text{Loading dose} = \frac{V_d \times \text{Target concentration}}{\text{Bioavailability}}$$

$$\text{Loading dose} = \frac{40 \text{ L} \times 4 \text{ mg/L}}{1.0} = 160 \text{ mg}$$

The answer is **D.**

3. Since the blood level for a drug with first-order kinetics drops by 50% during each half-life, the level will be 2 ng/mL after 1.6 days and 1 ng/mL after 3.2 days. The answer is **C.**

4. Verapamil is metabolized so readily that only the rate of delivery to the liver regulates its disappearance, ie, its elimination is blood flow-limited, not metabolism-limited. Therefore, further increases in liver enzymes could not increase its elimination. However, the rate of elimination of phenytoin is limited by its rate of metabolism since clearance is much less than hepatic blood flow. Therefore, the clearance of phenytoin can rise if some agent causes an increase in liver enzymes. The answer is **C.**

5. From the description given, if the minimum therapeutic plasma concentration of the hypothetical drug X is 100 units, the minimum toxic concentration is 150 units. If a dose is given that brings the plasma concentration to 150 units, it will fall to 75 units in 1 half-life (6 h). Because 75 units is less than the minimum therapeutic concentration, a 6-h dosing interval (four times a day) is too long. Thus, none of the intermittent dosing schedules listed would meet the requirement of the question. However, a constant intravenous infusion (which can be visualized as intermittent dosing at infinitely short intervals) would be appropriate. The answer is **E.**

6. By inspection of the data in the table, it is clear that the steady-state plasma concentration is approximately 4 mg/L. According to the table, 50% of this concentration was reached after 4 h of infusion. According to the constant infusion principle (Figure 3–3), 1 half-life is required to reach one half of the final concentration; therefore, the half-life of the drug is 4 h. Rearranging the equation for maintenance dosing (dosing rate = CL × Cp), it can be determined that the clearance = dosing rate/Cp, or 2 L/h. The volume of distribution can be calculated from the half-life equation ($t_{1/2} = 0.693 \times V_d/\text{CL}$) and is equal to 11.5 L. This drug follows first-order kinetics as indicated by the progressive approach to the steady-state plasma concentration. The answer is **B.**

7. Bioavailability is calculated from the ratio of the area under the curve after oral administration ($\text{AUC}_{(PO)}$) to the AUC after intravenous administration of the same dose ($\text{AUC}_{(IV)}$; Figure 3–4), not from peak concentration measurements. Many drugs given orally are incompletely absorbed or metabolized in the gut; they will have a bioavailability of less than 1.0 even if they are not metabolized in the liver. The FDA cannot mandate a particular bioavailability by any particular route, only that the bioavailability by that route be reasonably constant among preparations. Some drugs have a bioavailability of less than 1.0 even when given transdermally or intramuscularly. The answer is **D.**

8. The approach of the drug plasma concentration to steady-state concentration during continuous infusion follows a stereotypical curve (Figure 3–3) that rises rapidly at first and gradually levels off. It reaches 50% of steady state at 1 half-life, 75% at 2 half-lives, 87.5% at 3, 93.75% at 4, and progressively halves the difference between its current level and 100% of steady-state with each half-life. The answer is **E,** 32 h, or 4 half-lives.

9. The drug is being administered continuously; the steady-state concentration for a continuously administered drug is given by the equation in question 1. Thus,

$$\text{Dosage} = \text{Plasma level}_{ss} \times \text{Clearance}$$

$$1.92 \text{ mg/min} = Cp_{ss} \times \text{CL}$$

Rearranging:

$$Cp_{ss} = \frac{1.92 \text{ mg/min}}{\text{CL}}$$

$$Cp_{ss} = \frac{1.92 \text{ mg/min}}{640 \text{ mL/min}}$$

$$Cp_{ss} = 0.003 \text{ mg/mL or 3 mg/L}$$

The answer is **B.**

10. If the half-life is 1.4 h, the plasma concentration should approach steady state after 8 h (more than

4 half-lives). As indicated in question 9, the steady-state concentration is a function of dosage and clearance, not volume of distribution. If the plasma level is twice that predicted, the clearance in this patient must be half the average value. To reduce the risk of toxicity, the infusion should be halted until the concentration diminishes (1 half-life) and then restarted at half of the previous rate. The answer is **C**.

11. According to the curve that relates plasma concentration to infusion time (Figure 3–3), a drug will reach 50% of its final steady-state concentration in 1 half-life, 75% in 2 half-lives, etc. From 9 AM to 1 PM is 4 h, or 2 half-lives. Therefore, the measured concentration at 1 PM is 75% of the steady-state value ($0.75 \times Cp_{ss}$). The steady-state concentration will be 3 mg/L divided by 0.75, or 4 mg/L. The answer is **B**.

12. According to the curve that relates the decline of plasma concentration to time as the drug is eliminated (Figure 3–3), the plasma concentration of morphine was 4 times higher immediately after administration than at the time of the measurement, which occurred 6 h, or 2 half-lives, later. Therefore, the initial plasma concentration was 1 mg/L. Since the amount in the body at any time is equal to $V_d \times Cp$ (text Equation 1), the amount injected was 200 L × 1 mg/L, or 200 mg. The answer is **D**.

13. Half-life can be estimated from

$$t_{1/2} = V_d \frac{0.693}{CL} \text{ (text Equation 3)}$$

$$= 80 \text{ L} \times \frac{0.693}{1.386 \text{ L/h}}$$

$$= 80 \text{ L} \times \frac{1}{2 \text{ L/h}}$$

$$= 40 \text{ h}$$

The answer is **D**.

14. If the drug is cleared almost entirely by the kidney and creatinine clearance is reduced to one third of normal, the total daily dose should also be reduced to one third. The answer is **B**.

15. We are asked to determine the elimination half-life of the drug. The elimination phase of the graph of plasma concentration follows a straight line on the semilogarithmic graph, so we can conclude that the new drug follows first-order kinetics, the first requirement for determining the half-life. The straight-line portion of the graph shows a decline of 50% from the 2-h point (4 mg/L) to the 8-h sample (2 mg/L). Therefore, the half-life must be 8 minus 2 h, or 6 h. The answer is **D**, 6 h.

16. By definition, V_d is the amount of drug in the body divided by the plasma concentration. To determine the volume of distribution, the drug must have reached equilibrium in its diffusion into the volume of distribution. Equilibrium is not reached until the distribution phase is complete. Therefore, we cannot use any of the data points preceding the start of the elimination phase. On the other hand, the only point at which we know the amount of drug in the body with certainty is immediately after administration, when the amount is equal to the dose administered. This is the purpose of the extrapolated portion of the straight line that extends to zero time. The dashed line shows the plasma concentration curve that would have been obtained if distribution were instantaneous. From the intercept of the extrapolated line with the plasma concentration axis, we see that the plasma concentration would have been 5 mg/L. Therefore, $V_d = 100$ mg/5 mg/L, or 20 L. The answer is **E**, 20 L.

17. By definition, CL is equal to the rate of elimination divided by the plasma concentration. However, we are not given direct data for the rate of elimination. On the other hand, we have determined the half-life and the volume of distribution of the drug, so we can calculate the clearance from the relationship $t_{1/2} = 0.693 \times V_d \div CL$. Rearranging this equation, $CL = 0.693 \times V_d \div t_{1/2}$. Using the data from questions 16 and 17, we obtain 0.693×20 L ÷ 6 h, or 2.3 L/h (approximately). The answer is **D**.

SKILL KEEPER 1 ANSWER: ZERO-ORDER ELIMINATION (SEE CHAPTER 1)

The 3 important drugs that follow zero-order rather than first-order kinetics are ethanol, aspirin, and phenytoin.

SKILL KEEPER 2 ANSWER: FIRST-PASS EFFECT (SEE CHAPTER 1)

The oral route of administration entails passage of the drug through the liver before it enters the systemic circulation for distribution to the body. Therefore, this route results in the lowest bioavailability for most drugs.

CHECKLIST

When you complete this chapter, you should be able to:

☐ Compute the half-life of a drug based on its clearance and volume of distribution.

☐ Calculate loading and maintenance dosage regimens for oral or intravenous administration of a drug when given the following information: minimum therapeutic concentration; bioavailability; clearance; and volume of distribution.

☐ Calculate the dosage adjustment required for a patient with impaired renal function.

Drug Metabolism

All organisms are exposed to foreign chemical compounds (**xenobiotics**) in the air, water, and food. To ensure elimination of pharmacologically active xenobiotics as well as to terminate the action of many endogenous substances, metabolic pathways alter their activity and their susceptibility to excretion.

THE NEED FOR DRUG METABOLISM

Many cells that act as portals for entry of external molecules into the body (eg, pulmonary epithelium, intestinal epithelium) contain transporter molecules (P-glycoprotein family, others) that expel unwanted molecules immediately after absorption. However, some foreign molecules evade these gatekeepers and are absorbed. Therefore, all higher organisms, especially terrestrial animals, require mechanisms for ridding themselves of toxic foreign molecules after they are absorbed as well as mechanisms for excreting undesirable substances produced within the body. Biotransformation of drugs is one such process. It is an important mechanism by which the body terminates the action of some drugs; in other cases, it serves to activate prodrugs. Most drugs are relatively lipid soluble, a characteristic favorable to absorption across membranes. The same property would result in very slow removal from the body because the molecule would also be readily reabsorbed from the urine in the renal tubule. The body hastens excretion by transforming many drugs to less lipid-soluble, less readily reabsorbed forms.

TYPES OF METABOLIC REACTIONS

A. PHASE I REACTIONS

Phase I reactions include oxidation (especially by the **cytochrome P450** group of enzymes, also called **mixed-function oxidases**), reduction, deamination, and hydrolysis. Examples are listed in Table 4–1.

B. PHASE II REACTIONS

Phase II reactions are synthetic reactions that involve addition (conjugation) of subgroups to $-OH$, $-NH_2$, and $-SH$ functions on the drug molecule. The subgroups that are added include glucuronate, acetate, glutathione, glycine, sulfate, and methyl groups. Most of these groups are relatively polar and make the product less lipid soluble than the original drug molecule. Examples of phase II reactions are listed in Table 4–2. Drugs that are metabolized by both routes may undergo phase II metabolism before or after phase I.

SITES OF DRUG METABOLISM

The most important organ for drug metabolism is the liver. The kidneys play an important role in the metabolism of some drugs. A few drugs (eg, esters) are metabolized in many tissues (eg, liver, blood, intestinal wall) because of the broad distribution of their enzymes.

DETERMINANTS OF BIOTRANSFORMATION RATE

The rate of biotransformation of a drug may vary markedly among different individuals. This variation is most often due to genetic or drug-induced differences. For a few drugs, age or disease-related differences in drug metabolism are significant. Gender is important for only a few drugs (eg, ethanol). (First-pass metabolism of alcohol is greater in men than in women.) Because the rate of biotransformation is often the primary determinant of clearance, variations in drug metabolism must be considered carefully when designing a dosage regimen. Smoking, a common cause of enzyme induction in the liver and lung, may increase the metabolism of some drugs (eg, theophylline).

A. GENETIC FACTORS

Several drug-metabolizing systems have been shown to differ among families or populations in genetically determined ways.

1. Hydrolysis of esters—Succinylcholine is an ester that is metabolized by plasma cholinesterase ("pseudocholinesterase" or butyrylcholinesterase). In most individuals, this process occurs very rapidly, and a single dose of this neuromuscular blocking drug has a duration of action of about 5 min. Approximately 1 person in 2500 has an abnormal form of this enzyme that metabolizes succinylcholine and similar esters much more slowly. In such

---

HIGH-YIELD TERMS TO LEARN

Phase I reactions	Reactions that convert the parent drug to a more polar (water-soluble) or more reactive product by unmasking or inserting a polar functional group such as –OH, –SH, or –NH$_2$
Phase II reactions	Reactions that increase water solubility by conjugation of the drug molecule with a polar moiety such as glucuronate, acetate, or sulfate
CYP isozymes	Cytochrome P450 enzyme species (eg, CYP2D and CYP3A4) that are responsible for much of drug metabolism. Many isoforms of CYP have been recognized
Enzyme induction	Stimulation of drug-metabolizing capacity; usually manifested in the liver by increased synthesis of smooth endoplasmic reticulum (which contains high concentrations of phase I enzymes)
P-glycoprotein	An ATP-dependent transport molecule found in many epithelial and cancer cells. The transporter expels drug molecules from the cytoplasm into the extracellular space. In epithelial cells, expulsion is via the external or luminal face.

---

individuals, the neuromuscular paralysis produced by a single dose of succinylcholine may last many hours.

2. Acetylation of amines—Isoniazid and some other amines such as hydralazine and procainamide are metabolized by *N*-acetylation. Individuals deficient in acetylation capacity, termed *slow acetylators*, may have prolonged or toxic responses to normal doses of these drugs. Slow acetylators constitute about 50% of white and African-American persons in the United States and a much smaller fraction of Asian and Inuit (Eskimo) populations. The slow acetylation trait is inherited as an autosomal recessive gene.

3. Oxidation—The rate of oxidation of debrisoquin, sparteine, phenformin, dextromethorphan, metoprolol, and some tricyclic antidepressants by certain P450 isozymes has been shown to be genetically determined.

B. OTHER DRUGS

Coadministration of certain agents may alter the disposition of many drugs. Mechanisms include the following:

1. Enzyme induction—As indicated, induction usually results from increased synthesis of cytochrome P450-dependent drug-oxidizing enzymes in the liver. Many isozymes of the P450 family exist, and inducers

Table 4–1. Examples of phase I drug-metabolizing reactions.

Reaction Type	Typical Drug Substrates
Oxidations, P450 dependent	
Hydroxylation	Amphetamines, barbiturates, phenytoin
N-Dealkylation	Caffeine, morphine, theophylline
O-Dealkylation	Codeine
N-Oxidation	Acetaminophen, nicotine
S-Oxidation	Chlorpromazine, cimetidine, thioridazine
Deamination	Amphetamine, diazepam
Oxidations, P450 independent	
Amine oxidation	Epinephrine
Dehydrogenation	Chloral hydrate, ethanol
Reductions	Chloramphenicol, clonazepam, dantrolene, naloxone
Hydrolyses	
Esters	Aspirin, clofibrate, procaine, succinylcholine
Amides	Indomethacin, lidocaine, procainamide

Table 4–2. Examples of phase II drug-metabolizing reactions.

Reaction Type	Typical Drug Substrates
Glucuronidation	Acetaminophen, diazepam, digoxin, morphine, sulfamethiazole
Acetylation	Clonazepam, dapsone, isoniazid, mescaline, sulfonamides
Glutathione conjugation	Ethacrynic acid, reactive phase I metabolite of acetaminophen
Glycine conjugation	Deoxycholic acid, nicotinic acid (niacin), salicylic acid
Sulfation	Acetaminophen, estrone, methyldopa
Methylation	Dopamine, epinephrine, histamine, norepinephrine, thiouracil

Adapted, with permission, from Katzung BG, editor: *Basic & Clinical Pharmacology*, 9th ed. McGraw-Hill, 2004.

selectively increase subgroups of isozymes. Common inducers of a few of these isozymes and the drugs whose metabolism is increased are listed in Table 4–3. Several days are usually required to reach maximum induction; a similar amount of time is required to regress after withdrawal of the inducer. The most common strong inducers of drug metabolism are carbamazepine, phenobarbital, phenytoin, and rifampin.

2. Enzyme inhibition—A few common inhibitors and the drugs whose metabolism is diminished are listed in Table 4–4. The most likely inhibitors of drug metabolism to be involved in serious drug interactions are amiodarone, cimetidine, furanocoumarins present in grapefruit juice, ketoconazole, and the HIV protease inhibitor ritonavir. **Suicide inhibitors** are drugs that are metabolized to products that irreversibly inhibit the metabolizing enzyme. Such agents include ethinyl estradiol, norethindrone, spironolactone, secobarbital, allopurinol, fluroxene, and propylthiouracil. Metabolism may also be decreased by pharmacodynamic factors such as a reduction in blood flow to the metabolizing organ (eg, propranolol reduces hepatic blood flow).

3. Inhibitors of intestinal P-glycoprotein—P-glycoprotein (P-gp) has been identified as an important modulator of intestinal drug transport and usually functions to expel drugs from the intestinal mucosa into the

Table 4–3. A partial list of drugs that significantly induce P450-mediated drug metabolism in humans.

CYP Family Induced	Important Inducers	Drugs Whose Metabolism Is Induced
1A2	Benzo[*a*]pyrene (from tobacco smoke), carbamazepine, phenobarbital, rifampin, omeprazole	Acetaminophen, clozapine, haloperidol, theophylline, tricyclic antidepressants, *(R)*-warfarin
2C9	Barbiturates, especially phenobarbital, phenytoin, primidone, rifampin	Barbiturates, chloramphenicol, doxorubicin, ibuprofen, phenytoin, chlorpromazine, steroids, tolbutamide, *(S)*-warfarin
2C19	Carbamazepine, phenobarbital, phenytoin, rifampin	Tricyclic antidepressants, phenytoin, topiramate, *(R)*-warfarin
2E1	Ethanol, isoniazid	Acetaminophen, ethanol (minor), halothane
3A4	Barbiturates, carbamazepine, corticosteroids, efavirenz, phenytoin, rifampin, troglitazone	Antiarrhythmics, antidepressants, azole antifungals, benzodiazepines, calcium channel blockers, cyclosporine, delavirdine, doxorubicin, efavirenz, erythromycin, estrogens, HIV protease inhibitors, nefazodone, paclitaxel, proton pump inhibitors, HMG-CoA reductase inhibitors, rifabutin, rifampin, sildenafil, SSRIs, tamoxifen, trazodone, vinca alkaloids

Table 4–4. A partial list of drugs that significantly inhibit P450-mediated drug metabolism in humans.

CYP Family Inhibited	Inhibitors	Drugs Whose Metabolism Is Inhibited
1A2	Cimetidine, fluoroquinolones, grapefruit juice, macrolides, isoniazid, zileuton	Acetaminophen, clozapine, haloperidol, theophylline, tricyclic antidepressants, *(R)*-warfarin
2C9	Amiodarone, chloramphenicol, cimetidine, isoniazid, metronidazole, SSRIs, zafirlukast	Barbiturates, celecoxib, chloramphenicol, doxorubicin, ibuprofen, phenytoin, chlorpromazine, steroids, tolbutamide, *(S)*-warfarin
2C19	Fluconazole, omeprazole, SSRIs	Diazepam, phenytoin, topiramate, *(R)*-warfarin
2D6	Amiodarone, cimetidine, quinidine, SSRIs	Antidepressants, flecainide, lidocaine, mexiletine, opioids
3A4	Amiodarone, azole antifungals, cimetidine, clarithromycin, cyclosporine, diltiazem, erythromycin, fluoroquinolones, grapefruit juice, HIV protease inhibitors, metronidazole, quinine, SSRIs, tacrolimus	Antiarrhythmics, antidepressants, azole antifungals, benzodiazepines, calcium channel blockers, cyclosporine, delavirdine, doxorubicin, efavirenz, erythromycin, estrogens, HIV protease inhibitors, nefazodone, paclitaxel, proton pump inhibitors, HMG-CoA reductase inhibitors, rifabutin, rifampin, sildenafil, SSRIs, tamoxifen, trazodone, vinca alkaloids

lumen. (Other members of the P-gp family are found in the blood-brain barrier and in drug-resistant cancer cells.) Drugs that inhibit intestinal P-gp mimic drug metabolism inhibitors by increasing bioavailability and may result in toxic plasma concentrations of drugs given at normally nontoxic dosage. P-gp inhibitors include verapamil, mibefradil (a calcium channel blocker no longer on the market), and furanocoumarin components of grapefruit juice. Important drugs that are normally expelled by P-gp (and which are therefore potentially more toxic when given with a P-gp inhibitor) include digoxin, cyclosporine, and saquinavir.

TOXIC METABOLISM

Drug metabolism is not synonymous with drug inactivation. Some drugs are converted to active products by metabolism. If these products are toxic, severe injury may result under some circumstances. An important example is acetaminophen when taken in large overdoses (Figure 4–1). Acetaminophen is conjugated to harmless glucuronide and sulfate metabolites when it is taken in recommended doses by patients with normal liver function. If a large overdose is taken, however, the phase II metabolic pathways are overwhelmed, and a P450-dependent system converts some of the drug to a reactive intermediate (*N*-acetyl-*p*-benzoquinoneimine). This intermediate is conjugated with glutathione to a third harmless product if glutathione stores are adequate. If glutathione stores are exhausted, however, the reactive intermediate combines with essential hepatic cell proteins, resulting in cell death. Prompt administration of

other sulfhydryl donors (eg, acetylcysteine) may be life-saving after an overdose. In severe liver disease, stores of glucuronide, sulfate, and glutathione may be depleted, making the patient more susceptible to hepatic toxicity

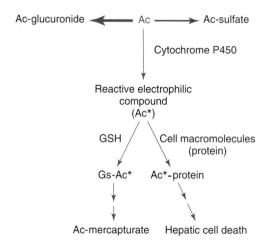

Figure 4–1. Metabolism of acetaminophen to harmless conjugates or to toxic metabolites. Acetaminophen glucuronide, acetaminophen sulfate, and the mercapturate conjugate of acetaminophen are all nontoxic phase II conjugates. Ac* is the toxic, reactive phase I metabolite (an epoxide). Transformation to the reactive metabolite occurs if hepatic stores of sulfate, glucuronide, and glutathione are depleted or overwhelmed or if phase I enzymes have been induced.

with near-normal doses of acetaminophen. Enzyme inducers (eg, ethanol) may increase acetaminophen toxicity because they increase phase I metabolism more than phase II metabolism, thus resulting in increased production of the reactive metabolite.

QUESTIONS

1. You are planning to treat asthma in a 19-year-old patient with recurrent, episodic attacks of bronchospasm with wheezing. You are concerned about drug interactions caused by changes in drug metabolism in this patient. Drug metabolism in humans usually results in a product that is
   (A) Less lipid soluble than the original drug
   (B) More likely to distribute intracellularly
   (C) More likely to be reabsorbed by kidney tubules
   (D) More lipid soluble than the original drug
   (E) Less water soluble than the original drug

2. If therapy with multiple drugs causes induction of drug metabolism in your asthma patient, it will
   (A) Be associated with increased smooth endoplasmic reticulum
   (B) Be associated with increased rough endoplasmic reticulum
   (C) Be associated with decreased enzymes in the soluble cytoplasmic fraction
   (D) Require 3–4 months to reach completion
   (E) Be irreversible

3. A factor that is likely to increase the duration of action of a drug that is metabolized by CYP3A4 in the liver is
   (A) Chronic administration of phenobarbital before and during therapy with the drug in question
   (B) Chronic therapy with cimetidine before and during therapy with the drug in question
   (C) Displacement from tissue binding sites by another drug
   (D) Increased cardiac output
   (E) Chronic administration of rifampin

4. Which of the following is a phase II drug-metabolizing reaction?
   (A) Acetylation
   (B) Deamination
   (C) Hydrolysis
   (D) Oxidation
   (E) Reduction

5. Reports of cardiac arrhythmias caused by unusually high blood levels of 2 antihistamines, terfenadine and astemizole, led to their removal from the market. These effects were best explained by
   (A) Concomitant treatment with phenobarbital
   (B) Use of these drugs by smokers

(C) A genetic predisposition to metabolize succinylcholine slowly
(D) Treatment of these patients with ketoconazole, an azole antifungal agent

6. Which of the following drugs is associated with slower metabolism in European-Americans and African-Americans than in most Asians?
   (A) Cimetidine
   (B) Procainamide
   (C) Quinidine
   (D) Rifampin
   (E) Succinylcholine

7. Which of the following drugs may inhibit the hepatic microsomal P450 responsible for warfarin metabolism?
   (A) Cimetidine
   (B) Ethanol
   (C) Phenobarbital
   (D) Procainamide
   (E) Rifampin

8. Which of the following drugs is hydrolyzed by a plasma esterase that is abnormally low in activity in about 1 of every 2500 humans?
   (A) Cimetidine
   (B) Ethanol
   (C) Procainamide
   (D) Rifampin
   (E) Succinylcholine

9. Chronic use of which of the following drugs may increase the toxicity of acetaminophen?
   (A) Cimetidine
   (B) Ethanol
   (C) Ketoconazole
   (D) Procainamide
   (E) Quinidine
   (F) Ritonavir
   (G) Succinylcholine
   (H) Verapamil

10. Which of the following drugs has higher first-pass metabolism in men than in women?
    (A) Cimetidine
    (B) Ethanol
    (C) Ketoconazole
    (D) Procainamide
    (E) Quinidine
    (F) Ritonavir
    (G) Succinylcholine
    (H) Verapamil

11. Which of the following drugs is an established inhibitor of P-glycoprotein (P-gp) drug transporters?
    (A) Cimetidine
    (B) Ethanol

(C) Ketoconazole
(D) Procainamide
(E) Quinidine
(F) Ritonavir
(G) Succinylcholine
(H) Verapamil

12. Which of the following agents, when used in combination with other anti-HIV drugs, permits dose reductions?
    (A) Cimetidine
    (B) Efavirenz
    (C) Ketoconazole
    (D) Procainamide
    (E) Quinidine
    (F) Ritonavir
    (G) Succinylcholine
    (H) Verapamil

ANSWERS

1. Biotransformation usually results in a product that is less lipid soluble. The answer is **A.**

2. The smooth endoplasmic reticulum, which contains the mixed-function oxidase drug-metabolizing enzymes, is selectively increased by inducers. The answer is **A.**

3. Phenobarbital can induce drug-metabolizing enzymes and thereby may reduce the duration of drug action. Displacement of drug from tissue may transiently increase the intensity of the effect but will decrease the volume of distribution and thereby reduce the half-life. Cimetidine is recognized as an inhibitor of P450 and may also decrease hepatic blood flow under some circumstances. The answer is **B.**

4. Acetylation is a phase II conjugation reaction. The answer is **A.**

5. Treatment with phenobarbital and smoking are associated with increased drug metabolism and lower, not higher, blood levels. Ketoconazole, itraconazole, erythromycin, and some substances in grapefruit juice slow the metabolism of certain older nonsedating antihistamines (Chapter 16). The answer is **D.**

6. Procainamide, like hydralazine and isoniazid, is metabolized by *N*-acetylation, an enzymatic process that is slow in about 20% of Asians and in about 50% of European-Americans and African-Americans. The answer is **B.**

7. Cimetidine is a commonly used drug and has well-documented ability to inhibit the hepatic metabolism of many drugs. The answer is **A.**

8. Succinylcholine is normally hydrolyzed quite rapidly by plasma cholinesterase (pseudocholinesterase). This enzyme is abnormal in about 1/2500 of the human population, resulting in an unusually long duration of action of succinylcholine in these patients. The answer is **E.**

9. Acetaminophen is normally eliminated by phase II conjugation reactions. The drug's toxicity is dependent on an oxidized reactive metabolite produced by phase I oxidizing P450 enzymes. Ethanol (and certain other drugs) induces P450 enzymes and thus reduces the hepatotoxic dose. The answer is **B.**

10. Ethanol is subject to metabolism in the stomach as well as in the liver. Independently of body weight and other factors, men have greater gastric ethanol metabolism and thus a lower bioavailability than women. The answer is **B.**

11. Verapamil is an inhibitor of P-glycoprotein drug transporters and has been used to enhance the cytotoxic actions of methotrexate in cancer chemotherapy. The answer is **H.**

12. Ritonavir inhibits hepatic drug metabolism, and its use at low doses in combination regimens has permitted dose reductions of other HIV protease inhibitors (eg, indinavir). The answer is **F.**

CHECKLIST

When you complete this chapter, you should be able to:

☐ List the major phase I and phase II metabolic reactions.

☐ Describe the mechanism of hepatic enzyme induction and list 3 drugs that are known to cause it.

☐ List 3 drugs that inhibit the metabolism of other drugs.

☐ List 3 drugs for which there are well-defined genetically determined differences in metabolism.

☐ Describe some of the effects of smoking, liver disease, and kidney disease on drug elimination.

☐ Describe the pathways by which acetaminophen is metabolized (1) to harmless products if normal doses are taken and (2) to hepatotoxic products if an overdose is taken.

Drug Evaluation & Regulation

Drugs are regulated in almost all countries by governmental agencies. In the United States, regulation is by the Food and Drug Administration (FDA). New drugs are developed in industrial or academic laboratories. Before a new drug can be approved for regular therapeutic use in humans, a series of animal and experimental human studies must be carried out.

New drugs may emerge from a variety of sources. Some are the result of identification of a new target for a disease, discovered through basic research in academic or industrial laboratories. Rational molecular design or screening is then used to find a molecule that selectively binds the target. In contrast, many (so-called "me-too" drugs) are the result of molecular manipulation that alters the pharmacokinetic properties of the original, prototype agent.

SAFETY & EFFICACY

Because society expects prescription drugs to be safe and effective, governments regulate the development and marketing of new drugs. The FDA is the regulatory body in the United States that proposes and administers these regulations. Current regulations require evidence of relative safety (derived from acute and subacute toxicity testing in animals) and probable therapeutic action (from the pharmacologic profile in animals) before human testing is permitted. Some information about the pharmacokinetics of a compound is also required before clinical evaluation is begun. Chronic toxicity test results are generally not required before human studies are started. The development of a new drug and its pathway through various levels of testing and regulation are illustrated in Figure 5–1. The cost of development of a new drug, including false starts and discarded molecules, is currently several hundred million dollars.

ANIMAL TESTING

The amount of animal testing required before human studies begin is a function of the proposed use and the urgency of the application. Thus, a drug proposed for occasional nonsystemic use requires less extensive testing than one destined for chronic systemic administration.

Anticancer drugs and drugs proposed for use in AIDS, because of the urgent need for new agents, require less evidence of safety than do drugs used in treatment of less threatening diseases and are often investigated and approved on an accelerated schedule.

A. ACUTE TOXICITY

Acute toxicity studies are required for all new drugs. These studies involve administration of single doses of the agent up to the lethal level in at least 2 species (eg, 1 rodent and 1 nonrodent).

B. SUBACUTE AND CHRONIC TOXICITY

Subacute and chronic toxicity testing are required for most agents, especially those intended for chronic use. Tests are usually conducted for a duration proportionate to the time proposed for human application, ie, 2–4 weeks (subacute) or 6–24 months (chronic), in at least 2 species.

TYPES OF ANIMAL TESTS

Tests done with animals often include general screening tests for pharmacologic effects, hepatic and renal function monitoring, blood and urine tests, gross and histopathologic examination of tissues, and tests of reproductive effects and carcinogenicity.

A. PHARMACOLOGIC PROFILE

The pharmacologic profile is a description of all the pharmacologic effects of a drug (eg, effects on blood pressure, gastrointestinal activity, respiration, renal function, endocrine function, CNS).

B. REPRODUCTIVE TOXICITY

Reproductive toxicity testing involves the study of the fertility effects of the candidate drug and its teratogenic and mutagenic effects. The FDA uses a 5-level descriptive scale to summarize information regarding the safety of drugs in pregnancy (Table 5–1). Unfortunately, this scale is frequently out of date and not always accurate. **Teratogenesis** can be defined as the induction of developmental defects in the somatic tissues of the fetus (eg, by exposure of the fetus to a chemical, infection, or radiation). Teratogenesis is studied by treating pregnant

HIGH-YIELD TERMS TO LEARN

Mutagenic	An effect on the inheritable characteristics of a cell or organism—a mutation in the DNA; usually tested in microorganisms with the Ames test
Carcinogenic	An effect of inducing malignant characteristics
Teratogenic	An effect on the in utero development of an organism resulting in abnormal structure or function; not generally heritable
Placebo	An inactive "dummy" medication made up to resemble the active investigational formulation as much as possible
Single-blind study	A clinical trial in which the investigators—but not the subjects—know which subjects are receiving active drug and which are receiving placebos
Double-blind study	A clinical trial in which neither the subjects nor the investigators know which subjects are receiving placebos; the code is held by a third party
IND	Investigational New Drug Exemption; an application for FDA approval to carry out new drug trials in humans; requires animal data
NDA	New Drug Application; seeks FDA approval to market a new drug for ordinary clinical use. Requires data from clinical trials as well as preclinical (animal) data.
Phases 1, 2, and 3 of clinical trials	Three parts of a clinical trial that are usually carried out before submitting an NDA to the FDA
Positive control	A known standard therapy, to be used along with placebo, to evaluate the superiority or inferiority of a new drug in relation to the others available
Orphan drugs	Drugs developed for diseases in which the expected number of patients is small. Some countries bestow certain commercial advantages on companies that develop drugs for uncommon diseases

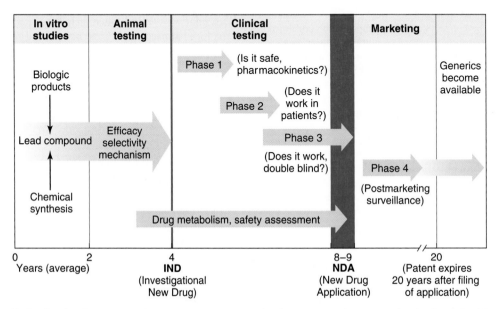

Figure 5–1. The development and testing process required to bring a new drug to market in the United States. Some requirements may be different for drugs used in life-threatening diseases. (Reproduced, with permission, from Katzung BG, editor: *Basic & Clinical Pharmacology,* 10th ed. McGraw-Hill, 2007.)

Table 5–1. FDA ratings of drug safety in pregnancy.

Category	Description
A	Controlled studies in women fail to demonstrate a risk to the fetus in the first trimester (and there is no evidence of a risk in later trimesters), and the possibility of fetal harm appears remote.
B	Either animal-reproduction studies have not demonstrated a fetal risk but there are no controlled studies in pregnant women, or animal-reproduction studies have shown an adverse effect (other than a decrease in fertility) that was not confirmed in controlled studies in women in the first trimester (and there is no evidence of a risk in later trimesters).
C	Either studies in animals have revealed adverse effects on the fetus (teratogenic or embryocidal or other) and there are no controlled studies in women or studies in women and animals are not available. Drugs should be given only if the potential benefit justifies the potential risk to the fetus.
D	There is positive evidence of human fetal risk, but the benefits from use in pregnant women may be acceptable despite the risk (eg, if the drug is needed in a life-threatening situation or for a serious disease for which safer drugs cannot be used or are ineffective).
X	Studies in animals or human beings have demonstrated fetal abnormalities or there is evidence of fetal risk based on human experience or both, and the risk of the use of the drug in pregnant women clearly outweighs any possible benefit. The drug is contraindicated in women who are or may become pregnant.

female animals of at least 2 species at selected times during early pregnancy when organogenesis is known to take place and later examining the fetuses or neonates for abnormalities. Examples of drugs known to have teratogenic effects include thalidomide, isotretinoin, valproic acid, ethanol, glucocorticoids, warfarin, lithium, and androgens. **Mutagenesis** is induction of changes in the genetic material of animals of any age and therefore induction of heritable abnormalities. The **Ames test,** the standard in vitro test for mutagenicity, uses a special strain of salmonella bacteria that naturally depends on specific nutrients in the culture medium. Loss of this dependence as a result of exposure to the test drug signals a mutation. The **dominant lethal test** is an in vivo mutagenicity test carried out in mice. Male animals are exposed to the test substance before mating. Abnormalities in the results of subsequent mating (eg, loss of embryos, deformed fetuses) signal a mutation in the male's germ cells. Many carcinogens (eg, aflatoxin, cancer chemotherapeutic drugs, and other agents that bind to DNA) have mutagenic effects and test positive in the Ames test.

C. CARCINOGENESIS

Carcinogenesis is the induction of malignant characteristics in cells. Because carcinogenicity is difficult and expensive to study, the Ames test is often used to screen chemicals, since there is a moderately high degree of correlation between mutagenicity in the Ames test and carcinogenicity in some animal tests. Agents with known

carcinogenic effects include coal tar, aflatoxin, dimethylnitrosamine and other nitrosamines, urethane, vinyl chloride, and the polycyclic aromatic hydrocarbons in tobacco smoke (eg, benzo[a]pyrene).

CLINICAL TRIALS

Human testing of new drugs in the United States requires approval by institutional committees that monitor the ethical (informed consent, patient safety) and scientific aspects (study design, statistical power) of the proposed tests. Such testing also requires the prior approval by the FDA of an **Investigational New Drug Exemption application (IND),** which is submitted by the manufacturer to the FDA (see Figure 5–1). The IND includes all of the preclinical data collected up to the time of submission and the detailed proposal for clinical trials. The major clinical testing process is informally divided into 3 phases that are carried out to provide information for a New Drug Application (NDA). The NDA constitutes the request for approval of general marketing of the new agent for prescription use and includes all of the results of preclinical and clinical testing. A fourth phase of study (the surveillance phase) follows NDA approval.

A. PHASE 1

A phase 1 trial consists of careful evaluation of the dose-response relationship in a small number of normal human volunteers (eg, 25–50). An exception is in phase

Table 5–2. Selected legislation pertaining to drugs in the United States.

Law	Purpose and Effect
Pure Food and Drug Act of 1906	Prohibited mislabeling and adulteration of foods and drugs (but no requirement for efficacy or safety)
Harrison Narcotics Act of 1914	Established regulations for the use of opium, opioids, and cocaine (marijuana added in 1937)
Food, Drug, and Cosmetics Act of 1938	Required that new drugs be tested for safety as well as purity
Kefauver-Harris Amendment (1962)	Required proof of efficacy as well as safety for new drugs
Dietary Supplement and Health Education Act (1994)	Amended the Food, Drug, and Cosmetics act of 1938 to establish standards for dietary supplements but prohibited the FDA from applying the same efficacy and safety standards applied to drugs

1 trials of cancer chemotherapeutic agents and other highly toxic drugs; these are carried out by administering the agents to patients with the target disease. In phase 1 studies, the acute effects of the agent are studied over a broad range of dosages, starting with one that produces no detectable effect and progressing to one that produces either a significant physiologic response or a very minor toxic effect.

B. PHASE 2

A phase 2 trial involves evaluation of a drug in a moderate number of patients (eg, 100–300) with the target disease. A placebo or positive control drug is included in a single-blind or double-blind design. The study is carried out under very carefully controlled conditions, and patients are very closely monitored, often in a hospital research ward. The goal is to determine whether the agent has the desired therapeutic effects at doses that are tolerated by sick patients.

C. PHASE 3

A phase 3 trial usually consists of a large design involving many patients (eg, 1000–5000 or more, in many centers) and many clinicians who are using the drug in the manner proposed for its ultimate general use (eg, in outpatients). Such studies usually include placebo and positive controls in a double-blind crossover design. The goals are to explore further the spectrum of beneficial actions of the new drug, to compare it with older therapies, and to discover toxicities, if any, that occur so infrequently as to be undetectable in phase 2 studies.

D. PHASE 4

Phase 4 represents the postmarketing surveillance phase of evaluation, in which it is hoped that toxicities that occur very infrequently will be detected and reported early enough to prevent major therapeutic disasters. Unlike the first 3 phases, phase 4 has not been rigidly regulated by the FDA. Because so many drugs have been found to be unacceptably toxic only after they have been marketed, there is considerable current interest in making phase 4 surveillance more consistent, effective, and informative.

DRUG LEGISLATION

In the United States, many laws regulating drugs were passed during the 20th century. Refer to Table 5–2 for a partial list of this legislation.

ORPHAN DRUGS

An orphan drug is a drug for a rare disease (one affecting fewer than 200,000 people in the United States). The study of such agents has often been neglected because the sales of an effective agent for an uncommon ailment might not pay the costs of development. In the United States, current legislation provides for tax relief and other incentives designed to encourage the development of orphan drugs.

QUESTIONS

1. With regard to clinical trials of most new drugs,
   (A) Phase 1 involves the study of a small number of normal volunteers by highly trained clinical pharmacologists
   (B) Phase 2 involves the use of the new drug in a large number of patients (1000–5000) who have the disease to be treated

(C) Phase 3 involves the determination of the drug's therapeutic index by the cautious induction of toxicity

(D) Phase 4 involves the detailed study of toxic effects that have been discovered in phase 3

(E) Phase 2 requires the use of a positive control (a known effective drug) and a placebo

2. Animal testing of potential new therapeutic agents
   (A) Extends over a time period of at least 3 years in order to discover late toxicities
   (B) Requires the use of at least 1 primate species (eg, rhesus monkey)
   (C) Requires the submission of histopathologic slides and specimens to the FDA for evaluation by government scientists
   (D) Has good predictability for drug allergy-type reactions
   (E) May be abbreviated in the case of some very toxic agents used in cancer

3. The "dominant lethal" test involves the treatment of a male adult animal with a chemical before mating; the pregnant female is later examined for fetal death and abnormalities. The dominant lethal test therefore is a test of
   (A) Teratogenicity
   (B) Mutagenicity
   (C) Carcinogenicity
   (D) All of the above
   (E) None of the above

4. An optimal phase 3 clinical trial of a new analgesic drug for mild pain would NOT include
   (A) A negative control (placebo)
   (B) A positive control (current standard therapy)
   (C) Double-blind protocol (neither the patient nor immediate observers of the patient know which agent is active)
   (D) A group of 2000–3000 subjects with a clinical condition requiring analgesia
   (E) Prior submission of an NDA (new drug application) to the FDA

5. In the testing of new compounds (eg, antihypertensive drugs) for potential therapeutic use
   (A) Animal tests cannot be used to predict the types of toxicities that may occur because there is no correlation with human toxicity
   (B) Human studies in normal individuals will be done before the drug is used in diseased individuals
   (C) Degree of risk must be assessed in at least 3 species of animals, including 1 primate species
   (D) The animal therapeutic index must be known before trial of the agents in humans

6. The Ames test is a method for detecting
   (A) Carcinogenesis in primates
   (B) Carcinogenesis in rodents
   (C) Mutagenesis in bacteria
   (D) Teratogenesis in any mammalian species
   (E) Teratogenesis in primates

ANSWERS

1. Except for known toxic drugs (eg, cancer chemotherapy drugs), phase 1 is carried out in 25–50 normal volunteers. Phase 2 is carried out in several hundred patients with the disease. The therapeutic index is rarely determined in any clinical trial. Phase 4 is the general surveillance phase that follows general marketing of the new drug. It is not targeted at specific effects. Positive controls and placebos are not a rigid requirement of any phase of clinical trials, although they are often used in phase 2 and phase 3 studies. The answer is **A.**

2. Drugs proposed for short-term use may not require long-term chronic testing. For some drugs, no primates are used; for other agents, only 1 species is used. The data from the tests, not the evidence itself, must be submitted to the FDA. Prediction of human drug allergy from animal testing is not very reliable. The answer is **E.**

3. The description of the test indicates that a chromosomal change (passed from father to fetus) is the toxicity detected. This is a mutation. The answer is **B.**

4. The first 4 items (**A–D**) are correct. An NDA cannot be acted upon until the first 3 phases of clinical trials have been completed. (The IND must be approved before clinical trials can be conducted.) The answer is **E.**

5. Animal tests in a single species do not always predict human toxicities; however, when these tests are carried out in several species, most acute toxicities that occur in humans will also appear in at least 1 animal species. According to current FDA rules, the "degree of risk" must be determined in at least 2 species. Use of primates is not always required. The therapeutic index is not required. Except for cancer chemotherapeutic agents and antivirals used in AIDs, phase 1 clinical trials are always carried out in normal subjects. The answer is **B.**

6. The Ames test is carried out in *Salmonella* and detects mutations in the bacterial DNA. Because mutagenic potential is associated with carcinogenic risk for many chemicals, the Ames test is often used to claim that a particular agent may be a carcinogen. However, the test itself only detects mutations. The answer is **C.**

CHECKLIST

When you complete this chapter, you should be able to:

☐ Describe the major animal and clinical studies carried out in drug development.

☐ Describe the purpose of the Investigational New Drug (IND) Exemption and the New Drug Application (NDA).

☐ Define carcinogenesis, mutagenesis, and teratogenesis.

PART II
Autonomic Drugs

Introduction to Autonomic Pharmacology

6

The autonomic nervous system (ANS) is the major involuntary, unconscious, automatic portion of the nervous system and contrasts in several ways with the somatic (voluntary) nervous system. The anatomy, neurotransmitter chemistry, receptor characteristics, and functional integration of the ANS are discussed in this chapter.

ANATOMIC ASPECTS OF THE ANS

The motor (efferent) portion of the ANS is the major pathway for information transmission from the CNS to the involuntary effector tissues (smooth muscle, cardiac muscle, and exocrine glands; Figure 6–1). Its 2 major subdivisions are the **parasympathetic** ANS **(PANS)** and the **sympathetic** ANS **(SANS)**. The **enteric nervous system (ENS)** is a semiautonomous part of the ANS located in the gastrointestinal tract, with specific functions for the control of this organ system. The ENS consists of the myenteric plexus (plexus of Auerbach) and the submucous plexus (plexus of Meissner); they send sensory input to the parasympathetic and sympathetic nervous systems and receive motor output from them.

There are many sensory (afferent) fibers in autonomic nerves. These are of considerable importance for the physiologic control of the involuntary organs but are directly influenced by only a few drugs.

A. CENTRAL ROOTS OF ORIGIN

The parasympathetic preganglionic motor fibers originate in cranial nerve nuclei III, VII, IX, and X and in sacral segments (usually S2–S4) of the spinal cord. The sympathetic preganglionic fibers originate in the thoracic (T1–T12) and lumbar (L1–L5) segments of the cord.

B. LOCATION OF GANGLIA

Most of the sympathetic ganglia are located in 2 paravertebral chains that lie along the spinal column. A few (the prevertebral ganglia) are located on the anterior aspect of the abdominal aorta. Most of the parasympathetic ganglia are located in the organs innervated, more distant from the spinal cord. Because of the locations of the ganglia, the preganglionic sympathetic fibers are short and the postganglionic fibers are long. The opposite is true for the parasympathetic system: preganglionic fibers are long and postganglionic fibers are short.

C. UNINNERVATED RECEPTORS

Some receptors that respond to autonomic transmitters and drugs receive no innervation. These include muscarinic receptors on the endothelium of blood vessels, some presynaptic receptors, and, in some species, the adrenoceptors on apocrine sweat glands and α_2 and β adrenoceptors in some blood vessels.

NEUROTRANSMITTER ASPECTS OF THE ANS

The synthesis, storage, release, receptor interactions, and termination of action of the neurotransmitters are very important in the action of autonomic drugs (Figure 6–2).

HIGH-YIELD TERMS TO LEARN

Adrenergic	A nerve ending that releases norepinephrine as the primary transmitter; also, a synapse in which norepinephrine is the primary transmitter
Adrenoceptor, adrenergic receptor	A receptor that binds, and is activated by, one of the catecholamine transmitters or hormones (norepinephrine, epinephrine, dopamine) and related drugs
Autonomic effector cells or tissues	Cells or tissues that have adrenoceptors or cholinoceptors which, when activated, alter the function of those cells or tissues, eg, smooth muscle, cardiac muscle, glands
Baroreceptor reflex	The neuronal homeostatic mechanism that maintains a constant arterial blood pressure; the sensory limb originates in the baroreceptors of the carotid sinus and aortic arch; efferent pathways run in parasympathetic and sympathetic nerves
Cholinergic	A nerve ending that releases acetylcholine; also, a synapse in which the primary transmitter is acetylcholine
Cholinoceptor, cholinergic receptor	A receptor that binds, and is activated by, acetylcholine and related drugs
Dopaminergic	A nerve ending that releases dopamine as the primary transmitter; also a synapse in which dopamine is the primary transmitter
Homeostatic reflex	A compensatory mechanism for maintaining a body function at a predetermined level, eg, the baroreceptor reflex for blood pressure
Parasympathetic	The part of the autonomic nervous system that originates in the cranial nerves and sacral part of the spinal cord; the craniosacral autonomic system
Postsynaptic receptor	A receptor located on the distal side of a synapse, eg, on a postganglionic neuron or an autonomic effector cell
Presynaptic receptor	A receptor located on the nerve ending from which the transmitter is released into the synapse; modulates the release of transmitter
Sympathetic	The part of the autonomic nervous system that originates in the thoracic and lumbar parts of the spinal cord

A. CHOLINERGIC TRANSMISSION

Acetylcholine (ACh) is the primary transmitter in all autonomic ganglia and at the parasympathetic postganglionic neuron-effector cell synapses. It is also the primary transmitter at the somatic (voluntary) skeletal muscle neuromuscular junction (Figure 6–1).

1. Synthesis and storage—ACh is synthesized from acetyl-CoA and choline by the enzyme choline acetyltransferase. The rate-limiting step is probably the transport of choline into the nerve terminal. This transport can be inhibited by the research drug **hemicholinium.** ACh is actively transported into its vesicles for storage by the vesicle-associated transporter, VAT. This process can be inhibited by another research drug, **vesamicol.**

2. Release of acetylcholine—Release of transmitter stores from vesicles in the nerve ending requires the entry of calcium through calcium channels and triggering of an interaction between proteins associated with the vesicles (**VAMPs, vesicle-associated membrane proteins: synaptobrevin, synaptotagmin**) and proteins associated with the nerve ending membrane (**SNAPs,**

synaptosome-associated proteins: SNAP25, syntaxin, and others). This interaction results in the fusion of the membranes of the vesicles with the nerve ending membranes, the opening of a pore to the extracellular space, and the release of the stored transmitter. The several types of **botulinum toxins** enzymatically alter synaptobrevin or one of the other docking or fusion proteins to prevent the release process.

3. Termination of action of ACh—The action of acetylcholine in the synapse is normally terminated by metabolism to acetate and choline by the enzyme acetylcholinesterase in the synaptic cleft. The products are not excreted but are recycled in the body. Inhibition of acetylcholinesterase is an important therapeutic (and potentially toxic) effect of several drugs.

4. Drug effects on synthesis, storage, release, and termination of action of ACh—Drugs that block the synthesis of ACh (eg, hemicholinium), its storage (eg, vesamicol), or its release (eg, botulinum toxin) are not very useful for systemic therapy because their effects are not sufficiently selective (ie, PANS and SANS ganglia

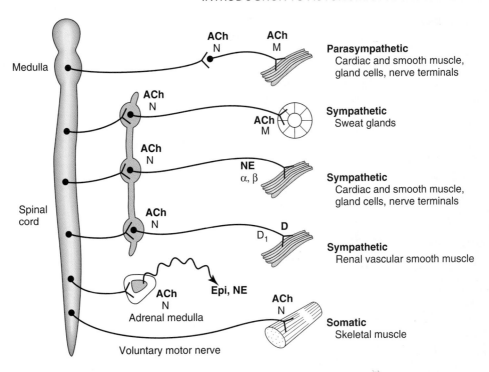

Figure 6–1. Schematic diagram comparing some features of the parasympathetic and sympathetic divisions of the autonomic nervous system with the somatic motor system. Parasympathetic ganglia are not shown as discrete structures because most of them are diffusely distributed in the walls of the organs innervated. ACh, acetylcholine; Epi, epinephrine; NE, norepinephrine; D, dopamine; N, nicotinic; M, muscarinic; α, β, alpha and beta adrenoceptors; D_1, dopamine$_1$ receptors. (Reproduced, with permission, from Katzung BG, editor: *Basic & Clinical Pharmacology*, 10th ed. McGraw-Hill, 2007.)

and somatic neuromuscular junctions may all be blocked). However, because botulinum toxin is a very large molecule and diffuses very slowly, it can be used by injection for local effects.

SKILL KEEPER: DRUG PERMEATION (SEE CHAPTER 1)

Botulinum toxin is a very large protein molecule and does not diffuse readily when injected into tissue. In spite of this property, it is able to enter cholinergic nerve endings from the extracellular space and block the release of acetylcholine. How might it cross the lipid membrane barrier? The Skill Keeper Answer appears at the end of the chapter.

B. Adrenergic Transmission

Norepinephrine (NE) is the primary transmitter at the sympathetic postganglionic neuron-effector cell

synapses in most tissues. Important exceptions include sympathetic fibers to thermoregulatory (eccrine) sweat glands and probably vasodilator sympathetic fibers in skeletal muscle, which release ACh. Dopamine may be a vasodilator transmitter in renal blood vessels.

1. Synthesis and storage—The synthesis of dopamine and NE is more complex than that of ACh (Figure 6–2). Tyrosine is hydroxylated by **tyrosine hydroxylase** (the rate-limiting step) to DOPA (dihydroxyphenylalanine), decarboxylated to dopamine, and (inside the vesicle) hydroxylated to norepinephrine. Tyrosine hydroxylase can be inhibited by **metyrosine**. NE and dopamine are transported into vesicles and stored there. Monoamine oxidase (MAO) is present on mitochondria in the adrenergic nerve ending and inactivates a portion of the dopamine and norepinephrine in the cytoplasm. Therefore, **MAO inhibitors** may increase the stores of these transmitters and other amines in the nerve endings (Chapter 30). The vesicular transporter can be inhibited by **reserpine**.

2. Release and termination of action—Dopamine and NE are released from their nerve endings by the same calcium-dependent mechanism responsible for

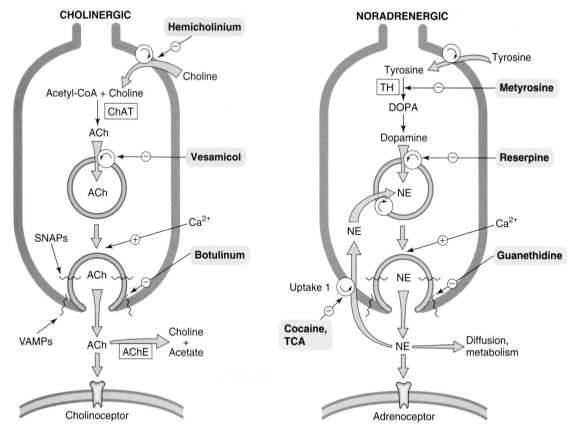

CHOLINERGIC

NORADRENERGIC

Figure 6–2. Characteristics of transmitter synthesis, storage, release, and termination of action at cholinergic and noradrenergic nerve terminals are shown from the top downward. Circles represent transporters; ACh, acetylcholine; AChE, acetylcholinesterase; ChAT, choline acetyltransferase; DOPA, dihydroxyphenylalanine; NE, norepinephrine; TCA, tricyclic antidepressant; TH, tyrosine hydroxylase.

ACh release (see prior discussion). Termination of action, however, is quite different. Metabolism is not responsible for termination of action of the catecholamine transmitters, norepinephrine and dopamine. Instead, **diffusion** and **reuptake** (especially uptake-1, Figure 6–2, by the norepinephrine transporter, NET) reduce their concentration in the synaptic cleft and stop their action. Outside the cleft, these transmitters can be metabolized—by **monoamine oxidase (MAO)** and **catechol-*O*-methyltransferase (COMT)**—and the products of these enzymatic reactions are excreted. Determination of the 24-h excretion of **metanephrine, normetanephrine, 3-methoxy-4-hydroxymandelic acid (VMA),** and other metabolites provides a measure of the total body production of catecholamines, a determination useful in diagnosing conditions such as pheochromocytoma. Inhibition of MAO increases stores of catecholamines and has both therapeutic and toxic potential.

3. Drug effects on adrenergic transmission—Drugs that block norepinephrine synthesis (eg, metyrosine) or catecholamine storage (eg, reserpine) or release (eg, guanethidine) have been used in several diseases (eg, pheochromocytoma, hypertension) because they block sympathetic but not parasympathetic functions. Other drugs *promote* catecholamine release, (eg, the amphetamine-like agents).

C. COTRANSMITTERS

Many (probably all) autonomic nerves have transmitter vesicles that contain other transmitter molecules in addition to the primary agents (ACh or NE) described above. These cotransmitters may be localized in the same vesicles as the primary transmitter or in a separate population of vesicles. Substances recognized to date as cotransmitters include **ATP, enkephalins, vasoactive intestinal peptide (VIP), neuropeptide Y, substance**

P, **neurotensin, somatostatin,** and others. Their main role in autonomic function appears to involve modulation of synaptic transmission. The same substances function as primary transmitters in other synapses.

RECEPTOR CHARACTERISTICS

The major receptor systems in the ANS include cholinoceptors, adrenoceptors, and dopamine receptors, which have been described in some detail. The numerous receptors for cotransmitter substances have not been as fully defined.

A. Cholinoceptors

Also referred to as cholinergic receptors, these molecules respond to acetylcholine and its analogs. Cholinoceptors are subdivided as follows (Table 6–1):

1. Muscarinic receptors—As their name suggests, these receptors respond to muscarine (an alkaloid) as well as to acetylcholine. The effects of activation of these receptors resemble those of postganglionic parasympathetic nerve stimulation. Muscarinic receptors are located primarily on autonomic effector cells (including heart, vascular endothelium, smooth muscle, presynaptic nerve terminals, and exocrine glands). Evidence (including their genes) has been found for 5 subtypes, of which 3 appear to be important in peripheral autonomic transmission. All 5 are G protein-coupled receptors (Chapter 2).

2. Nicotinic receptors—These receptors are parts of ion channels and respond to acetylcholine and nicotine, another acetylcholine mimic, but not to muscarine. The 2 major nicotinic subtypes are located in ganglia and in skeletal muscle end plates. The nicotinic receptors are the primary receptors for transmission at these sites.

B. Adrenoceptors

Also referred to as adrenergic receptors, adrenoceptors are divided into several subtypes (Table 6–2).

1. Alpha receptors—These are located on vascular smooth muscle, presynaptic nerve terminals, blood platelets, fat cells (lipocytes), and neurons in the brain. Alpha receptors are further divided into 2 major types, α_1 and α_2. These 2 subtypes constitute different families and utilize different G coupling proteins.

2. Beta receptors—These receptors are located on most types of smooth muscle, cardiac muscle, some presynaptic nerve terminals, and lipocytes as well as in the brain. Beta receptors are divided into 3 major subtypes, β_1, β_2, and β_3. These subtypes are rather similar and utilize the same G coupling protein.

C. Dopamine Receptors

Dopamine (D, DA) receptors are a subclass of adrenoceptors but with rather different distribution and function. Dopamine receptors are especially important in the renal and splanchnic vessels and in the brain. Although at least 5 subtypes exist, the D_1 subtype appears to be the most important peripheral effector-cell dopamine receptor. D_2 receptors are found on presynaptic nerve terminals. D_1, D_2, and other types of dopamine receptors also occur in the CNS.

EFFECTS OF ACTIVATING AUTONOMIC NERVES

Each division of the ANS has specific effects on organ systems. These effects, summarized in Table 6–3, should be memorized.

Dually innervated organs such as the iris of the eye and the sinoatrial node of the heart receive both sympathetic and parasympathetic innervation. The pupil has a natural, intrinsic diameter to which it returns if the influence of both divisions of the ANS is removed. Pharmacologic ganglionic blockade will, therefore, cause it to move to its intrinsic size. Similarly, the cardiac sinus node pacemaker rate has an intrinsic value (about 100—110/min) in the absence of both ANS inputs. How will these variables change (increase or

Table 6–1. Characteristics of the most important cholinoceptors in the peripheral nervous system.

Receptor	Location	Mechanism	Major Functions
M_1	Nerve endings	G_q-coupled	↑ IP_3, DAG cascade
M_2	Heart, some nerve endings	G_i-coupled	↓ cAMP, activates K^+ channels
M_3	Effector cells: smooth muscle, glands, endothelium	G_q-coupled	↑ IP_3, DAG cascade
N_N	ANS ganglia	Ion channel	Depolarizes, evokes action potential
N_M	Neuromuscular end plate	Ion channel	Depolarizes, evokes action potential

Table 6–2. Characteristics of some important adrenoceptors in the ANS.

Receptor	Location	G Protein	Second Messenger	Major Functions
Alpha$_1$ (α_1)	Effector tissues: smooth muscle, glands	G$_q$	↑ IP$_3$, DAG	↑ Ca^{2+}, causes contraction, secretion
Alpha$_2$ (α_2)	Nerve endings, some smooth muscle	G$_i$	↓ cAMP	↓ Transmitter release, causes contraction
Beta$_1$ (β_1)	Cardiac muscle, juxtaglomerular apparatus	G$_s$	↑ cAMP	↑ Heart rate, ↑ force; ↑ renin release
Beta$_2$ (β_2)	Smooth muscle, liver, heart	G$_s$	↑ cAMP	Relax smooth muscle; ↑ glycogenolysis; ↑ heart rate, force
Beta$_3$ (β_3)	Adipose cells	G$_s$	↑ cAMP	↑ Lipolysis
Dopamine$_1$ (D$_1$)	Smooth muscle	G$_s$	↑ cAMP	Relax renal vascular smooth muscle

decrease) if the ganglia are blocked? The answer is predictable if one knows which system is dominant. For example, both the pupil and, at rest, the SA node are dominated by the parasympathetic system. The resting pupil diameter and sinus rate are therefore under considerable PANS influence. Thus, blockade of both systems, with removal of the dominant PANS and nondominant SANS effects, will result in mydriasis and tachycardia.

NONADRENERGIC, NONCHOLINERGIC (NANC) TRANSMISSION

Some nerve fibers in autonomic effector tissues do not show the histochemical characteristics of either cholinergic or adrenergic fibers. Some of these are motor fibers that cause the release of ATP and other purines related to it. Purine-evoked responses have been identified in the bronchi, gastrointestinal tract, and urinary tract. Other motor fibers are peptidergic, ie, they release peptides as the primary transmitters (see list in prior Cotransmitters section).

Other nonadrenergic, noncholinergic fibers have the anatomic characteristics of sensory fibers and contain peptides such as substance P that are stored in and released from the fiber terminals. These fibers have been termed "sensory-efferent" or "sensory-local effector" fibers because when activated by a sensory input they are capable of releasing transmitter peptides from the sensory ending itself, from local axon branches, and from collaterals that terminate in the autonomic ganglia. These peptides are potent agonists in many autonomic effector tissues.

SITES OF AUTONOMIC DRUG ACTION

Because of the number of steps in the transmission of autonomic commands from the CNS to the effectors, there are many sites at which autonomic drugs may act. These sites include the CNS centers, the ganglia, the postganglionic nerve terminals, the effector cell receptors, and the mechanisms responsible for transmitter synthesis, storage, release, and termination of action. The most selective effect is achieved by drugs acting at receptors that mediate very selective actions (Table 6–4). Many natural and synthetic toxins have significant effects on autonomic and somatic nerve function.

INTEGRATION OF AUTONOMIC FUNCTION

Functional integration in the autonomic nervous system is provided mainly through the mechanism of negative feedback and is extremely important in determining the overall response to endogenous and exogenous ANS molecules. This process utilizes modulatory pre- and postsynaptic receptors at the local level and homeostatic reflexes at the systemic level.

A. LOCAL INTEGRATION

Local feedback control has been found at the level of the nerve endings in all systems investigated. The best documented of these is the negative feedback of norepinephrine upon its own release from adrenergic nerve terminals. This effect is mediated by α_2 receptors located on the presynaptic nerve membrane (Figure 6–3).

Table 6–3. Direct effects of autonomic nerve activity on some organ systems.

Organ	Effect of			
	Sympathetic		Parasympathetic	
	Action[a]	Receptor[b]	Action	Receptor[b]
Eye				
Iris				
Radial muscle	Contracts	α_1	...	...
Circular muscle	...	...	Contracts	M_3
Ciliary muscle	[Relaxes]	β	Contracts	M_3
Heart				
Sinoatrial node	Accelerates	β_1, β_2	Decelerates	M_2
Ectopic pacemakers	Accelerates	β_1, β_2	...	...
Contractility	Increases	β_1, β_2	Decreases (atria)	$[M_2]$
Blood vessels				
Skin, splanchnic vessels	Contracts	α	...	...
Skeletal muscle vessels	Relaxes	β_2	...	...
	Contracts	α	...	...
	[Relaxes]	$[M^c]$	...	...
Bronchiolar smooth muscle	Relaxes	β_2	Contracts	M_3
Gastrointestinal tract				
Smooth muscle				
Walls	Relaxes	$\alpha_2,^d \beta_2$	Contracts	M_3
Sphincters	Contracts	α_1	Relaxes	M_3
Secretion	Inhibits	α_2	Increases	M_3
Myenteric plexus	...	...	Activates	M_1
Genitourinary smooth muscle				
Bladder wall	Relaxes	β_2	Contracts	M_3
Sphincter	Contracts	α_1	Relaxes	M_3
Uterus, pregnant	Relaxes	β_2	...	...
	Contracts	α	Contracts	M_3
Penis, seminal vesicles	Ejaculation	α	Erection	M
Skin				
Pilomotor smooth muscle	Contracts	α	...	...
Sweat glands			...	...
Thermoregulatory	Increases	M	...	...
Apocrine (stress)	Increases	α	...	...
Metabolic functions				
Liver	Gluconeogenesis	β_2, α	...	...
Liver	Glycogenolysis	β_2, α	...	...
Fat cells	Lipolysis	β_3	...	...
Kidney	Renin release	β_1	...	...
Autonomic nerve endings				
Sympathetic	...	...	Decreases NE release	M^e
Parasympathetic	Decreases ACh release	α	...	...

Reproduced, with permission, from Katzung BG, editor: *Basic & Clinical Pharmacology,* 9th ed. McGraw-Hill, 2004.

[a]Less important actions are shown in brackets.

[b]Specific receptor type: α = alpha, β = beta, M = muscarinic.

[c]Vascular smooth muscle in skeletal muscle has sympathetic cholinergic dilator fibers.

[d]Probably through presynaptic inhibition of parasympathetic activity.

[e]Probably M_1, but M_2 may participate in some locations.

Table 6–4. Steps in autonomic transmission: effects of drugs.

Process	Drug Example	Site	Action
Action potential propagation	Local anesthetics, tetrodotoxin,[a] saxitoxin[b]	Nerve axons	Block sodium channels; block conduction
Transmitter synthesis	Hemicholinium	Cholinergic nerve terminals: membrane	Blocks uptake of choline and slows synthesis
	α-Methyltyrosine (metyrosine)	Adrenergic nerve terminals and adrenal medulla: cytoplasm	Blocks synthesis
Transmitter storage	Vesamicol	Cholinergic terminals: vesicles	Prevents storage, depletes
	Reserpine	Adrenergic terminals: vesicles	Prevents storage, depletes
Transmitter release	Many[c]	Nerve terminal membrane receptors	Modulate release
	ω-Conotoxin GVIA[d]	Nerve terminal calcium channels	Reduces transmitter release
	Botulinum toxin	Cholinergic vesicles	Prevents release
	Alpha-latrotoxin[e]	Cholinergic and adrenergic vesicles	Causes explosive release
	Tyramine, amphetamine	Adrenergic nerve terminals	Promote transmitter release
Transmitter uptake after release	Cocaine, tricyclic antidepressants	Adrenergic nerve terminals	Inhibit uptake; increase transmitter effect on post-synaptic receptors
	6-Hydroxydopamine	Adrenergic nerve terminals	Destroys the terminals
Receptor activation or blockade	Norepinephrine	Receptors at adrenergic junctions	Binds α receptors; causes activation
	Phentolamine	Receptors at adrenergic junctions	Binds α receptors; prevents activation
	Isoproterenol	Receptors at adrenergic junctions	Binds β receptors; activates adenylyl cyclase
	Propranolol	Receptors at adrenergic junctions	Binds β receptors; prevents activation
	Nicotine	Receptors at nicotinic cholinergic junctions (autonomic ganglia, neuromuscular end plates	Binds nicotinic receptors; opens ion channel in postsynaptic membrane
	Tubocurarine	Neuromuscular end plates	Prevents activation
	Bethanechol	Receptors, parasympathetic effector cells (smooth muscle, glands)	Binds and activates muscarinic receptors
	Atropine	Receptors, parasympathetic effector cells	Binds muscarinic receptors; prevents activation
Enzymatic activation of transmitter	Neostigmine	Cholinergic synapses (acetylcholinesterase)	Inhibits enzyme; prolongs and intensifies transmitter action
	Tranylcypromine	Adrenergic nerve terminals (monoamine oxidase)	Inhibits enzyme; increases stored transmitter pool

Reproduced, with permission, from Katzung BG, editor: *Basic & Clinical Pharmacology*, 9th ed. McGraw-Hill, 2004.

[a]Toxin of puffer fish, California newt.
[b]Toxin of *Gonyaulax* (red tide organism).
[c]Norepinephrine, dopamine, acetylcholine, angiotensin II, various prostaglandins, etc.
[d]Toxin of marine snails of the genus *Conus*.
[e]Black widow spider venom.

Noradrenergic nerve terminal

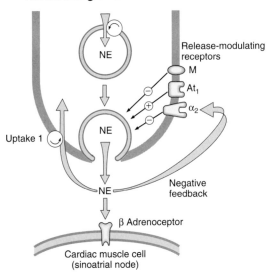

Figure 6–3. Local control of ANS function via modulation of transmitter release. In the example shown, release of norepinephrine from a sympathetic nerve ending is modulated by norepinephrine itself, acting on presynaptic α_2 autoreceptors, and by acetylcholine and angiotensin II. Many other modulators (see text) influence the release process.

Presynaptic receptors that bind the primary transmitter substance and thereby regulate its release are called *autoreceptors*. Transmitter release is also modulated by other receptors *(heteroreceptors)*; in the case of adrenergic nerve terminals, receptors for acetylcholine, histamine, serotonin, prostaglandins, peptides, and other substances have been found. Presynaptic regulation by a variety of endogenous chemicals probably occurs in all nerve fibers.

Postsynaptic modulatory receptors, including 2 types of muscarinic receptors and at least 1 type of peptidergic receptor, have been found in ganglionic synapses, where nicotinic transmission is primary. These receptors may facilitate or inhibit transmission by evoking slow excitatory or inhibitory postsynaptic potentials (EPSPs or IPSPs).

B. Systemic Reflexes

Systemic reflexes include mechanisms that regulate blood pressure, gastrointestinal motility, bladder tone, airway smooth muscle, and other processes. The control of blood pressure—by the baroreceptor neural reflex and the renin-angiotensin-aldosterone hormonal response—is especially important (Figure 6–4). These homeostatic mechanisms have evolved to maintain mean arterial blood pressure at a level determined by the vasomotor center and renal sensors. Any deviation from this blood pressure "set point" causes a change in ANS activity and renin-angiotensin-aldosterone levels. These changes are very important in determining the response to conditions or drugs that alter blood pressure. For example, a decrease in blood pressure caused by hemorrhage causes increased SANS discharge and renin release. As a result, peripheral vascular resistance, venous tone, heart rate, and cardiac force are increased by norepinephrine released from sympathetic nerves. Blood volume is replenished by retention of salt and water in the kidney under the influence of increased levels of aldosterone. These compensatory responses may be large enough to overcome some of the actions of drugs. For example, the treatment of hypertension with a vasodilator such as hydralazine will be unsuccessful if the compensatory tachycardia (via the baroreceptor reflex) and the salt and water retention (via the renin system response) are not prevented through the use of additional drugs. It is therefore essential that the student understand this homeostatic system.

C. Complex Organ Control: The Eye

The eye contains multiple tissues with various functions, several of them under autonomic control (Figure 6–5).

KEY DRUGS

The following drugs or metabolites mentioned in this chapter are of special significance. It is important to know which ones occur in the normal ANS and what their functions are. For those not normally found in the ANS, it is important to know the effects of their administration.

Acetylcholine

Botulinum toxin

Cocaine

Dopamine

Epinephrine

Metanephrine

Norepinephrine

Saxitoxin

Tetrodotoxin

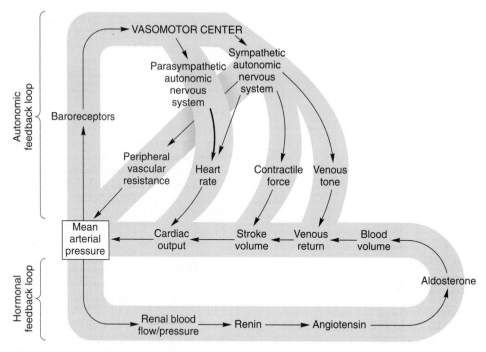

Figure 6–4. Autonomic and hormonal control of cardiovascular function. Note that 2 feedback loops are present: the autonomic nervous system loop and the hormonal loop. Each major loop has several components. In the neuronal loop, sensory input to the vasomotor center is via afferent fibers in the ninth and tenth cranial (PANS) nerves. On the efferent side, the sympathetic nervous system directly influences 4 major variables: peripheral vascular resistance, heart rate, contractile force, and venous tone. The parasympathetic nervous system directly influences heart rate. In addition, angiotensin II directly increases peripheral vascular resistance (not shown), and the sympathetic nervous system directly increases renin secretion (not shown). Because these control mechanisms have evolved to maintain normal blood pressure, the net feedback effect of each loop is negative; feedback tends to compensate for the change in arterial blood pressure that evoked the response. Thus, decreased blood pressure due to blood loss would be compensated by increased sympathetic outflow and renin release. Conversely, elevated pressure due to the administration of a vasoconstrictor drug would cause reduced sympathetic outflow and renin release and increased parasympathetic (vagal) outflow.

The pupil, discussed previously, is under reciprocal control by the SANS (via α receptors on the pupillary dilator muscle) and the PANS (via muscarinic receptors on the pupillary constrictor). The ciliary muscle, which controls accommodation, is under primary control of muscarinic receptors innervated by the PANS, with insignificant contributions from the SANS. The ciliary *epithelium*, on the other hand, has important β receptors that have a permissive effect on aqueous humor secretion. Each of these receptors is an important target of drugs that are discussed in the following chapters.

QUESTIONS

1. In the autonomic regulation of blood pressure
   (A) Cardiac output is maintained constant at the expense of other hemodynamic variables
   (B) Elevation of blood pressure results in elevated aldosterone secretion
   (C) Baroreceptor sensory nerve fibers travel in the sympathetic nerves
   (D) Stroke volume and mean arterial blood pressure are the primary direct determinants of cardiac output
   (E) A condition that reduces the sensitivity of the sensory baroreceptor nerve endings will cause an increase in sympathetic discharge

2. A child has swallowed the contents of 2 bottles of a nasal decongestant whose primary ingredient is a potent, selective α adrenoceptor agonist drug. The signs of alpha activation that may occur in this patient include
   (A) Bronchodilation
   (B) Cardioacceleration (tachycardia)

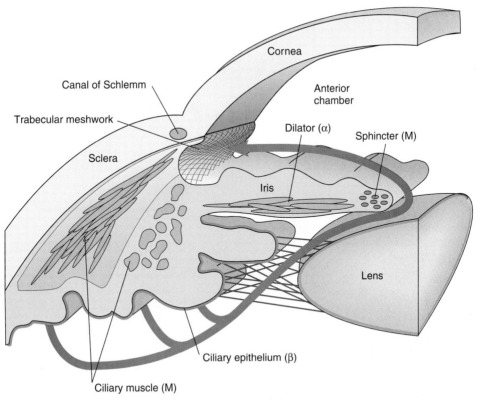

Figure 6–5. Some pharmacologic targets in the eye. The diagram illustrates clinically important structures and their receptors. The heavy arrow (color) illustrates the flow of aqueous humor from its secretion by the ciliary epithelium to its drainage through the canal of Schlemm. (M, muscarinic; α, alpha receptor; β, beta receptor.

(C) Pupillary dilation (mydriasis)
(D) Renin release
(E) Vasodilation

3. Ms Green has severe hypertension and is to receive minoxidil. Minoxidil is a powerful arteriolar vasodilator that does not act on autonomic receptors. When used in severe hypertension, its effects would probably include
(A) Tachycardia and increased cardiac contractility
(B) Tachycardia and decreased cardiac output
(C) Decreased mean arterial pressure and decreased cardiac contractility
(D) Decreased mean arterial pressure and increased salt and water excretion by the kidney
(E) No change in mean arterial pressure and decreased cardiac contractility

4. Full activation of the sympathetic nervous system, as in maximal exercise, can produce all of the following responses EXCEPT

(A) Bronchodilation
(B) Decreased intestinal motility
(C) Increased renal blood flow
(D) Mydriasis
(E) Increased heart rate (tachycardia)

Questions 5–8. For these questions, use the accompanying diagram. Assume that the diagram can represent either the sympathetic or the parasympathetic system.

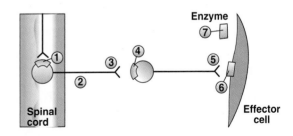

5. Which of the following drugs acts at site 3?
   (A) Botulinum toxin
   (B) Cocaine
   (C) Reserpine
   (D) Tyramine

6. Acetylcholine does *not* interact at which one of the following sites in the diagram?
   (A) Site 2
   (B) Site 4
   (C) Site 5
   (D) Site 6
   (E) Site 7

7. Atropine, a muscarinic receptor blocking drug, is useful for dilating the pupil and paralyzing accommodation. These effects of atropine occur at which one of the following sites on the diagram?
   (A) Site 3
   (B) Site 4
   (C) Site 5
   (D) Site 6
   (E) Site 7

8. If the effector cell in the diagram is a thermoregulatory sweat gland, which of the following compounds is released from structure 5?
   (A) Acetylcholine
   (B) Dopamine
   (C) Epinephrine
   (D) Norepinephrine

9. Nicotinic receptor sites do NOT include
   (A) Bronchial smooth muscle
   (B) Adrenal medullary cells
   (C) Parasympathetic ganglia
   (D) Skeletal muscle
   (E) Sympathetic ganglia

10. Several children at a summer camp were hospitalized with symptoms thought to be due to ingestion of food containing botulinum toxin. The effects of botulinum toxin are likely to include
    (A) Bronchospasm
    (B) Cycloplegia
    (C) Diarrhea
    (D) Skeletal muscle spasms
    (E) Hyperventilation

11. The neurotransmitter agent that is normally released in the sinoatrial node of the heart in response to a blood pressure increase is
    (A) Acetylcholine
    (B) Dopamine
    (C) Epinephrine
    (D) Glutamate
    (E) Norepinephrine

12–14. Assume that the diagram below represents a sympathetic postganglionic nerve ending

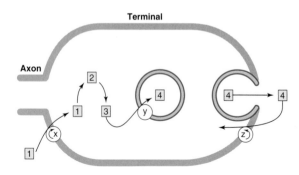

12. The carrier represented by "y" in the diagram can be blocked by
    (A) Botulinum toxin
    (B) Cocaine
    (C) Guanethidine
    (D) Reserpine

13. The conversion of the intermediate "1" to "2" in the diagram can be inhibited by
    (A) Botulinum toxin
    (B) Cocaine
    (C) Metyrosine
    (D) Reserpine
    (E) Vesamicol

14. The carrier denoted "z" in the diagram can be inhibited by
    (A) Cocaine
    (B) Dopamine
    (C) Metyrosine
    (D) Reserpine

15. A drug that facilitates catecholamine transmitter release from adrenergic nerve endings is
    (A) Acetylcholine
    (B) Amphetamine
    (C) Botulinum toxin
    (D) Dopamine
    (E) Epinephrine
    (F) Metyrosine
    (G) Norepinephrine
    (H) Reserpine
    (I) Tetrodotoxin
    (J) Vesamicol

ANSWERS

1. A decrease in baroreceptor sensitivity would decrease input to the vasomotor center, which would be interpreted by the vasomotor center as a

decrease in blood pressure. This would lead to an increase in sympathetic outflow. The answer is **E**.

2. Mydriasis can be caused by contraction of the radial fibers of the iris; these smooth muscle cells have α receptors. All the other responses are mediated by β adrenoceptors (Table 6–4). The answer is **C**.

3. Because of the baroreceptor reflex, a drug that directly decreases peripheral vascular resistance will cause a reflex increase in sympathetic outflow, an increase in renin release, and a decrease in parasympathetic outflow. As a result, heart rate and cardiac force will increase. In addition, salt and water retention will occur. The answer is **A**.

4. Sympathetic discharge causes constriction of the renal resistance vessels and a fall in renal blood flow. This is the typical response in severe exercise or hypotension. The answer is **C**.

5. Each of these agents has a different mechanism of action, yet all but 1 act on the sympathetic postganglionic nerve terminal (site 5). Site 3 is a cholinergic nerve ending. The answer is **A**.

6. Acetylcholine acts at both the nicotinic ganglionic receptor (site 4) and at muscarinic receptors on effector cells (site 6) and presynaptic nerve endings (site 5). ACh also interacts with acetylcholinesterase (site 7) but does not influence electrical transmission in axons (site 2). The answer is **A**.

7. In the simplified diagram, the muscarinic receptors blocked by atropine are located only at the smooth muscle effector cells and postganglionic nerve terminals. This type of receptor is also found in ganglia, but higher concentrations of atropine are required to block it. Blocking presynaptic muscarinic receptors would not produce mydriasis and cycloplegia. The answer is **D**.

8. The nerves innervating the thermoregulatory (eccrine) sweat glands are sympathetic *cholinergic* nerves. The answer is **A**.

9. Both types of ganglia and the skeletal muscle neuromuscular junction have nicotinic cholinoceptors, as does the adrenal medulla (a modified form of sympathetic postganglionic neuron tissue). Bronchial smooth muscle contains muscarinic cholinoceptors. The answer is **A**.

10. Botulinum toxin impairs all types of cholinergic transmission, including transmission at ganglionic synapses and somatic motor nerve endings. Botulinum toxin prevents discharge of vesicular transmitter content from cholinergic nerve endings. All of the signs listed except cycloplegia indicate increased muscle contraction; cycloplegia (paralysis of accommodation) results in blurred near vision. The answer is **B**.

11. Acetylcholine is the transmitter at parasympathetic nerve endings innervating the sinus node (the vagus nerve). When blood pressure increases, the vasomotor center tries to return it to normal by slowing the heart rate. The answer is **A**.

12. The vesicular carrier in the diagram transports dopamine and norepinephrine into the vesicles for storage. It can be blocked by reserpine. The answer is **D**.

13. The intermediate "1" in the diagram is tyrosine. It is converted to DOPA ("2"). This rate-limiting step in catecholamine synthesis can be inhibited by the tyrosine analog metyrosine (see Figure 6–2). The answer is **C**.

14. The reuptake carrier in sympathetic postganglionic nerve endings can be blocked by cocaine or tricyclic antidepressants. The answer is **A**.

15. Amphetamine facilitates the release of catecholamine transmitters from sympathetic nerve endings (Table 6–4). The answer is **B**.

 SKILL KEEPER ANSWER: DRUG PERMEATION (SEE CHAPTER 1)

Botulinum toxin is too large to cross membranes by means of lipid or aqueous diffusion. It must bind to membrane receptors and enter by endocytosis. Botulinum-binding receptors for endocytosis are present on cholinergic neurons but not adrenergic ones.

CHECKLIST

When you complete this chapter, you should be able to:

☐ Describe the steps in the synthesis, storage, release, and termination of action of the major autonomic transmitters.

☐ Name 2 cotransmitter substances.

☐ Name the major types of autonomic receptors and the tissues in which they are found.

☐ Describe the organ system effects of stimulation of the parasympathetic and sympathetic systems.

☐ Name examples of inhibitors of acetylcholine and norepinephrine synthesis, storage, and release. Predict the effects of these inhibitors on the function of the major organ systems.

☐ List the determinants of blood pressure and describe the baroreceptor reflex response for the following perturbations: (1) blood loss, (2) administration of a vasodilator, (3) a vasoconstrictor, (4) a cardiac stimulant, (5) a cardiac depressant.

☐ Describe the effects of loss of sympathetic output to the face (Horner's syndrome) and list the transmitters involved.

☐ Describe the results of transplantation of the heart with interruption of its autonomic nerves on cardiac function.

☐ Describe the actions of several toxins that affect nerve function: tetrodotoxin, saxitoxin, botulinum toxins, and latrotoxin.

Cholinoceptor-Activating & Cholinesterase-Inhibiting Drugs

Cholinomimetic drugs are drugs that mimic acetylcholine by directly or indirectly activating the receptors with which acetylcholine interacts. The directly acting agents combine with the cholinoceptor in the same way as acetylcholine. The indirect-acting cholinesterase inhibitors have many effects like those of the direct-acting agonists but act by inhibiting the enzyme that terminates the action of endogenous acetylcholine.

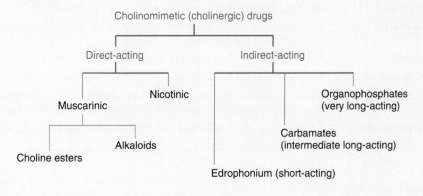

Drugs with acetylcholine-like effects (cholinomimetics) are subdivided in 2 ways: on the basis of their mode of action (ie, whether they act directly at the acetylcholine receptor or indirectly through inhibition of cholinesterase); and for those that act directly, on the basis of their spectrum of action (ie, whether they act on muscarinic or nicotinic cholinoceptors).

Acetylcholine may be considered the prototype that acts directly at both muscarinic and nicotinic receptors. Neostigmine is a prototype for the indirect-acting cholinesterase inhibitors.

DIRECT-ACTING CHOLINOMIMETIC AGONISTS

A group of choline esters (acetylcholine, methacholine, carbachol, and bethanechol) and a second group of naturally occurring alkaloids (muscarine, pilocarpine, nicotine,

lobeline) comprise this subclass. Newer drugs are occasionally introduced for special applications. The members differ in their spectrum of action (amount of muscarinic versus nicotinic stimulation) and in their pharmacokinetics (Table 7–1). Both factors influence their clinical use.

A. CLASSIFICATION

Muscarinic agonists are parasympathomimetic, ie, they mimic the actions of parasympathetic nerve stimulation, in addition to other effects. Five subgroups of muscarinic receptors have been identified (Table 7–2), but the muscarinic agonists available for clinical use activate them nonselectively. Nicotinic agonists are classified on the basis of whether ganglionic or neuromuscular stimulation predominates; however, agonist selectivity is very limited. On the other hand, relatively selective *antagonists* are available for the two nicotinic receptor types (Chapter 8).

HIGH-YIELD TERMS TO LEARN

Choline ester	A cholinomimetic drug consisting of choline (an alcohol) esterified with an acidic substance, (eg, acetic or carbamic acid); usually poorly lipid soluble
Cholinergic crisis	The clinical condition of excessive activation of cholinoceptors; it may include muscle weakness as well as parasympathetic signs
Cholinomimetic alkaloid	A drug with weakly basic properties (usually of plant origin) whose effects resemble those of acetylcholine; usually lipid soluble
Cyclospasm	Marked contraction of the ciliary muscle; maximum accommodation for close vision
Direct-acting cholinomimetic	A drug that binds and activates cholinoceptors; the effects mimic those of acetylcholine
Endothelium-derived relaxing factor (EDRF)	A potent vasodilator substance, largely nitric oxide (NO), that is released from vascular endothelial cells
Indirect-acting cholinomimetic	A drug that amplifies the effects of endogenous acetylcholine by inhibiting acetylcholinesterase
Muscarinic agonist	A cholinomimetic drug with primarily muscarine-like actions
Myasthenic crisis	In patients with myasthenia, an acute worsening of symptoms; often caused by inadequate cholinomimetic treatment
Nicotinic agonist	A cholinomimetic drug with primarily nicotine-like actions
Organophosphate	An ester of phosphoric acid and an organic alcohol that inhibits cholinesterase
Organophosphate aging	A process whereby the organophosphate, after binding to cholinesterase, is chemically modified and becomes more firmly bound to the enzyme
Parasympathomimetic	A drug whose effects resemble those of stimulating the parasympathetic nerves

SKILL KEEPER: DRUG METABOLISM (SEE CHAPTER 4)

Acetylcholine is metabolized in the body by hydrolysis of the ester bond. Is this a phase I or phase II metabolic reaction? The Skill Keeper Answer appears at the end of the chapter.

B. MOLECULAR MECHANISMS OF ACTION

1. Muscarinic mechanism—Several molecular mechanisms of muscarinic action have been defined (Table 7–2). One involves G_q protein coupling of muscarinic receptors (especially M_1 and M_3 receptors) to phospholipase C, a membrane-bound enzyme, leading to the release of the second messengers diacylglycerol (DAG) and inositol-1,4,5-trisphosphate (IP_3). DAG modulates the action of protein kinase C, an enzyme important in secretion, while IP_3 evokes the release of calcium from intracellular storage sites, which results in

contraction in smooth muscle. A second mechanism couples muscarinic receptors (especially M_2 receptors) to adenylyl cyclase through the inhibitory G_i coupling protein. A third mechanism couples the same M_2 receptors via the βγ subunit of the G protein to potassium channels in the heart and elsewhere; muscarinic agonists facilitate opening of these channels. M_4 and M_5 receptors may be important in the CNS but have not been shown to play major roles in peripheral organs.

2. Nicotinic mechanism—The mechanism of nicotinic action has been clearly defined. The nicotinic ACh receptor is located on a channel protein that is selective for sodium and potassium. When the receptor is activated, the channel opens and depolarization of the cell occurs as a direct result of the influx of sodium, causing an excitatory postsynaptic potential (EPSP). If large enough, the EPSP evokes a propagated action potential in the surrounding membrane. The nicotinic receptors present on sympathetic and parasympathetic ganglion cells (N_N) differ slightly from those on neuromuscular end plates (N_M).

C. TISSUE AND ORGAN EFFECTS

The tissue and organ system effects are summarized in Table 7–3. Note that vasodilation (and decreased blood

Table 7–1. Cholinomimetics: spectrum of action and pharmacokinetics.

Drug	Spectrum of Action[a]	Pharmacokinetic Features
Direct-acting		
Acetylcholine	B	Rapidly hydrolyzed by cholinesterase (ChE); duration of action 5–30 s; poor lipid solubility
Bethanechol	M	Resistant to ChE; orally active, poor lipid solubility; duration of action 30 min to 2 h
Carbachol	B	Like bethanechol
Pilocarpine	M	Not an ester, good lipid solubility; duration of action 30 min to 2 h
Nicotine	N	Like pilocarpine; duration of action 1–6 h; high lipid solubility
Indirect-acting		
Edrophonium	B	Alcohol, quaternary amine, poor lipid solubility, not orally active; duration of action 5–15 min
Neostigmine	B	Carbamate, quaternary amine, poor lipid solubility, orally active; duration of action 30 min to 2 h or more
Physostigmine	B	Carbamate, tertiary amine, good lipid solubility, orally active; duration of action 30 min to 2 h
Pyridostigmine	B	Carbamate like neostigmine, but longer duration of action (4–8 h)
Echothiophate	B	Organophosphate, moderate lipid solubility; duration of action 2–7 days
Parathion	B	Organophosphate, high lipid solubility; duration of action 7–30 days

[a]M, muscarinic; N, nicotinic; B, both.

pressure) is not a parasympathomimetic response (ie, it is not evoked by parasympathetic nerve discharge, even though directly acting cholinomimetics cause vasodilation). This action results from the release of endothelium-derived relaxing factor (EDRF; nitric oxide and possibly other substances) in the vessels, mediated by *uninnervated* muscarinic receptors on the endothelial cells. Note also that decreased blood pressure evokes the baroreceptor reflex, resulting in strong compensatory sympathetic discharge to the heart. As a result, injections of small to moderate amounts of direct-acting muscarinic cholinomimetics often cause *tachycardia*, whereas parasympathetic (vagal) nerve discharge to the heart causes *bradycardia*. Another effect seen with cholinomimetic drugs but not with parasympathetic nerve stimulation is thermoregulatory sweating; this is a *sympathetic* cholinergic effect (see Chapter 6).

The tissue and organ level effects of nicotinic ganglionic stimulation depend on the autonomic innervation of the organ involved. The blood vessels are dominated by sympathetic innervation; therefore, nicotinic receptor activation results in vasoconstriction mediated by sympathetic postganglionic nerve discharge. The gut is dominated by parasympathetic control; nicotinic drugs increase motility and secretion because of increased parasympathetic postganglionic neuron discharge. Nicotinic neuromuscular end plate activation by direct-acting drugs results in fasciculations and spasm of the muscles involved. Prolonged activation

Table 7–2. Cholinoceptor types and their postreceptor mechanisms.

Receptor Type	G Protein	Postreceptor Mechanisms
M_1	G_q	↑ IP_3, DAG cascade
M_2	G_i	↓ cAMP synthesis
M_3	G_q	↑ IP_3, DAG cascade
M_4	G_i	↓ cAMP synthesis
M_5	G_q	↑ IP_3, DAG cascade
N_M	None	Na^+, K^+ depolarizing current
N_N	None	Na^+, K^+ depolarizing current

Table 7–3. Effects of cholinomimetics on major organ systems.

Organ	Response[a]
CNS	Complex stimulatory effects, eg, nicotine (elevation of mood, alerting), physostigmine (convulsions); excessive concentrations may cause coma
Eye	
Sphincter muscle of iris	Contraction (miosis)
Ciliary muscle	Contraction (accommodation for near vision), cyclospasm
Heart	
Sinoatrial node	Decrease in rate (negative chronotropy), but note important reflex response in intact subject (see text)
Atria	Decrease in contractile force (negative inotropy); decrease in refractory period
Atrioventricular node	Decrease in conduction velocity (negative dromotropy), increase in refractory period
Ventricles	Small decrease in contractile force
Blood vessels	Dilation via release of EDRF[b] from endothelium
Bronchi	Contraction (bronchoconstriction)
Gastrointestinal tract	
Motility	Increase in smooth muscle contraction, peristalsis
Sphincters	Decrease in tone, relaxation
Urinary bladder	
Detrusor	Increase in contraction
Trigone and sphincter	Relaxation; voiding
Skeletal muscle	Activation of neuromuscular end plates, contraction
Glands (exocrine)	Increased secretion (thermoregulatory sweating, lacrimation, salivation, bronchial secretion, gastrointestinal glands)

[a]Only the direct effects are indicated; homeostatic responses to these direct actions may be important (see text).
[b]EDRF, endothelium-derived relaxing factor (primarily nitric oxide).

results in paralysis (see Chapter 27), which is an important hazard of exposure to nicotine-containing and organophosphate insecticides.

D. CLINICAL USE

Several clinical conditions benefit from an increase in cholinergic activity. They are summarized in Table 7–4. Direct-acting nicotinic agonists have no therapeutic applications except in producing skeletal muscle paralysis (succinylcholine, Chapter 27); indirect-acting agents are used when increased nicotinic activation is needed at the neuromuscular junction (see later discussion).

E. TOXICITY

The signs and symptoms of overdosage are readily predicted from the general pharmacology of acetylcholine.

1. Muscarinic toxicity—These effects include CNS stimulation (uncommon with choline esters and pilocarpine), miosis, spasm of accommodation, bronchoconstriction, increased gastrointestinal and genitourinary smooth muscle activity, increased secretory activity (sweat glands, airway, gastrointestinal tract, lacrimal glands), and vasodilation. Transient bradycardia occurs, followed by reflex tachycardia if the drug is administered as an intravenous bolus; reflex tachycardia otherwise.

2. Nicotinic toxicity—Toxic effects include CNS stimulation (including convulsions) followed by depression, ganglionic stimulation and block, and neuromuscular end plate depolarization leading to fasciculations and then paralysis.

Table 7–4. Clinical applications of some cholinomimetics.

Drug	Clinical Applications	Action
Direct-acting agonists		
Bethanechol	Postoperative and neurogenic ileus and urinary retention; oral or parenteral	Activates bowel and bladder smooth muscle
Carbachol	Glaucoma; topical[a]	Activates pupillary sphincter and ciliary muscle
Pilocarpine	Glaucoma, Sjögren's syndrome; topical	Activates pupillary sphincter and ciliary muscle; stimulates salivation
Nicotine	Smoking deterrence (patch, chewing gum)	Replaces rapid-onset (cigarettes) with slower action
Indirect-acting agents		
Neostigmine	Postoperative and neurogenic ileus and urinary retention; oral or parenteral	Amplifies endogenous acetylcholine; see bethanechol
Neostigmine, edrophonium, pyridostigmine	Myasthenia gravis, reversal of neuromuscular blocking drugs; oral or parenteral (edrophonium, parenteral only)	Amplifies endogenous acetylcholine; useful effect at skeletal muscle neuro-muscular end plates
Physostigmine	Glaucoma; topical[a]	Amplifies effects of endogenous acetylcholine

[a]The current treatment of glaucoma is summarized in Table 10–3.

INDIRECT-ACTING AGONISTS

A. CLASSIFICATION AND PROTOTYPES

Hundreds of indirect-acting cholinomimetic drugs have been synthesized in 2 major chemical classes: carbamic acid esters (carbamates; neostigmine is a prototype) and phosphoric acid esters (phosphates, organophosphates; parathion is a prototype). A third class has only one member: edrophonium is an alcohol (not an ester) with a very short duration of action.

B. MECHANISM OF ACTION

Both carbamate and organophosphate inhibitors bind to cholinesterase and undergo prompt hydrolysis. The alcohol portion of the molecule is then released. The acidic portion (carbamate ion or phosphate ion) is released much more slowly, and this retained portion prevents the binding and hydrolysis of endogenous acetylcholine, thus **amplifying** ACh effects wherever the transmitter is released.

1. Carbamates—After hydrolysis, the carbamate residue is released by cholinesterase over a period of 2–8 h.

2. Organophosphates—Organophosphates are long-acting drugs; they form an extremely stable phosphate complex with the enzyme. After initial hydrolysis, the phosphoric acid residue is released over periods of days to weeks.

C. EFFECTS

By inhibiting cholinesterase, these agents cause an increase in the concentration, half-life, and actions of acetylcholine in synapses where ACh is released physiologically. Therefore, the indirect agents have muscarinic or nicotinic effects depending on which organ system is under consideration. Cholinesterase inhibitors do not have significant actions at uninnervated sites where acetylcholine is not normally released (eg, vascular endothelial cells).

D. CLINICAL USE

The clinical applications of the indirect-acting cholinomimetics are predictable from a consideration of the organs and the diseases that benefit from an amplification of cholinergic activity. The effects are summarized in Table 7–4. Carbamates, which include neostigmine, physostigmine, ambenonium, and pyridostigmine, are used far more commonly in therapeutics than are organophosphates. The treatment of myasthenia is especially important. Some carbamates (eg, carbaryl) are used in agriculture as insecticides. Two organophosphates used in medicine are malathion (a scabicide), and metrifonate (an anthelmintic agent).

Edrophonium is used for the rapid reversal of non-depolarizing neuromuscular blockade (Chapter 27), in the diagnosis of myasthenia, and in differentiating myasthenic from cholinergic crisis in patients with this

KEY DRUGS		
Subclass	**Prototypes**	**Other Significant Drugs**
Direct-acting drugs		
Muscarinic agonists	Acetylcholine	Muscarine, bethanechol, carbachol, pilocarpine
Nicotinic agonists	Acetylcholine	Nicotine, carbachol, succinylcholine
Indirect-acting drugs		
Alcohol	Edrophonium	
Carbamates	Neostigmine	Pyridostigmine, physostigmine
Organophosphates	Parathion	Malathion, sarin

disease. Because cholinergic crisis can result in muscle weakness like that of myasthenic crisis, distinguishing the two conditions may be difficult. Administration of a short-acting cholinomimetic such as edrophonium will improve muscle strength in myasthenic crisis but weaken it in cholinergic crisis.

E. TOXICITY

In addition to their therapeutic uses, some indirect-acting agents (especially organophosphates) have clinical importance because of accidental exposures to toxic amounts of pesticides. The most toxic of these drugs (eg, parathion) can be rapidly fatal if exposure is not immediately recognized and treated. The treatment of first choice is the antimuscarinic agent atropine, but this drug has no effect on the nicotinic signs of toxicity. After first binding to cholinesterase, most organophosphate inhibitors can be removed from the enzyme by the use of "regenerator" compounds such as pralidoxime (see Chapter 8), and this may reverse the nicotinic signs. If the enzyme-inhibitor binding is allowed to persist, however, aging (a further chemical change) occurs and regenerator drugs can no longer remove the inhibitor. Treatment is described in more detail in Chapter 8. Because of their toxicity and short persistence in the environment, organophosphates are used extensively in agriculture as insecticides and anthelmintic agents; examples include malathion and parathion. Some of these agents (eg, malathion, dichlorvos) are relatively safe in humans because they are metabolized rapidly to inactive products in mammals (and birds) but not in insects. Some are prodrugs (eg, malathion, parathion) and must be metabolized to the active product (malaoxon from malathion, paraoxon from parathion). The signs and symptoms of poisoning are the same as those described for the direct-acting agents, with the following exceptions: vasodilation is a late and uncommon effect; bradycardia is more common than tachycardia; CNS stimulation is common with organophosphate and physostigmine overdosage and

includes convulsions, followed by respiratory and cardiovascular depression. The spectrum of toxicity can be remembered with the aid of the mnemonic DUMBBELSS (diarrhea, urination, miosis, bronchoconstriction, bradycardia, excitation [of skeletal muscle and CNS], lacrimation, and salivation and sweating).

QUESTIONS

1. A patient requires mild cholinomimetic stimulation following surgery. Neostigmine and bethanechol in moderate doses have significantly *different* effects on which one of the following?
   (A) Gastric secretion
   (B) Neuromuscular end plate
   (C) Salivary glands
   (D) Sweat glands
   (E) Ureteral tone

2. Parathion has which one of the following characteristics?
   (A) It is inactivated by conversion to paraoxon
   (B) It is less toxic to humans than malathion
   (C) It is more persistent in the environment than DDT
   (D) It is poorly absorbed through skin and lungs
   (E) Its toxicity, if treated early, may be partly reversed by pralidoxime

3. Ms Brown has had myasthenia gravis for several years. She reports to the emergency department complaining of rapid onset of weakness of her hands, diplopia, and difficulty swallowing. She may be suffering from a change in response to her myasthenia therapy, ie, a cholinergic or a myasthenic crisis. The best drug for distinguishing between myasthenic crisis (insufficient therapy) and cholinergic crisis (excessive therapy) is
   (A) Atropine
   (B) Pyridostigmine

(C) Edrophonium
(D) Physostigmine
(E) Pralidoxime

4. A crop duster pilot has been accidentally exposed to a high concentration of an agricultural organophosphate insecticide. If untreated, the cause of death from such a poisoning would probably be
   (A) Cardiac arrhythmia
   (B) Gastrointestinal bleeding
   (C) Heart failure
   (D) Hypertension
   (E) Respiratory failure

5. Mr Green has just been diagnosed with myasthenia gravis. You are considering different therapies for his disease. Pyridostigmine and neostigmine may cause which one of the following?
   (A) Bronchodilation
   (B) Cycloplegia
   (C) Diarrhea
   (D) Irreversible inhibition of acetylcholinesterase
   (E) Reduced gastric acid secretion

6. Parasympathetic nerve stimulation and a slow infusion of bethanechol will each:
   (A) Increase bladder tone
   (B) Cause ganglion cell depolarization
   (C) Increase heart rate
   (D) Cause skeletal muscle end plate depolarization
   (E) Cause vasodilation

7. In the bronchi, pilocarpine activates which one of the following receptors?
   (A) M_1
   (B) M_2
   (C) M_3
   (D) M_4
   (E) M_5

8. In the comparison of bethanechol and pilocarpine, which one of the following is correct?
   (A) Both are hydrolyzed by acetylcholinesterase
   (B) Both inhibit nicotinic receptors
   (C) Both may decrease sweating
   (D) Both may increase gastrointestinal motility
   (E) Neither causes tachycardia

9. Actions and clinical uses of muscarinic cholinoceptor agonists include which one of the following?
   (A) Bronchodilation (asthma)
   (B) Cycloplegia, improved aqueous humor drainage (glaucoma)
   (C) Increased gastrointestinal motility (abdominal surgery)
   (D) Decreased neuromuscular transmission and relaxation of skeletal muscle (surgical anesthesia)

10. A direct-acting cholinomimetic that is lipid soluble and has been used in the treatment of glaucoma and Sjögren's syndrome is
    (A) Acetylcholine
    (B) Bethanechol
    (C) Physostigmine
    (D) Pilocarpine
    (E) Neostigmine

11. Which one of the following is an indirect-acting carbamate cholinomimetic with poor lipid solubility and a duration of action of about 2–4 h?
    (A) Acetylcholine
    (B) Bethanechol
    (C) Physostigmine
    (D) Pilocarpine
    (E) Neostigmine

12. Which of the following agents is a prodrug that is much less toxic in mammals than in insects?
    (A) Malathion
    (B) Nicotine
    (C) Parathion
    (D) Physostigmine
    (E) Pilocarpine

13. Which one of the following is a direct-acting cholinomimetic used for its mood-elevating action and as an insecticide?
    (A) Bethanechol
    (B) Neostigmine
    (C) Nicotine
    (D) Physostigmine
    (E) Pilocarpine

14. An indirect-acting cholinomimetic that readily enters the CNS is
    (A) Bethanechol
    (B) Muscarine
    (C) Neostigmine
    (D) Nicotine
    (E) Physostigmine

15. The primary second messenger process involved in the contraction of the ciliary muscle when focusing on near objects involves:
    (A) cAMP (Cyclic adenosine monophosphate)
    (B) DAG (Diacylglycerol)
    (C) Depolarizing influx of sodium ions via a channel
    (D) IP_3 (Inositol 1,4,5-trisphosphate)
    (E) NO (Nitric oxide)

ANSWERS

1. Because neostigmine acts on the enzyme cholinesterase which is present at all cholinergic

synapses, this drug increases acetylcholine effects at the nicotinic junctions as well as muscarinic ones. Bethanechol, on the other hand, is a direct-acting agent that is selective for muscarinic receptors and has no effect on nicotinic junctions such as the skeletal muscle end plate. The answer is **B**.

2. The "-thion" organophosphates (those containing the P=S bond) are activated, not inactivated, by conversion to "-oxon" (P=O) derivatives. They are less stable than halogenated hydrocarbon insecticides of the DDT type; therefore, they are less persistent in the environment. Parathion is more toxic than malathion. It is very lipid soluble and rapidly absorbed through the lungs and skin. The answer is **E**.

3. Because cholinergic crisis will be worsened by a cholinomimetic, we choose the shortest-acting cholinesterase inhibitor, edrophonium. The answer is **C**.

4. Respiratory failure, from neuromuscular paralysis or CNS depression, is the most important cause of acute deaths in cholinesterase inhibitor toxicity. The answer is **E**.

5. Cholinesterase inhibition is typically associated with increased (never decreased) bowel activity. (Fortunately, many patients become tolerant to this effect.) The answer is **C**.

6. Choice (C) is not correct because the vagus slows the heart. Parasympathetic nerve stimulation does not cause vasodilation. Ganglion cells and the end plate contain nicotinic receptors. The answer is **A**.

7. Muscarinic receptors M_1 through M_3 are mainly responsible for the peripheral effects of cholinomimetics. M_3 is the subtype involved in smooth muscle contraction. The answer is **C**.

8. Both bethanechol and pilocarpine may increase gastrointestinal motility. The answer is **D**.

9. Cholinomimetics cause cyclospasm, the opposite of paralysis of accommodation (cycloplegia). In open-angle glaucoma, this results in increased outflow of aqueous and decreased intraocular pressure. The answer is **C**.

10. Pilocarpine is the only direct-acting cholinomimetic on the list that is lipid soluble and frequently used in the treatment of glaucoma. Physostigmine is also lipid soluble and used in glaucoma, but it is indirect-acting. The answer is **D**.

11. Neostigmine is the prototypical indirect-acting cholinomimetic; it is a quaternary (charged) substance with poor lipid solubility; its duration of action is about 2–4 h. The answer is **E**.

12. Malathion and parathion are prodrug insecticides, but malathion is much less toxic than parathion in mammals. The answer is A.

13. Nicotine is a direct-acting cholinomimetic alkaloid with the properties noted. The answer is **C**.

14. Physostigmine is a plant alkaloid and, like most such compounds, is lipid soluble and enters the CNS readily. The answer is **E**.

15. Cholinomimetics cause smooth muscle contraction mainly through the release of intracellular calcium. This release is triggered by an increase in IP_3. The answer is **D**.

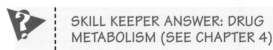

SKILL KEEPER ANSWER: DRUG METABOLISM (SEE CHAPTER 4)

The esters acetylcholine and methacholine are hydrolyzed by acetylcholinesterase. Hydrolytic drug metabolism reactions are classified as phase I.

CHECKLIST

When you complete this chapter, you should be able to:

☐ List the locations and types of acetylcholine receptors in the major organ systems (CNS, autonomic ganglia, eye, heart, vessels, bronchi, gut, genitourinary tract, skeletal muscle, exocrine glands).

☐ Describe the second messengers involved and the effects of acetylcholine on the major organs.

☐ List the major clinical uses of cholinomimetic agonists.

☐ Describe the pharmacodynamic differences between direct-acting and indirect-acting cholinomimetic agents.

☐ Relate the different pharmacokinetic properties of the various choline esters and cholinomimetic alkaloids to their chemical properties.

☐ List the major signs and symptoms of (1) organophosphate insecticide poisoning and (2) acute nicotine toxicity.

Cholinoceptor Blockers & Cholinesterase Regenerators

8

The cholinoceptor antagonists are readily grouped into subclasses on the basis of their spectrum of action (ie, whether they block muscarinic or nicotinic receptors). These drugs are pharmacologic antagonists. A special subgroup, the cholinesterase regenerators, are not receptor blockers but rather are chemical antagonists of organophosphate cholinesterase inhibitors.

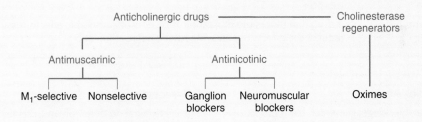

MUSCARINIC ANTAGONISTS

A. CLASSIFICATION AND PHARMACOKINETICS

1. Classification of the muscarinic antagonists— Muscarinic antagonists can be subdivided according to their selectivity for specific M receptors or their lack of such selectivity. Although the division of muscarinic receptors into subgroups is well documented (Chapters 6, 7), only a few receptor-selective M_1 antagonists have reached clinical trials (eg, pirenzepine). Most of the drugs in general use in the United States at present are relatively nonspecific, but darifenacin is somewhat selective for the M_3 subtype. The muscarinic blockers can also be subdivided on the basis of their primary clinical target organs (CNS, eye, bronchi, or gastrointestinal and genitourinary tracts). Drugs used for their effects on the CNS or the eye must be sufficiently lipid soluble to cross lipid barriers. A major determinant of this property is the presence or absence of a permanently charged (quaternary) amine group in the drug molecule. This is because charged molecules are more polar and therefore less likely to penetrate a lipid barrier such as the blood-brain barrier or the cornea of the eye.

2. Pharmacokinetics of atropine—Atropine is the prototypical nonselective muscarinic blocker. This alkaloid is found in *Atropa belladonna* and many other plants. Because it is a tertiary amine, atropine is relatively lipid soluble and readily crosses membrane barriers. The drug is well distributed into the CNS and other organs and is eliminated partially by metabolism in the liver and partially by renal excretion. The elimination half-life is approximately 2 h, and the duration of action of normal doses is 4–8 h except in the eye, where effects last for 72 h or longer.

3. Pharmacokinetics of other muscarinic blockers— In ophthalmology, topical activity (the ability to enter the eye after conjunctival administration) and duration of action are important in determining the usefulness of several antimuscarinic drugs (see Clinical Uses). Similar ability to cross lipid barriers is important for the agents used in parkinsonism. In contrast, the drugs used for their antisecretory or antispastic actions in the gut and the bronchi are often selected for minimum CNS activity; these drugs may incorporate quaternary amine groups to limit penetration through the blood-brain barrier.

HIGH-YIELD TERMS TO LEARN

Anticholinergic	A drug that blocks muscarinic or nicotinic receptors
Atropine fever	Hyperthermia induced by antimuscarinic drugs; caused mainly by inhibition of sweating
Atropine flush	Marked cutaneous vasodilation of the arms and upper torso and head by antimuscarinic drugs; mechanism unknown
Cholinesterase regenerator	A chemical antagonist that binds the phosphorus of organophosphates and displaces acetylcholinesterase
Cycloplegia	Paralysis of accommodation
Depolarizing blockade	Flaccid skeletal muscle paralysis caused by persistent depolarization of the neuromuscular end plate
Miotic	A drug that constricts the pupil
Mydriatic	A drug that dilates the pupil
Nondepolarizing blockade	Flaccid skeletal muscle paralysis caused by blockade of the nicotinic end plate receptor
Parasympatholytic	A drug that blocks the muscarinic receptors of autonomic effector tissues and reduces the effects of parasympathetic nerve stimulation

B. Mechanism of Action

The muscarinic blocking agents act like competitive (surmountable) pharmacologic antagonists; their blocking effects can be overcome by increased concentrations of muscarinic agonists.

C. Effects

The peripheral actions of muscarinic blockers are mostly predictable effects derived from cholinoceptor blockade (Table 8–1). These include the ocular, gastrointestinal, genitourinary, and secretory effects. The

Table 8–1. Effects of muscarinic blocking drugs.

Organ	Effect	Mechanism
CNS	Sedation, antimotion sickness action, antiparkinson action, amnesia, delirium	Block of muscarinic receptors, several subtypes
Eye	Cycloplegia, mydriasis	Block of M_3 receptors
Bronchi	Bronchodilation, especially if constricted	Block of M_3 receptors
Gastrointestinal tract	Relaxation, slowed peristalsis	Block of M_1, M_3 receptors
Genitourinary tract	Relaxation of bladder wall, urinary retention	Block of M_3 and possibly M_1 receptors
Heart	Initial bradycardia, especially at low doses, then tachycardia	Tachycardia from block of M_2 receptors in the SA node
Blood vessels	Block of muscarinic vasodilation; not manifest unless a muscarinic agonist is present	Block of M_3 receptors on endothelium of vessels
Glands	Marked reduction of salivation; moderate reduction of lacrimation, sweating; less reduction of gastric secretion	Block of M_1, M_3 receptors
Skeletal muscle	None	

CNS effects are less predictable. Those seen at therapeutic concentrations include sedation, reduction of motion sickness, and, as noted above, reduction of some of the signs of parkinsonism. Cardiovascular effects at therapeutic doses include an initial slowing of heart rate caused by central or (more likely) presynaptic vagal effects followed by the tachycardia and decreased atrioventricular conduction time that would be predicted from peripheral vagal blockade. It has been claimed that the M_1-selective agents (not available in the United States) are somewhat selective for the GI tract.

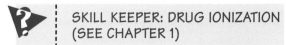

SKILL KEEPER: DRUG IONIZATION (SEE CHAPTER 1)

The pK_a of atropine is 9.7. What fraction of atropine (an amine) is in the lipid-soluble form in urine of pH 7.7? The Skill Keeper Answer appears at the end of the chapter.

D. CLINICAL USES

The muscarinic blockers have several useful therapeutic applications in the central nervous system, eye, bronchi, gut, and urinary bladder. These uses are summarized in Table 8–2.

1. CNS—Scopolamine is standard therapy for motion sickness; it is one of the most effective agents available for this condition. A transdermal patch formulation is available. Benztropine, biperiden, and trihexyphenidyl are representative of several antimuscarinic agents used in parkinsonism. Although not as effective as levodopa (see Chapter 28), these agents may be useful as adjuncts

or when patients become unresponsive to levodopa. Benztropine is sometimes used parenterally to treat acute dystonias caused by antipsychotic medications.

2. Eye—Antimuscarinic drugs are used to cause mydriasis, as indicated by the origin of the name belladonna ("beautiful lady") from the ancient cosmetic use of extracts of the *Atropa belladonna* plant to dilate the pupils. They also paralyze accommodation. The drugs include (in descending order of duration of action) atropine (>72 h), homatropine (24 h), cyclopentolate (2–12 h), and tropicamide (0.5–4 h). These agents are all well absorbed from the conjunctival sac into the eye.

3. Bronchi—Parenteral atropine has long been used to reduce airway secretions during general anesthesia. Ipratropium is a quaternary antimuscarinic agent used by inhalation to promote bronchodilation in asthma and chronic obstructive pulmonary disease (COPD). Although not as efficacious as beta agonists, ipratropium is less likely to cause tachycardia and cardiac arrhythmias in sensitive patients. It has very few antimuscarinic effects outside the lungs because it is poorly absorbed and rapidly metabolized.

4. Gut—Atropine, methscopolamine, and propantheline were used in the past to reduce acid secretion in acid-peptic disease, but are now obsolete for this indication because they are not as effective as H_2 blockers (Chapter 16) and proton pump inhibitors (Chapter 60), and they cause far more frequent and severe adverse effects. The M_1-selective inhibitor pirenzepine is available in Europe for the treatment of peptic ulcer. Muscarinic blockers can also be used to reduce cramping and hypermotility in transient diarrheas, but drugs such as diphenoxylate and loperamide (Chapter 31) are more effective.

5. Bladder—Oxybutynin, tolterodine, darifenacin, or similar agents may be used to reduce urgency in mild cystitis and to reduce bladder spasms following urologic

Table 8–2. Some clinical applications of antimuscarinic drugs.

Organ System	Drugs[a]	Application
CNS	Benztropine, trihexyphenidyl, biperiden	To reduce symptoms of Parkinson's disease
	Scopolamine	To reduce symptoms of motion sickness
Eye	Atropine, homatropine, cyclopentolate, tropicamide	To produce mydriasis and cycloplegia
Bronchi	Ipratropium, tiotropium	To reduce symptoms of asthma and chronic obstructive pulmonary disease
Gastrointestinal tract	Glycopyrrolate, dicyclomine, methscopolamine	To reduce transient hypermotility
Genitourinary tract	Oxybutynin, tolterodine, darifenacin	To reduce urgency, spasm, and incontinence
All	Atropine (IV)	Antidote in organophosphate poisoning

[a]Only a few of many drugs are listed.

surgery. Tolterodine and darifenacin are promoted for the treatment of stress incontinence.

E. Toxicity

A traditional mnemonic for atropine toxicity is "Dry as a bone, red as a beet, mad as a hatter." This description reflects both predictable antimuscarinic effects and some unpredictable actions.

1. Predictable toxicities—Antimuscarinic actions lead to several important and potentially dangerous effects. Blockade of thermoregulatory sweating may result in hyperthermia or "atropine fever." This is the most dangerous effect of the antimuscarinic drugs in children and is potentially lethal in infants. Atropine toxicity is described as feeling "dry as a bone" because sweating, salivation, and lacrimation are all significantly reduced or stopped. Moderate tachycardia is common, and severe tachycardia or arrhythmias may occur. In the elderly, important additional targets of toxicity include the eye (acute angle-closure glaucoma may occur) and the bladder (urinary retention is possible, especially in men with prostatic hyperplasia). Constipation and blurred vision are common adverse effects in all age groups.

2. Other toxicities—Toxicities not predictable from peripheral autonomic actions include the following.

a. CNS effects—CNS toxicity includes sedation, amnesia, and delirium or hallucinations ("mad as a hatter"); convulsions may also occur. Central muscarinic receptors are probably involved. Other drug groups with antimuscarinic effects, eg, tricyclic antidepressants, may cause hallucinations or delirium in the elderly.

b. Cardiovascular effects—At toxic doses, intraventricular conduction may be blocked; this action is probably not mediated by muscarinic blockade and is difficult to treat. Dilation of the cutaneous vessels of the arms, head, neck, and trunk also occurs at these doses; the resulting "atropine flush" ("red as a beet") may be diagnostic of overdose with these drugs.

F. Contraindications

The antimuscarinic agents should be used cautiously in infants because of the danger of hyperthermia. The drugs are relatively contraindicated in persons with glaucoma, especially the closed-angle form, and in men with prostatic hyperplasia.

NICOTINIC ANTAGONISTS

A. Classification

Nicotinic receptor antagonists are divided into ganglion-blocking drugs and neuromuscular-blocking drugs.

B. Ganglion-Blocking Drugs

Blockers of ganglionic nicotinic receptors act like competitive pharmacologic antagonists, though there is

evidence that some also block the pore of the nicotinic channel itself. These drugs were the first successful agents for the treatment of hypertension. Hexamethonium (C6, a prototype), mecamylamine, and several other ganglion blockers were extensively used for this disease. Unfortunately, the adverse effects of ganglion blockade in hypertension are so severe (both sympathetic and parasympathetic divisions are blocked) that patients were unable to tolerate them for long periods (Table 8–3). Trimethaphan was the ganglion blocker most recently used in clinical practice, but it too has been almost abandoned. It is poorly lipid soluble, inactive orally, and has a short half-life. It was used intravenously to treat severe accelerated hypertension (malignant hypertension) and to produce controlled hypotension.

Recent interest has focused on nicotinic receptors in the CNS and their relation to nicotine addiction and to Tourette's syndrome. Paradoxically, both nicotine (in the form of nicotine patches) and mecamylamine, a nicotinic ganglion blocker that enters the CNS, have been shown to have some benefit in these applications.

Because ganglion blockers interrupt sympathetic control of venous tone, they cause marked venous pooling; postural hypotension is a major manifestation of this effect. Other toxicities of ganglion-blocking drugs include dry mouth, blurred vision, constipation, and severe sexual dysfunction (see Table 8–3). As a result, ganglion blockers are rarely used.

C. Neuromuscular-Blocking Drugs

Neuromuscular-blocking drugs are important for producing complete skeletal muscle relaxation in surgery; new ones are introduced regularly. They are discussed in greater detail in Chapter 27.

1. Nondepolarizing group—**Tubocurarine** is the prototype. It produces a competitive block at the end plate nicotinic receptor, causing flaccid paralysis that lasts 30–60 minutes (longer if large doses have been given). Pancuronium, atracurium, vecuronium, and several newer drugs are shorter-acting, nondepolarizing blockers (see Chapter 27).

2. Depolarizing group—Although these drugs are nicotinic agonists, not antagonists, they also cause flaccid paralysis (see Chapter 27). **Succinylcholine**, the only member of this group used in the United States, produces fasciculations during induction of paralysis; patients may complain of muscle pain after its use. The drug is hydrolyzed by butyrylcholinesterase (also known as plasma cholinesterase or pseudocholinesterase) and has a half-life of a few minutes in persons with normal plasma cholinesterase. Approximately one in 2500 individuals produces a genetically determined form of abnormal cholinesterase that does not metabolize succinylcholine effectively. The drug's duration of action is grossly prolonged in such individuals.

Table 8–3. Effects of ganglion-blocking drugs.

Organ	Effects
CNS	Antinicotinic action may include reduction of nicotine craving and amelioration of Tourette's syndrome (mecamylamine only)
Eye	Moderate mydriasis and cycloplegia
Bronchi	Little effect; asthmatics may note some bronchodilation
Gastrointestinal tract	Marked reduction of motility, constipation may be severe
Genitourinary tract	Reduced contractility of the bladder; impairment of erection and ejaculation
Heart	Moderate tachycardia; reduction in force and cardiac output
Vessels	Reduction in arteriolar and venous tone, dose-dependent reduction in blood pressure; orthostatic hypotension usually marked
Glands	Reductions in salivation, lacrimation, sweating, and gastric secretion
Skeletal muscle	No significant effect

3. Toxicity—The toxicity of neuromuscular blockers is discussed in Chapter 27.

CHOLINESTERASE REGENERATORS

Pralidoxime is the prototype cholinesterase regenerator. These agents are not receptor antagonists but belong to a class of *chemical* antagonists. These molecules contain an oxime group, which has an extremely high affinity for the phosphorus atom in organophosphate insecticides. Because the affinity of the oxime group for phosphorus exceeds the affinity of the enzyme active site for phosphorus, these agents are able to bind the inhibitor and displace the enzyme (if aging has not occurred). The active enzyme is thus regenerated. Pralidoxime, the oxime currently available in the United States, may be used to treat patients exposed to insecticides, such as parathion, or to nerve gases.

QUESTIONS

1–2. A 3-year-old child has been admitted to the emergency room. Antimuscarinic drug overdose is suspected.

1. Atropine overdose may cause which one of the following?
   (A) Gastrointestinal smooth muscle cramping
   (B) Increased cardiac rate
   (C) Increased gastric secretion
   (D) Pupillary constriction
   (E) Urinary frequency

2. In infants, the most dangerous effect of belladonna alkaloids is
   (A) Dehydration
   (B) Hallucinations
   (C) Hypertension
   (D) Hyperthermia
   (E) Intraventricular heart block

KEY DRUGS		
Subclass	**Prototype**	**Other Significant Agents**
Muscarinic blockers	Atropine	Scopolamine, glycopyrrolate, ipratropium, tropicamide, oxybutynin, benztropine
Nicotinic blockers		
Ganglion blockers	Hexamethonium	Trimethaphan, mecamylamine
Neuromuscular blockers	Tubocurarine	See Chapter 27
Cholinesterase regenerator	Pralidoxime	

3. Which of the following pairs of drugs and properties is most correct?
   (A) Atropine: poorly absorbed after oral administration
   (B) Benztropine: quaternary amine, poor CNS penetration
   (C) Cyclopentolate: well absorbed from conjunctival sac into the eye
   (D) Ipratropium: well-absorbed, long elimination half-life
   (E) Scopolamine: short duration of action when used as anti-motion sickness agent

4. Which one of the following can be blocked by atropine?
   (A) Decreased blood pressure caused by hexamethonium
   (B) Increased blood pressure caused by nicotine
   (C) Increased skeletal muscle strength caused by neostigmine
   (D) Tachycardia caused by exercise
   (E) Tachycardia caused by infusion of acetylcholine

5. Which of the following best describes the mechanism of action of scopolamine?
   (A) Chemical antagonist at muscarinic receptors
   (B) Irreversible antagonist at muscarinic receptors
   (C) Physiologic antagonist at muscarinic receptors
   (D) Reversible antagonist at muscarinic receptors
   (E) Reversible antagonist at nicotinic receptors

6–7. Two new synthetic drugs (X and Y) are to be studied for their cardiovascular effects. The drugs are given to three anesthetized animals while the blood pressure is recorded. The first animal has received no pretreatment (control), the second has received an effective dose of a long-acting ganglion blocker, and the third has received an effective dose of a long-acting muscarinic antagonist.

6. Drug X caused a 50 mm Hg rise in mean blood pressure in the control animal, no blood pressure change in the ganglion-blocked animal, and a 75 mm mean blood pressure rise in the atropine-pretreated animal. Drug X is probably a drug similar to
   (A) Acetylcholine
   (B) Atropine
   (C) Epinephrine
   (D) Hexamethonium
   (E) Nicotine

7. The net changes induced by drug Y in these experiments are shown in the following graph. Drug Y is probably a drug similar to
   (A) Acetylcholine
   (B) Edrophonium
   (C) Hexamethonium
   (D) Nicotine
   (E) Pralidoxime

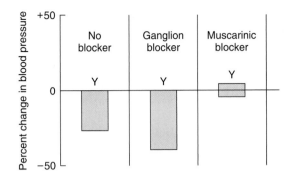

8. A 30-year-old man has been treated with several autonomic drugs for 4 weeks. He is now admitted to the emergency department showing signs of drug toxicity. Which of the following signs would distinguish between an overdose of a ganglion blocker versus a muscarinic blocker?
   (A) Blurred vision
   (B) Dry mouth, constipation
   (C) Mydriasis
   (D) Postural hypotension
   (E) Tachycardia

9. Which one of the following does NOT cause cycloplegia (paralysis of accommodation) when used topically in the eye?
   (A) Atropine
   (B) Cyclopentolate
   (C) Physostigmine
   (D) Scopolamine
   (E) Tropicamide

10. You have been asked to consult in the treatment of an 80-year-old woman. An antimuscarinic drug is being considered. Ordinary doses of atropine may be hazardous in the elderly because
   (A) Atropine can elevate intraocular pressure in patients with glaucoma
   (B) Atropine frequently causes ventricular arrhythmias
   (C) Urinary retention is often precipitated by atropine in women
   (D) The elderly are particularly prone to develop dangerous hyperthermia when given atropine
   (E) Atropine often causes excessive vasodilation and hypotension in the elderly

11. Accepted therapeutic indications for the use of antimuscarinic drugs include all of the following EXCEPT
   (A) Hypertension
   (B) Motion sickness
   (C) Parkinson's disease
   (D) Postoperative bladder spasm
   (E) To antidote parathion poisoning

12. Which of the following is an expected effect of a therapeutic dose of an antimuscarinic drug?
    (A) Decreased cAMP in cardiac muscle
    (B) Decreased DAG in salivary gland tissue
    (C) Increased IP_3 in intestinal smooth muscle
    (D) Increased potassium efflux from smooth muscle
    (E) Increased sodium influx into the skeletal muscle end plate

13. Which one of the following drugs causes vasodilation that can be blocked by atropine?
    (A) Atropine
    (B) Benztropine
    (C) Bethanechol
    (D) Botulinum
    (E) Cyclopentolate
    (F) Neostigmine
    (G) Pralidoxime

14. Which one of the following drugs has a very high affinity for the phosphorus atom in parathion and is often used to treat life-threatening insecticide toxicity
    (A) Atropine
    (B) Benztropine
    (C) Bethanechol
    (D) Botulinum
    (E) Cyclopentolate
    (F) Neostigmine
    (G) Pralidoxime

ANSWERS

1. Tachycardia is a characteristic atropine overdose effect. The answer is **B.**

2. Choices **B, D,** and **E** are all possible effects of the atropine group. In infants, however, the most dangerous effect is hyperthermia. Deaths with body temperatures in excess of 42°C have occurred after the use of atropine-containing eye drops in children. The answer is **D.**

3. Atropine is very well absorbed. Scopolamine has a relatively long duration of action, especially when used as an anti-motion sickness transdermal patch. Ipratropium is a quaternary amine (and therefore permanently charged) and poorly absorbed from the airways. Benztropine is tertiary, lipid soluble, and penetrates into the CNS well. Only **C** is correct.

4. Atropine blocks muscarinic receptors and inhibits parasympathomimetic effects. Nicotine can induce both parasympathomimetic and sympathomimetic effects by virtue of its ganglion-stimulating action. Hypertension and exercise-induced tachycardia reflect sympathetic discharge and therefore would not be blocked by atropine. The answer is **E.**

5. All of the muscarinic blockers, including scopolamine, act as reversible, competitive pharmacologic antagonists. The answer is **D.**

6. Drug X causes an increase in blood pressure that is blocked by a ganglion blocker but not by a muscarinic blocker. The pressor response is actually increased by pretreatment with atropine, a muscarinic blocker, suggesting that compensatory vagal discharge might have blunted the full response. This description fits a ganglion stimulant like nicotine but not epinephrine, since epinephrine's pressor effects are produced at α receptors, not in the ganglia. The answer is **E.**

7. Drug Y causes a decrease in blood pressure that is blocked by a muscarinic blocker but not by a ganglion blocker. Therefore, the depressor effect must be evoked at a site distal to the ganglia. In fact, the drop in blood pressure is actually greater in the presence of ganglion blockade, suggesting that compensatory sympathetic discharge might have blunted the full depressor action of drug Y in the untreated animal. The description fits a direct-acting muscarinic stimulant such as acetylcholine (given in high dosage). Indirect-acting cholinomimetics (cholinesterase inhibitors) would not produce this pattern because the vascular muscarinic receptors involved in the depressor response are not innervated and are, therefore, unresponsive to indirectly acting agents. The answer is **A.**

8. Ganglion blockers and muscarinic blockers can both cause mydriasis, increase resting heart rate, blur vision, and cause dry mouth and constipation, because these are determined largely by parasympathetic tone. Postural hypotension, on the other hand, is a sign of sympathetic blockade, which would occur with ganglion blockers but not muscarinic blockers (Chapter 6). The answer is **D.**

9. All antimuscarinic agents are, in theory, capable of causing cycloplegia. (Ganglion blockers also cause cycloplegia.) Physostigmine, on the other hand, is an indirect-acting cholinomimetic and has the opposite effect. The answer is **C.**

10. The elderly have a much higher incidence of glaucoma than younger people (and may be unaware of the disease until late in its course). Antimuscarinic agents may increase intraocular pressure in individuals with glaucoma. Elderly men (not women) have a much higher probability of developing urinary retention—because they have a high incidence of prostatic hyperplasia. Hypotensive and hyperthermic reactions to ordinary doses of atropine are not common in the elderly. The answer is **A.**

11. Hypertension is not responsive to antimuscarinic agents. The answer is **A.**

12. Muscarinic M_1 and M_3 receptors mediate increases in IP_3 and DAG in target tissues (intestine, salivary glands). M_2 receptors (heart) mediate a decrease in cAMP and an increase in potassium permeability. Antimuscarinic agents block these effects. The answer is **B**.

13. Bethanechol (Chapter 7) causes vasodilation by activating muscarinic receptors on the endothelium of blood vessels. This effect can be blocked by atropine. The answer is **C**.

14. Pralidoxime has a very high affinity for the phosphorus atom in organophosphate insecticides. The answer is **G**.

SKILL KEEPER ANSWER: DRUG IONIZATION (SEE CHAPTER 1)

The pK_a of atropine is 9.7. According to the Henderson-Hasselbalch equation,

$$Log\ (protonated/unprotonated) = pK_a - pH$$
$$Log\ (P/U) = 9.7 - 7.7$$
$$Log\ (P/U) = 2$$
$$P/U = antilog\ (2)$$
$$= 100/1$$

Therefore, about 99% of the drug is in the protonated form, 1% in the unprotonated form. Since atropine is a weak base, it is the unprotonated form that is lipid soluble. Therefore, about 1% of the atropine in the urine is lipid soluble.

CHECKLIST

When you complete this chapter, you should be able to:

☐ Describe the effects of atropine on the major organ systems (CNS, eye, heart, vessels, bronchi, gut, genitourinary tract, exocrine glands, skeletal muscle).

☐ List the signs, symptoms, and treatment of atropine overdose.

☐ List the major clinical indications and contraindications for the use of muscarinic antagonists.

☐ Describe the effects of the ganglion-blocking nicotinic antagonists.

☐ List one antimuscarinic agent promoted for each of the following uses: to produce mydriasis and cycloplegia; to treat parkinsonism, asthma, bladder spasm, and the muscarinic effects of insecticides.

☐ Describe the mechanism of action and clinical use of pralidoxime.

Sympathomimetics

9

The sympathomimetics constitute a very important group of drugs used for cardiovascular, respiratory, and other conditions. They are readily divided into subgroups on the basis of their spectrum of action (α, β, or dopamine receptor affinity) or mode of action (direct or indirect).

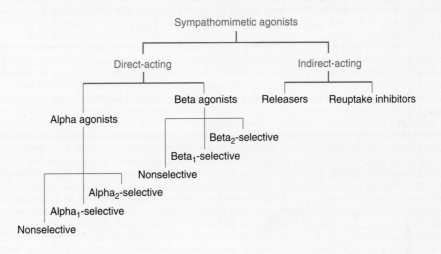

CLASSIFICATION

A. MODE OF ACTION

Sympathomimetic agonists may directly activate their adrenoceptors, or they may act indirectly to increase the concentration of catecholamine transmitter in the synapse. Amphetamine derivatives and tyramine cause the release of stored catecholamines; these sympathomimetics are therefore mainly indirect in their mode of action. Another form of indirect action is seen with cocaine and the tricyclic antidepressants; these drugs inhibit reuptake of catecholamines by the norepinephrine transporter (NET) in nerve terminals (see Figure 6–2) and thus increase the synaptic activity of released transmitter.

Blockade of metabolism (ie, block of catechol-*O*-methyltransferase [COMT] and monoamine oxidase [MAO]) has little direct effect on autonomic activity, but MAO inhibition increases the stores of catecholamines and related molecules in adrenergic synaptic vesicles and thus may potentiate the action of indirectly acting sympathomimetics.

B. SPECTRUM OF ACTION

Adrenoceptors are classified as α or β receptors; both groups are further subdivided into subgroups. The distribution of these receptors is set forth in Table 9–1. Epinephrine may be considered a single prototype agonist with effects at all receptor types (α_1, α_2, β_1, β_2, and β_3). Alternatively, separate prototypes, phenylephrine (an alpha agonist) and isoproterenol (beta) may be defined. Dopamine receptors constitute a third class of adrenoceptors. The just-mentioned drugs have relatively little effect on dopamine receptors, but dopamine itself is a potent dopamine receptor agonist and when given

HIGH-YIELD TERMS TO LEARN

Anorexiant	A drug that decreases appetite (causes anorexia)
Catecholamine	A dihydroxyphenylethylamine derivative (eg, norepinephrine, epinephrine)
Decongestant	A drug that reduces nasal or oropharyngeal mucosal swelling, usually by constricting blood vessels in the submucosal tissue
Mydriatic	A drug that causes dilation of the pupil; opposite of miotic
Phenylisopropylamine	A derivative of phenylisopropylamine (eg, amphetamine, ephedrine). Unlike catecholamines, phenylisopropylamines usually have oral activity, a long half-life, some CNS activity, and an indirect mode of action.
Selective α-agonist, β-agonist	Drugs that have relatively greater effects on α or β adrenoceptors; none are *absolutely* selective or specific
Sympathomimetic	A drug that mimics stimulation of the sympathetic autonomic nervous system
Reuptake inhibitor	An indirectly acting drug that increases the activity of transmitters in the synapse by inhibiting their reuptake into the presynaptic nerve ending. May act selectively on noradrenergic, serotonergic, or both types of nerve endings

Table 9–1. Types of adrenoceptors, some of the peripheral tissues in which they are found, and their major effects.

Type	Tissue	Actions
α_1	Most vascular smooth muscle	Contracts ($\uparrow$ vascular resistance)
	Pupillary dilator muscle	Contracts (mydriasis)
	Pilomotor smooth muscle	Contracts (erects hair)
	Liver (in some species, eg, rat)	Stimulates glycogenolysis
α_2	Adrenergic and cholinergic nerve terminals	Inhibits transmitter release
	Platelets	Stimulates aggregation
	Some vascular smooth muscle	Contracts
	Fat cells	Inhibits lipolysis
	Pancreatic B (β) cells	Inhibits insulin release
β_1	Heart	Stimulates rate and force
	Juxtaglomerular cells	Stimulates renin release
β_2	Airways, uterine, and vascular smooth muscle	Relaxes
	Liver (human)	Stimulates glycogenolysis
	Pancreatic B (β) cells	Stimulates insulin release
	Somatic motor neuron terminals (voluntary muscle)	Causes tremor
β_3	Fat cells	Stimulates lipolysis
Dopamine$_1$ (D$_1$)	Renal and other splanchnic blood vessels	Dilates ($\downarrow$ resistance)
Dopamine$_2$ (D$_2$)	Nerve terminals	Inhibits adenylyl cyclase

as a drug can also activate β receptors (intermediate doses) and α receptors (larger doses).

CHEMISTRY & PHARMACOKINETICS

The endogenous adrenoceptor agonists (epinephrine, norepinephrine, and dopamine) are catecholamines and are rapidly metabolized by COMT and MAO. If used as drugs, these adrenoceptor agonists are inactive by the oral route and must be given parenterally. When released from nerve endings, they are subsequently taken up into nerve endings and into perisynaptic cells; this uptake may also occur with norepinephrine, epinephrine, and dopamine given as drugs. These agonists have a short duration of action. When given parenterally, they do not enter the CNS in significant amounts. Isoproterenol, a synthetic catecholamine, is similar to the endogenous transmitters but is not readily taken up into nerve endings. Phenylisopropylamines, eg, amphetamines, are resistant to MAO; most of them are not catecholamines and are therefore also resistant to COMT. These agents are orally active; they enter the CNS, and their effects last much longer than do those of catecholamines. Tyramine, which is not a phenylisopropylamine, is rapidly metabolized by MAO except in patients who are taking an MAO inhibitor drug. MAO inhibitors are sometimes used in the treatment of depression (Chapter 30).

MECHANISMS OF ACTION

A. ALPHA₁ RECEPTOR EFFECTS

Alpha₁ receptor effects are mediated primarily by the trimeric coupling protein G_q. When G_q is activated, the alpha moiety of this protein activates the phosphoinositide cascade and causes the release of inositol-1,4, 5-trisphosphate (IP_3) and diacylglycerol (DAG) from membrane lipids. Calcium is subsequently released from stores in smooth muscle cells, and enzymes are activated. Direct gating of calcium channels may also play a role in increasing intracellular calcium concentration.

B. ALPHA₂ RECEPTOR EFFECTS

Alpha₂ receptor activation results in inhibition of adenylyl cyclase via the coupling protein G_i.

C. BETA RECEPTOR EFFECTS

Beta receptors (β_1, β_2, and β_3) stimulate adenylyl cyclase via the coupling protein G_s, which leads to an increase in cAMP concentration in the cell.

D. DOPAMINE RECEPTOR EFFECTS

Dopamine D_1 receptors activate adenylyl cyclase via G_s in neurons and vascular smooth muscle. Dopamine D_2 receptors are more important in the brain but probably also play a significant role as presynaptic receptors on peripheral nerves. These receptors act via G_i and reduce the synthesis of cAMP.

ORGAN SYSTEM EFFECTS

A. CNS

Catecholamines do not enter the CNS effectively. Sympathomimetics that do enter the CNS (eg, amphetamines) have a spectrum of stimulant effects, beginning with mild alerting or reduction of fatigue, and progressing to anorexia, euphoria, and insomnia. Some of these central effects probably reflect the release of dopamine in certain dopaminergic tracts. Very high doses lead to marked anxiety or aggressiveness, paranoia, and, less commonly, convulsions.

B. EYE

The smooth muscle of the pupillary dilator responds to topical phenylephrine and similar α agonists with contraction and mydriasis. Accommodation is not significantly affected. Outflow of aqueous humor may be facilitated by nonselective α agonists, with a subsequent reduction of intraocular pressure. Alpha₂-selective agonists also reduce intraocular pressure, apparently by reducing synthesis of aqueous humor.

C. BRONCHI

The smooth muscle of the bronchi relaxes markedly in response to β₂ agonists. These agents are the most efficacious and reliable drugs available for reversing bronchospasm.

D. GASTROINTESTINAL TRACT

The gastrointestinal tract is well endowed with both α and β receptors, located on both smooth muscle and on neurons of the enteric nervous system. Activation of either α or β receptors leads to relaxation of the smooth muscle. Alpha₂ agonists may also decrease salt and water secretion into the intestine.

E. GENITOURINARY TRACT

The genitourinary tract contains α receptors in the bladder trigone and sphincter area; these receptors mediate contraction of the sphincter. In men, α_1 receptors mediate prostatic smooth muscle contraction. Sympathomimetics are sometimes used to increase sphincter tone. Beta₂ agonists may cause significant uterine relaxation in pregnant women near term, but the doses required also cause significant tachycardia.

F. VASCULAR SYSTEM

Different vascular beds respond differently, depending on their dominant receptor type (Tables 9–1 and 9–2).

1. Alpha₁ agonists—Alpha₁ agonists (eg, phenylephrine) constrict skin and splanchnic blood vessels and increase peripheral vascular resistance and venous pressure. Because these drugs increase blood pressure, they often evoke a compensatory reflex bradycardia.

Table 9–2. Effects of prototypical sympathomimetics on vascular resistance, blood pressure, and heart rate.

	Effect on				
Drug	**Skin, Splanchnic Vessel Resistance**	**Skeletal Muscle Vascular Resistance**	**Renal Vascular Resistance**	**Mean Blood Pressure**	**Heart Rate**
Phenylephrine	↑↑↑	↑	↑	↑↑	↓
Isoproterenol	—	↓↓	—	↓↓	↑↑
Norepinephrine	↑↑↑↑	↑↑	↑	↑↑↑	↓

2. Alpha₂ agonists—Alpha$_2$ agonists (eg, clonidine) cause vasoconstriction when administered intravenously or topically (eg, as a nasal spray), but when given orally they accumulate in the CNS and *reduce* sympathetic outflow and blood pressure as described in Chapter 11.

3. Beta agonists—Beta$_2$ agonists (eg, albuterol) cause significant reduction in arteriolar tone in the skeletal muscle vascular bed and can reduce peripheral vascular resistance and arterial blood pressure. Beta$_1$ agonists have relatively little effect on vessels.

4. Dopamine—Dopamine causes vasodilation in the splanchnic and renal vascular beds by activating D$_1$ receptors. This effect can be very useful in the treatment of renal failure associated with shock. At higher doses, dopamine activates β receptors in the heart and elsewhere; at still higher doses, α receptors are activated.

G. HEART

The heart is well supplied with β$_1$ and β$_2$ receptors. The β$_1$ receptors predominate in some parts of the heart; both β receptors mediate increased rate of cardiac pacemakers (normal and abnormal), increased AV node conduction velocity, and increased cardiac force.

H. NET CARDIOVASCULAR ACTIONS

Sympathomimetics with both α and β$_1$ effects (eg, norepinephrine) may cause a reflex increase in vagal outflow because they increase blood pressure and evoke the baroreceptor reflex. This reflex vagal effect may dominate any direct beta effects on the heart rate, so that a slow infusion of norepinephrine typically causes increased blood pressure and bradycardia (Figure 9–1; Table 9–2). If the reflex is blocked (eg, by a ganglion blocker),

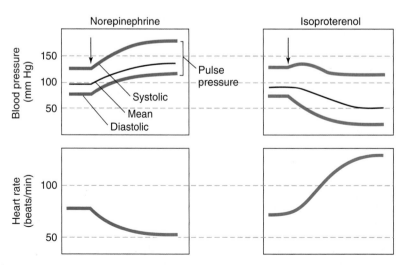

Figure 9–1. Typical effects of norepinephrine and isoproterenol on blood pressure and heart rate. Note that the pulse pressure is only slightly increased by norepinephrine but is markedly increased by isoproterenol. The reduction in heart rate caused by norepinephrine is the result of baroreceptor reflex activation of vagal outflow to the heart.

norepinephrine will cause a direct β_1-mediated tachycardia. A pure α agonist (eg, phenylephrine) will routinely slow heart rate via the baroreceptor reflex, while a pure β agonist (eg, isoproterenol) will almost always increase the rate.

The diastolic blood pressure is affected mainly by peripheral vascular resistance and the heart rate. The adrenoceptors with the greatest effects on vascular resistance are α and β_2 receptors. The pulse pressure (the systolic minus the diastolic pressure) is determined mainly by the stroke volume (a function of force of cardiac contraction), which is influenced by β_1 receptors. The systolic pressure is the sum of the diastolic and the pulse pressures and is therefore a function of both α and β effects.

I. Metabolic & Hormonal Effects

Beta$_1$ agonists increase renin secretion. Beta$_2$ agonists increase insulin secretion by the pancreas. They also increase glycogenolysis in the liver. The resulting hyperglycemia is countered by the increased insulin levels. Transport of glucose out of the liver is associated initially with hyperkalemia; transport into peripheral organs (especially skeletal muscle) is accompanied by movement of potassium into these cells, resulting in a later hypokalemia. All β agonists appear to stimulate lipolysis via the β_3 receptor.

SKILL KEEPER: BLOOD PRESSURE CONTROL MECHANISMS IN PHEOCHROMOCYTOMA (SEE CHAPTER 6)

Patients with pheochromocytoma may have this tumor for several months or even years before symptoms or signs lead to a diagnosis. Predict the probable compensatory responses to a chronic increase in blood pressure caused by a tumor releasing large amounts of norepinephrine. The Skill Keeper Answer appears at the end of the chapter.

CLINICAL USES

Pharmacokinetic characteristics and clinical applications of selected sympathomimetics are shown in Table 9–3.

A. Anaphylaxis

Epinephrine is the **drug of choice** for the immediate treatment of anaphylactic shock. The catecholamine is sometimes supplemented with antihistamines and corticosteroids, but these agents are neither as efficacious as epinephrine nor as rapid acting.

B. CNS

The phenylisopropylamines such as amphetamine are widely used and abused for their CNS effects. Legitimate indications include narcolepsy, attention deficit disorder, and, with appropriate controls, weight reduction. The anorexiant effect may be helpful in initiating weight loss but is insufficient to maintain the loss unless patients also receive intensive dietary and psychological counseling and support. The drugs are abused or misused for the purpose of deferring sleep and for their mood-elevating, euphoria-producing action (see Chapter 32).

C. Eye

The α agonists, especially phenylephrine, are often used topically to produce mydriasis and to reduce the conjunctival itching and congestion caused by irritation or allergy. These drugs do not cause cycloplegia. Epinephrine and a prodrug, dipivefrin, now obsolete, were used topically in the treatment of glaucoma. Phenylephrine has also been used for glaucoma, mainly outside the United States. Newer α_2 agonists are in current use for glaucoma and include apraclonidine and brimonidine. As noted, the α_2-selective agonists appear to reduce aqueous synthesis. See Table 10–3 for a summary of drugs used in glaucoma.

D. Bronchi

The β agonists, especially the β_2-selective agonists, are drugs of choice in the treatment of acute asthmatic bronchoconstriction. The short-acting β_2-selective agonists (eg, albuterol, metaproterenol, terbutaline) are not recommended for prophylaxis, but they are safe and effective and may be lifesaving in the treatment of bronchospasm. Much longer acting β_2-selective agonists, salmeterol and formoterol, are recommended for prophylaxis (and not for the treatment of acute symptoms), see Chapter 20.

E. Cardiovascular Applications

1. Conditions in which an *increase* in blood flow is desired—In acute heart failure and some types of shock, an increase in cardiac output and blood flow to the tissues is needed. Beta$_1$ agonists may be useful in this situation because they increase cardiac contractility and reduce (to some degree) afterload by decreasing the impedance to ventricular ejection through a small β_2 effect. Dobutamine and dopamine are used.

2. Conditions in which a *decrease* in blood flow or increase in blood pressure is desired—Alpha$_1$ agonists are useful in situations in which vasoconstriction is appropriate. These include local hemostatic (epinephrine) and decongestant effects (phenylephrine) as well as spinal shock (norepinephrine, phenylephrine), in which temporary maintenance of blood pressure may help maintain perfusion of the brain, heart, and kidneys. Shock due to septicemia or myocardial infarction, on

Table 9–3. Pharmacokinetics and clinical applications of some sympathomimetics.

Drug	Oral Activity	Duration of Action	Clinical Application
Catecholamines			
Epinephrine	No	Minutes	To treat anaphylaxis, asthma, glaucoma; to cause vasoconstriction
Norepinephrine	No	Minutes	Emergency treatment of neurogenic or severe hypotension
Isoproterenol	Poor	Minutes	To treat asthma, AV blockade (rare)
Dopamine	No	Minutes	To treat shock, heart failure
Dobutamine	No	Minutes	To treat shock, heart failure
Other sympathomimetics			
Amphetamine, methylphenidate, others	Yes	Hours	To treat narcolepsy, attention deficit hyperkinetic disorder, obesity
Ephedrine	Yes	Hours	To treat urinary incontinence, neurogenic hypotension, asthma (obsolete)
Phenylephrine	Poor	Minutes to hours	To cause mydriasis, vasoconstriction, decongestion
Albuterol, metaproterenol, terbutaline	Moderate (used by inhalation or systemic)	Minutes to hours	To treat asthma
Oxymetazoline, xylometazoline	Yes	Hours	To produce nasal decongestion (long duration)
Cocaine	Poor	Minutes-hours	To produce local anesthesia with vasoconstriction

the other hand, is usually made worse by vasoconstrictors, because sympathetic discharge is usually already increased. Alpha agonists are often mixed with local anesthetics to reduce the loss of anesthetic from the area of injection into the circulation. Chronic orthostatic hypotension due to inadequate sympathetic tone can be treated with oral ephedrine or a newer orally active α_1 agonist, midodrine.

F. GENITOURINARY TRACT

Beta$_2$ agonists (ritodrine, terbutaline) are sometimes used to suppress premature labor, but the cardiac stimulant effect may be hazardous to both mother and fetus. Nonsteroidal anti-inflammatory drugs, calcium channel blockers, and magnesium are also used for this indication.

Long-acting oral sympathomimetics such as ephedrine are sometimes used to improve urinary continence in children with enuresis and in the elderly. This action is mediated by α receptors in the trigone of the bladder and, in men, the smooth muscle of the prostate.

TOXICITY

A. CATECHOLAMINES

Because of their limited penetration into the brain, these drugs have little CNS toxicity when given systemically. In the periphery, their adverse effects are extensions of their pharmacologic alpha or beta actions: excessive vasoconstriction, cardiac arrhythmias, myocardial infarction, hemorrhagic stroke, and pulmonary edema or hemorrhage.

B. OTHER SYMPATHOMIMETICS

The phenylisopropylamines may produce mild to severe CNS toxicity, depending on dosage. In small doses, they induce nervousness, anorexia, and insomnia; in higher doses, they may cause anxiety, aggressiveness, or paranoid behavior. Convulsions may occur. Peripherally acting agents have toxicities that are predictable on the basis of the receptors they activate. Thus, α_1 agonists cause hypertension and β_1 agonists cause sinus tachycardia and serious arrhythmias. Beta$_2$ agonists cause skeletal muscle tremor. It is important to note that none of these drugs

KEY DRUGS		
Subclass	**Prototype**	**Other Significant Agents**
General agonists		
Direct ($\alpha_1, \alpha_2, \beta_1, \beta_2$)	Epinephrine	
Indirect, releasers	Amphetamine	Ephedrine, tyramine
Indirect, uptake inhibitors	Cocaine	Tricyclic antidepressants
Selective agonists		
$\alpha_1, \alpha_2, \beta_1$	Norepinephrine	
$\alpha_1 > \alpha_2$	Midodrine	Phenylephrine[a]
$\alpha_1 < \alpha_2$	Clonidine	Oxymetazoline
$\beta_1 = \beta_2$	Isoproterenol	
$\beta_1 > \beta_2$	Dobutamine	
$\beta_1 < \beta_2$	Albuterol	Metaproterenol, terbutaline
Dopamine agonist	Dopamine	Bromocriptine[b]

[a]Moderate selectivity.
[b]Ergot derivative; see Chapter 28.

is perfectly selective; at high doses, β_1-selective agents have β_2 actions and vice versa. Cocaine is of special importance as a drug of abuse: its major toxicities include cardiac arrhythmias or infarction and convulsions. A fatal outcome is more common with acute cocaine overdose than with any other sympathomimetic.

QUESTIONS

1. Dilation of vessels in skeletal muscle, constriction of cutaneous vessels, and positive inotropic and chronotropic effects on the heart are all actions of
   (A) Acetylcholine
   (B) Epinephrine
   (C) Isoproterenol
   (D) Metaproterenol
   (E) Norepinephrine

2. A 7-year-old boy has a significant bed-wetting problem. A long-acting indirect sympathomimetic agent which has been used by the oral route for this and other indications is
   (A) Dobutamine
   (B) Ephedrine
   (C) Epinephrine
   (D) Isoproterenol
   (E) Phenylephrine

3. When pupillary dilation—but not cycloplegia—is desired, a good choice is
   (A) Isoproterenol
   (B) Norepinephrine
   (C) Phenylephrine
   (D) Pilocarpine
   (E) Tropicamide

4. Which one of the following acts primarily on receptors located on the membrane of the autonomic effector cell (ie, muscle or glandular tissue)?
   (A) Amphetamine
   (B) Clonidine
   (C) Cocaine
   (D) Norepinephrine
   (E) Tyramine

5. When a moderate pressor dose of norepinephrine is given after pretreatment with a large dose of atropine, which of the following is the most probable response to the norepinephrine?
   (A) A decrease in heart rate caused by direct cardiac effect
   (B) A decrease in heart rate caused by indirect reflex effect
   (C) An increase in heart rate caused by direct cardiac action
   (D) An increase in heart rate caused by indirect reflex action
   (E) No change in heart rate

6. Which of the following drugs will prevent tachycardia evoked by isoproterenol?
   (A) Atropine
   (B) Hexamethonium
   (C) Phentolamine (an α–blocker)
   (D) Physostigmine
   (E) Propranolol (a β–blocker)

7–8: Your patient is to receive a selective β_2 stimulant drug.

7. Beta$_2$-selective stimulants are often effective in
(A) Angina due to coronary insufficiency
(B) Asthma
(C) Chronic heart failure
(D) Delayed or insufficiently strong labor
(E) Raynaud's syndrome

8. In considering possible drug effects in this patient, you would note that β_2 stimulants frequently cause
(A) Direct stimulation of renin release
(B) Hypoglycemia
(C) Increased cGMP in mast cells
(D) Skeletal muscle tremor
(E) Vasodilation in the skin

9. Epinephrine causes a decrease in:
(A) cAMP in heart muscle
(B) Free fatty acids in blood
(C) Glucose in blood
(D) Lactate in blood
(E) Triglycerides in fat cells

10. Phenylephrine causes
(A) Constriction of vessels in the nasal mucosa
(B) Increased gastric secretion and motility
(C) Increased skin temperature
(D) Miosis
(E) Thermoregulatory sweating

11–12. Autonomic drugs X and Y were given in moderate doses as IV boluses to normal volunteers. The systolic and diastolic blood pressures changed as shown in the diagram below.

11. Which of the following drugs most resembles drug X?
(A) Acetylcholine
(B) Atropine
(C) Epinephrine
(D) Isoproterenol
(E) Norepinephrine

12. Which of the following most resembles drug Y?
(A) Acetylcholine
(B) Atropine
(C) Epinephrine
(D) Isoproterenol
(E) Norepinephrine

13. A new drug was given by subcutaneous injection to 25 normal subjects in a phase 1 clinical trial. The cardiovascular effects are summarized in the table below. Which of the following drugs does the new experimental agent most resemble?

Variable	Control	Peak Drug Effect
Systolic BP (mm Hg)	116	144
Diastolic BP (mm Hg)	76	96
Cardiac output (L/min)	5.4	4.7
Heart rate (beats/min)	71.2	54.3

(A) Bethanechol
(B) Epinephrine
(C) Isoproterenol
(D) Phenylephrine
(E) Physostigmine

ANSWERS

1. The actions describe the effects of activating α, β_1, and β_2 receptors. Of the drugs listed, only epinephrine has all of these actions. The answer is **B.**

2. Phenylephrine and ephedrine are the only orally effective agents listed. Phenylephrine has a direct and relatively short action. Ephedrine also occurs in the herb Ma-huang and in "energy" supplements. The answer is **B.**

3. Antimuscarinics (tropicamide) are mydriatic and cycloplegic; α-sympathomimetic agonists are only

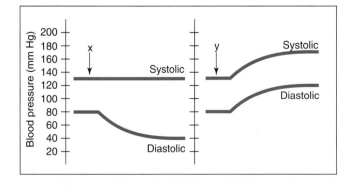

mydriatic. Norepinephrine penetrates the conjunctiva poorly and would produce intense vasoconstriction. Pilocarpine causes *miosis.* The answer is **C.**

4. The indirect-acting agents (amphetamine, cocaine, and tyramine) act through catecholamines in or released from the nerve terminal. Clonidine acts primarily on presynaptic nerve endings although it can activate α_2 receptors located elsewhere. The answer is **D.**

5. Atropine will prevent the normal reflex bradycardia, since that requires integrity of the vagal pathway. The direct action of norepinephrine on the sinus node will be unmasked. The answer is **C.**

6. In considering questions that may involve reflex homeostatic responses, it helps to recall the pathway and receptors involved in the baroceptor reflex. In the case of isoproterenol-induced tachycardia, a reflex is evoked by the decrease in blood pressure. This reflex will be processed by the vasomotor center and result in increased SANS outflow to the sinus node to increase heart rate. This reflex would be blocked by a ganglion blocker such as hexamethonium. However, isoproterenol *also* causes tachycardia directly by activating the β receptors in the sinus node, an effect not blocked by ganglion blockers. Only a β–blocker (propranolol) will prevent both the reflex and indirectly induced isoproterenol tachycardia. The answer is **E.**

7. Beta agonists increase cardiac rate and force and increase myocardial oxygen demand; they are generally contraindicated in angina. In chronic heart failure, the heart is already subject to excessive sympathetic drive. The absence of β_2 receptors in the cutaneous vascular bed makes β agonists useless in conditions involving reduced skin blood flow. Uterine and bronchiolar smooth muscle are relaxed by β_2 agonists. The answer is **B.**

8. Tremor is a common β_2 effect. Blood vessels in the skin have almost exclusively α (vasoconstrictor) receptors. Stimulation of renin release is a β_1 effect. Beta$_2$ agonists cause *hyper*glycemia. The answer is **D.**

9. Epinephrine increases plasma free fatty acids by activating lipolysis of triglycerides in fat cells. The answer is **E.**

10. Vasoconstriction in the nasal mucosa is the basis for the widespread use of α agonists as topical decongestants. The answer is **A.**

11. The drug X dose caused a decrease in diastolic blood pressure and little change in systolic pressure. Thus, there was a large increase in pulse pressure. The decrease in diastolic pressure suggests that the drug decreased vascular resistance, ie, it must have significant muscarinic or β agonist effects. The fact that it also markedly increased pulse pressure suggests that it strongly increased stroke volume, also a β-agonist effect. The drug with these beta effects is isoproterenol (Figure 9–1). The answer is **D.**

12. Drug Y caused a marked increase in diastolic pressure, suggesting strong alpha vasoconstrictor effects. It also caused a small increase in pulse pressure, suggesting some β-agonist action. The drug that best matches this description in norepinephrine. The answer is **E.**

SKILL KEEPER ANSWER: BLOOD PRESSURE CONTROL MECHANISMS IN PHEOCHROMOCYTOMA (SEE CHAPTER 6)

Because the control mechanisms that attempt to maintain blood pressure constant are intact in patients with pheochromocytoma (they are reset in patients with ordinary hypertension), a number of compensatory changes are observed in pheochromocytoma patients (see Figure 6–4). These include reduced renin, angiotensin, and aldosterone levels in the blood. With the reduced aldosterone effect on the kidney, more salt and water is excreted, reducing blood volume. Since the red cell mass is not affected, hematocrit is often increased. If the tumor releases only norepinephrine, a compensatory bradycardia may also be present, but most patients release enough epinephrine to maintain heart rate at a normal or even increased level.

13. The investigational agent caused a marked increase in diastolic pressure but little increase in pulse pressure (from 40 mm Hg to 48 mm Hg). These changes suggest a strong alpha effect on vessels but little β–agonist action in the heart. The heart rate decreased markedly, reflecting a baroreceptor reflex compensatory response. Note that the stroke volume increased slightly (cardiac output divided by heart rate; from 75.8 mL to 86.6 mL). This is to be expected even in the absence of beta effects if bradycardia causes increased diastolic filling time. The drug behaves most like a pure α agonist. The answer is **D.**

CHECKLIST

When you complete this chapter, you should be able to:

☐ List tissues that contain significant numbers of α_1 or α_2 receptors.

☐ List tissues that contain significant numbers of β_1 or β_2 receptors.

☐ Describe the major organ system effects of a pure α agonist, a pure β agonist, and a mixed α and β agonist. Give examples of each type of drug.

☐ Describe a clinical situation in which the effects of an indirect sympathomimetic would differ from those of a direct agonist.

☐ List the major clinical applications of the adrenoceptor agonists.

Adrenoceptor Blockers

10

Alpha and β adrenoceptor-blocking agents are divided into primary subgroups on the basis of their receptor selectivity. All of these agents are pharmacologic antagonists. Because α- and β-blockers differ markedly in their effects and clinical applications, these drugs are considered separately in the following discussion.

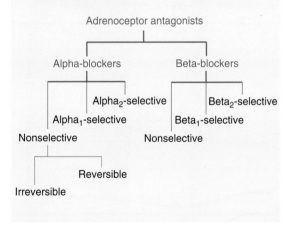

ALPHA-BLOCKING DRUGS

A. CLASSIFICATION

Subdivisions of the α-blockers are based on selective affinity for α_1 versus α_2 receptors or a lack thereof. Other features used to classify the α-blocking drugs are their reversibility and duration of action.

1. Alpha$_1$ selective—**Prazosin** is a selective, reversible pharmacologic α_1-blocker. Doxazosin, terazosin, and tamsulosin are similar drugs. The advantage of α_1 selectivity is discussed below.

2. Alpha$_2$ selective—**Yohimbine** and **rauwolscine** are α_2-selective competitive pharmacologic antagonists. They are used primarily in research applications.

3. Irreversible, long acting—**Phenoxybenzamine** is the prototypical long-acting, irreversible α-blocker. It is slightly α_1 selective.

4. Reversible, shorter acting—**Phentolamine** is a competitive, reversible blocking agent that does not distinguish between α_1 and α_2 receptors.

B. PHARMACOKINETICS

These drugs are all active by the oral as well as the parenteral route, though phentolamine is rarely given orally. Phenoxybenzamine has a short elimination half-life but a long duration of action—about 48 h—because it binds covalently to its receptor. Phentolamine has a duration of action of 2–4 h when used orally and 20–40 min when given parenterally. Prazosin and the other α_1-selective blockers act for 8–24 h.

C. MECHANISM OF ACTION

Phenoxybenzamine binds covalently to the α receptor, thereby producing an irreversible (insurmountable) blockade. The other agents are competitive pharmacologic antagonists—ie, their effects can be surmounted by increased concentrations of agonist. This difference may be important in the treatment of pheochromocytoma because a massive release of catecholamines from the tumor may overcome a reversible blockade.

D. EFFECTS

1. Nonselective blockers—These agents cause a predictable blockade of α-mediated responses to sympathetic nervous system discharge and exogenous sympathomimetics (ie, the α responses listed in Table 9–1). The most important effects of nonselective α-blockers are those on the cardiovascular system: a reduction in vascular tone with a reduction of both arterial and venous pressures. There are no significant direct cardiac effects. However, the nonselective α-blockers do cause baroreceptor reflex-mediated tachycardia as a result of the drop in mean arterial pressure (Figure 6–4). This tachycardia may be exaggerated because the α_2 receptors on adrenergic nerve terminals in the heart, which normally reduce the net release of norepinephrine, are also blocked (Figure 6–3).

HIGH-YIELD TERMS TO LEARN

Competitive blocker	A surmountable antagonist; one (eg, phentolamine) that can be overcome by increasing the dose of agonist
Epinephrine reversal	Conversion of the pressor response to epinephrine (typical of large doses) to a blood pressure-lowering effect; caused by α-blockers
Intrinsic sympathomimetic activity (ISA)	Partial agonist action by adrenoceptor blockers; typical of several β-blockers (eg, pindolol, acebutolol)
Irreversible blocker	A nonsurmountable inhibitor, usually because of covalent bond formation (eg, phenoxybenzamine)
Membrane stabilizing activity (MSA)	Local anesthetic action; typical of several β-blockers (eg, propranolol)
Orthostatic hypotension	Hypotension that is most marked in the upright position; caused by venous pooling or inadequate blood volume; typical of α-blockade
Partial agonist	A drug (eg, pindolol) that produces a smaller maximal effect than a full agonist and therefore can inhibit the effect of a full agonist
Pheochromocytoma	A tumor that resembles the adrenal medulla; consisting of cells that release varying amounts of norepinephrine and epinephrine into the circulation

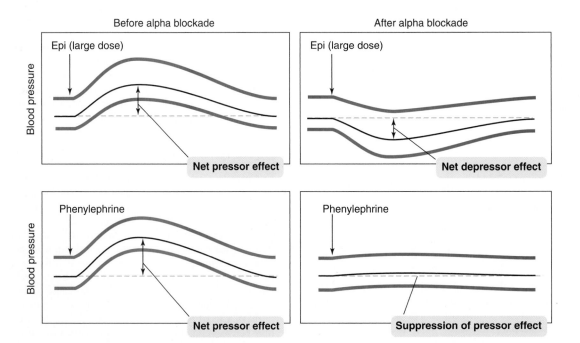

Figure 10–1. The effects of an α-blocker, eg, phentolamine, on the blood pressure responses to epinephrine and phenylephrine. The epinephrine response exhibits reversal of the mean blood pressure change from a net increase (the α response) to a net decrease (the β₂ response). The response to phenylephrine is suppressed but not reversed, because phenylephrine is a "pure" α agonist without β action.

Epinephrine reversal is a predictable result of the use of this agonist in a patient who has received an α-blocker. The term refers to a reversal in the blood pressure effect of large doses of epinephrine, from a pressor response (mediated by α receptors) to a depressor response (mediated by β_2-receptors) (Figure 10–1). The effect is not observed with phenylephrine or norepinephrine because these drugs lack sufficient β_2 effects. Epinephrine reversal is occasionally seen as an unexpected (but predictable) effect of drugs for which α blockade is an adverse effect (eg, some phenothiazine tranquilizers, antihistamines).

2. Selective α-blockers—Because prazosin and its analogs block vascular α_1 receptors much more effectively than the α_2-modulatory receptors associated with cardiac sympathetic nerve endings, these drugs cause much less reflex tachycardia than the nonselective α-blockers when reducing blood pressure.

E. Clinical Uses

1. Nonselective α-blockers—Nonselective α-blockers have limited clinical applications. The best-documented application is in the presurgical management of pheochromocytoma. Such patients may have severe hypertension and reduced blood volume, which should be corrected before subjecting the patient to the stress of surgery. Phenoxybenzamine is usually used during this preparatory phase; phentolamine is sometimes used during surgery. Phenoxybenzamine also has serotonin receptor-blocking effects, which justify its occasional use in carcinoid tumor; and H_1 antihistamine effects, which lead to its use in mastocytosis.

Accidental local infiltration of potent α agonists such as norepinephrine may lead to tissue ischemia and necrosis if not promptly reversed; infiltration of the ischemic area with phentolamine is sometimes used to prevent tissue damage. Overdose with drugs of abuse such as amphetamine, cocaine, or phenylpropanolamine may lead to severe hypertension because of their indirect sympathomimetic actions. This hypertension will usually respond well to α-blockers. Sudden cessation of clonidine therapy leads to rebound hypertension (Chapter 11); this phenomenon is often treated with phentolamine.

Raynaud's phenomenon sometimes responds to α-blockers, but their efficacy is not well documented in this condition. Phentolamine or yohimbine has been used by direct injection to cause penile erection in men with erectile dysfunction.

2. Selective α-blockers—Prazosin, doxazosin, and terazosin are used in hypertension (see Chapter 11). These α_1-blockers and tamsulosin are also extensively used in the management of urinary hesitancy and prevention of urinary retention in men with benign prostatic hyperplasia.

F. Toxicity

The most important toxicities of the α-blockers are simple extensions of their α-blocking effects. The main manifestations are orthostatic hypotension and, in the case of the nonselective agents, marked reflex tachycardia. Tachycardia is less common and less severe with α_1-selective blockers. Phentolamine also has some non-alpha-mediated vasodilating effects. In patients with coronary disease, angina may be precipitated by the tachycardia. Oral administration of some of these drugs can cause nausea and vomiting. The α_1-selective agents are associated with an exaggerated orthostatic hypotensive response to the first dose in some patients. Therefore, the first dose is usually small and taken just before going to bed.

BETA-BLOCKING DRUGS

A. Classification, Subgroups, and Mechanisms

All of the clinically used β-blockers are competitive pharmacologic antagonists. **Propranolol** is the prototype. Drugs in this group are usually classified into subgroups on the basis of β_1 selectivity, partial agonist activity, local anesthetic action, and lipid solubility (Table 10–1).

1. Receptor selectivity—Beta$_1$ receptor selectivity (β_1 block > β_2 block) is a property of **acebutolol, atenolol, esmolol, metoprolol,** and several other β-blockers. This property may be an advantage when treating patients with asthma. Nadolol, propranolol, and timolol are typical nonselective β-blockers.

Labetalol and **carvedilol** have combined α- and β-blocking actions. These drugs are optically active, and different isomers have α- or β-blocking action.

2. Partial agonist activity—Partial agonist activity ("intrinsic sympathomimetic activity") may be an advantage in treating patients with asthma because these drugs (eg, **pindolol, acebutolol**)—at least in theory—are less likely to cause bronchospasm. In contrast, the full antagonists such as propranolol often cause severe bronchospasm in patients with airway disease.

SKILL KEEPER: PARTIAL AGONIST ACTION (SEE CHAPTER 2)

Draw a concentration-response graph showing the effect of increasing concentrations of albuterol on airway diameter (as a percentage of maximum) in the presence of a large concentration of pindolol. On the same graph, draw the curves for the percentage of receptors bound to albuterol and to pindolol at each concentration. The Skill Keeper Answer appears at the end of the chapter.

Table 10–1. Properties of several β-adrenoceptor blocking drugs.

Drug	Selectivity	Partial Agonist Activity	Local Anesthetic Activity	Lipid Solubility	Elimination Half-Life
Acebutolol	β$_1$	Yes	Yes	Low	3–4 h
Atenolol	β$_1$	No	No	Low	6–9 h
Carvedilol[a]	None	No	No	Moderate	7–10 h
Esmolol	β$_1$	No	No	Low	10 min
Labetalol[a]	None	Yes[b]	Yes	Low	5 h
Metoprolol	β$_1$	No	Yes	Moderate	3–4 h
Nadolol	None	No	No	Low	14–24 h
Pindolol	None	Yes	Yes	Moderate	3–4 h
Propranolol	None	No	Yes	High	3.5–6 h
Timolol	None	No	No	Moderate	4–5 h

[a]Also causes α receptor blockade.
[b]Partial agonist effect at β$_2$ receptors
Modified, with permission, from Katzung BG, editor: *Basic & Clinical Pharmacology*, 10th ed., McGraw-Hill, 2007.

3. Local anesthetic activity—Local anesthetic activity ("membrane stabilizing activity") is a disadvantage when β-blockers are used topically in the eye because it decreases protective reflexes and increases the risk of corneal ulceration. Local anesthetic effects are absent from **timolol** and several other β-blockers.

4. Pharmacokinetics—Most of the systemic agents have been developed for chronic oral use, but bioavailability

Table 10–2. Clinical applications of β-blockers.

Application	Drugs	Effect
Hypertension	Atenolol, propranolol, metoprolol, timolol, others	Reduced cardiac output, reduced renin secretion, other
Angina pectoris	Propranolol, others	Reduced cardiac rate and force
Arrhythmia prophylaxis after myocardial infarction	Propranolol, metoprolol, timolol	Reduced automaticity of all cardiac pacemakers
Supraventricular tachycardia	Propranolol, esmolol, acebutolol	Slowed or blocked AV conduction velocity; blocked reentry
Heart failure	Carvedilol, labetalol, metoprolol	Decreased mortality, mechanism poorly understood
Hypertrophic cardiomyopathy	Propranolol	Slowed rate of cardiac contraction
Migraine prophylaxis	Propranolol	Mechanism not understood
Familial tremor, other types of tremor, "stage fright"	Propranolol	Reduced β$_2$ alteration of neuromuscular transmission; possible CNS effects
Thyroid storm, thyrotoxicosis	Propranolol, esmolol	Reduced cardiac rate and arrhythmogenesis; reduced conversion of T$_4$ to T$_3$
Glaucoma[a]	Timolol, others (topical)	Reduced secretion of aqueous humor

[a]See Table 10–3 for other drugs used in glaucoma.

Table 10–3. Drugs used in glaucoma.

Group, Drugs	Mechanism	Methods of Administration
Beta-blockers Timolol, others	Decreased secretion of aqueous humor from the ciliary epithelium	Topical drops
Prostaglandins Latanoprost, others	Increased aqueous outflow	Topical drops
Cholinomimetics Pilocarpine, physostigmine	Ciliary muscle contraction, opening of trabecular meshwork, increased outflow	Topical drops or gel, plastic film slow-release insert
Alpha agonists Nonselective: epinephrine	Increased outflow via uveoscleral veins	Topical drops (obsolete)
Alpha$_2$ selective agonists Apraclonidine, brimonidine	Decreased aqueous secretion	Topical drops
Diuretics Acetazolamide, dorzolamide	Decreased aqueous secretion due to lack of HCO_3^-	Oral (acetazolamide) or topical (others)

Modified and reproduced, with permission, from Katzung BG, editor: *Basic & Clinical Pharmacology*, 10th ed. McGraw-Hill, 2007.

and duration of action vary widely (Table 10–1). Esmolol is a short-acting ester β-blocker that is only used parenterally. Nadolol is the longest acting β-blocker. Acebutolol, atenolol, and nadolol are less lipid soluble than other β-blockers and probably enter the CNS to a lesser extent.

B. EFFECTS AND CLINICAL USES

Most of the organ-level effects of β-blockers are predictable from blockade of the β receptor-mediated effects of sympathetic discharge. The clinical applications of β blockade are remarkably broad (Table 10–2). The treatment of open-angle glaucoma involves the use of several groups of autonomic drugs as well as other agents (Table 10–3). The cardiovascular applications of β-blockers—especially in hypertension, angina, and arrhythmias—are extremely important. Treatment of chronic (not acute) heart failure has become an important application of β-blockers. Several large clinical trials have shown that that some, but not all, β-blockers can reduce morbidity and mortality when used properly (Chapter 13). Labetalol, carvedilol, and metoprolol appear to be beneficial in this application. Pheochromocytoma is sometimes treated with combined α- and β-blocking agents (eg, labetalol), especially if the tumor is producing large amounts of epinephrine as well as norepinephrine.

KEY DRUGS

Subgroup	Prototype	Other Significant Agents

Alpha-blockers
  Nonselective
  Alpha$_1$ selective
  Alpha$_2$ selective
	
	Phentolamine
	Prazosin
	Yohimbine
		
		Phenoxybenzamine[a]
		Terazosin, doxazosin

Beta-blockers
  Nonselective
 	
  Beta$_1$ selective
	
	Propranolol
	
	Metoprolol
		
		Carvedilol, labetalol, nadolol, timolol
		Atenolol, esmolol

[a]Compared with prazosin, phenoxybenzamine is only slightly α_1 selective.

C. TOXICITY

Cardiovascular adverse effects, which are extensions of the β blockade induced by these agents, include bradycardia, atrioventricular blockade, and heart failure. Patients with airway disease may suffer severe asthma attacks. Beta-blockers have been shown experimentally to reduce insulin secretion but this does not appear to be a clinically important effect. However, pre-monitory symptoms of hypoglycemia from insulin overdosage, eg, tachycardia, tremor, and anxiety, may be masked by β-blockers, and mobilization of glucose from the liver may be impaired. CNS adverse effects include sedation, fatigue, and sleep alterations. Atenolol, nadolol, and several other less lipid-soluble β-blockers are claimed to have less marked CNS action because they do not enter the CNS as readily as other members of this group.

QUESTIONS

1. Which of the following effects of epinephrine would be blocked by phentolamine but not by metoprolol?
    (A) Cardiac stimulation
    (B) Contraction of radial smooth muscle in the iris
    (C) Increase of cAMP in fat
    (D) Relaxation of bronchial smooth muscle
    (E) Relaxation of the uterus

2. Both phentolamine and phenoxybenzamine
    (A) Are inactive by the oral route
    (B) Block both α and β receptors
    (C) Cause hypertension
    (D) Cause tachycardia
    (E) Induce vasospasm in large doses

3. Propranolol is *not* useful in the treatment of which one of the following?
    (A) Angina
    (B) Familial tremor
    (C) Hypertension
    (D) Idiopathic hypertrophic subaortic cardiomyopathy
    (E) Partial atrioventricular heart block

4. Adverse effects that limit the use of adrenoceptor blockers include
    (A) Bronchoconstriction from α-blocking agents
    (B) Heart failure exacerbation from β-blockers
    (C) Impaired blood sugar response with α-blockers
    (D) Increased intraocular pressure with β-blockers
    (E) Sleep disturbances from α-blocking drugs

5–8. Four new synthetic drugs (designated W, X, Y, and Z) are to be studied for their cardiovascular effects. They are given to four anesthetized rats while the heart rate is recorded. The first animal has received no pretreatment ("control"); the second

has received an effective dose of hexamethonium; the third has received an effective dose of atropine; and the fourth has received an effective dose of phenoxybenzamine. The net changes induced by the new drugs (not by the blocking drugs) are described in the following questions.

5. Drug W increased heart rate in the control animal, the atropine-pretreated animal, and the phenoxybenzamine-pretreated animal. However, Drug W had no effect on heart rate in the hexamethonium-pretreated animal. Drug W is probably a drug similar to
    (A) Acetylcholine
    (B) Edrophonium
    (C) Isoproterenol
    (D) Nitric oxide
    (E) Norepinephrine

6. Drug X had the effects shown in the table below.

In the Rat Receiving	Heart Rate Response to Drug X Was
No pretreatment	↓
Hexamethonium	↑
Atropine	↑
Phenoxybenzamine	↑

Drug X is probably a drug similar to
    (A) Acetylcholine
    (B) Edrophonium
    (C) Isoproterenol
    (D) Nitric oxide
    (E) Norepinephrine

7. Drug Y had the effects shown in the table below.

In the Rat Receiving	Heart Rate Response to Drug Y Was
No pretreatment	↑
Hexamethonium	↑
Atropine	↑
Phenoxybenzamine	↑

Drug Y is probably a drug similar to
    (A) Acetylcholine
    (B) Edrophonium
    (C) Isoproterenol
    (D) Nitric oxide
    (E) Norepinephrine

8. The results of the test of Drug Z are shown in the graph.

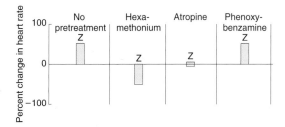

Drug Z is probably a drug similar to
(A) Acetylcholine
(B) Edrophonium
(C) Isoproterenol
(D) Nitric oxide
(E) Norepinephrine

9. A traveler to your city visits you with a request for a renewal of his prescription for phenoxybenzamine. While preparing to telephone his physician, you recall that phenoxybenzamine is relatively *contraindicated* in which of the following?
(A) Carcinoid
(B) Essential hypertension
(C) Mastocytosis
(D) Pheochromocytoma
(E) Raynaud's phenomenon

10. When given to a patient, phentolamine blocks which one of the following?
(A) Bradycardia induced by phenylephrine
(B) Bronchodilation induced by epinephrine
(C) Increased cardiac contractile force induced by norepinephrine
(D) Miosis induced by acetylcholine
(E) Vasodilation induced by isoproterenol

11. Pretreatment with propranolol will block which one of the following?
(A) Methacholine-induced tachycardia
(B) Nicotine-induced hypertension
(C) Norepinephrine-induced bradycardia
(D) Phenylephrine-induced mydriasis
(E) Pilocarpine-induced miosis

12. Your 75-year-old patient with angina and glaucoma is to receive a β-blocking drug. Regarding β-blocking drugs
(A) Esmolol's pharmacokinetics are compatible with chronic topical use
(B) Metoprolol blocks β_2 receptors selectively
(C) Nadolol lacks β_2-blocking action
(D) Pindolol is a β antagonist with high membrane-stabilizing (local anesthetic) activity
(E) Timolol lacks the local anesthetic effects of propranolol

13. Which of the following binds covalently to the site specified?
(A) Atenolol—β receptor
(B) Carvedilol—cardiac β receptors
(C) Labetalol—α and β receptors
(D) Phenoxybenzamine—α receptor
(E) Pindolol—β receptor

14. A new drug was administered to an anesthetized animal with the results shown. A large dose of epinephrine was administered before and after the new agent for comparison. Which of the following agents does the new drug most closely resemble?
(A) Atenolol
(B) Atropine
(C) Labetalol
(D) Phenoxybenzamine
(E) Propranolol

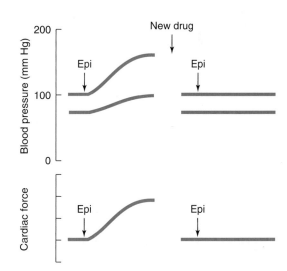

ANSWERS

1. Contraction of the pupillary dilator radial smooth muscle is mediated by α receptors. All the other effects are mediated by β receptors. The answer is **B.**

2. These α-blockers cause hypotension and significant reflex tachycardia. They have no β-blocking action and never cause vasospasm. The answer is **D.**

3. Atrioventricular block is an important contraindication to the use of β-blockers. The answer is **E.**

4. Although *chronic* heart failure is often treated with β–blockers, acute heart failure can be precipitated by these drugs. Choices **A, C,** and **E** reverse the correct pairing of receptor subtype (α versus β) with effect. Choice **D** reverses the direction of change of intraocular pressure. The answer is **B.**

5. In developing a strategy for this type of question, consider first the actions of the known blocking drugs. Hexamethonium blocks reflexes as well as the direct action of nicotine. Atropine would block direct muscarinic effects of an unknown drug (if it had any) or reflex slowing of the heart mediated by the vagus. Phenoxybenzamine blocks only α-receptor-mediated processes. If the response produced in the nonpretreated animal is blocked or reversed by hexamethonium, it is probably a reflex response. In that case, consider all the receptors involved in mediating the reflex. Drug W causes tachycardia that is prevented by ganglion blockade and therefore is probably a compensatory reflex tachycardia. We do not have information about β blockade, but a reflex tachycardia must be mediated by β receptors in the heart. Two of the choices may cause reflex tachycardia: acetylcholine and nitric oxide. However, the reflex tachycardia evoked by acetylcholine would be blocked by atropine (atropine would prevent the vasodilation that elicited the tachycardia). Thus, drug W must be nitric oxide. The answer is **D**.

6. Drug X causes slowing of the heart rate, but this is converted into tachycardia by hexamethonium and atropine—ie, the bradycardia is caused by reflex vagal discharge. Phenoxybenzamine also reverses the bradycardia to tachycardia, suggesting that α receptors are needed to induce the reflex bradycardia and that X has direct β agonist actions. The choices that evoke a vagal reflex bradycardia but can also cause direct tachycardia are limited; the answer is **E**.

7. Drug Y causes tachycardia that is not significantly influenced by any of the blockers; therefore, drug Y must have a direct β agonist effect on the heart. The answer is **C**.

8. Drug Z causes tachycardia that is converted to bradycardia by hexamethonium and blocked completely by atropine. This indicates that the tachycardia is a reflex evoked by vasodilation. Drug Z causes bradycardia when the ganglia are blocked, indicating that it also has a direct muscarinic action on the heart. This is confirmed by the ability of atropine to block both the tachycardia and the bradycardia. The answer is **A**.

9. Phenoxybenzamine is not useful in essential hypertension because it causes severe tachycardia and marked orthostatic hypotension. The drug is used in Raynaud's phenomenon, although efficacy in this application is controversial. The answer is **B**.

10. Phenylephrine induces bradycardia through the baroreceptor reflex. Blockade of this drug's alpha-mediated vasoconstrictor effect will prevent the bradycardia. The answer is **A**.

11. The β-blocker will not block the vagal slowing induced by norepinephrine hypertension. Nicotine-induced hypertension and phenylephrine-induced mydriasis are mediated by α receptors. Pilocarpine is a muscarinic agonist. The answer is **A**.

12. Esmolol is a short-acting β-blocker for parenteral use only. Nadolol is a nonselective β-blocker, and metoprolol is a β_1-selective blocker. Timolol is useful in glaucoma because it does not anesthetize the cornea. The answer is **E**.

13. Phenoxybenzamine is the only autonomic receptor blocker in clinical use that binds covalently with its receptor. The answer is **D**.

14. The new drug blocks both the α-mediated effects (increased diastolic and mean arterial blood pressure) and β-mediated action (increased cardiac force). In addition, it does not cause epinephrine reversal. The drug must have *both α- and β-blocking effects.* The answer is **C**.

SKILL KEEPER ANSWER: PARTIAL AGONIST ACTION (SEE CHAPTER 2)

Because pindolol is a partial agonist at β receptors, the concentration-response curve will show a bronchodilating effect at zero albuterol concentration. As albuterol concentration increases, the airway diameter will also increase. The binding curves will show pindolol binding starting at 100% of receptors and going to zero as albuterol concentration increases, with albuterol binding starting at zero and going to 100%.

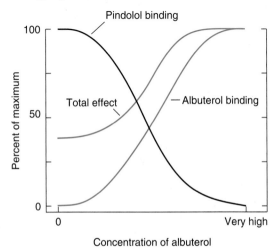

CHECKLIST

When you complete this chapter, you should be able to:

☐ Describe and compare the effects of an α-blocker on the hemodynamic responses to epinephrine, norepinephrine, and phenylephrine.

☐ Compare the effects of propranolol, labetalol, metoprolol, and pindolol.

☐ Compare the pharmacokinetics of propranolol, atenolol, esmolol, and nadolol.

☐ Describe the clinical indications and toxicities of typical α- and β-blockers.

PART III

Cardiovascular Drugs

Drugs Used in Hypertension

Antihypertensive drugs are organized around a clinical indication—the need to treat a disease—rather than a receptor type. The drugs covered in this unit have a variety of mechanisms of action, including diuresis, sympathoplegia, vasodilation, and antagonism of angiotensin.

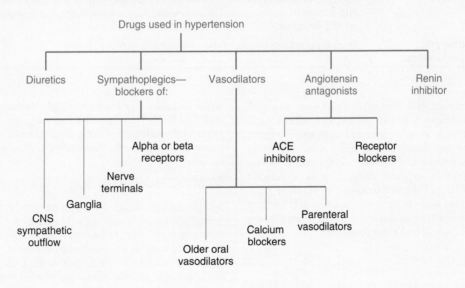

Fewer than 20% of cases of hypertension are due to ("secondary" to) factors that can be clearly defined and corrected. This type of hypertension is associated with pheochromocytoma, coarctation of the aorta, renal

vascular disease, adrenal cortical tumors, and a few other rare conditions. Most cases of hypertension are idiopathic or "primary." The strategies for treating idiopathic high blood pressure are based on the determinants of

HIGH-YIELD TERMS TO LEARN	
Baroreceptor reflex	Primary autonomic mechanism for blood pressure homeostasis; involves sensory input from carotid sinus and aorta to the vasomotor center and output via the parasympathetic and sympathetic motor nerves
Catecholamine reuptake pump	Nerve terminal transporter responsible for recycling catecholamine transmitters after release into the synapse
Catecholamine vesicle pump	Storage vesicle transporter that pumps amine from cytoplasm into vesicle
End-organ damage	Vascular damage in heart, kidney, retina, or brain
Essential hypertension	Hypertension of unknown etiology; also called "primary" hypertension
False transmitter	Substance stored in vesicles and released into synaptic cleft but lacking the effect of the true transmitter
Malignant hypertension	Accelerated hypertension causing rapid damage to vessels in end organs; a medical emergency
Orthostatic hypotension	Hypotension on assuming upright posture; postural hypotension
Postganglionic neuron blocker	Drug that blocks transmission by an action in the postganglionic nerve terminal
Rebound hypertension	Elevated blood pressure (usually above pretreatment levels) resulting from loss of antihypertensive drug effect
Reflex tachycardia	Tachycardia resulting from lowering of blood pressure; mediated by the baroreceptor reflex
Stepped care	Progressive addition of drugs to a regimen, starting with one (usually a diuretic) and adding in stepwise fashion a sympatholytic, a vasodilator, and (sometimes) an ACE inhibitor
Sympatholytic, sympathoplegic	Drug that reduces effects of the sympathetic nervous system

arterial pressure (see Figure 6–4). These strategies include reductions of blood volume, sympathetic tone, vascular smooth muscle tone, and angiotensin effects. Because of the baroreceptor reflex and the renin response to lower blood pressure, compensatory homeostatic responses to these drugs may be significant (Table 11–1). As indicated in Figure 11–1, some compensatory responses can be counteracted with β-blockers or reserpine (for tachycardia) and diuretics or angiotensin antagonists (for salt and water retention).

DIURETICS

Diuretics are covered in greater detail in Chapter 15 but are mentioned here because of their importance in hypertension. These drugs lower blood pressure by reduction of blood volume and probably also by a direct vascular effect that is not fully understood. The diuretics most important for treating hypertension are the **thiazides** (eg, hydrochlorothiazide) and the **loop diuretics** (eg, furosemide). Thiazides may be adequate in mild hypertension, but the loop agents are often used in moderate, severe, and malignant hypertension. Compensatory responses to blood pressure lowering by diuretics are minimal (Table 11–1). When thiazides are given, the maximum antihypertensive effect is often achieved with doses below those required for the maximum diuretic effect.

SYMPATHOPLEGICS

Sympathoplegic drugs can interfere with sympathetic nerve function in several ways. The result is a reduction of one or more of the following: venous tone, heart rate, contractile force of the heart, cardiac output, and total peripheral resistance (see Figure 6–4). Compensatory responses and adverse effects are marked for some of these agents (Table 11–1). Sympathoplegics are subdivided by anatomic site of action (Figure 11–2).

A. BARORECEPTOR-SENSITIZING AGENTS

No currently available drugs act at this site.

B. CNS-ACTIVE AGENTS

Alpha$_2$-selective agonists (eg, **clonidine, methyldopa**) cause a decrease in sympathetic outflow by activation of α_2 receptors in the CNS. These drugs readily enter the

Table 11–1. Compensatory responses to antihypertensive drugs and some of their adverse effects.

Class and Drug	Compensatory Responses	Adverse Effects
Diuretics		
Hydrochlorothiazide	Minimal	Hypokalemia, slight hyperlipidemia, hyperuricemia, hyperglycemia, lassitude, weakness, impotence
Furosemide	Minimal	Hypokalemia, hypovolemia, ototoxicity
Sympathoplegics		
Clonidine	Salt and water retention	Dry mouth, severe rebound hypertension if drug is suddenly stopped
Methyldopa	Salt and water retention	Sedation, positive Coombs test, hemolytic anemia (rare)
Ganglion blockers (obsolete)	Salt and water retention	Severe orthostatic hypotension, constipation, blurred vision, sexual dysfunction
Reserpine (low dose)	Minimal	Diarrhea, nasal stuffiness, sedation, depression
Alpha₁-selective blockers	Salt and water retention, slight tachycardia	Orthostatic hypotension (usually limited to first few doses)
Beta-blockers	Minimal	Sleep disturbances, sedation, impotence, cardiac disturbances, asthma
Vasodilators		
Hydralazine	Salt and water retention, marked tachycardia	Reversible lupus-like syndrome (but lacking renal effects)
Minoxidil	Marked salt and water retention, marked tachycardia	Hirsutism, pericardial effusion
Nifedipine	Minor salt and water retention	Constipation, cardiac disturbances, flushing
Nitroprusside	Salt and water retention	Cyanide, thiocyanate toxicity
Angiotensin antagonists		
ACE inhibitors	Minimal	Cough, renal damage in the fetus and in preexisting renal disease
Angiotensin receptor blockers	Minimal	Renal damage in the fetus and in preexisting renal disease

CNS when given orally. Methyldopa is a prodrug; it is converted to **methylnorepinephrine** in the brain. Clonidine and methyldopa both reduce blood pressure by reducing cardiac output, vascular resistance, or both. The major compensatory response is salt retention. Sudden discontinuation of clonidine causes rebound hypertension, which may be quite severe. This rebound increase in blood pressure can be controlled by reinstitution of clonidine therapy or administration of α-blockers such as phentolamine. Methyldopa occasionally causes hematologic immunotoxicity, detected initially by test tube agglutination of red blood cells (positive Coombs test) and in some patients progressing to hemolytic anemia. Both drugs may cause sedation—methyldopa more so.

C. GANGLION-BLOCKING DRUGS

Nicotinic blockers that act in the ganglia are very efficacious but because their adverse effects (Table 11–1) are severe, they are now considered obsolete. **Hexamethonium** and **trimethaphan** are extremely powerful blood pressure-lowering drugs. The major compensatory response is salt retention. Toxicities reflect parasympathetic blockade (blurred vision, constipation, urinary hesitancy, sexual dysfunction) and sympathetic blockade (sexual dysfunction, orthostatic hypotension).

D. POSTGANGLIONIC SYMPATHETIC NERVE TERMINAL BLOCKERS

Drugs that deplete the adrenergic nerve terminal of its norepinephrine stores (eg, **reserpine**) or that deplete and block release of the stores (eg, **guanethidine**) can lower blood pressure. The major compensatory response is salt and water retention. In high dosages, both reserpine and guanethidine are very efficacious but produce severe adverse effects. Reserpine is still occasionally used in low doses as an adjunct to other agents. Guanethidine is rarely

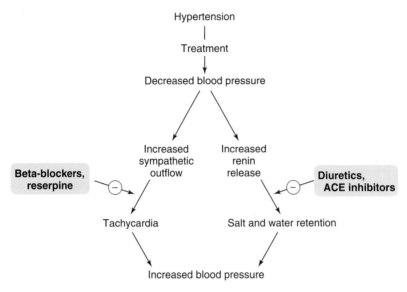

Figure 11–1. Compensatory responses to decreased blood pressure when treating hypertension. Arrows with minus signs indicate drugs used to minimize the compensatory responses.

used. Reserpine readily enters the CNS; guanethidine does not. Both have long durations of action (days to weeks). The most serious toxicity of reserpine is behavioral depression, which may require discontinuation of the drug. The major toxicities of guanethidine are orthostatic hypotension and sexual dysfunction. Guanethidine requires the catecholamine reuptake pump (uptake 1; see Figure 6–2) to reach its intracellular site of action. Therefore, drugs that inhibit this pump (eg, cocaine, tricyclic antidepressants) will interfere with the action of guanethidine.

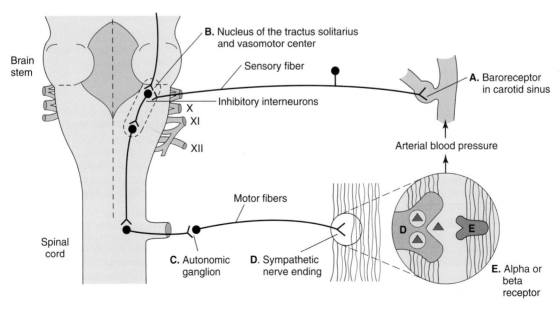

Figure 11–2. Baroreceptor reflex arc and sites of action of sympathoplegic drugs. The letters (A–E) indicate potential sites of action of subgroups of sympathoplegics.

MAO inhibitors were once used in hypertension because they cause the formation of a false transmitter (octopamine) in sympathetic postganglionic neuron terminals and lower blood pressure. Octopamine is stored in the adrenergic vesicles along with reduced amounts (per vesicle) of norepinephrine. Normal nerve action potentials release this weak false transmitter with norepinephrine, resulting in diminished vascular and cardiac responses. However, large doses of indirect-acting sympathomimetics (eg, the tyramine in a meal of fermented foods) may cause release of large amounts of stored norepinephrine and result in a hypertensive crisis. Because of this risk and the availability of better drugs, MAO inhibitors are no longer used in hypertension. However, they are still occasionally used for treatment of severe depressive disorder (Chapter 30).

E. ADRENOCEPTOR BLOCKERS

Alpha$_1$-selective agents (eg, **prazosin**) and β-blockers (eg, **propranolol**) are popular antihypertensive drugs. Alpha-blockers reduce vascular resistance and venous return. The nonselective α-blockers (phentolamine, phenoxybenzamine) are of no value in chronic hypertension because of excessive compensatory responses, especially tachycardia. Alpha$_1$-selective adrenoceptor blockers are relatively free of the severe adverse effects of the nonselective α-blockers and postganglionic nerve terminal sympathoplegic agents.

Beta-blockers initially reduce cardiac output, but after a few days their action may include a decrease in vascular resistance as a contributing effect. The latter effect may result from reduced angiotensin levels (β-blockers reduce renin release from the kidney). The β-blockers are among the most heavily used antihypertensive drugs, although there is increasing evidence that not all members of the β-blocker class are equally efficacious. Beta-blocker therapy is associated with slightly elevated glucose, LDL, and triglyceride concentrations and diminished HDL levels in the blood; other potential adverse effects are listed in Table 11–1.

VASODILATORS

Drugs that dilate blood vessels by acting directly on smooth muscle cells through nonautonomic mechanisms are useful in treating some hypertensive patients. Four major mechanisms are utilized by vasodilators: release of nitric oxide, opening of potassium channels (which leads to hyperpolarization), blockade of calcium channels, and activation of D$_1$ dopamine receptors (Table 11–2). Compensatory responses are marked for some vasodilators (especially hydralazine and minoxidil) and include salt retention and tachycardia (Table 11–1).

A. HYDRALAZINE AND MINOXIDIL

These older vasodilators have more effect on arterioles than on veins. They are orally active and suitable for chronic therapy. Hydralazine apparently acts through the release of nitric oxide from endothelial cells. However, it is rarely used at high dosage because of its toxicity; therefore, its efficacy is limited. Its toxicities include compensatory responses (tachycardia, salt and water retention; Table 11–1) and drug-induced lupus erythematosus, which is reversible upon stopping the drug. However, drug-induced lupus is uncommon at dosages below 200 mg/d.

Minoxidil is extremely efficacious and is thus reserved for severe hypertension. Minoxidil is a prodrug; its metabolite, minoxidil sulfate, is a potassium channel opener that hyperpolarizes and relaxes vascular smooth muscle. The toxicity of minoxidil consists of severe compensatory responses (Table 11–1, Figure 11–1), hirsutism, and pericardial abnormalities.

B. CALCIUM CHANNEL-BLOCKING AGENTS

Calcium channel blockers (eg, **nifedipine, verapamil, diltiazem**) are effective vasodilators; because they are orally active, these drugs are suitable for chronic use in hypertension of any severity. Many dihydropyridine analogs of nifedipine are also available. Because they produce fewer compensatory responses, the calcium channel blockers are usually preferred to hydralazine and minoxidil. Their mechanism of action and toxicities are discussed in greater detail in Chapter 12.

C. NITROPRUSSIDE AND DIAZOXIDE

These parenteral vasodilators are used in hypertensive emergencies. Nitroprusside is a short-acting agent

Table 11–2. Mechanisms of action of vasodilators.

Mechanism	Examples
Release of nitric oxide from drug or endothelium	Nitroprusside, hydralazine
Hyperpolarization of vascular smooth muscle through opening of potassium channels	Minoxidil sulfate, diazoxide
Reduction of calcium influx	Verapamil, diltiazem, nifedipine
Activation of dopamine$_1$ receptors	Fenoldopam

(duration of action is a few minutes) that must be infused continuously. The drug's mechanism of action involves the release of nitric oxide (from the drug molecule itself), which stimulates guanylyl cyclase and increases cGMP concentration in smooth muscle. The toxicity of nitroprusside includes excessive hypotension, tachycardia, and, if infusion is continued over several days, accumulation of cyanide or thiocyanate in the blood.

Diazoxide is a thiazide derivative but lacks diuretic properties. It is given as intravenous boluses or as an infusion and has a duration of action of several hours. Diazoxide opens potassium channels, thus hyperpolarizing and relaxing smooth muscle cells. This drug also reduces insulin release and can be used to treat hypoglycemia caused by insulin-producing tumors. The toxicity of diazoxide includes hypotension, hyperglycemia, and salt and water retention.

D. FENOLDOPAM

Dopamine D_1 receptor activation by fenoldopam causes prompt, marked arteriolar vasodilation. This drug is given by intravenous infusion. It has a short duration of action (10 min) and is used for hypertensive emergencies.

ANGIOTENSIN ANTAGONISTS AND A RENIN INHIBITOR

The two primary groups of angiotensin antagonists are the **ACE inhibitors (ACEIs)** and the **angiotensin II receptor blockers (ARBs).** Of these, the more extensively used are the ACE inhibitors (eg, **captopril**), which inhibit the enzyme variously known as angiotensin-converting enzyme, kininase II, and peptidyl dipeptidase. The result is a **reduction** in blood levels of angiotensin II and aldosterone and an **increase** in endogenous vasodilators of the kinin family (bradykinin; Figure 11–3). ACE inhibitors have a low incidence of serious adverse effects when given in normal dosage (except in pregnancy) and produce minimal compensatory responses (Table 11–1). The toxicities of ACE inhibitors include cough (up to 30% of patients), renal damage in occasional patients with preexisting renal vascular disease (although they *protect* the diabetic kidney), and renal damage in the fetus. These drugs are absolutely contraindicated in pregnancy.

The second group of angiotensin antagonists, the receptor blockers, are represented by the orally active agents **losartan** and its several analogs, which competitively inhibit angiotensin II at its AT_1 receptor site. Losartan, valsartan, irbesartan, candesartan, and other analogs appear to be as effective in lowering blood pressure as the ACE inhibitors and have the advantage of a lower incidence of cough. However, they do cause fetal renal toxicity like that of the ACE inhibitors and are thus contraindicated in pregnancy.

The newest drug in the antihypertensive group is **aliskiren**, an inhibitor of renin's action on its substrate, angiotensinogen. It thus reduces the formation of angiotensin I and, in consequence, angiotensin II. Toxicities include headache and diarrhea. It does not appear to cause cough but it is not yet known whether it has the other toxicities of the angiotensin antagonists. Angiotensin antagonists and renin inhibitors reduce aldosterone levels (angiotensin II is a major stimulant of aldosterone release) and cause potassium retention. Potassium accumulation may be

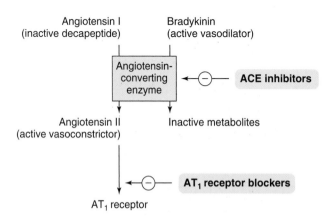

Figure 11–3. Actions of angiotensin-converting enzyme inhibitors and AT_1 receptor blockers. The enzyme is responsible for activating angiotensin by conversion of angiotensin I to angiotensin II and for inactivating bradykinin, a vasodilator normally present in very low concentrations. Block of the enzyme thus decreases the concentration of a vasoconstrictor and increases the concentration of a vasodilator. The AT_1 receptor antagonists lack the effect on bradykinin levels, which may explain the lower incidence of cough observed with these agents.

marked, especially if the patient has renal impairment, is consuming a high-potassium diet, or is taking other drugs that tend to conserve potassium, eg, potassium-sparing diuretics. Under these circumstances, potassium concentrations may reach toxic levels.

SKILL KEEPER: COMPENSATORY RESPONSES TO ANTIHYPERTENSIVE DRUGS (SEE CHAPTER 6)

If hydralazine in moderate dosage is administered for several weeks, compensatory cardiac and renal responses will be observed. Specify the exact mechanisms and structures involved in these responses. The Skill Keeper Answer appears at the end of the chapter.

CLINICAL USES OF ANTIHYPERTENSIVE DRUGS

A. "STEPPED CARE"

Therapy of hypertension is complex because the disease is symptomless until far advanced and because the drugs can be expensive and sometimes cause major compensatory responses and significant toxicities. However, overall toxicity can be reduced and compensatory responses minimized by the use of multiple drugs at lower dosages. This approach is usually used in patients with severe hypertension. Typically, drugs are added to a patient's regimen in stepwise fashion; each additional agent is chosen from a different subgroup until adequate blood pressure control has been achieved. The usual steps include (1) lifestyle measures such as salt restriction and weight reduction, (2) diuretics, (3) sympathoplegics, (4) ACE inhibitors, and (5) vasodilators. The sympathoplegic chosen first is usually a β-blocker or combined β- and α-blocker such as carvedilol. The vasodilator chosen first is usually a calcium channel blocker. The ability of drugs in steps 2 and 3 to control the compensatory responses induced by the others should be noted (eg, propranolol reduces the tachycardia induced by hydralazine). Thus, rational polypharmacy minimizes toxicities while producing additive or supra-additive therapeutic effects.

B. MONOTHERAPY

It has been found in large clinical studies that many patients do well on a single drug (eg, an ACE inhibitor, calcium channel blocker, or combined α- and β-blocker). This approach to the treatment of mild and moderate hypertension has become more popular than stepped care because of its simplicity, better patient compliance, and—with modern drugs—a relatively low incidence of toxicity.

C. AGE AND ETHNICITY

Older patients of most races respond better to diuretics and β-blockers than to ACE inhibitors. African-Americans of all ages respond better to diuretics and calcium channel blockers, less well to ACE inhibitors.

KEY DRUGS

Subgroups	Prototypes	Other Significant Agents
Diuretics	Thiazides, loop diuretics (see Chapter 15)	
Sympathoplegics		
CNS action	Clonidine, methyldopa	
Ganglion blockers	Hexamethonium	Trimethaphan
Postganglionic neuron blockers	Reserpine, guanethidine	
Receptor blockers	Prazosin, propranolol	
Vasodilators	Hydralazine, nifedipine, nitroprusside, fenoldopam	Minoxidil, verapamil, diazoxide
Angiotensin antagonists		
ACE inhibitors	Captopril	Enalapril, fosinopril
Angiotensin receptor blockers	Losartan	Valsartan
Renin inhibitor	Aliskiren	

D. MALIGNANT HYPERTENSION

Malignant hypertension is an accelerated form of severe hypertension associated with rising blood pressure and rapidly progressing damage to vessels and end organs. This condition may be signaled by deterioration of renal function, encephalopathy, and retinal hemorrhages or by angina, stroke, or myocardial infarction. Management of malignant hypertension must be carried out on an emergency basis in the hospital. Powerful vasodilators (nitroprusside, fenoldopam, or diazoxide) are combined with diuretics (furosemide) and β-blockers to lower blood pressure to the 140–160/90–110 mm Hg range promptly (within a few hours). Further reduction is then pursued more slowly.

QUESTIONS

1. A friend has very severe hypertension and asks about a drug her doctor wishes to prescribe. Her physician has explained that this drug is associated with tachycardia and fluid retention (which may be marked) and increased hair growth. Which of the following is most likely to produce the effects that your friend has described?
    (A) Captopril
    (B) Guanethidine
    (C) Minoxidil
    (D) Prazosin
    (E) Propranolol

2. A patient is admitted to the emergency department with severe bradycardia following a drug overdose. His family reports that he has been depressed about his hypertension. Which one of the following drugs does NOT slow the heart rate?
    (A) Clonidine
    (B) Guanethidine
    (C) Hydralazine
    (D) Propranolol
    (E) Reserpine

3. In comparing clonidine and prazosin, which one of the following is correct?
    (A) Prazosin—but not clonidine—results in salt and water retention if used alone
    (B) Prazosin causes fewer CNS adverse effects (such as sedation) than clonidine
    (C) Clonidine causes immunologic adverse effects (eg, hemolytic anemia), whereas prazosin is free of this effect
    (D) Clonidine causes more orthostatic hypotension than prazosin

4. Which one of the following is characteristic of captopril treatment in patients with essential hypertension?

    (A) Competitively blocks angiotensin II at its receptor
    (B) Decreases angiotensin II concentration in the blood
    (C) Decreases renin concentration in the blood
    (D) Increases sodium and decreases potassium in the blood
    (E) Decreases sodium and increases potassium in the urine

5. A pregnant patient is admitted to the hematology service with moderately severe hemolytic anemia. After a thorough workup, the only positive finding is a history of treatment with an antihypertensive drug since 2 months after beginning the pregnancy. The most likely cause of the patient's blood disorder is
    (A) Atenolol
    (B) Captopril
    (C) Hydralazine
    (D) Methyldopa
    (E) Minoxidil

6. Postural hypotension is a common adverse effect of which one of the following types of drugs?
    (A) ACE inhibitors
    (B) Alpha receptor blockers
    (C) Arteriolar dilators
    (D) Beta$_1$-selective receptor blockers
    (E) Nonselective β-blockers

7. A visitor from another city comes to your office complaining of incessant cough. He has diabetes and hypertension and has recently started taking a different antihypertensive medication. The most likely cause of his cough is
    (A) Captopril
    (B) Losartan
    (C) Minoxidil
    (D) Propranolol
    (E) Verapamil

8. Which one of the following is a significant effect of the drug named?
    (A) Cyanide toxicity with hydralazine
    (B) Hyperglycemia with diazoxide
    (C) Lupus erythematosus with nitroprusside
    (D) Pericardial abnormalities with verapamil
    (E) Atrioventricular block with minoxidil

9. Comparison of prazosin with propranolol shows that
    (A) Both decrease cardiac output
    (B) Both decrease renin secretion
    (C) Both increase heart rate
    (D) Both increase sympathetic outflow from the CNS
    (E) Both produce orthostatic hypotension

10. Verapamil is associated with which one of the following?
    (A) Constipation
    (B) Decreased PR interval
    (C) Hypoglycemia
    (D) Tachycardia
    (E) Thyrotoxicosis

11. Which of the following is used in severe hypertensive emergencies; is very short acting; and must be given by intravenous infusion?
    (A) Atenolol
    (B) Captopril
    (C) Diazoxide
    (D) Hydralazine
    (E) Labetalol
    (F) Minoxidil
    (G) Nifedipine
    (H) Nitroprusside
    (I) Prazosin
    (J) Propranolol

12. Which of the following is NOT a prodrug and acts by opening potassium channels?
    (A) Atenolol
    (B) Captopril
    (C) Diazoxide
    (D) Fenoldopam
    (E) Hydralazine
    (F) Minoxidil
    (G) Nifedipine
    (H) Nitroprusside
    (I) Prazosin
    (J) Propranolol

13. A drug that can cause renal damage in the fetus if given during pregnancy
    (A) Captopril
    (B) Diazoxide
    (C) Fenoldopam
    (D) Guanethidine
    (E) Hydralazine

ANSWERS

1. Marked tachycardia and fluid retention are compensatory responses usually seen with strong vasodilators. The fact that the unknown drug also increases hair growth points strongly at minoxidil. The answer is **C.**

2. Except for α-blockers, any sympathoplegic can, in sufficient dosage, cause bradycardia. Conversely, any vasodilator may induce tachycardia and, unless it is also sympathoplegic or a calcium channel blocker, will never slow the heart rate. The answer is **C.**

3. Prazosin is a relatively selective drug and essentially all of its effects can be ascribed to blockade of peripheral α_1 adrenoceptors. Like other peripherally acting sympathoplegics, it can cause salt and water retention and orthostatic hypotension. It is relatively free of CNS effects. Clonidine causes some sedation (it has even been used as "knock-out drops"), but it is not associated with hemolytic anemia. The answer is **B.**

4. Converting enzyme inhibitors act on the enzyme, not on the angiotensin receptor. The plasma renin level may increase as a result of the compensatory response to reduced angiotensin II. The answer is **B.**

5. Methyldopa is the only antihypertensive drug associated with hemolytic anemia (usually preceded by a positive Coombs test). It is still used in some obstetrical practices because of its history of relative safety. Hydralazine is also associated with autoimmune toxicity, but this takes the form of a lupus-like syndrome with butterfly facial rash, fever, joint and muscle pains, and antinuclear antibodies. The answer is **D.**

6. Orthostatic hypotension is usually due to venous pooling. Venous pooling is normally prevented by α receptor activation. The answer is **B.**

7. Chronic cough is a common adverse effect of captopril and other ACE inhibitors. It may be relieved by prior administration of aspirin. These drugs are very commonly used in hypertensive diabetic patients because of their proven benefits in diabetes. Angiotensin II receptor blockers such as losartan and valsartan have a lower incidence of cough but do cause renal damage in the fetus. The answer is **A.**

8. Diazoxide may cause hyperglycemia. It is sometimes used to *treat* hypoglycemia (eg, caused by insulinoma) because it can inhibit insulin release. The answer is **B.**

9. Propranolol—but not prazosin—may decrease cardiac output. Prazosin may increase renin output (a compensatory response), but β-blockers inhibit its release by the kidney. By reducing blood pressure, both may increase central sympathetic outflow (a compensatory response). Propranolol does not cause orthostatic hypotension. The answer is **D.**

10. Verapamil is associated with constipation, probably through inhibition of calcium influx in intestinal smooth muscle. The answer is **A.**

11. Diazoxide, nitroprusside, and labetalol are the drugs in the list that are used in hypertensive emergencies. (Fenoldopam is also used.) Diazoxide has a long duration of action and is usually given by intermittent

injection. Labetalol also has a long duration of effect (hours) and can be given orally or parenterally. The answer is **H.**

12. Diazoxide is a potassium channel opener as given. Minoxidil sulfate, a metabolite of minoxidil, also acts by this mechanism. The answer is **C.**

13. All ACE inhibitors can cause renal damage in patients with preexisting renal vascular disease and in the developing fetus. (The angiotensin II receptor antagonists appear to have similar renal toxicity.) The answer is **A.**

SKILL KEEPER ANSWER: COMPENSATORY RESPONSES TO ANTIHYPERTENSIVE DRUGS (SEE CHAPTER 6)

The compensatory responses to hydralazine use are tachycardia and salt and water retention. These responses are generated by the baroreceptor and renin-angiotensin-aldosterone mechanisms summarized in Figure 6–4. The motor limb of the sympathetic response consists of outflow from the vasomotor center to the heart and vessels, as shown in Figure 11–2. You should be able to reproduce these diagrams from memory.

CHECKLIST

When you complete this chapter, you should be able to:

☐ List the 4 major groups of antihypertensive drugs and give examples of drugs in each group. (Renin inhibitors are not yet considered a "major group.")

☐ Describe the compensatory responses, if any, to each of the 4 major types of antihypertensive drugs.

☐ List the major sites of action of sympathoplegic drugs and give examples of drugs that act at each site.

☐ List the 4 mechanisms of action of vasodilator drugs.

☐ List the major antihypertensive vasodilator drugs and describe their effects.

☐ Describe the differences between the 2 types of angiotensin antagonists.

☐ List the major toxicities of the prototype antihypertensive agents.

Drugs Used in the Treatment of Angina Pectoris

12

Angina pectoris refers to a strangling or pressure-like pain caused by cardiac ischemia. The pain is usually located substernally but is sometimes perceived in the neck, shoulder, or epigastrium. Drugs used in angina exploit two main strategies: reduction of oxygen demand and increase of the oxygen delivery to the myocardium.

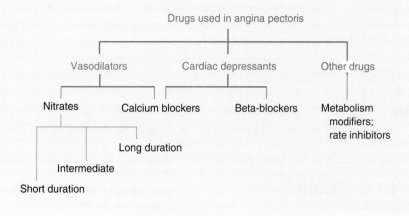

PATHOPHYSIOLOGY OF ANGINA

A. TYPES OF ANGINA

1. Atherosclerotic angina—Atherosclerotic angina is also known as angina of effort or classic angina. It is associated with atheromatous plaques that partially occlude 1 or more coronaries. When cardiac work increases (eg, in exercise), the obstruction of flow and inadequate oxygen delivery results in the accumulation of acidic metabolites and ischemic changes that stimulate myocardial pain endings. Rest usually leads to relief of the pain within 15 min. Atherosclerotic angina constitutes about 90% of angina cases.

2. Vasospastic angina—Vasospastic angina is also known as rest angina, variant angina, or Prinzmetal's angina. It involves reversible spasm of coronaries, usually at the site of an atherosclerotic plaque. Spasm may occur at any time, even during sleep. Vasospastic angina may deteriorate into unstable angina.

3. Unstable angina—The third type of angina—unstable or crescendo angina, also known as **acute coronary syndrome**—is characterized by increased frequency and severity of attacks that result from a combination of atherosclerotic plaques, platelet aggregation at fractured plaques, and vasospasm. Unstable angina is thought to be the immediate precursor of a myocardial infarction and is treated as a medical emergency.

HIGH-YIELD TERMS TO LEARN

Angina of effort, classic angina, atherosclerotic angina	Angina (crushing, strangling, chest pain) that is precipitated by exertion, ie, increased O_2 demand that cannot be met because of irreversible atherosclerotic obstruction of coronary arteries
Vasospastic angina, variant angina, Prinzmetal's angina	Angina precipitated by reversible spasm of coronary vessels
Coronary vasodilator	Older, incorrect name for drugs useful in angina; drugs that relieve angina of effort do not usually act primarily through coronary vasodilation; some potent coronary vasodilators are ineffective in angina
"Monday disease"	Industrial disease caused by chronic exposure to vasodilating concentrations of organic nitrates in the workplace; characterized by headache, dizziness, and tachycardia on return to work after 2 days absence
Nitrate tolerance, tachyphylaxis	Loss of effect of a nitrate vasodilator when exposure is prolonged beyond 10–12 h
Unstable angina	Rapidly progressing increase in frequency and severity of anginal attacks, especially pain at rest; an acute coronary syndrome and probably heralds imminent myocardial infarction
Preload	Filling pressure of the heart; determines end-diastolic fiber length and tension
Afterload	Resistance to ejection of stroke volume; determined by arterial blood pressure and arterial stiffness
Intramyocardial fiber tension	Force exerted by myocardial fibers, especially ventricular fibers at any given time; a primary determinant of O_2 requirement
Double product	The product of heart rate and systolic blood pressure; an estimate of cardiac work
Myocardial revascularization	Mechanical intervention to improve O_2 delivery to the myocardium by angioplasty or bypass grafting

DETERMINANTS OF CARDIAC OXYGEN REQUIREMENT

The pharmacologic treatment of coronary insufficiency is based on the physiologic factors that control myocardial oxygen requirement. A major determinant is **myocardial fiber tension** (the higher the tension, the greater the oxygen requirement).

Several variables contribute to fiber tension (Figure 12–1), as discussed next.

A. PRELOAD AND AFTERLOAD

Preload (diastolic filling pressure) is a function of blood volume and venous tone. Venous tone is mainly controlled by sympathetic outflow. **Afterload** is determined

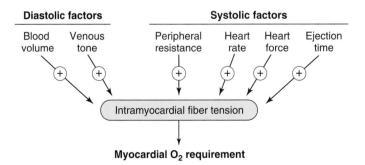

Figure 12–1. Determinants of the volume of oxygen required by the heart. Both diastolic and systolic factors contribute to the oxygen requirement; most of these factors are directly influenced by sympathetic discharge (venous tone, peripheral resistance, heart rate, and heart force).

by arterial blood pressure and large artery stiffness. It is one of the systolic determinants of oxygen requirement.

B. HEART RATE

Heart rate contributes to time-integrated fiber tension because at fast heart rates, fibers spend more time at systolic tension levels. Furthermore, at faster rates, diastole is abbreviated, and diastole constitutes the time available for coronary flow (coronary blood flow is low or nil during systole). Systolic blood pressure and heart rate may be multiplied to yield the **double product,** a measure of cardiac work and therefore of oxygen requirement. In patients with atherosclerotic angina, effective drugs reduce the double product.

C. CARDIAC CONTRACTILITY

Force of cardiac contraction is another systolic factor controlled mainly by sympathetic outflow to the heart. **Ejection time** for ventricular contraction is inversely related to force of contraction but is also influenced by impedance to outflow. Increased ejection time (prolonged systole) increases oxygen requirement.

THERAPEUTIC STRATEGIES

The defect that causes anginal pain is inadequate coronary oxygen delivery relative to the myocardial oxygen requirement. This defect can be corrected—at present—in 2 ways: by **increasing oxygen delivery** and by **reducing oxygen requirement** (Figure 12–2). Currently available pharmacologic therapies include the **nitrates,** the **calcium channel blockers,** and the **β-blockers.**

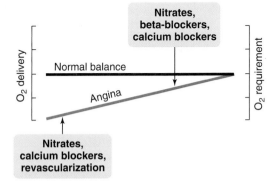

Figure 12–2. Strategies for the treatment of angina pectoris. Angina is characterized by reduced coronary oxygen delivery versus oxygen requirement. In some cases, this can be corrected by increasing oxygen delivery (box on left: revascularization or, in the case of reversible vasospasm, nitrates and calcium channel blockers). More often, drugs are used to reduce oxygen requirement (box on right: nitrates, β-blockers, and calcium channel blockers).

A newer group of drugs attempts to increase the **efficiency of oxygen utilization** by shifting the energy substrate preference of the heart from fatty acids to glucose. Drugs that may act by this mechanism are termed partial fatty acid oxidation inhibitors (pFOX inhibitors) and include **ranolazine** and trimetazidine. However, more recent evidence suggests that a major mechanism of action of ranolazine is inhibition of late sodium current. Another new group of antianginal drugs selectively reduces heart rate with no other detectable hemodynamic effects. These investigational drugs (**ivabradine** is the prototype) act by inhibition of the sinoatrial pacemaker current, I_f.

The nitrates, calcium blockers, and β-blockers all reduce the oxygen requirement in atherosclerotic angina; nitrates and calcium channel blockers (but not β-blockers) can also increase oxygen delivery by reducing vasospasm. **Myocardial revascularization** corrects coronary obstruction either by bypass grafting or by angioplasty (enlargement of the lumen by means of a special catheter). Therapy of unstable angina differs from that of stable angina because urgent angioplasty is the treatment of choice in most patients and platelet clotting is the major target of drug therapy. The platelet glycoprotein IIb/IIIa inhibitors—abciximab, eptifibatide, and tirofiban—are used in this condition (see Chapter 34). Intravenous nitroglycerin is sometimes of value.

NITRATES

A. CLASSIFICATION AND PHARMACOKINETICS

Nitroglycerin (the active ingredient in dynamite) is the most important of the therapeutic nitrates and is available in forms that provide a range of durations of action from 10–20 min (sublingual) to 8–10 h (transdermal) (Table 12–1). Because treatment of acute attacks and prevention of attacks are both important aspects of therapy, the pharmacokinetics of these different dosage forms are clinically significant.

Nitroglycerin (glyceryl trinitrate) is rapidly denitrated in the liver and in smooth muscle—first to the dinitrate (glyceryl dinitrate), which retains a significant vasodilating effect; and more slowly to the mononitrate, which is much less active. Because of the high enzyme activity in the liver, the first-pass effect for nitroglycerin is large—about 90%. The efficacy of oral (swallowed) nitroglycerin probably results from the high levels of glyceryl dinitrate in the blood. The effects of sublingual nitroglycerin are mainly the result of the unchanged drug because this route avoids the first-pass effect (see Chapters 1 and 3).

Other nitrates are similar to nitroglycerin in their pharmacokinetics and pharmacodynamics. Isosorbide dinitrate is another commonly used nitrate; it is available in sublingual and oral forms. Isosorbide dinitrate is rapidly denitrated in the liver and smooth muscle to

Table 12–1. Pharmacokinetically distinct forms of nitrates and nitrites used in angina.

Category	Example	Duration of Action
Very short acting	Inhaled amyl nitrite[a]	3–5 min
Short	Sublingual nitroglycerin or isosorbide dinitrate	10–30 min (isosorbide dinitrate has a somewhat longer half-life than nitroglycerin)
Intermediate	Oral regular or sustained release nitroglycerin or isosorbide dinitrate or mononitrate	4–5 h (much of the effect is due to active metabolites)
Long	Transdermal nitroglycerin patch	8–10 h (blood levels may persist for 24 h but tolerance limits the duration of action)

[a]Obsolete for use in angina.

isosorbide mononitrate, which is also active. Isosorbide mononitrate is available as a separate drug for oral use. Several other nitrates are available for oral use and, like the oral nitroglycerin preparation, have an intermediate duration of action (4–6 h). Amyl nitrite is a volatile and rapidly acting vasodilator that was used for angina by the inhalational route but is now rarely prescribed.

B. MECHANISM OF ACTION

Denitration of the nitrates within smooth muscle cells releases nitric oxide (NO), which stimulates guanylyl cyclase, and causes an increase of the second messenger cGMP; the latter results in smooth muscle relaxation by dephosphorylation of myosin light chain phosphate. Note that this mechanism is identical to that of nitroprusside (see Chapter 11).

C. ORGAN SYSTEM EFFECTS

1. Cardiovascular—Smooth muscle relaxation leads to an important degree of venodilation, which results in reduced cardiac size and cardiac output through reduced preload. Relaxation of arterial smooth muscle may increase flow through partially occluded epicardial coronary vessels. Reduced afterload, from arteriolar dilation, may contribute to an increase in ejection and a further decrease in cardiac size. Some studies suggest that of the vascular beds, the veins are the most sensitive, arteries less so, and arterioles least sensitive. Venodilation leads to decreased diastolic heart size and fiber tension. Arteriolar dilation leads to reduced peripheral resistance and blood pressure. These changes contribute to an overall reduction in myocardial fiber tension, oxygen consumption, and the double product. Thus, the primary mechanism of therapeutic benefit in atherosclerotic angina is reduction of the oxygen requirement. A secondary mechanism—namely, an increase in coronary flow via collateral vessels in ischemic areas—has also been proposed. In vasospastic angina, a reversal of coronary spasm and increased flow can be demonstrated.

Nitrates have no direct effects on cardiac muscle, but a significant reflex tachycardia and increased force of contraction are predictable when nitroglycerin reduces the blood pressure.

2. Other organs—Nitrates relax the smooth muscle of the bronchi, gastrointestinal tract, and genitourinary tract, but these effects are too small to be clinically useful. Intravenous nitroglycerin (sometimes used in unstable angina) reduces platelet aggregation. There are no significant effects on other tissues.

D. CLINICAL USES

As previously noted, nitroglycerin is available in several formulations (Table 12–1). The standard form for treatment of acute anginal pain is the sublingual tablet or spray, which has a duration of action of 10–20 min. Isosorbide dinitrate is similar with a duration of 30 min. Oral (swallowed) normal-release nitroglycerin has a duration of action of 4–6 h. Sustained-release oral forms have a somewhat longer duration of action. Transdermal formulations (ointment or patch) can maintain blood levels for up to 24 h. Tolerance develops after 8–10 h, however, with rapidly diminishing effectiveness thereafter. It is therefore recommended that nitroglycerin patches be removed after 10–12 h to allow recovery of sensitivity to the drug.

E. TOXICITY OF NITRATES AND NITRITES

The most common toxic effects of nitrates are the responses evoked by vasodilation. These include tachycardia (from the baroreceptor reflex), orthostatic hypotension (a direct extension of the venodilator effect), and throbbing headache from meningeal artery vasodilation.

Nitrates interact with sildenafil and similar drugs promoted for erectile dysfunction. These agents inhibit a phosphodiesterase isoform (PDE 5) that metabolizes cGMP in smooth muscle (Figure 12–3). The increased cGMP in erectile smooth muscle relaxes it, allowing for

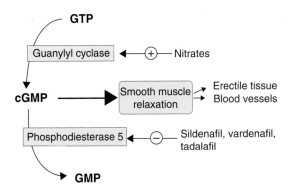

Figure 12–3. Mechanism of the interaction between nitrates and drugs used in erectile dysfunction. Because these drug groups increase cGMP by complementary mechanisms, they can have a synergistic effect on blood pressure.

greater inflow of blood and more effective and prolonged erection. This effect also occurs in vascular smooth muscle. As a result, the combination of nitrates (through increased production of cGMP) and a PDE 5 inhibitor (through decreased breakdown of cGMP) causes a synergistic relaxation of vascular smooth muscle with potentially dangerous hypotension and hypoperfusion of critical organs.

Nitrites are of significant toxicologic importance because they cause methemoglobinemia at high blood concentrations. This same effect has a potential antidotal action in cyanide poisoning (see later discussion). The nitrates do not cause methemoglobinemia. In the past, the nitrates were responsible for several occupational diseases in munitions factories in which workplace contamination by these volatile chemicals was severe. The most common of these diseases was "Monday disease," ie, the alternating development of tolerance (during the work week) and loss of tolerance (over the weekend) for the vasodilating action and its associated tachycardia and headache, resulting in headache, tachycardia, and dizziness every Monday.

F. Nitrites in the Treatment of Cyanide Poisoning

Cyanide ion rapidly complexes with the iron in cytochrome oxidase, resulting in a block of oxidative metabolism and cell death. Fortunately, the iron in methemoglobin has a higher affinity for cyanide than does the iron in cytochrome oxidase. Nitrites convert the ferrous iron in hemoglobin to the ferric form, yielding methemoglobin. Therefore, cyanide poisoning can be treated by a 3-step procedure: (1) immediate exposure to amyl nitrite, followed by (2) intravenous administration of sodium nitrite, which rapidly increases the methemoglobin level to the degree necessary to remove a significant amount of cyanide from cytochrome oxidase.

This is followed by (3) intravenous sodium thiosulfate, which converts cyanomethemoglobin resulting from step 2 to thiocyanate and methemoglobin. Thiocyanate is much less toxic than cyanide and is excreted by the kidney. (It should be noted that excessive methemoglobinemia is fatal because methemoglobin is a very poor oxygen carrier.)

CALCIUM CHANNEL-BLOCKING DRUGS

A. Classification and Pharmacokinetics

Several types of calcium channel blockers are approved for use in angina; these drugs are typified by **nifedipine,** a **dihydropyridine,** and several other dihydropyridines; **diltiazem**; and **verapamil.** Although calcium channel blockers differ markedly in structure, all are orally active and most have half-lives of 3–6 h. Nimodipine is another member of the dihydropyridine family with similar properties, but it is approved only for the management of stroke associated with subarachnoid hemorrhage.

B. Mechanism of Action

These drugs block voltage-gated L-type calcium channels, the calcium channels most important in cardiac and smooth muscle. By decreasing calcium influx during action potentials in a frequency- and voltage-dependent manner, these agents reduce intracellular calcium concentration and muscle contractility. None of these channel blockers interfere with calcium-dependent neurotransmission or hormone release because these processes utilize different types of calcium channels that are not blocked by these agents.

C. Effects

Calcium blockers relax blood vessels and, to a lesser extent, the uterus, bronchi, and gut. The rate and contractility of the heart are reduced by diltiazem and verapamil. Because they block calcium-dependent conduction in the AV node, verapamil and diltiazem may be used to treat AV nodal arrhythmias (see Chapter 14). Nifedipine and other dihydropyridines evoke greater vasodilation, and the resulting sympathetic reflex prevents bradycardia and may actually increase the heart rate. All the calcium channel blockers reduce blood pressure and reduce the double product in patients with angina.

D. Clinical Use

Calcium blockers are effective as prophylactic therapy in both effort and vasospastic angina; nifedipine has also been used to abort acute anginal attacks. In severe atherosclerotic angina, these drugs are particularly valuable when combined with nitrates (Table 12–2). In addition to well-established uses in angina, hypertension, and supraventricular tachycardia, some of these agents are used in migraine, preterm labor, stroke, and

Table 12–2. Effects of nitrates alone or with beta-blockers or calcium channel blockers in angina pectoris.[a]

	Nitrates Alone	Beta-Blockers or Calcium Channel Blockers Alone	Combined Nitrate and Beta-Blocker or Calcium Channel Blocker
Heart rate	*Reflex increase*	**Decrease**	**Decrease**
Arterial pressure	Decrease	**Decrease**	**Decrease**
End-diastolic pressure	**Decrease**	*Increase*	**Decrease**
Contractility	*Reflex increase*	**Decrease**	No effect or decrease
Ejection time	Reflex decrease	*Increase*	No effect
Net myocardial oxygen requirement	**Decrease**	**Decrease**	**Decrease**

[a]Undesirable effects (effects that increase oxygen requirement) are shown in *italics;* major beneficial effects are shown in **bold.**

Raynaud's phenomenon. As noted, nimodipine is approved for use in hemorrhagic stroke.

E. TOXICITY

The calcium channel blockers cause constipation, pretibial edema, nausea, flushing, and dizziness. More serious adverse effects include heart failure, atrioventricular blockade, and sinus node depression; these are more common with verapamil than with the dihydropyridines.

> **SKILL KEEPER: NIFEDIPINE CARDIOTOXICITY (SEE CHAPTER 6)**
>
> *A pair of studies during the 1990s suggested that use of nifedipine was associated with an increased risk of myocardial infarction. What effects of nifedipine might lead to this result? The Skill Keeper Answer appears at the end of the chapter.*

BETA-BLOCKING DRUGS

A. CLASSIFICATION AND MECHANISM OF ACTION

These drugs are described in detail in Chapter 10. All β-blockers are effective in the prophylaxis of atherosclerotic angina attacks.

B. EFFECTS

Actions include both beneficial antianginal effects (decreased heart rate, cardiac force, blood pressure) and detrimental effects (increased heart size, longer ejection period; Table 12–2). Like the nitrates and calcium channel blockers, the β-blockers reduce cardiac work and the double product.

C. CLINICAL USE

Beta-blockers are used only for prophylactic therapy of angina; they are of no value in an acute attack. They are effective in preventing exercise-induced angina but are ineffective against the vasospastic form. The combination of β-blockers with nitrates is useful because the adverse undesirable compensatory effects evoked by the nitrates (tachycardia and increased cardiac force) are prevented or reduced by β-blockade. See Table 12–2.

D. TOXICITY

See Chapter 10.

NONPHARMACOLOGIC THERAPY

Myocardial revascularization by coronary artery bypass grafting (CABG) and percutaneous transluminal coronary angioplasty (PTCA) are extremely important in the treatment of severe angina. These are the only methods capable of consistently increasing coronary flow in atherosclerotic angina and increasing the double product.

QUESTIONS

1–3. Mr Green, 60 years old, has severe chest pain when he walks uphill in cold weather to his home. The pain disappears when he rests. A decision is made to treat him with nitroglycerin.

1. Nitroglycerin, either directly or through reflexes, results in which one of the following effects?

KEY DRUGS		
Subclass	**Prototypes**	**Other Significant Agents**
Nitrates	Nitroglycerin	Different dosage forms, isosorbide dinitrate, amyl nitrite
Calcium channel blockers	Nifedipine, verapamil, diltiazem	Nimodipine
Beta-blockers	Propranolol	See Chapter 10

(A) Decreased heart rate
(B) Decreased venous capacitance
(C) Increased afterload
(D) Increased cardiac force
(E) Increased diastolic intramyocardial fiber tension

2. In advising Mr Green about the adverse effects he may notice, you point out that nitroglycerin in moderate doses often produces certain symptoms. Which of the following effects might occur due to the mechanism listed?
(A) Headache due to meningeal vasodilation
(B) Hypertension due to reflex tachycardia
(C) Dizziness due to meningeal vasodilation
(D) Dizziness due to reduced cardiac force of contraction
(E) Diuresis due to sympathetic discharge

3. Two years later, Mr Green returns complaining that his nitroglycerin works well when he takes it for an acute attack but that he is having frequent attacks now and would like something to *prevent* them. Useful drugs for the *prophylaxis* of angina of effort include which one of the following?
(A) Amyl nitrite
(B) Diltiazem
(C) Esmolol
(D) Sublingual isosorbide dinitrate
(E) Sublingual nitroglycerin

4. The antianginal effect of propranolol may be attributed to which one of the following?
(A) Block of exercise-induced tachycardia
(B) Decreased end-diastolic ventricular volume
(C) Dilation of constricted coronary vessels
(D) Increased cardiac force
(E) Decreased ventricular ejection time

5. The major common determinant of myocardial oxygen consumption is
(A) Blood volume
(B) Cardiac output
(C) Diastolic blood pressure
(D) Heart rate
(E) Myocardial fiber tension

6. M.A. is a new patient who presents with hypertension and angina. In considering adverse effects of possible drugs, you note that an adverse effect that nitroglycerin, prazosin, and ganglion blockers have in common is
(A) Bradycardia
(B) Impaired sexual function
(C) Lupus erythematosus syndrome
(D) Orthostatic hypotension
(E) Throbbing headache

7. Which of the following is most likely to cause methemoglobinemia?
(A) Sodium cyanide
(B) Amyl nitrite
(C) Isosorbide mononitrate
(D) Isosorbide dinitrate
(E) Nitroglycerin

8. A patient is admitted to the emergency department following a drug overdose. He is noted to have severe tachycardia. He has been receiving therapy for hypertension and angina. A drug that often causes tachycardia is
(A) Diltiazem
(B) Guanethidine
(C) Isosorbide dinitrate
(D) Propranolol
(E) Verapamil

9. A patient being treated for another condition complains that whenever he takes that medication, his angina becomes worse. Drugs that may precipitate angina when used for other indications do NOT include
(A) Amphetamine
(B) Hydralazine
(C) Isoproterenol
(D) Metoprolol
(E) Terbutaline

10. When nitrates are used in combination with other drugs for the treatment of angina, which one of the following combinations results in additive effects on the variable specified?

(A) Beta-blockers and nitrates on end-diastolic cardiac size
(B) Beta-blockers and nitrates on heart rate
(C) Calcium channel blockers and β-blockers on cardiac force
(D) Calcium channel blockers and nitrates on cardiac ejection time
(E) Calcium channel blockers and nitrates on heart rate

11. Which of the following is approved for the treatment of hemorrhagic stroke?
(A) Amyl nitrite
(B) Hydralazine
(C) Isosorbide mononitrate
(D) Nifedipine
(E) Nimodipine
(F) Nitroglycerin (sublingual)
(G) Nitroglycerin (transdermal)
(H) Propranolol
(I) Terbutaline
(J) Verapamil

12. Which of the following drugs interacts with nitroglycerin by inhibiting the metabolism of cGMP?
(A) Amyl nitrite
(B) Hydralazine
(C) Isosorbide mononitrate
(D) Nifedipine
(E) Propranolol
(F) Sildenafil
(G) Terbutaline

ANSWERS

1. Nitroglycerin increases cardiac force because the decrease in blood pressure evokes a compensatory increase in sympathetic discharge. The answer is **D.**

2. Nitroglycerin causes hypotension as a result of arterial and venous dilation. Dilation of meningeal arteries has no effect on CNS function but does cause headache. The answer is **A.**

3. The calcium channel blockers and the β-blockers are generally effective in reducing the number of attacks of angina of effort, and most have durations of 4–8 h. Oral and transdermal nitrates have similar or longer durations. Amyl nitrite, the sublingual nitrates, and esmolol (an intravenous β-blocker) have short durations of action and are of no value in prophylaxis. The answer is **B.**

4. Propranolol blocks tachycardia but has none of the other effects listed. The answer is **A.**

5. The answer is **E,** fiber tension. The other variables contribute to this determinant.

6. These drugs all reduce venous return sufficiently to cause some degree of postural hypotension. Throbbing headache is a problem only with the nitrates, sexual problems only with ganglion blockers, and bradycardia and lupus with none of them. The answer is **D.**

7. Nitrites, not nitrates, cause methemoglobinemia in adults. Methemoglobinemia is deliberately induced in one of the treatments of cyanide poisoning. The answer is **B.**

8. Isosorbide dinitrate (like all the nitrates) can cause reflex tachycardia, but all the other drugs listed here slow heart rate. The answer is **C.**

9. In general, drugs that cause hypertension or tachycardia—whether directly or by reflex—tend to precipitate angina in individuals with coronary obstruction unless cardiac work is greatly reduced (as in the case of the nitrates). The answer is **D.** (***Note:*** "all . . . except" and "do not include" type questions are no longer used in USMLE examinations but may be encountered elsewhere.)

10. The effects of β-blockers (or calcium channel blockers) and nitrates on heart size, force, ejection time, and rate are opposite. The answer is **C.**

11. Nimodipine, a dihydropyridine calcium channel blocker, is approved only for the treatment of hemorrhagic stroke. The answer is **E.**

12. Sildenafil inhibits phosphodiesterase 5, an enzyme that inactivates cGMP. The answer is **F.**

SKILL KEEPER ANSWER: NIFEDIPINE CARDIOTOXICITY (SEE CHAPTER 6)

Long-term studies have suggested that patients receiving prompt-release nifedipine may have an increased risk of myocardial infarction. Slow-release formulations do not seem to impose this risk. These observations have been explained as follows: Rapidly acting vasodilators—such as nifedipine in its prompt-release formulation—cause significant and sudden reduction in blood pressure. The drop in blood pressure evokes increased sympathetic outflow to the cardiovascular system and increases heart rate and force of contraction as shown in Figure 6–4. These changes can markedly increase cardiac oxygen requirement. If coronary blood flow does not increase sufficiently to match the increased requirement, ischemia and necrosis can result.

CHECKLIST

When you complete this chapter, you should be able to:

☐ Describe the pathophysiology of effort angina and vasospastic angina.

☐ List the major determinants of cardiac oxygen consumption.

☐ List the strategies for relief of anginal pain.

☐ Contrast the therapeutic and adverse effects of nitrates, β-blockers, and calcium channel blockers when used for angina.

☐ Explain why the combination of a nitrate with a β-blocker or a calcium channel blocker may be more effective than either alone.

☐ Explain why the combination of a nitrate and sildenafil is potentially dangerous.

☐ Contrast the effects of medical therapy and surgical therapy of angina.

Drugs Used in Heart Failure

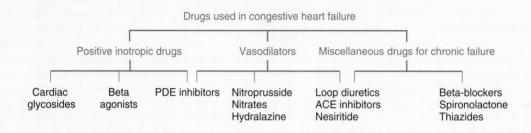

Heart failure results when cardiac output is inadequate for the needs of the body. A defect in cardiac contractility is complicated by multiple compensatory processes that further weaken the failing heart. The drugs used in heart failure vary broadly in their targets and actions.

Drugs used in congestive heart failure

Positive inotropic drugs — Vasodilators — Miscellaneous drugs for chronic failure

Cardiac glycosides | Beta agonists | PDE inhibitors

Nitroprusside
Nitrates
Hydralazine

Loop diuretics
ACE inhibitors
Nesiritide

Beta-blockers
Spironolactone
Thiazides

PATHOPHYSIOLOGY

Heart failure is an extremely serious cardiac condition associated with a high mortality rate. The fundamental physiologic defect in heart failure is a decrease in cardiac output relative to the needs of the body. The cause of this defect is still not completely understood. In some cases it can be ascribed to simple loss of functional myocardium, as in myocardial infarction. It is frequently associated with chronic hypertension, valvular disease, coronary artery disease, and a variety of cardiomyopathies. In most cases of heart failure, a reduction of cardiac contractile force can be detected during systole. In other cases, stiffening of the ventricles prevents adequate filling during diastole. The natural history of heart failure is characterized by a slow deterioration of cardiac function, punctuated by episodes of acute cardiac decompensation that are often associated with pulmonary or peripheral edema or both (congestion).

The reduction in cardiac output is best shown by the ventricular function curve (Frank-Starling curve; Figure 13–1). The changes in the ventricular function curve reflect some compensatory responses of the body and may also be used to demonstrate the response to

drugs. As ventricular ejection decreases, the end-diastolic fiber length increases as shown by the shift from point A to point B in Figure 13–1. Operation at point B is intrinsically less efficient than operation at shorter fiber lengths because of the increase in myocardial oxygen requirement associated with increased fiber stretch (see Figure 12–1).

The homeostatic responses of the body to depressed cardiac output are extremely important and are mediated mainly by the sympathetic nervous system and the renin-angiotensin-aldosterone system. They are summarized in Figure 13–2. The major responses include the following: (1) Tachycardia—an early manifestation of increased sympathetic tone. (2) Increased peripheral vascular resistance—another early response, also mediated by increased sympathetic tone. (3) Retention of salt and water by the kidney—an early compensatory response, mediated by the renin-angiotensin-aldosterone system and facilitated by increased sympathetic outflow. Increased blood volume results in edema and pulmonary congestion and contributes to the increased end-diastolic fiber length. (4) Cardiomegaly (enlargement of the heart)—a slower compensatory response, mediated at least in part by sympathetic discharge and angiotensin II. Although these compensatory responses can temporarily

---

HIGH-YIELD TERMS TO LEARN

Bigeminy	An arrhythmia consisting of normal sinus beats coupled with ventricular extrasystoles, ie, "twinned beats" (Figure 13–4)
End-diastolic fiber length	The length of the ventricular fibers at the end of diastole; a determinant of the force of the following contraction
Heart failure	A condition in which the cardiac output is insufficient for the needs of the body. Low-output failure is the more common form and is more responsive to positive inotropic drugs than high-output failure
PDE inhibitor	Phosphodiesterase inhibitor; a drug that inhibits one or more enzymes that degrade cAMP (and other cyclic nucleotides). Example: high concentrations of theophylline, aminophylline, amrinone
Premature ventricular beats	An abnormal beat arising from a cell below the AV node—often from a Purkinje fiber, sometimes from a ventricular fiber
Sodium pump (Na$^+$/K$^+$ ATPase)	A transport molecule in the membranes of all vertebrate cells; responsible for the maintenance of normal low intracellular sodium and high intracellular potassium concentrations
Sodium-calcium exchanger	A transport molecule in the membrane of many cells that pumps one calcium atom outward against its concentration gradient in exchange for three sodium ions moving inward down their concentration gradient
Ventricular function curve	The graph that relates cardiac output, stroke volume, etc, to filling pressure or end-diastolic fiber length; also known as the Frank-Starling curve
Ventricular tachycardia	An arrhythmia consisting entirely or largely of beats originating below the AV node

---

improve cardiac output, they also increase the load on the heart and the increased load contributes to further long-term decline in cardiac function. (5) Apoptosis occurs, resulting in a reduction in the number of functioning myocytes and their replacement by connective tissue. Evidence suggests that catecholamines, angiotensin II, and aldosterone play a direct role in these changes.

THERAPEUTIC STRATEGIES

Pharmacologic therapies for heart failure include the removal of retained salt and water with diuretics; reduction of afterload and salt and water retention by means of angiotensin-converting enzyme inhibitors; reduction of excessive sympathetic stimulation by β-blockers; reduction of preload or afterload with vasodilators; and direct augmentation of depressed cardiac contractility with positive inotropic drugs such as digitalis glycosides. In addition, considerable evidence suggests that angiotensin antagonists, some β adrenoceptor blockers, and the aldosterone antagonists spironolactone and eplerenone also have long-term beneficial effects. The use of diuretics is discussed in Chapter 15.

Current clinical evidence suggests that acute heart failure should be treated with a loop diuretic; if very severe, a prompt-acting positive inotropic agent such as a β agonist or phosphodiesterase inhibitor, and vasodilators as required to optimize filling pressures and blood pressure may also be needed. Chronic failure is best treated with diuretics (often a loop agent plus spironolactone) plus an ACE inhibitor and, if tolerated, a β-blocker. Digitalis may be helpful if systolic dysfunction is prominent. Nesiritide, a recombinant form of brain natriuretic peptide, has vasodilating and diuretic properties and has been heavily promoted for use in acute failure.

CARDIAC GLYCOSIDES

Digitalis glycosides are no longer considered first-line drugs in the treatment of heart failure. However, because they are not discussed elsewhere in this book, we begin our discussion with this group.

A. PROTOTYPES AND PHARMACOKINETICS

All cardiac glycosides include a steroid nucleus and a lactone ring; most also have one or more sugar residues. The cardiac glycosides are often called "digitalis" because several come from the digitalis (foxglove) plant. **Digoxin** is the prototype agent and the only one commonly used

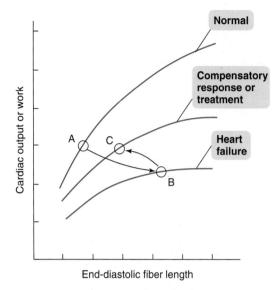

Figure 13–1. Ventricular function (Frank-Starling) curves. The abscissa can be any measure of preload-fiber length, filling pressure, pulmonary capillary wedge pressure, etc. The ordinate is a measure of useful external cardiac work-stroke volume, cardiac output, etc. In heart failure, output is reduced at all fiber lengths and the heart expands because ejection fraction is decreased. As a result, the heart moves from point A to point B. Compensatory sympathetic discharge or effective treatment allows the heart to eject more blood, and the heart moves to point C on the middle curve.

in the United States. A very similar molecule, digitoxin, which also comes from the foxglove, is no longer available in the United States. The pharmacokinetics of digoxin are summarized in Table 13–1.

B. MECHANISM OF ACTION

Inhibition of Na^+/K^+ ATPase of the cell membrane by digitalis is well documented and is considered to be the primary biochemical mechanism of action of digitalis (Figure 13–3). Inhibition of Na^+/K^+ ATPase results in a small increase in intracellular sodium. The increased sodium alters the driving force for sodium-calcium exchange by the exchanger, NaxC, so that less calcium is removed from the cell. The increased intracellular calcium is stored in the sarcoplasmic reticulum and upon release increases contractile force. Other mechanisms of action for digitalis have been proposed, but they are probably not as important as the inhibition of ATPase. The consequences of Na^+/K^+ ATPase inhibition are seen in both the mechanical and the electrical function of the heart. Digitalis also modifies autonomic outflow, and this action has effects on the electrical properties of the heart.

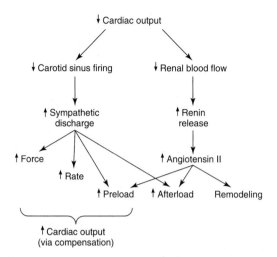

Figure 13–2. Compensatory responses that occur in heart failure. These responses play an important role in the progression of the disease. (Reproduced, with permission, from Katzung BG, editor: *Basic & Clinical Pharmacology,* 10th ed. McGraw-Hill, 2007.)

C. CARDIAC EFFECTS

1. Mechanical effects—The increase in contractility evoked by digitalis results in increased ventricular ejection, decreased end-systolic and end-diastolic size, increased cardiac output, and increased renal perfusion. These beneficial effects permit a decrease in the compensatory sympathetic and renal responses previously described. The decrease in sympathetic tone is especially beneficial: reduced heart rate, preload, and afterload permit the heart to function more efficiently (point C in Figure 13–1).

2. Electrical effects—Electrical effects include early cardiac parasympathomimetic responses and later arrhythmogenic responses. They are summarized in Table 13–2.

Table 13–1. Pharmacokinetic parameters of digoxin, the only cardiac glycoside used in the United States.

Oral bioavailability	60–85%
Primary organs of elimination	Kidney (60%), liver (40%)
Volume of distribution	6–8 L/kg body weight
Clearance	0.1 L/h/kg body weight
Half-life	36–40 h
Protein bound in plasma	20–40%

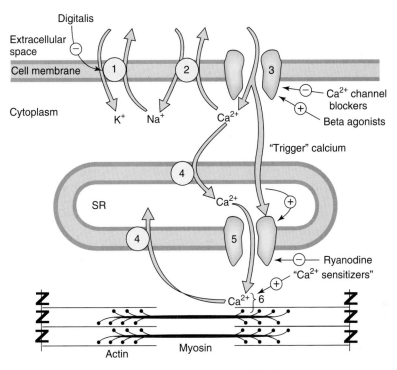

Figure 13–3. Schematic diagram of a cardiac sarcomere with the cellular components involved in excitation-contraction coupling. Factors involved in excitation-contraction coupling are numbered. 1: Na^+/K^+ ATPase; 2: $Na–Ca^{2+}$ exchanger, NaxC; 3: voltage-gated calcium channel; 4: calcium transporter (SERCA) in the wall of the sarcoplasmic reticulum (SR); 5: calcium release channel in the SR, RyR; 6: site of calcium interaction with the troponin-tropomyosin system. (Reproduced, with permission, from Katzung BG, editor: *Basic & Clinical Pharmacology,* 9th ed. McGraw-Hill, 2004.)

Table 13–2. Major actions of cardiac glycosides on cardiac electrical function.

	Tissue		
Variable	**Atrial Muscle**	**AV Node**	**Purkinje System, Ventricles**
Effective refractory period	↓(PANS)	↑(PANS)	↓(Direct)
Conduction velocity	↑(PANS)	↓(PANS)	Negligible
Automaticity	↑(Direct)	↑(Direct)	↑(Direct)
Electrocardiogram Before arrhythmias	Negligible	↑PR interval	↓QT interval; T-wave inversion; ST-segment depression
Arrhythmias	Atrial tachycardia, fibrillation	AV nodal tachycardia, AV blockade	Premature ventricular beats, bigeminy, ventricular tachycardia, ventricular fibrillation

PANS, parasympathomimetic actions; direct, direct membrane actions.

a. Early responses—Increased PR interval, caused by the decrease in atrioventricular conduction velocity, and flattening of the T wave are common effects. The effects on the atria and AV node are largely parasympathetic in origin and can be partially blocked by atropine. The increase in the atrioventricular nodal refractory period is particularly important when atrial flutter or fibrillation is present because the refractoriness of the AV node determines the ventricular rate in these arrhythmias. The effect of digitalis is to slow ventricular rate. Shortened QT, inversion of the T, and ST depression may occur later.

b. Toxic responses—Increased automaticity, caused by intracellular calcium overload, is the most important manifestation of toxicity. Intracellular calcium overload results in delayed afterdepolarizations, which may evoke extrasystoles, tachycardia, or fibrillation in any part of the heart. In the ventricles, the extrasystoles are recognized as premature ventricular beats (PVBs). When PVBs are coupled to normal beats in a 1:1 fashion, the rhythm is called bigeminy (Figure 13–4).

D. CLINICAL USES

1. Congestive heart failure—Digitalis is the traditional positive inotropic agent used in the treatment of chronic heart failure. However, careful clinical studies indicate that while digitalis improves functional status (reducing symptoms), it does not prolong life. Other agents (diuretics, ACE inhibitors, vasodilators) may be equally effective and less toxic, and some of these alternative therapies do prolong life (see later discussion). Because the half-lives of cardiac glycosides are long, the drugs accumulate significantly in the body, and dosing regimens must be carefully designed and monitored.

2. Atrial fibrillation—In atrial flutter and fibrillation, it is desirable to reduce the conduction velocity or increase the refractory period of the atrioventricular node so that ventricular rate is controlled within a range compatible with efficient filling and ejection. The parasympathomimetic action of digitalis often accomplishes this therapeutic objective, although high doses may be required. Alternative drugs for rate control include β-blockers and calcium channel blockers, but these drugs have negative inotropic effects.

E. INTERACTIONS

Quinidine causes a well-documented reduction in digoxin clearance and can increase the serum digoxin level if digoxin dosage is not adjusted. Several other drugs have been shown to have the same effect (amiodarone, verapamil, others), but the interactions with these drugs are not clinically significant. Digitalis effects are inhibited by extracellular potassium and magnesium and facilitated by extracellular calcium. Loop diuretics and thiazides, often used in treating heart failure, may significantly reduce serum potassium and thus precipitate digitalis toxicity. Digitalis-induced vomiting may deplete serum magnesium and similarly facilitate toxicity. These ion interactions are important in treating digitalis toxicity (see later discussion).

F. DIGITALIS TOXICITY

The major signs of digitalis toxicity are arrhythmias, nausea, vomiting, and diarrhea. Rarely, confusion or hallucinations and visual aberrations may occur. The treatment of arrhythmias is important because this manifestation of digitalis toxicity is common and dangerous. Chronic intoxication is an extension of the therapeutic effect of the drug and is caused by excessive calcium accumulation in cardiac cells (calcium overload). This overload triggers abnormal automaticity and the arrhythmias noted in Table 13–2. Digitalis arrhythmia is more likely if serum potassium or magnesium is lower than normal or if serum calcium is higher than normal.

Severe, acute intoxication caused by suicidal or accidental extreme overdose results in cardiac depression leading to cardiac arrest rather than tachycardia or fibrillation.

Treatment of digitalis toxicity includes several steps, as follows.

1. Correction of potassium or magnesium deficiency—Correction of potassium deficiency (caused, for example, by diuretic use) is useful in chronic digitalis intoxication. Mild toxicity may often be managed by omitting one or two doses of digitalis and giving oral or parenteral K⁺ supplements. Potassium should not be raised above the level of 5 meq/L. Similarly, if hypomagnesemia is present, it should be treated by normalizing serum magnesium. Severe acute intoxication (as in suicidal overdoses) usually causes marked hyperkalemia and should not be treated with supplemental potassium.

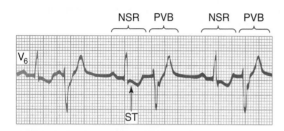

Figure 13–4. Electrocardiographic record showing digitalis-induced bigeminy. The complexes marked NSR are normal sinus rhythm beats; an inverted T wave and depressed ST segment are present. The complexes marked PVB are premature ventricular beats.

2. Antiarrhythmic drugs—Antiarrhythmic drugs may be useful if increased automaticity is prominent and does not respond to normalization of serum potassium. Agents that do not severely impair cardiac contractility (eg, lidocaine or phenytoin) are favored, but drugs such as propranolol have also been used successfully. Severe acute digitalis overdose usually causes marked *inhibition* of all cardiac pacemakers. Antiarrhythmic drugs are dangerous in such patients and an electronic pacemaker may be required.

3. Digoxin antibodies—Digoxin antibodies (Fab fragments; Digibind) are extremely effective and should always be used if other therapies appear to be failing. They are effective for poisoning with many cardiac glycosides in addition to digoxin and may save patients who would otherwise die.

> ### SKILL KEEPER: MAINTENANCE DOSE CALCULATIONS (SEE CHAPTER 3)
>
> *Digoxin has a narrow therapeutic window, and its dosing must be carefully managed. The drug's minimum effective concentration is about 1 ng/mL. About 60% is excreted in the urine; the rest is metabolized in the liver. The normal clearance of digoxin is 7 L/h/70 kg; volume of distribution is 500 L/70 kg; and bioavailability is 70%. If your 70-kg patient's renal function is only 30% of normal, what daily oral maintenance dosage should be used to achieve a safe plasma concentration of 1 ng/mL?* The Skill Keeper Answer appears at the end of the chapter.

OTHER DRUGS USED IN CONGESTIVE HEART FAILURE

The other major agents used in heart failure include diuretics, ACE inhibitors, β_1-selective sympathomimetics, β-blockers, phosphodiesterase inhibitors, and vasodilators.

A. DIURETICS

Diuretics are commonly used in heart failure before digitalis and other drugs are considered. **Furosemide** is a very useful agent for immediate reduction of the pulmonary congestion and severe edema associated with acute heart failure and moderate or severe chronic failure. Thiazides such as **hydrochlorothiazide** are sometimes sufficient for mild chronic failure. Clinical studies suggest that **spironolactone** and eplerenone (aldosterone antagonist diuretics) have significant long-term

benefits and can reduce mortality in chronic failure. The pharmacology of the diuretics is discussed in Chapter 15.

B. ANGIOTENSIN ANTAGONISTS

These agents have been shown to reduce morbidity and mortality in chronic heart failure. Although they have no direct positive inotropic action, angiotensin antagonists reduce aldosterone secretion, salt and water retention, and vascular resistance. They are now considered, along with diuretics, to be first-line drugs for chronic heart failure. The angiotensin receptor blockers (ARBs, eg, **losartan**) appear to have the same benefits as ACE inhibitors (eg, **captopril**), although experience with ARBs is not as extensive as with ACE inhibitors.

C. BETA₁-ADRENOCEPTOR AGONISTS

Dobutamine (β_1-selective) and **dopamine** are often useful in acute failure in which systolic function is markedly depressed. However, they are not appropriate for chronic failure because of tolerance, lack of oral efficacy, and significant arrhythmogenic effects.

D. BETA-ADRENOCEPTOR ANTAGONISTS

Several β-blockers (**carvedilol, labetalol, metoprolol)** have been shown in long-term studies to reduce progression of *chronic* heart failure. This benefit of β-blockers had long been recognized in patients with hypertrophic cardiomyopathy but has now been shown to occur also in patients without cardiomyopathy. Beta-blockers are not of value in acute failure and may be detrimental if systolic dysfunction is marked.

E. PHOSPHODIESTERASE INHIBITORS

Amrinone and **milrinone** are the major representatives of this infrequently used group, although theophylline (in the form of its salt, **aminophylline**) was commonly used in the past. These drugs increase cAMP by inhibiting its breakdown by phosphodiesterase and cause an increase in cardiac intracellular calcium similar to that produced by β-adrenoceptor agonists. Phosphodiesterase inhibitors also cause vasodilation, which may be responsible for a major part of their beneficial effect. At sufficiently high concentrations, these agents may increase the sensitivity of the contractile protein system to calcium (site 6 in Figure 13–3). These agents should not be used in chronic failure: they have been shown to increase morbidity and mortality.

F. VASODILATORS

Vasodilator therapy with **nitroprusside** or **nitroglycerin** is often used for acute severe failure with congestion. The use of these vasodilator drugs is based on the reduction in cardiac size and improved efficiency that can be realized with proper adjustment of venous return (preload) and reduction of resistance to ventricular ejection (afterload). Vasodilator therapy can be dramatically

---

KEY DRUGS

Subclass	Prototype	Other Significant Agents
Cardiac glycosides	Digoxin	
Other positive inotropic drugs	Dobutamine, amrinone	Dopamine
Angiotensin antagonists	Captopril, losartan	
Diuretics	Furosemide, spironolactone	Hydrochlorothiazide
Vasodilators	Nitroprusside, hydralazine	Nitroglycerin, nesiritide

---

effective, especially in cases in which increased afterload is a major factor in causing the failure (eg, continuing hypertension in an individual who has just had an infarct). The natriuretic peptide **nesiritide** acts chiefly by causing vasodilation although it does have natriuretic effects as well. It is given by IV infusion for acute failure only. Nesiritide has significant renal toxicity and renal function must be monitored. Chronic heart failure sometimes responds favorably to oral vasodilators such as hydralazine or isosorbide dinitrate (or both) but calcium channel blockers (eg, verapamil) are of no value.

QUESTIONS

1. The drugs that have been found to be *least* useful in heart failure are the
   (A) Na⁺/K⁺ ATPase inhibitors

   (B) Calcium channel blockers
   (C) Beta-adrenoceptor agonists
   (D) Beta-adrenoceptor antagonists
   (E) ACE inhibitors

2. The mechanism of action of digitalis glycosides is associated with
   (A) A decrease in calcium uptake by the sarcoplasmic reticulum
   (B) An increase in ATP synthesis
   (C) A modification of the actin molecule
   (D) An increase in systolic cytoplasmic calcium levels
   (E) A block of cardiac β adrenoceptors

3. A patient who has been taking digoxin for several years for chronic heart failure is about to receive atropine for another condition. A common effect of digoxin (at therapeutic blood levels) that can be almost entirely blocked by atropine is
   (A) Decreased appetite
   (B) Increased atrial contractility
   (C) Increased PR interval on the ECG
   (D) Headaches
   (E) Tachycardia

4. A 65-year-old woman has been admitted to the coronary care unit with a left ventricular myocardial infarction. If this patient develops acute severe heart failure with marked pulmonary edema, which one of the following would be most useful?
   (A) Digoxin
   (B) Furosemide
   (C) Minoxidil
   (D) Propranolol
   (E) Spironolactone

5. Which one of the following is most likely to contribute to the arrhythmogenic effect of digoxin?
   (A) Increased vagal discharge
   (B) Increased intracellular calcium
   (C) Decreased sympathetic discharge
   (D) Increased extracellular magnesium
   (E) Increased extracellular potassium

6. Which of the following situations constitutes an added risk of digoxin toxicity even if serum potassium is maintained constant?
   (A) Administration of captopril
   (B) Administration of quinidine
   (C) Administration of lidocaine
   (D) Administration of losartan
   (E) Hypocalcemia

7. Which one of the following drugs does NOT reduce mortality in chronic congestive heart failure?
   (A) Captopril
   (B) Carvedilol
   (C) Digoxin
   (D) Enalapril
   (E) Spironolactone

8. Which row in the following table correctly shows the major effects of full therapeutic doses of digoxin on the AV node and the ECG?

Row	AV Refractory Period	QT Interval	T Wave
(A)	Increased	Increased	Upright
(B)	Increased	Decreased	Inverted
(C)	Decreased	Increased	Upright
(D)	Decreased	Decreased	Upright
(E)	Decreased	Increased	Inverted

9. Which one of the following drugs is associated with clinically useful or physiologically important positive inotropic effect?
(A) Captopril
(B) Dobutamine
(C) Enalapril
(D) Losartan
(E) Nesiritide

10. Successful therapy of heart failure with digoxin will result in which one of the following?
(A) Decreased heart rate
(B) Decreased parasympathetic outflow
(C) Increased aldosterone
(D) Increased renin secretion
(E) Increased sympathetic outflow to the heart

11. Which of the following is a monovalent cation that will decrease or reverse a mild to moderate digitalis-induced arrhythmia?
(A) Digibind antibodies
(B) Digitoxin
(C) Digoxin
(D) Dobutamine
(E) Enalapril
(F) Furosemide
(G) Lidocaine
(H) Magnesium
(I) Potassium
(J) Quinidine

12. Which of the following has been shown to prolong life in patients with chronic congestive failure but has a negative inotropic effect on cardiac contractility?
(A) Carvedilol
(B) Digoxin
(C) Dobutamine
(D) Enalapril
(E) Furosemide

13. Which of the following is a β_1-selective agonist sometimes used in acute heart failure?
(A) Atenolol
(B) Digoxin
(C) Dobutamine

(D) Enalapril
(E) Furosemide
(F) Quinidine
(G) Spironolactone

14. Which of the following is the drug of choice in treating suicidal overdose of digitoxin?
(A) Digoxin antibodies
(B) Lidocaine
(C) Magnesium
(D) Phenytoin
(E) Potassium

ANSWERS

1. All the drug groups listed are commonly used in heart failure except calcium channel blockers. Although these drugs reduce afterload, they cause too much cardiac depression. The answer is **B**.

2. Digitalis does not alter calcium uptake or ATP synthesis; it does not modify actin. Cardiac adrenoceptors are not blocked. The most accurate description of digitalis's mechanism in this list is that it increases intracellular calcium. The answer is **D**.

3. The parasympathomimetic effects of digitalis can be blocked by muscarinic blockers such as atropine. The only parasympathomimetic effect in the list provided is increased PR interval, representing slowing of AV conduction. The answer is **C**.

4. Acute severe congestive failure with pulmonary edema often requires a vasodilator that reduces intravascular pressures in the lungs. Furosemide has such vasodilating actions in the context of acute failure. Minoxidil would decrease arterial pressure and increase the heart rate excessively. Digoxin has a slow onset of action and lacks vasodilating effects. Spironolactone is useful in chronic failure but not in acute pulmonary edema. The answer is **B**.

5. The effects of digitalis include increased vagal action on the heart and increased intracellular calcium, including calcium overload, the most important manifestation of toxicity. Decreased sympathetic

discharge and increased extracellular potassium and magnesium reduce digitalis arrhythmogenesis. The answer is **B**.

6. Digitalis toxicity is facilitated by hypercalcemia, hypokalemia, or hypomagnesemia. It is also more likely if a patient begins taking quinidine after being stabilized on a dose of digitalis, because quinidine reduces the clearance of digoxin. Lidocaine does not have this effect. The answer is **B**.

7. All the groups listed *except* digitalis have been shown to reduce mortality. Cardiac glycosides reduce symptoms but not mortality. The answer is **C**.

8. Digitalis increases the AV node refractory period—a parasympathomimetic action. Its effects on the ventricles include shortened action potential and QT interval, and a change in repolarization with flattening or inversion of the T wave. The answer is **B**.

9. Although they are extremely useful in heart failure, ACE inhibitors (eg, captopril, enalapril), and ARBs (eg, losartan) have no positive inotropic effect on the heart. Nesiritide is a vasodilator with diuretic and renotoxic effects. The answer is **B**.

10. Digoxin reduces sympathetic outflow to the heart and vessels and reduces renin secretion (because the drug replaces the need for compensatory responses). It increases parasympathetic outflow. The answer is **A**.

11. Potassium is the only monovalent cation in the list, and it is used for reversing mild to moderate digitalis toxicity if hypokalemia is present. The answer is **I**.

12. Several β-blockers, including carvedilol, have been shown to prolong life in heart failure patients even though these drugs have a negative inotropic action on the heart. Their benefits presumably result from some other effect and at least one has failed to show a mortality benefit. The answer is **A**.

13. Dobutamine is a β_1-selective agonist used in acute heart failure. The answer is **C**.

14. The drug of choice in severe, massive overdose with any cardiac glycoside is digoxin antibody, Digibind. These antibodies are sufficiently nonselective to bind a variety of cardiac glycosides. The other drugs listed are used in moderate overdosage associated with increased automaticity. The answer is **A**.

SKILL KEEPER ANSWER: MAINTENANCE DOSE CALCULATIONS (SEE CHAPTER 3)

Maintenance dosage is equal to $CL \times Cp \div F$, so

Maintenance dosage for a patient with normal renal function

$= 7 \text{ L/h} \times 1 \text{ ng/mL} \div 0.7 = 7 \text{ L/h} \times 1 \text{ mcg/L} \div 0.7$

$= 10 \text{ mcg/h} = 240 \text{ mcg/d}$

But this patient has only 30% of normal renal function, so

$CL \text{ (total)} = 0.3 \times CL \text{ (renal [60% of total])}$
$\qquad\qquad + CL \text{ (liver [40% of total])}$

$CL \text{ (total)} = 0.3 \times 0.6 \times 7 \text{ L/h} + 0.4 \times 7 \text{ L/h, and}$

$CL \text{ (total)} = 1.26 \text{ L/h} + 2.8 \text{ L/h} = 4.06 \text{ L/h, and}$

Maintenance dosage $= 4.06 \text{ L/h} \times 1 \text{ mcg/L} \div 0.7$
$\qquad\qquad\qquad = 5.8 \text{ mcg/h} = 139 \text{ mcg/d}$

CHECKLIST

When you complete this chapter, you should be able to:

☐ Describe the strategies and list the major drug groups used in the treatment of heart failure.

☐ Describe the probable mechanism of action of digitalis and its major effects. Indicate why digitalis is no longer considered a first-line therapy for chronic heart failure.

☐ Describe the nature and mechanism of digitalis's toxic effects on the heart.

☐ List some positive inotropic drugs other than digitalis that have been used in heart failure.

☐ Describe the beneficial effects of diuretics, vasodilators, ACE inhibitors, and other drugs that lack positive inotropic effects in heart failure.

Antiarrhythmic Drugs

14

Cardiac arrhythmias commonly occur in the presence of preexisting heart disease. They are the most common cause of death in patients with a myocardial infarction or terminal heart failure. They are also the most serious manifestation of digitalis toxicity and are often associated with anesthesia, hyperthyroidism, and electrolyte disorders. The drugs used for arrhythmias fall into five major groups or classes, but most have very low therapeutic indices and when feasible, non-drug therapies (cardioversion, pacemakers, implanted defibrillators) are preferred.

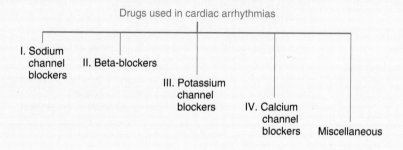

Drugs used in cardiac arrhythmias

I. Sodium channel blockers
II. Beta-blockers
III. Potassium channel blockers
IV. Calcium channel blockers
Miscellaneous

PATHOPHYSIOLOGY

A. WHAT IS AN ARRHYTHMIA?

Normal electrical cardiac function (normal sinus rhythm, NSR) is dependent on generation of an impulse in the normal pacemaker (the sinoatrial [SA] node) and its conduction through the atrial muscle, through the atrioventricular (AV) node, through the Purkinje conduction system, to the ventricular muscle (Figure 14–1). Normal pacemaking and conduction require normal action potentials (dependent on sodium, calcium, and potassium channel activity) under appropriate autonomic control. Arrhythmias (also called dysrhythmias) are therefore defined by exclusion, ie, any rhythm that is not a normal sinus rhythm is an arrhythmia.

B. ARRHYTHMOGENIC MECHANISMS

Abnormal **automaticity** and abnormal (reentrant) **conduction** are the 2 major mechanisms for arrhythmias. A few of the clinically important arrhythmias are **atrial flutter, atrial fibrillation** (AF), **atrioventricular nodal**

reentry (a common type of supraventricular tachycardia [SVT]), **premature ventricular beats** (PVBs), **ventricular tachycardia** (VT), and **ventricular fibrillation** (VF). Examples of electrocardiographic recordings of normal sinus rhythm and some of these common arrhythmias are shown in Figure 14–2. **Torsade de pointes** is a ventricular arrhythmia of great pharmacologic importance because it is often *induced* by antiarrhythmic and other drugs that prolong the QT interval. It has the electrocardiographic morphology of a polymorphic ventricular tachycardia, often displaying waxing and waning QRS amplitude. Torsade is also associated with **long QT syndrome,** a heritable abnormal prolongation of the QT interval caused by mutations in the I_K or I_{Na} channel molecules.

C. NORMAL ELECTRICAL ACTIVITY IN THE CARDIAC CELL

The cellular action potentials shown in Figure 14–1 are the result of ion fluxes through voltage-gated channels and carrier mechanisms. These processes are diagrammed

---

HIGH-YIELD TERMS TO LEARN

Abnormal automaticity	Pacemaker activity that originates anywhere other than in the sinoatrial node
Abnormal conduction	Conduction of an impulse that does not follow the path defined in Figure 14–1 or reenters tissue previously excited
Atrial, ventricular fibrillation	Arrhythmias involving rapid reentry and chaotic movement of impulses through the tissue of the atria or ventricles; ventricular, but not atrial, fibrillation is fatal if not terminated within a few minutes
Class (group) I, II, III, and IV drugs	A method for classifying antiarrhythmic drugs, sometimes called the Singh-Vaughan Williams classification; based loosely on the channel or receptor affected
Reentrant arrhythmias	Arrhythmias of abnormal conduction; they involve the repetitive movement of an impulse through tissue previously excited by the same impulse
Effective refractory period	The period that must pass after the upstroke of a conducted impulse in a part of the heart before a new action potential can be propagated in that cell or tissue
Selective depression	The ability of certain drugs to selectively depress areas of excitable membrane that are most susceptible, leaving other areas relatively unaffected
Supraventricular tachycardia	A reentrant arrhythmia that travels through the AV node; it may also be conducted through atrial and ventricular tissue as part of the reentrant circuit
Ventricular tachycardia	A very common arrhythmia, often associated with myocardial infarction; ventricular tachycardia may involve abnormal automaticity or abnormal conduction, usually impairs cardiac output, and may deteriorate into ventricular fibrillation; for these reasons it requires prompt management

---

in Figure 14–3. In most parts of the heart, sodium current (I_{Na}) dominates the upstroke (phase 0) of the action potential (AP) and is the most important determinant of its conduction velocity. After a very brief activation, the sodium current enters a more prolonged period of inactivation. In the AV node, calcium current (I_{Ca}) dominates the upstroke and the AP conduction velocity. The plateau of the AP (phase 2) is dominated by calcium current (I_{Ca}) and a potassium repolarizing current (I_K). At the end of the plateau, I_K causes rapid repolarization (phase 3).

The refractory period of the cardiac cell is a function of how rapidly sodium channels recover from inactivation. Recovery from inactivation depends on both the membrane potential, which varies with repolarization time and the extracellular potassium concentration, and the actions of drugs that bind to the sodium channel (ie, sodium channel blockers). The carrier processes (sodium pump and sodium–calcium exchanger) contribute little to the shape of the AP (but they are critical for the maintenance of the ion gradients on which the sodium, calcium, and potassium currents depend). Antiarrhythmic drugs act on 1 or more of the 3 major currents (I_{Na}, I_{Ca}, I_K) or on the β adrenoceptors that modulate these currents.

D. DRUG CLASSIFICATION

The antiarrhythmic agents are usually classified using a system loosely based on the channel or receptor involved. This system specifies 4 classes or groups, usually denoted by Roman numerals I–IV, plus 1 miscellaneous group.

  I. Sodium channel blockers
  II. Beta adrenoceptor blockers
  III. Potassium channel blockers
  IV. Calcium channel blockers

The **miscellaneous** group includes adenosine, potassium ion, and magnesium ion.

CLASS I ANTIARRHYTHMICS (LOCAL ANESTHETICS)

A. PROTOTYPES

The class I drugs are further subdivided on the basis of their effects on action potential duration. Class IA agents (prototype **procainamide**) prolong the AP. Class IB drugs (prototype **lidocaine**) shorten the AP in some cardiac tissues. Class IC drugs (prototype **flecainide**) have no effect on AP duration.

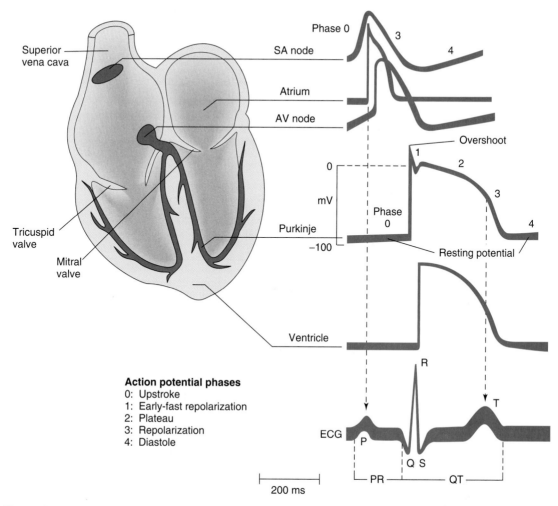

Action potential phases
0: Upstroke
1: Early-fast repolarization
2: Plateau
3: Repolarization
4: Diastole

Figure 14–1. Schematic representation of the heart and normal cardiac electrical activity (intracellular recordings from areas indicated and ECG). The ECG is the body surface manifestation of the depolarization and repolarization waves of the heart. The P wave is generated by atrial depolarization, the QRS by ventricular muscle depolarization, and the T wave by ventricular repolarization. The PR interval is a measure of conduction time from atrium to ventricle through the AV node, and the QRS duration indicates the time required for all of the ventricular cells to be activated (ie, the intraventricular conduction time). The QT interval reflects the duration of the ventricular action potential.

B. Mechanism of Action

All class I drugs slow or block conduction in ischemic and depolarized cells and slow or abolish abnormal pacemakers wherever these processes depend on sodium channels. The most selective agents (those in class IB) have significant effects on sodium channels in ischemic tissue but minimal effect on channels in normal cells. In contrast, less selective class I drugs (classes IA and IC) cause some reduction of I_{Na} even in normal cells.

Useful sodium channel-blocking drugs bind to their receptors much more readily when the channel is open or inactivated than when it is fully repolarized and recovered from its previous activity. Ion channels in arrhythmic tissue spend more time in the open or inactivated states than do channels in normal tissue. Therefore, these antiarrhythmic drugs block channels in abnormal tissue more effectively than channels in normal tissue. As a result, antiarrhythmic sodium channel blockers are **use dependent** or **state dependent** in their action (ie, they selectively depress tissue that is frequently depolarizing, eg, during a fast tachycardia; or tissue that is relatively depolarized during rest, eg, by

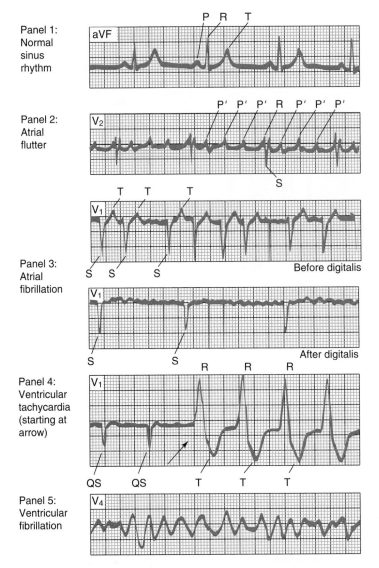

Figure 14–2. Typical ECGs of normal sinus rhythm and some common arrhythmias. Major waves (P, Q, R, S, and T) are labeled in each electrocardiographic record except in panel 5, in which electrical activity is completely disorganized and none of these deflections are recognizable. (Modified and reproduced, with permission, from Goldman MJ: *Principles of Clinical Electrocardiography,* 11th ed. McGraw-Hill, 1982.)

hypoxia). The effects of the major class I drugs are summarized in Table 14–1 and in Figure 14–4.

1. Drugs with class IA action—Procainamide is a class IA prototype. Other drugs with class IA actions include quinidine and disopyramide. **Amiodarone,** often classified as class III, also has typical class IA actions. These drugs affect both atrial and ventricular arrhythmias. They block I_{Na}, and therefore slow conduction velocity in the atria, Purkinje fibers, and ventricular cells. At high doses they also slow AV conduction. The reduction in ventricular conduction results in increased QRS duration in the ECG. In addition, these drugs block I_K. Therefore, they increase AP duration and the effective refractory period (ERP) in addition to slowing conduction velocity and ectopic pacemakers. The increase in AP duration generates an increase in QT interval (Table 14–1). Amiodarone has similar effects on sodium current and has the greatest AP-prolonging effect.

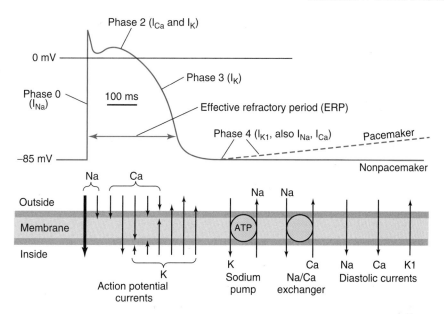

Figure 14–3. Components of the membrane action potential (AP) in a typical Purkinje or ventricular cardiac cell. The deflections of the AP, designated as phases 0–3, are generated by several ionic currents. The actions of the sodium pump and sodium–calcium exchanger are mainly involved in maintaining ionic steady state during repetitive activity. Note that small but significant currents occur during diastole (phase 4) in addition to the pump and exchanger activity. In nonpacemaker cells, the outward potassium current during phase 4 is sufficient to maintain a stable negative resting potential as shown by the solid line at the right end of the tracing. In pacemaker cells, however, the potassium current is smaller and the depolarizing currents (sodium, calcium, or both) during phase 4 are large enough to gradually depolarize the cell during diastole (shown by the dashed line).

2. Drugs with class IB actions—**Lidocaine** is the prototype IB drug and is used exclusively by the IV or IM routes. **Mexiletine** is an orally active IB agent. Lidocaine selectively affects ischemic or depolarized Purkinje and ventricular tissue and has little effect on atrial tissue; the drug reduces AP duration in some cells, but because it slows recovery of sodium channels from inactivation it does not shorten (and may even prolong) the effective refractory period. Mexiletine has similar effects. Because these agents have little effect on normal cardiac cells, they have little effect on the ECG (Table 14–1). **Phenytoin**, an anticonvulsant and not a true local anesthetic, is sometimes classified with the class IB antiarrhythmic agents because it can be used to reverse digitalis-induced arrhythmias. It resembles lidocaine in lacking significant effects on the normal ECG.

3. Drugs with class IC action—**Flecainide** is the prototype drug with class IC actions. **Encainide** and **propafenone** are also members of this class. These drugs have no effect on ventricular AP duration or the QT interval. They are powerful depressants of sodium current, however, and can markedly slow conduction velocity in atrial and ventricular cells. They increase the QRS duration of the ECG.

C. PHARMACOKINETICS

See Table 14–1.

D. CLINICAL USES AND TOXICITIES

1. Class IA drugs—Procainamide can be used in all types of arrhythmias: atrial and ventricular arrhythmias may be responsive. Quinidine and disopyramide have similar effects but are used much less frequently. Procainamide is also commonly used in arrhythmias during the acute phase of myocardial infarction.

Procainamide may cause hypotension (especially when used parenterally) and a reversible syndrome similar to lupus erythematosus. Quinidine causes cinchonism (headache, vertigo, tinnitus); cardiac depression; gastrointestinal upset; and autoimmune reactions (eg, thrombocytopenic purpura). As noted in Chapter 13, quinidine reduces the clearance of digoxin and may increase the serum concentration of the glycoside

Table 14–1. Properties of the prototype antiarrhythmic drugs.

Drug	Class	Half-life	Route	PR Interval	QRS Duration	QT Interval
Adenosine	Misc	3 s	IV	↑↑↑	—	—
Amiodarone	III, I A	1–10 weeks	Oral, parenteral	↑	↑↑	↑↑↑↑
Disopyramide	I A	6–8 h	Oral	↓ or ↑[a]	↑↑	↑↑
Esmolol	II	10 min	IV	↑↑	—	—
Flecainide	I C	20 h	Oral	↑ (slight)	↑↑	—
Ibutilide	III	6 h	IV	—	—	↑↑↑
Lidocaine	I B	1–2 h	IV	—	—[b]	—
Mexiletine	I B	12 h	Oral	—	—[b]	—
Procainamide	I A	3–4 h	Oral, IV	↑ or ↓[a]	↑↑	↑↑
Propranolol	II	3.5–6 h	Oral, IV	↑↑	—	—
Quinidine	I A	6 h	Oral, IV	↓ or ↑[a]	↑↑	↑↑↑
Sotalol	III, II	7 h	Oral	↑↑	—	↑↑↑
Verapamil	IV	7 h	Oral, IV	↑↑	—	—

[a]PR interval may decrease due to antimuscarinic action or increase due to channel blocking action.
[b]Lidocaine, mexiletine, and some other class I B drugs slow conduction through ischemic, depolarized ventricular cells but not in normal tissue.

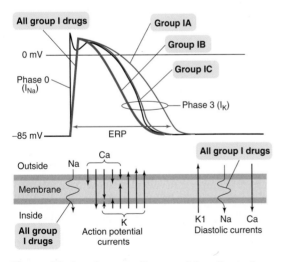

Figure 14–4. Schematic diagram of the effects of class I agents. Note that all class I drugs reduce both phase 0 and phase 4 sodium currents in susceptible cells (shown as wavy lines). Class IA drugs also reduce potassium current (I_K) and prolong the AP duration. This results in significant prolongation of the effective refractory period. Class IB and class IC drugs have different (or no) effects on potassium current and thus shorten or have no effect on the AP duration.

significantly. Disopyramide has marked antimuscarinic effects and may precipitate heart failure. All class IA drugs may precipitate new arrhythmias. Torsade de pointes is particularly associated with quinidine and other drugs that prolong AP duration (except amiodarone). The toxicities of amiodarone are discussed below.

Hyperkalemia usually exacerbates the cardiac toxicity of class I drugs. Treatment of overdose with these agents is often carried out with sodium lactate (to reverse drug-induced arrhythmias) and pressor sympathomimetics (to reverse drug-induced hypotension) if indicated.

2. Class IB drugs—Lidocaine is useful in acute ischemic ventricular arrhythmias, eg, following myocardial infarction. Atrial arrhythmias are not responsive unless caused by digitalis. Mexiletine has similar actions and is given orally. Lidocaine is usually given intravenously, but intramuscular administration is also possible. It is never given orally because it has a very high first-pass effect and its metabolites are potentially cardiotoxic.

Lidocaine and mexiletine rarely cause typical local anesthetic toxicity (ie, CNS stimulation, including convulsions); cardiovascular depression (usually minor); and allergy (usually rashes but may extend to anaphylaxis). These drugs may also precipitate arrhythmias, but this is much less common than with class IA drugs. Hyperkalemia increases cardiac toxicity.

3. Class IC drugs—Flecainide is effective in both atrial and ventricular arrhythmias but is approved only for refractory ventricular tachycardias and for certain intractable supraventricular arrhythmias. Flecainide and its congeners are more likely than other antiarrhythmic drugs to exacerbate or precipitate arrhythmias (*proarrhythmic* effect). This toxicity was dramatically demonstrated by the Cardiac Arrhythmia Suppression Trial (CAST), a large clinical trial of the prophylactic use of class IC drugs in myocardial infarction survivors. The trial results showed that class IC drugs caused greater mortality than placebo. For this reason, the class IC drugs are now restricted to use in persistent arrhythmias that fail to respond to other drugs. These drugs also cause local anesthetic-like CNS toxicity. Hyperkalemia increases the cardiac toxicity of these agents.

CLASS II ANTIARRHYTHMICS (BETA-BLOCKERS)

A. PROTOTYPES, MECHANISMS, AND EFFECTS

Beta-blockers are discussed in more detail in Chapter 10. **Propranolol** and **esmolol** are prototype antiarrhythmic β-blockers. Their mechanism in arrhythmias is primarily cardiac β-adrenoceptor blockade and reduction in cAMP, which results in the reduction of both sodium and calcium currents and the suppression of abnormal pacemakers. The AV node is particularly sensitive to β-blockers; the PR interval is usually prolonged by class II drugs (Table 14–1). Under some conditions, these drugs may have some direct local anesthetic (sodium channel-blocking) effect in the heart, but this is probably rare at the concentrations achieved clinically. Sotalol and amiodarone, generally classified as class III drugs, also have class II β-blocking effects.

B. CLINICAL USES AND TOXICITIES

Esmolol, a very short-acting β-blocker for intravenous administration, is used exclusively in acute arrhythmias. Propranolol, metoprolol, and timolol are commonly used as prophylactic drugs in patients who have had a myocardial infarction. These drugs provide a protective effect for 2 years or longer after the infarct.

SKILL KEEPER:
CHARACTERISTICS OF
β-BLOCKERS (SEE CHAPTER 10)

Describe the important subgroups of β-blockers and their major pharmacokinetic and pharmacodynamic features. The Skill Keeper Answer appears at the end of the chapter.

The toxicities of β-blockers are the same in patients with arrhythmias as in patients with other conditions. While patients with arrhythmias are often more prone to β-blocker-induced depression of cardiac output than are patients with normal hearts, it must be noted that judicious use of these drugs reduces progression of chronic heart failure (Chapter 13) and reduces the incidence of potentially fatal arrhythmias in this condition.

CLASS III ANTIARRHYTHMICS (POTASSIUM I_K CHANNEL BLOCKERS)

A. PROTOTYPES

Sotalol and **ibutilide** are typical class III drugs. Sotalol is a chiral compound (ie, it has 2 optical isomers). One isomer is an effective β-blocker, and both isomers contribute to the antiarrhythmic action. The clinical preparation contains both isomers. **Dofetilide** is a newer potassium channel-blocking drug. **Amiodarone** is usually classified as a class III drug because it markedly prolongs AP duration as well as blocking sodium channels.

B. MECHANISM AND EFFECTS

The hallmark of class III drugs is prolongation of the AP duration. This AP prolongation is caused by blockade of I_K potassium channels that are responsible for the repolarization of the AP (Figure 14–5). AP prolongation

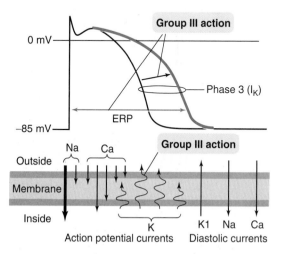

Figure 14–5. Schematic diagram of the effects of class III agents. All class III drugs prolong the AP duration in susceptible cardiac cells by reducing the outward (repolarizing) phase 3 potassium current (I_K, wavy lines). The main effect is to prolong the effective refractory period. Note that the phase 4 diastolic potassium current (I_{K1}) is not affected by these drugs.

results in an increase in effective refractory period and reduces the ability of the heart to respond to rapid tachycardias. Sotalol, ibutilide, dofetilide, and amiodarone (and quinidine; see prior discussion) produce this effect on most cardiac cells; the action of these drugs is, therefore, apparent in the ECG as an increase in QT interval. *N*-Acetylprocainamide (NAPA), a metabolite of procainamide, also significantly prolongs the AP and the QT interval.

C. CLINICAL USES AND TOXICITIES

Sotalol is commonly used and is available by the oral route (Table 14–1). Sotalol may precipitate torsade de pointes arrhythmia as well as signs of excessive β-blockade such as sinus bradycardia or asthma. Ibutilide and dofetilide are recommended for atrial flutter and fibrillation. Their most important toxicity is induction of torsade de pointes. The toxicities of class IA drugs (which share the I_K potassium channel-blocking action of class III agents) are discussed with the class IA drugs.

D. AMIODARONE: A SPECIAL CASE

Amiodarone is effective in most types of arrhythmias and is considered the most efficacious of all antiarrhythmic drugs. This may be because it has a broad spectrum: It blocks sodium, calcium, and potassium channels and β adrenoceptors. Because of its toxicities, however, amiodarone is approved for use mainly in arrhythmias that are resistant to other drugs. Nevertheless, it is used very extensively, off label, in a wide variety of arrhythmias because of its superior efficacy.

Amiodarone causes microcrystalline deposits in the cornea and skin, thyroid dysfunction (hyper- or hypothyroidism), paresthesias, tremor, and pulmonary fibrosis. Amiodarone rarely causes new arrhythmias, perhaps because it blocks calcium channels and β receptors as well as sodium and potassium channels. **Dronedarone**, an amiodarone analog that may be less toxic, is investigational.

CLASS IV ANTIARRHYTHMICS (CALCIUM CHANNEL BLOCKERS)

A. PROTOTYPE

Verapamil is the prototype. **Diltiazem** is also an effective antiarrhythmic drug, although it is not approved for this purpose. Nifedipine and the other dihydropyridines are *not* useful as antiarrhythmics, probably because they decrease arterial pressure sufficiently to evoke a compensatory sympathetic discharge to the heart. The latter effect facilitates rather than suppresses arrhythmias.

B. MECHANISM AND EFFECTS

Verapamil and diltiazem are effective in arrhythmias that must traverse calcium-dependent cardiac tissue (eg, the atrioventricular node). These agents cause a state- and use-dependent selective depression of calcium current in tissues that require the participation of L-type calcium channels (Figure 14–6). AV conduction velocity is decreased and effective refractory period increased by these drugs. PR interval is consistently increased (Table 14–1).

C. CLINICAL USE AND TOXICITIES

Calcium channel blockers are effective for converting atrioventricular nodal reentry (also known as nodal tachycardia) to normal sinus rhythm. Their major use is in the prevention of these nodal arrhythmias in patients prone to recurrence. These drugs are orally active; verapamil (Table 14–1) and diltiazem are also available for parenteral use. The most important toxicity of these drugs is excessive pharmacologic effect, because cardiac contractility, AV conduction, and blood pressure can be significantly depressed. See Chapter 12 for additional discussion of toxicity. Amiodarone has moderate calcium channel-blocking activity.

MISCELLANEOUS ANTIARRHYTHMIC DRUGS

A. ADENOSINE

Adenosine is a normal component of the body, but when it is given in high doses (6–12 mg) as an intravenous bolus the drug markedly slows or completely blocks conduction in the atrioventricular node (Table 14–1), probably by hyperpolarizing this tissue (through increased I_{K1}) and by reducing calcium current. Adenosine is extremely effective in abolishing AV nodal arrhythmias, and because of its very low toxicity it has become the drug of choice for this arrhythmia. Adenosine has an extremely short duration of action (about 15 s). Toxicity includes flushing and hypotension, but because of their short duration these effects do not limit the use of the drug. Transient chest pain and dyspnea (probably due to bronchoconstriction) may also occur.

B. POTASSIUM ION

Potassium depresses ectopic pacemakers, including those caused by digitalis toxicity. Hypokalemia is associated with an increased incidence of arrhythmias, especially in patients receiving digitalis. Conversely, excessive potassium levels depress conduction and can cause reentry arrhythmias. Therefore, when treating arrhythmias, serum potassium should be measured and normalized if abnormal.

C. MAGNESIUM ION

Magnesium appears to have similar depressant effects as potassium on digitalis-induced arrhythmias. Magnesium

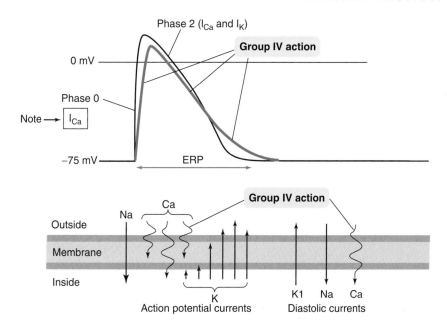

Figure 14–6. Schematic diagram of the effects of class IV drugs in a calcium-dependent cardiac cell in the AV node (note that the AP upstroke in this figure is due mainly to calcium current). Class IV drugs reduce inward calcium current during the AP and during phase 4 (wavy lines). As a result, conduction velocity is slowed in the AV node and refractoriness is prolonged. Pacemaker depolarization during phase 4 is slowed as well if caused by excessive calcium current.

also appears to be effective in some cases of torsade de pointes arrhythmia.

NONPHARMACOLOGIC TREATMENT OF ARRHYTHMIAS

It should be noted that electrical methods of treatment of arrhythmias have become very important. These methods include (1) external defibrillation, (2) implanted defibrillators, (3) implanted pacemakers, and (4) radiofrequency ablation of arrhythmogenic foci via a catheter.

QUESTIONS

1–3. An elderly patient with rheumatoid arthritis and chronic heart disease is being considered for treatment with procainamide. She is already receiving digoxin, hydrochlorothiazide, and potassium supplements for her cardiac condition.

KEY DRUGS		
Subclass	**Prototypes**	**Other Significant Agents**
IA	Procainamide	Amiodarone, quinidine
IB	Lidocaine	Mexiletine
IC	Flecainide	Propafenone
II	Propranolol	Esmolol, sotalol
III	Sotalol, amiodarone	Ibutilide, dofetilide
IV	Verapamil	Diltiazem
Miscellaneous	Adenosine	Potassium, magnesium

1. In making your decision to treat with procainamide, which of the following statements would be most relevant?
   (A) Procainamide may worsen or precipitate hyperthyroidism
   (B) Procainamide is not effective for atrial arrhythmias
   (C) Procainamide prolongs the action potential and may precipitate torsade de pointes arrhythmia
   (D) Procainamide commonly induces thrombocytopenia
   (E) Procainamide commonly induces headache and tinnitus

2. In deciding on a treatment regimen with procainamide for this patient, which of the following statements is MOST correct?
   (A) A possible drug interaction with digoxin suggests that digoxin blood levels should be obtained before and after starting procainamide
   (B) Hyperkalemia should be avoided to reduce the likelihood of procainamide toxicity
   (C) Procainamide cannot be used if the patient has asthma because it has a β-blocking effect
   (D) Procainamide has a duration of action of 20–30 h
   (E) Procainamide is not active by the oral route

3. If this patient should manifest severe acute procainamide toxicity from an overdose, rational therapy would entail the immediate administration of
   (A) A calcium chelator such as EDTA
   (B) Digitalis
   (C) KCl
   (D) Nitroprusside
   (E) Sodium lactate

4. When used as an antiarrhythmic drug, lidocaine typically
   (A) Increases action potential duration
   (B) Increases contractility
   (C) Increases PR interval
   (D) Reduces abnormal automaticity
   (E) Reduces resting potential

5. Which of the following drugs is NOT suitable for chronic oral therapy of arrhythmias?
   (A) Amiodarone
   (B) Disopyramide
   (C) Esmolol
   (D) Quinidine
   (E) Verapamil

6. A 16-year-old girl is found to have paroxysmal attacks of rapid heart rate. The antiarrhythmic of choice in most cases of *acute* AV nodal tachycardia is

   (A) Adenosine
   (B) Amiodarone
   (C) Flecainide
   (D) Propranolol
   (E) Quinidine

7. A patient is admitted to the emergency department for evaluation of an abnormal ECG. Overdose of an antiarrhythmic drug is considered. Which of the following drugs is correctly paired with its ECG effects?
   (A) Quinidine: increased PR and decreased QT intervals
   (B) Flecainide: increased PR, QRS, and QT intervals
   (C) Verapamil: increased PR interval
   (D) Lidocaine: decreased QRS and PR interval
   (E) Metoprolol: increased QRS duration

8. Which of the following drugs does NOT consistently reduce the potassium (I_K) repolarizing current and thereby prolong the action potential duration?
   (A) Amiodarone
   (B) Ibutilide
   (C) Lidocaine
   (D) Quinidine
   (E) Sotalol

9. Recognized adverse effects of quinidine include which one of the following?
   (A) Cinchonism
   (B) Constipation
   (C) Lupus erythematosus
   (D) Increase in digoxin clearance
   (E) Pulmonary fibrosis

10. A drug that hyperpolarizes and prevents conduction of impulses in the AV node is
    (A) Adenosine
    (B) Digoxin
    (C) Lidocaine
    (D) Quinidine
    (E) Verapamil

11. Which of the following drugs is used by the oral route, blocks sodium channels, and decreases action potential duration in ischemic tissue?
    (A) Adenosine
    (B) Amiodarone
    (C) Disopyramide
    (D) Esmolol
    (E) Flecainide
    (F) Lidocaine
    (G) Mexiletine
    (H) Procainamide
    (I) Quinidine
    (J) Verapamil

12. Which of the following slows conduction through the atrioventricular node and has its primary action directly on L-type calcium channels?
    (A) Adenosine
    (B) Amiodarone
    (C) Disopyramide
    (D) Esmolol
    (E) Flecainide
    (F) Lidocaine
    (G) Mexiletine
    (H) Procainamide
    (I) Quinidine
    (J) Verapamil

13. Which of the following has the longest half-life of all antiarrhythmic drugs?
    (A) Adenosine
    (B) Amiodarone
    (C) Disopyramide
    (D) Esmolol
    (E) Flecainide
    (F) Lidocaine
    (G) Mexiletine
    (H) Procainamide
    (I) Quinidine
    (J) Verapamil

14. A drug was tested in the electrophysiology laboratory to determine its effects on the cardiac action potential in ventricular cells. The results are shown in the diagram. Which of the following drugs does this agent most resemble?

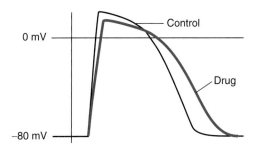

    (A) Adenosine
    (B) Flecainide
    (C) Lidocaine
    (D) Procainamide
    (E) Verapamil

ANSWERS

1. Procainamide prolongs refractory period by blocking sodium channels and by prolonging the AP. All of the other statements are false. The answer is **C**.

2. Hyperkalemia facilitates procainamide toxicity. Procainamide is active by the oral route and has a duration of action of 2–4 h (in the prompt-release form). Procainamide has no documented interaction with digoxin and little or no β-blocking action. The answer is **B**.

3. The most effective therapy for procainamide toxicity appears to be concentrated sodium lactate. This drug may (1) increase sodium current by increasing the ionic gradient and (2) reduce drug-receptor binding by alkalinizing the tissue. The answer is **E**.

4. Lidocaine reduces automaticity in the ventricles; the drug does not alter resting potential or AP duration and does not increase contractility. The answer is **D**.

5. Esmolol is an ester that is rapidly metabolized even when given intravenously; it is inactive by the oral route. Therefore, esmolol would not be suitable for chronic therapy. The answer is **C**.

6. Calcium channel blockers are effective in supraventricular tachycardias. However, adenosine is just as effective in most acute nodal tachycardias and is less toxic because of its extremely short duration of action. The answer is **A**.

7. All the associations listed are incorrect except verapamil. This class IV drug increases PR interval. The answer is **C**.

8. All of the IA drugs and class III agents reduce potassium current during phase 3 and prolong the AP. Lidocaine, the prototype IB drug, actually shortens the duration under some circumstances. The answer is **C**.

9. Quinidine, derived from the bark of the cinchona tree, has a wide spectrum of adverse effects but causes increased—not decreased—gastrointestinal motility and often results in diarrhea. Procainamide causes lupus; quinidine causes thrombocytopenia; amiodarone causes pulmonary fibrosis. The answer is **A**.

10. The only antiarrhythmic agent that consistently alters the resting potential of the AV node is adenosine. It apparently activates I_{K1} potassium channels in the AV node, thus forcing the membrane potential closer to the Nernst potassium potential; thus, adenosine significantly hyperpolarizes this tissue, preventing the conduction of action potentials. The answer is **A**.

11. Class IB drugs such as lidocaine and mexiletine typically block sodium channels and decrease the AP duration. Mexiletine—but not lidocaine—is orally active. The answer is **G**.

12. Verapamil is the calcium channel blocker in this list. (Adenosine and β-blockers also slow AV conduction

but do not act directly on calcium channels.) The answer is **J**.

13. Amiodarone has the longest half-life of all the antiarrhythmics (Table 14–1). The answer is **B**.

14. The drug effect shown in the diagram includes slowing of the upstroke of the AP and prolongation of repolarization. This is most typical of class IA drugs. The answer is **D,** procainamide.

SKILL KEEPER ANSWER: CHARACTERISTICS OF β-BLOCKERS (SEE CHAPTER 10)

The major subgroups of β-blockers and their pharmacologic features are conveniently listed in a table:

β-Blocker Subgroup, Features	Examples
Nonselective	Propranolol and timolol are typical
β₁-selective	Atenolol, acebutolol, and metoprolol are typical; possibly less hazardous in asthmatic patients
Partial agonist	Acebutolol and pindolol are typical; possibly less hazardous in asthmatic patients
Lacking local anesthetic effect	Timolol is the prototype; important for use in glaucoma
Low lipid solubility	Atenolol is the prototype; may reduce CNS toxicity
Very short and long acting	Esmolol (an ester) is the shortest-acting and used only IV; nadolol is the longest-acting
Combined β and α blockade	Carvedilol, labetalol

CHECKLIST

When you complete this chapter, you should be able to:

☐ Describe the distinguishing electrophysiologic and ECG features of the 4 major classes of antiarrhythmic drugs and adenosine.

☐ List 2 or 3 of the most important drugs in each of the 4 classes.

☐ List the major toxicities of those drugs.

☐ Describe the mechanism of selective depression by local anesthetic antiarrhythmic agents.

☐ Explain how hyperkalemia, hypokalemia, or an antiarrhythmic drug can cause an arrhythmia.

Diuretic Agents

Each segment of the nephron—proximal convoluted tubule (PCT), thick ascending limb of the loop of Henle (TAL), distal convoluted tubule (DCT), and cortical collecting tubule (CCT)—has a different mechanism for reabsorbing sodium and other ions. The subgroups of the sodium-excreting diuretics are based on these sites and processes in the nephron. Several other drugs alter water excretion predominantly. The effects of the diuretic agents are predictable from a knowledge of the function of the segment of the nephron in which they act.

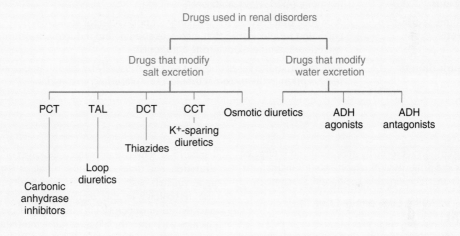

RENAL TRANSPORT MECHANISMS & DIURETIC DRUG GROUPS

The major transport mechanisms in the various segments of the nephron are shown in Figure 15–1.

A. PROXIMAL CONVOLUTED TUBULE (PCT)

This segment carries out isosmotic reabsorption of amino acids, glucose, and numerous cations. It is also the major site for sodium chloride and sodium bicarbonate reabsorption. The proximal tubule is responsible for 60–70% of the total reabsorption of sodium. No currently available drug directly acts on NaCl reabsorption in the PCT. The mechanism for bicarbonate reabsorption is shown in Figure 15–2. Bicarbonate itself is poorly reabsorbed through the luminal membrane, but conversion of bicarbonate to carbon dioxide via carbonic acid permits rapid reabsorption of the carbon dioxide. Bicarbonate can then be regenerated from carbon dioxide within the tubular cell and transported into the interstitium. Sodium is separately reabsorbed from the lumen in exchange for hydrogen ions and transported into the interstitial space by the sodium pump. Carbonic anhydrase, the enzyme required for the bicarbonate reabsorption process on the brush border and in the cytoplasm, is the target of **carbonic anhydrase inhibitor diuretic drugs.** Active secretion and reabsorption of weak acids and bases also occurs in the proximal tubule. Most weak acid transport occurs in the straight S_2 segment, distal to the convoluted part.

HIGH-YIELD TERMS TO LEARN

Bicarbonate diuretic	A diuretic that selectively increases sodium bicarbonate excretion. Example: a carbonic anhydrase inhibitor.
Diluting segment	A segment of the nephron that removes solute without water; the thick ascending limb and the distal convoluted tubule are active salt-absorbing segments that are not permeant to water
Hyperchloremic metabolic acidosis	A shift in body electrolyte and pH balance involving elevated chloride, diminished bicarbonate concentration, and a decrease in pH in the blood. Typical result of bicarbonate diuresis.
Hypokalemic metabolic alkalosis	A shift in body electrolyte balance and pH involving a decrease in serum potassium and an increase in blood pH. Typical result of loop and thiazide diuretic actions.
Nephrogenic diabetes insipidus	Loss of urine-concentrating ability in the kidney caused by lack of responsiveness to antidiuretic hormone (ADH is normal or high)
Pituitary diabetes insipidus	Loss of urine-concentrating ability in the kidney caused by lack of antidiuretic hormone (ADH is low or absent)
Potassium-sparing diuretic	A diuretic that reduces the exchange of potassium for sodium in the collecting tubule; a drug that increases sodium and reduces potassium excretion. Example: aldosterone antagonists.
Uricosuric diuretic	A diuretic that increases uric acid excretion, usually by inhibiting uric acid reabsorption in the proximal tubule. Example: ethacrynic acid.

Uric acid transport is especially important and is targeted by some of the drugs used in treating gout (Chapter 36). Weak bases are transported in the S_1 and S_2 segments.

B. Thick Ascending Limb of the Loop of Henle (TAL)

This segment pumps sodium, potassium, and chloride out of the lumen into the interstitium of the kidney. It is also a major site of calcium and magnesium reabsorption, as shown in Figure 15–3. Reabsorption of sodium, potassium, and chloride are all accomplished by a single carrier, which is the target of the **loop diuretics.** This cotransporter provides part of the concentration gradient for the countercurrent concentrating mechanism in the kidney and is responsible for the reabsorption of 20–30% of the sodium filtered at the glomerulus. Because potassium is pumped into the cell from both the luminal and basal sides, an escape route must be provided; this occurs into the lumen via a potassium-selective channel. Because the potassium diffusing through these channels is not accompanied by an anion, a net positive charge is set up in the lumen. This positive potential drives the reabsorption of calcium and magnesium.

C. Distal Convoluted Tubule (DCT)

This segment actively pumps sodium and chloride out of the lumen of the nephron via the carrier shown in

Figure 15–4. This cotransporter is the target of the **thiazide diuretics.** The distal convoluted tubule is responsible for approximately 5–8% of sodium reabsorption. Calcium is also reabsorbed in this segment under the control of parathyroid hormone (PTH). Removal of the reabsorbed calcium back into the blood requires the sodium-calcium exchange process discussed in Chapter 13.

D. Cortical Collecting Tubule (CCT)

The final segment of the nephron is the last tubular site of sodium reabsorption and is controlled by aldosterone (Figure 15–5). This segment is responsible for reabsorbing 2–5% of the total filtered sodium. The reabsorption of sodium occurs via channels (not a transporter) and is accompanied by an equivalent loss of potassium or hydrogen ions. The collecting tubule is thus the primary site of acidification of the urine and of potassium excretion. The aldosterone receptor and the sodium channels are sites of action of the **potassium-sparing diuretics.** Reabsorption of water occurs in the medullary collecting tubule under the control of antidiuretic hormone (ADH).

E. Diuretic Drug Groups

Because the mechanisms for reabsorption of salt and water differ in each of the 4 segments discussed above, the diuretics acting in these segments each have differing

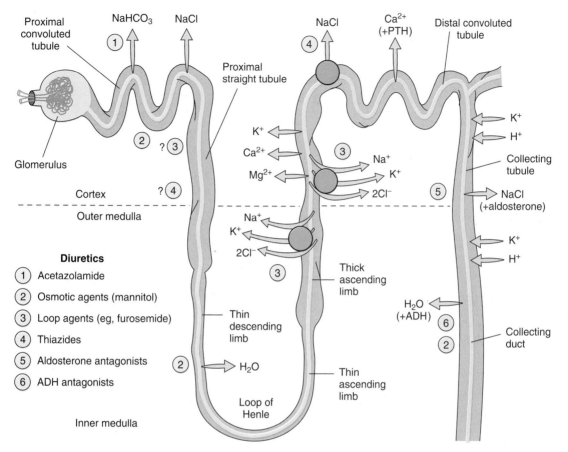

Figure 15–1. Tubule transport systems and sites of action of diuretics. Circles with arrows denote known ion cotransporters that are targets of the diuretics indicated by the numerals. Question marks denote preliminary or incompletely documented suggestions for the location of certain drug effects. (Reproduced, with permission, from Katzung BG, editor: *Basic & Clinical Pharmacology*, 10th ed. McGraw-Hill, 2007.)

mechanisms of action. Most diuretics act from the luminal side of the membrane and must be present in the urine. They are filtered at the glomerulus and some are also secreted by the weak acid-secretory carrier in the proximal tubule. An exception is the aldosterone receptor antagonist group (eg, spironolactone and eplerenone), drugs that enter the collecting tubule cell from the basolateral side and bind to the cytoplasmic aldosterone receptor.

CARBONIC ANHYDRASE INHIBITORS

A. PROTOTYPES AND MECHANISM OF ACTION

Acetazolamide is the prototypical agent. These diuretics are sulfonamide derivatives. The mechanism of action is inhibition of carbonic anhydrase in the brush border and intracellular carbonic anhydrase in the PCT cells

(Figure 15–2). Inhibition of carbonic anhydrase by acetazolamide also occurs in other tissues of the body.

B. EFFECTS

The major renal effect is bicarbonate diuresis (ie, sodium bicarbonate is excreted); body bicarbonate is thus depleted, and metabolic acidosis results. As increased sodium is presented to the cortical collecting tubule, some of the excess sodium is reabsorbed and potassium is secreted, resulting in significant potassium "wasting" (Table 15–1). As a result of bicarbonate depletion, sodium bicarbonate excretion slows—even with continued diuretic administration—and the diuresis is self-limiting within 2–3 days. The inhibitory effect of acetazolamide occurs throughout the body; secretion of bicarbonate into aqueous humor by the ciliary epithelium in the eye and into the cerebrospinal fluid by the choroid plexus is

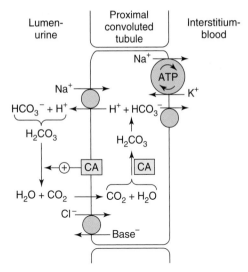

Figure 15–2. Mechanism of sodium bicarbonate reabsorption in the proximal tubule cell. CA, carbonic anhydrase. (Reproduced, with permission, from Katzung BG, editor: *Basic & Clinical Pharmacology*, 10th ed. McGraw-Hill, 2007.)

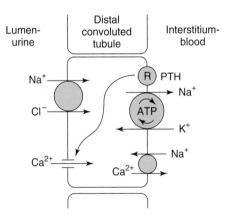

Figure 15–4. Mechanism of sodium and chloride reabsorption by the transporter NCC in the distal convoluted tubule. A separate reabsorptive mechanism, modulated by parathyroid hormone, is present for movement of calcium into the cell from the urine. This calcium must be transported via the sodium-calcium exchanger back into the blood. (Reproduced, with permission, from Katzung BG, editor: *Basic & Clinical Pharmacology*, 10th ed. McGraw-Hill, 2007.)

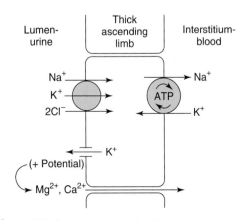

Figure 15–3. Mechanism of sodium, potassium, and chloride reabsorption by the transporter NKCC2 in the thick ascending limb of the loop of Henle. Note that pumping of potassium into the cell from both the lumen and the interstitium would result in unphysiologically high intracellular K^+ concentration. This is avoided by movement of K^+ down its concentration gradient back into the lumen, carrying with it excess positive charge. This positive charge drives the reabsorption of calcium and magnesium. (Reproduced, with permission, from Katzung BG, editor: *Basic & Clinical Pharmacology*, 10th ed. McGraw-Hill, 2007.)

reduced. In the eye, a useful reduction in intraocular pressure can be achieved. This effect is not self-limiting. In the CNS, acidosis of the cerebrospinal fluid results in hyperventilation, which can protect against high-altitude sickness.

C. CLINICAL USES

The major application of carbonic anhydrase inhibitors is in the treatment of glaucoma (Table 10–3). Acetazolamide must be administered orally, but topical analogs are now available (dorzolamide, brinzolamide) for use in the eye. Carbonic anhydrase inhibitors are also used to prevent acute mountain (high-altitude) sickness. These agents are used for their diuretic effect only if edema is accompanied by significant metabolic alkalosis.

D. TOXICITY

Drowsiness and paresthesias are commonly reported after oral therapy. Cross allergenicity between these and all other sulfonamide derivatives (other sulfonamide diuretics, hypoglycemic agents, antibacterial sulfonamides) is uncommon but does occur. Alkalinization of the urine by these drugs may cause precipitation of calcium salts and formation of renal stones. Renal potassium wasting may be marked. Patients with hepatic impairment may develop hepatic encephalopathy because of increased ammonia reabsorption.

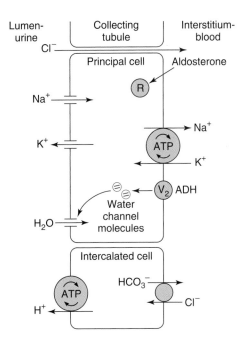

Figure 15–5. Mechanism of sodium, potassium, and hydrogen ion movement in the collecting tubule cells. Synthesis of Na$^+$/K$^+$ ATPase, and the epithelial sodium channels (ENaC) and potassium channels is under the control of aldosterone, which combines with an intracellular receptor, *R*, before entering the nucleus. (Reproduced, with permission, from Katzung BG, editor: *Basic & Clinical Pharmacology*, 10th ed. McGraw-Hill, 2007.)

LOOP DIURETICS

A. PROTOTYPES AND MECHANISM OF ACTION

Furosemide is the prototypical loop agent. Furosemide, bumetanide, and torsemide are sulfonamide derivatives. **Ethacrynic acid** is a phenoxyacetic acid derivative; it is not a sulfonamide but acts by the same mechanism.

Loop diuretics inhibit the cotransport of sodium, potassium, and chloride (Figure 15–3). The loop diuretics are relatively short acting (diuresis usually occurs over a 4-h period following a dose).

B. EFFECTS

The loop of Henle is responsible for a significant fraction of total renal sodium chloride reabsorption; therefore, a full dose of a loop diuretic produces a massive sodium chloride diuresis. If tissue perfusion is adequate, edema fluid is rapidly excreted and blood volume may be significantly reduced. The diluting ability of the nephron is reduced because the loop of Henle is the site of significant dilution of urine. Inhibition of the Na$^+$/K$^+$/2Cl$^-$ transporter also results in loss of the lumen-positive potential, which reduces reabsorption of divalent cations as well. As a result, calcium excretion is significantly increased. Ethacrynic acid is a moderately effective uricosuric drug if blood volume is maintained. The presentation of large amounts of sodium to the collecting tubule may result in significant potassium wasting and excretion of protons; hypokalemic alkalosis may result (Table 15–1). The loop diuretics also have potent pulmonary vasodilating effects; the mechanism is not known.

Prostaglandins are important in maintaining glomerular filtration. When synthesis of prostaglandins is inhibited, as with nonsteroidal anti-inflammatory drugs (chapter 36), the efficacy of diuretics—especially loop diuretics—decreases.

C. CLINICAL USE

The major application of loop diuretics is in the treatment of edematous states (eg, heart failure, ascites). They are particularly valuable in acute pulmonary edema, in which the pulmonary vasodilating action plays a useful role. They are sometimes used in hypertension if response to thiazides is inadequate, but the short duration of action of loop diuretics is a disadvantage in this condition. A less common but important application is in the treatment of severe hypercalcemia (eg, that induced by malignancy). This life-threatening condition can often be managed with large doses of furosemide coupled with parenteral

Table 15–1. Electrolyte changes produced by diuretic drugs.

Group	Amount in Urine			Body pH
	NaCl	NaHCO$_3$	K$^+$	
Carbonic anhydrase inhibitors	↑	↑↑↑	↑	Acidosis
Loop diuretics	↑↑↑↑	—	↑	Alkalosis
Thiazides	↑↑	↑,—	↑	Alkalosis
K$^+$-sparing diuretics	↑	—	↓	Acidosis

volume and electrolyte (sodium and potassium chloride) supplementation. It should be noted that diuresis *without* volume replacement will result in hemoconcentration; serum calcium concentration then will not diminish and may even increase further.

D. TOXICITY

Loop diuretics usually induce hypokalemic metabolic alkalosis. Because large amounts of sodium are presented to the collecting tubules, wasting of potassium (which is excreted by the kidney in an effort to conserve sodium) may be severe. Because they are so efficacious, the loop diuretics can cause hypovolemia and cardiovascular complications. Ototoxicity is an important toxic effect of the loop agents. The sulfonamides in this group may cause typical sulfonamide allergy.

THIAZIDE DIURETICS

A. PROTOTYPES AND MECHANISM OF ACTION

Hydrochlorothiazide, the prototypical agent, and all the other members of this group are sulfonamide derivatives. A few derivatives that lack the typical thiazide ring in their structure nevertheless have effects identical to those of thiazides and are therefore considered thiazide-like. Thiazides are active by the oral route and have a duration of action of 6–12 h, considerably longer than most loop diuretics. The major action of thiazides is to inhibit sodium chloride transport in the early segment of the distal convoluted tubule (Figure 15–4).

B. EFFECTS

In full doses, thiazides produce moderate but sustained sodium and chloride diuresis. Hypokalemic metabolic alkalosis may occur (Table 15–1). Reduction in the transport of sodium from the lumen into the tubular cell reduces intracellular sodium and promotes sodium-calcium exchange at the basolateral membrane. As a result, reabsorption of calcium from the urine is increased and urine calcium content is decreased—the *opposite* of the effect of loop diuretics. Because they act in a diluting segment of the nephron, thiazides may reduce the excretion of water and cause dilutional hyponatremia. Thiazides also reduce blood pressure, and the maximal pressure-lowering effect occurs at doses lower than the maximal diuretic doses (Chapter 11).

When a thiazide is used with a loop diuretic, a synergistic effect occurs with marked diuresis.

C. CLINICAL USE

The major application of thiazides is in hypertension, for which their long duration and moderate intensity of action are particularly useful. Chronic therapy of edematous conditions such as mild heart failure is another application, although loop diuretics are usually preferred. Chronic renal calcium stone formation can sometimes be controlled with thiazides because of their ability to reduce urine calcium concentration.

D. TOXICITY

Massive sodium diuresis with hyponatremia is an uncommon but dangerous early effect of thiazides. Chronic therapy is often associated with potassium wasting, since an increased sodium load is presented to the collecting tubules. Diabetic patients may have significant hyperglycemia. Serum uric acid and lipid levels are also increased in some individuals. Thiazides are sulfonamides and share potential sulfonamide allergenicity.

POTASSIUM-SPARING DIURETICS

A. PROTOTYPES AND MECHANISM OF ACTION

Spironolactone and **eplerenone** are steroid derivatives and act as pharmacologic antagonists of aldosterone in the collecting tubules. By combining with and blocking the intracellular aldosterone receptor, these drugs reduce the expression of genes controlling synthesis of epithelial sodium ion channels and Na^+/K^+ ATPase. **Amiloride** and **triamterene** act by blocking the epithelial sodium channels in the same portion of the nephron (Figure 15–5). (These drugs do *not* block I_{Na} channels in excitable membranes.) Spironolactone and eplerenone have slow onsets and offsets of action (24–72 h). Amiloride and triamterene have durations of action of 12–24 h.

B. EFFECTS

All drugs in this class cause an increase in sodium clearance and a decrease in potassium and hydrogen ion excretion and therefore qualify as potassium-sparing diuretics. They may cause hyperkalemic metabolic acidosis (Table 15–1).

C. CLINICAL USE

Potassium wasting caused by chronic therapy with loop or thiazide diuretics, if not controlled by dietary potassium supplements, will usually respond to these drugs. The most common use is in the form of products that combine a thiazide with a potassium-sparing agent in a single pill.

Aldosteronism (eg, the elevated serum aldosterone levels that occur in cirrhosis) is an important indication for spironolactone. Aldosteronism is also a feature of heart failure, and spironolactone and eplerenone have been shown to have significant long-term benefits in this condition (Chapter 13). Some of this effect may occur in the heart, an action that is not yet understood.

D. TOXICITY

The most important toxic effect is hyperkalemia. These drugs should never be given with potassium supplements. Other aldosterone antagonists (such as ACE inhibitors and angiotensin receptor blockers), if used at all, should be used with caution. Spironolactone can cause endocrine abnormalities, including gynecomastia and antiandrogenic effects. Eplerenone appears to have less endocrine effect.

 SKILL KEEPER: DIURETIC COMBINATIONS AND ELECTROLYTES (SEE CHAPTER 13)

Describe the possible interactions of cardiac glycosides (digoxin) with the major classes of diuretics. The Skill Keeper Answer appears at the end of the chapter.

OSMOTIC DIURETICS

A. PROTOTYPES AND MECHANISM OF ACTION

Mannitol, the prototypical osmotic diuretic, is given intravenously. Other drugs often classified with mannitol (but rarely used) include glycerin, isosorbide, and urea. Because it is freely filtered at the glomerulus but poorly reabsorbed from the tubule, mannitol remains in the lumen and "holds" water by virtue of its osmotic effect. The major location for this action is the proximal convoluted tubule, where the bulk of isosmotic reabsorption normally occurs. Reabsorption of water is also reduced in the descending limb of the loop of Henle and the collecting tubule.

B. EFFECTS

The volume of urine is increased. Most filtered solutes will be excreted in larger amounts unless they are actively reabsorbed. Sodium excretion is usually increased because the rate of urine flow through the tubule is greatly accelerated and sodium transporters cannot handle the volume rapidly enough. Mannitol can also reduce brain volume and intracranial pressure by osmotically extracting water from the tissue into the blood. A similar effect occurs in the eye.

C. CLINICAL USE

These drugs are used to maintain high urine flow (eg, when renal blood flow is reduced and in conditions of solute overload from severe hemolysis or rhabdomyolysis). Mannitol and several other osmotic agents are useful in reducing intraocular pressure in acute glaucoma and intracranial pressure in neurologic conditions.

D. TOXICITY

Removal of water from the intracellular compartment may cause hyponatremia and pulmonary edema. As the water is excreted, hypernatremia may follow. Headache, nausea, and vomiting are common.

ANTIDIURETIC HORMONE AGONISTS & ANTAGONISTS

A. PROTOTYPES AND MECHANISM OF ACTION

Antidiuretic hormone (ADH) and **desmopressin** are prototypical ADH agonists. They are peptides and must be given parenterally. **Demeclocycline** and **conivaptan** are ADH *antagonists.* Lithium has ADH-antagonist effects but is never used for this purpose.

ADH facilitates water reabsorption from the collecting tubule by activation of V_2 receptors, which stimulate adenylyl cyclase via G_s. The increased cAMP causes the insertion of additional aquaporin AQP2 water channels into the luminal membrane in this part of the tubule (Figure 15–6). Conivaptan is an ADH inhibitor at V_{1a} and V_2 receptors. Demeclocycline and lithium inhibit the action of ADH at some point distal to the generation of cAMP and presumably interfere with the insertion of water channels into the membrane.

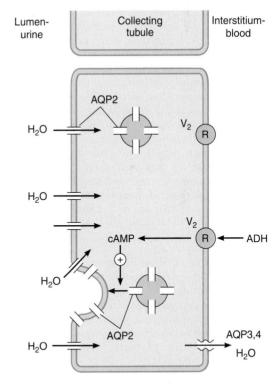

Figure 15–6. Mechanism of water transport across the membranes of collecting duct cells. Aquaporins 3 and 4 (AQP3, 4) are normally present in the basolateral membranes, but the luminal water channel, AQP2, is inserted only in the presence of ADH or similar antidiuretic peptides acting on the vasopressin V_2 receptor. (Reproduced, with permission, from Katzung BG, editor: *Basic & Clinical Pharmacology,* 10th ed. McGraw-Hill, 2007.)

KEY DRUGS		
Subclass	**Prototypes**	**Other Significant Drugs**
Carbonic anhydrase inhibitors	Acetazolamide	
Loop diuretics	Furosemide, ethacrynic acid	
Thiazides and thiazide-like drugs	Hydrochlorothiazide	Metolazone
Potassium-sparing diuretics	Spironolactone, amiloride	Eplerenone
Osmotic diuretics	Mannitol	
ADH agonists	Vasopressin (ADH)	Desmopressin
ADH antagonists	Demeclocycline, conivaptan	Lithium

B. Effects and Clinical Uses

ADH and desmopressin reduce urine volume and increase its concentration. ADH and desmopressin are useful in pituitary diabetes insipidus. They are of no value in the nephrogenic form of the disease, but salt restriction, thiazides, and loop diuretics may be used. These therapies reduce blood volume, a very strong stimulus to proximal tubular reabsorption. The proximal tubule thus substitutes—in part—for the deficient concentrating function of the collecting tubule.

ADH antagonists oppose the actions of ADH and other naturally occurring peptides that act on the same V_2 receptor. Such peptides are produced by certain tumors (eg, small cell carcinoma of the lung) and can cause significant water retention and dangerous hyponatremia. This **syndrome of inappropriate ADH secretion (SIADH)** can be treated with demeclocycline and conivaptan. Lithium also works but has greater toxicity.

C. Toxicity

In the presence of ADH or desmopressin, a large water load may cause dangerous hyponatremia. Large doses of either peptide may cause hypertension in some individuals.

In children younger than 8 years, demeclocycline (like other tetracyclines) causes bone and teeth abnormalities. Lithium causes nephrogenic diabetes insipidus as a toxic effect; because of its other toxicities, the drug is never used to treat SIADH.

QUESTIONS

1. A 70-year-old man is admitted with a history of heart failure and an acute left ventricular myocardial infarction. He has severe pulmonary edema. Which of the following drugs is MOST likely to prove useful in the treatment of acute pulmonary edema?
   (A) Acetazolamide
   (B) Furosemide
   (C) Hydrochlorothiazide
   (D) Mannitol
   (E) Spironolactone

2. A 50-year-old man has a history of frequent episodes of renal colic with high-calcium renal stones. The most useful diuretic agent in the treatment of recurrent calcium stones is
   (A) Acetazolamide
   (B) Furosemide
   (C) Hydrochlorothiazide
   (D) Mannitol
   (E) Spironolactone

3. When used chronically, thiazide diuretics have all of the following properties or effects EXCEPT
   (A) Decreased urinary excretion of calcium
   (B) Elevation of blood cholesterol
   (C) Elevation of blood glucose
   (D) Elevation of plasma uric acid
   (E) Ototoxicity

4. Which of the following drugs is correctly associated with its site of action and maximal diuretic efficacy?
   (A) Acetazolamide—collecting duct—15% of filtered Na^+
   (B) Furosemide—thick ascending limb—20–30%
   (C) Metolazone—collecting tubule—2%
   (D) Thiazides—distal convoluted tubule—25%
   (E) Spironolactone—proximal convoluted tubule—40%

5. A patient with long-standing diabetic renal disease and hyperkalemia and recent-onset heart failure requires a diuretic. Which of the following agents would be the safest in a patient with severe hyperkalemia?
   (A) Amiloride
   (B) Hydrochlorothiazide

(C) Losartan
(D) Spironolactone
(E) Triamterene

6. Which of the following diuretics would be most useful in a comatose patient with cerebral edema?
(A) Acetazolamide
(B) Amiloride
(C) Ethacrynic acid
(D) Furosemide
(E) Mannitol

7. Which of the following is associated with use of thiazide diuretics?
(A) Hypocalciuria
(B) Hypernatremia
(C) Hyperkalemia
(D) Hypouricemia
(E) Metabolic acidosis

8. Which of the following therapies would be most useful in the management of severe hypercalcemia?
(A) Amiloride plus saline infusion
(B) Furosemide plus saline infusion
(C) Hydrochlorothiazide plus saline infusion
(D) Mannitol plus saline infusion
(E) Spironolactone plus saline infusion

9. A 60-year-old patient complains of paresthesias and occasional nausea associated with one of her drugs. She is found to have hyperchloremic metabolic acidosis. She is probably taking
(A) Acetazolamide for glaucoma
(B) Amiloride for edema associated with aldosteronism
(C) Furosemide for severe hypertension and heart failure
(D) Hydrochlorothiazide for hypertension
(E) Mannitol for cerebral edema

10. A 70-year-old woman is admitted to the emergency department because of a "fainting spell" at home. She appears to have suffered no trauma from her fall, but her blood pressure is 110/60 when lying down and 60/40 when she sits up. Neurologic examination and an ECG are within normal limits when she is lying down. Questioning reveals that she has recently started taking "water pills" (diuretics) for a heart condition. Which of the following drugs is the most likely cause of her fainting spell?
(A) Acetazolamide
(B) Amiloride
(C) Furosemide
(D) Hydrochlorothiazide
(E) Spironolactone

11. A 55-year-old patient with severe posthepatitis cirrhosis is started on a diuretic for another condition. Two days later he is found in a coma. The drug most likely to cause coma in a patient with cirrhosis is
(A) Acetazolamide
(B) Amiloride
(C) Furosemide
(D) Hydrochlorothiazide
(E) Spironolactone

12. A drug that has its major effect in the distal convoluted tubule is
(A) Acetazolamide
(B) Amiloride
(C) Demeclocycline
(D) Desmopressin
(E) Ethacrynic acid
(F) Furosemide
(G) Hydrochlorothiazide
(H) Mannitol
(I) Spironolactone
(J) Triamterene

13. A drug that increases the formation of dilute urine in water-loaded subjects and is used to treat SIADH is
(A) Acetazolamide
(B) Amiloride
(C) Conivaptan
(D) Desmopressin
(E) Ethacrynic acid
(F) Furosemide
(G) Hydrochlorothiazide
(H) Mannitol
(I) Spironolactone
(J) Triamterene

14. A drug that is useful in acute glaucoma and high-altitude sickness is
(A) Acetazolamide
(B) Amiloride
(C) Demeclocycline
(D) Desmopressin
(E) Ethacrynic acid

ANSWERS

1. Loop diuretics have a rapid onset of action, are very efficacious, and appear to have significant direct smooth muscle-relaxing effects in the pulmonary vessels. They are therefore drugs of choice in acute pulmonary edema. The only drug in the list that is a loop agent is furosemide. The answer is **B**.

2. The thiazides are useful in the prevention of calcium stones because these drugs inhibit the renal excretion of calcium. In contrast, the loop agents facilitate calcium excretion. The answer is **C**.

3. Thiazides do not cause ototoxicity; loop diuretics do. The answer is **E**.

4. Spironolactone acts in the collecting tubule, not the proximal convoluted tubule. Furosemide, a loop diuretic, can produce a 20–30% increase in sodium excretion. Metolazone, a thiazide-like drug, acts in the distal convoluted tubule, not in the collecting tubule. The answer is **B.**

5. Hyperkalemia should not be treated with drugs that interfere with aldosterone production (eg, losartan, an angiotensin II receptor blocker) or collecting tubule potassium excretion (eg, amiloride, spironolactone, triamterene). These agents are all capable of increasing serum potassium. Hydrochlorothiazide would not reduce serum potassium rapidly, but it would not increase it. The answer is **B.**

6. An osmotic agent is needed to remove water from the cells of the edematous brain and reduce intracranial pressure rapidly. The answer is **E.**

7. Thiazides produce hypocalciuria and are sometimes used to reduce the frequency of calcium kidney stones. The answer is **A.**

8. Diuretic therapy of hypercalcemia requires a reduction in calcium reabsorption in the thick ascending limb. However, a loop diuretic alone would reduce blood volume around the remaining calcium so that serum calcium would not decrease appropriately. Therefore, saline infusion should accompany the loop diuretic. The answer is **B.**

9. Paresthesias and gastrointestinal distress are common adverse effects of acetazolamide, especially when it is taken chronically, as in glaucoma. The observation that the patient has metabolic acidosis also suggests the use of acetazolamide. The answer is **A.**

10. The case history suggests that the syncope (fainting) is associated with diuretic use. Complications of diuretics that can result in syncope include both postural hypotension (which this patient exhibits) due to excessive reduction of blood volume and arrhythmias due to excessive potassium loss. Potassium wasting is more common with thiazides (because of their long duration of action), but these drugs rarely cause reduction of blood volume sufficient to result in orthostatic hypotension. The answer is **C,** furosemide.

11. The carbonic anhydrase inhibitors cause metabolic acidosis and urinary alkalosis. Patients with severe impairment of liver function are unable to synthesize urea efficiently and become dependent on renal excretion of ammonium ion to rid the body of nitrogenous wastes. However, in alkaline urine the ammonium ion is rapidly converted to ammonia gas, which is very rapidly reabsorbed. Hyperammonemia results, with severe neurologic consequences. The answer is **A.**

12. Hydrochlorothiazide and all other thiazides and thiazide-like diuretics (eg, metolazone), act in the distal convoluted tubule. The answer is **G.**

13. Inability to form dilute urine in the fully hydrated condition is characteristic of SIADH. Antagonists of ADH are needed to treat this condition. The answer is **C.**

14. Carbonic anhydrase inhibitors are useful in glaucoma and altitude sickness. The answer is **A.**

SKILL KEEPER ANSWER: DIGITALIS AND DIURETICS (SEE CHAPTER 13)

Digoxin toxicity is facilitated by hypokalemia. Therefore, potassium-wasting diuretics (eg, loop agents, thiazides), which are often needed in heart failure, can increase the risk of a fatal digitalis arrhythmia. Carbonic anhydrase inhibitors, although also potassium-wasting agents, are rarely used for their systemic and diuretic effects and are therefore less likely to be involved in digitalis toxicity. The K^+-sparing diuretics, in contrast to the other groups, can be useful in preventing such interactions.

CHECKLIST

When you complete this chapter, you should be able to:

☐ List 5 major types of diuretics and relate them to their sites of action.

☐ Describe 2 drugs that reduce potassium loss during sodium diuresis.

☐ Describe a therapy that will reduce calcium excretion in patients who have recurrent urinary stones.

☐ Describe a treatment for severe hypercalcemia in a patient with advanced carcinoma.

☐ Describe a method for reducing urine volume in nephrogenic diabetes insipidus.

☐ List the major applications and the toxicities of thiazides, loop diuretics, and potassium-sparing diuretics.

PART IV
Drugs with Important Actions on Smooth Muscle

Histamine, Serotonin, & the Ergot Alkaloids

16

Autacoids are endogenous molecules with powerful pharmacologic effects that do not fall into traditional autonomic groups. Histamine and serotonin (5-hydroxytryptamine; 5-HT) are the most important amine autacoids. The ergot alkaloids are a heterogeneous group of drugs (not autacoids) that interact with serotonin receptors, dopamine receptors, and α receptors. They are included in this chapter because of their effects on serotonin receptors and on smooth muscle. Peptide and eicosanoid autacoids are discussed in chapters 17 and 18. Nitric oxide is discussed in Chapter 19.

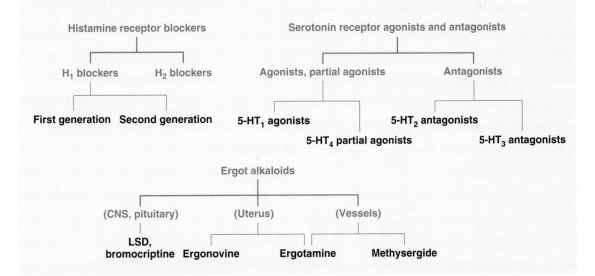

HIGH-YIELD TERMS TO LEARN

Acid-peptic disease	Disease of the upper digestive tract caused by acid and pepsin; includes erosions and ulcers
Autacoids	Endogenous substances with complex physiologic and pathophysiologic functions; commonly understood to include histamine, serotonin, prostaglandins, and vasoactive peptides
Carcinoid	A neoplasm of the bronchi or gastrointestinal tract that may secrete serotonin and a variety of peptides
Ergotism ("St. Anthony's fire")	Disease caused by excess ingestion of ergot alkaloids; classically an epidemic caused by consumption of grain (eg, in bread) that is contaminated by the ergot fungus
Gastrinoma	A tumor that produces large amounts of gastrin; associated with hypersecretion of gastric acid and pepsin leading to ulceration
IgE-mediated immediate reaction	An allergic response caused by interaction of an antigen with IgE antibodies on mast cells; results in the release of histamine and other mediators of allergy
Oxytocic	A drug that causes contraction of the uterus
Zollinger-Ellison syndrome	Syndrome of hypersecretion of gastric acid and pepsin, often caused by gastrinoma; it is associated with severe acid-peptic ulceration and diarrhea

---

HISTAMINE

Histamine is formed from the amino acid histidine and is stored in high concentrations in vesicles in mast cells, some neurons, and a few other cell types. Histamine is metabolized by the enzymes monoamine oxidase and diamine oxidase. Excess production of histamine in the body (eg, in systemic mastocytosis) can be detected by measurement of imidazoleacetic acid (its major metabolite) in the urine. Because it is released from mast cells in response to IgE-mediated (immediate) allergic reactions, this autacoid plays an important pathophysiologic role in seasonal rhinitis (hay fever), urticaria, and angioneurotic edema. Histamine also plays an important physiologic role in the control of acid secretion in the stomach and as a neurotransmitter.

A. RECEPTORS AND EFFECTS

Two receptors for histamine, H_1 and H_2, mediate most of the peripheral actions; 2 others (H_3, H_4) have also been identified (Table 16–1).

1. H_1 receptor—This G_q-coupled receptor is important in smooth muscle effects, especially those caused by IgE-mediated responses. IP_3 and DAG are the second messengers. Typical responses include bronchoconstriction and vasodilation, the latter by release of nitric oxide. Capillary endothelial cells, in addition to releasing NO and other vasodilating substances, also contract, opening gaps in the permeability barrier and leading to

the formation of local edema. These effects are manifest in allergic reactions and in mastocytosis.

2. H_2 receptor—This G_s-coupled receptor mediates gastric acid secretion by parietal cells in the stomach. It also has a cardiac stimulant effect. A third action is to reduce histamine release from mast cells—a negative feedback effect. These actions are mediated by activation of adenylyl cyclase, which increases intracellular cAMP.

3. H_3 receptor—This receptor appears to be involved mainly in presynaptic modulation of histaminergic neurotransmission in the CNS. In the periphery, it appears to be a presynaptic heteroreceptor with modulatory effects on the release of other transmitters (see Chapter 6).

4. H_4 receptor—The H_4 receptor is located on leukocytes (especially eosinophils) and mast cells and is involved in chemotactic responses by these cells.

B. CLINICAL USE

Histamine has no therapeutic applications, but drugs that block its effects at H_1 and at H_2 receptors are very important in clinical medicine. No antagonists of H_3 or H_4 receptors are currently available.

HISTAMINE H_1 ANTAGONISTS

A. CLASSIFICATION AND PROTOTYPES

A wide variety of antihistaminic H_1 blockers are available from several different chemical families. Two major

Table 16–1. Some histamine and serotonin receptor subtypes.[a]

Receptor Subtype	Distribution	Postreceptor Mechanisms	Prototype Antagonist
H_1	Smooth muscle	$G_q; \uparrow IP_3,$ DAG	Diphenhydramine
H_2	Stomach, heart, mast cells	$G_s; \uparrow$ cAMP	Cimetidine
H_3	Nerve endings, CNS	$G_i; \downarrow$ cAMP	—
H_4	Leukocytes	$G_i; \downarrow$ cAMP	—
5-HT_{1D}	Brain	$G_i; \downarrow$ cAMP	—
5-HT_2	Smooth muscle, platelets	$G_q; \uparrow IP_3,$ DAG	Ketanserin
5-HT_3	Area postrema (CNS), sensory and enteric nerves	Ligand-gated cation channel	Ondansetron
5-HT_4	Presynaptic nerve terminals in the enteric nervous sytem	$G_s; \uparrow$ cAMP	Tegaserod (partial agonist)

[a]Many other serotonin receptor subtypes are recognized in the CNS. They are discussed in Chapter 21.

subgroups or "generations" have been developed (see the drug classification at the beginning of the chapter). The older members of the first-generation agents, typified by **diphenhydramine,** are highly sedating agents with significant autonomic receptor-blocking effects. A newer subgroup of first-generation agents are less sedating and have much less autonomic effect. **Chlorpheniramine** and **cyclizine** may be considered prototypes. The second-generation H_1 blockers, typified by **fexofenadine, loratadine,** and **cetirizine,** are far less lipid soluble than the first-generation agents and have reduced sedating and autonomic effects. Because they have been developed for use in chronic conditions, all H_1 blockers are active by the oral route. Most are metabolized extensively in the liver. Half-lives of the older H_1 blockers vary from 4 h to 12 h. Most newer agents (eg, fexofenadine, cetirizine, loratadine) have half-lives of 12–24 h.

B. MECHANISM AND EFFECTS

H_1 blockers are competitive pharmacologic antagonists at the H_1 receptor; these drugs have no effect on histamine release from storage sites. They are more effective if given before histamine release occurs.

Because their structure closely resembles that of muscarinic blockers and α adrenoceptor blockers, many of the first-generation agents are potent pharmacologic antagonists at these autonomic receptors. A few also block serotonin receptors. As noted, most older first-generation agents are sedating, and some—not all—first-generation agents have anti-motion sickness effects. Many H_1 blockers are potent local anesthetics.

H_1-blocking drugs have negligible effects at H_2 receptors.

C. CLINICAL USE

H_1 blockers have major applications in allergies of the immediate type (ie, those caused by antigens acting on IgE antibody-sensitized mast cells). These conditions include hay fever and urticaria.

Diphenhydramine, dimenhydrinate, cyclizine, meclizine, and promethazine are used as anti-motion sickness drugs. Diphenhydramine is also used for management of chemotherapy-induced vomiting.

Adverse effects of the drugs are sometimes exploited therapeutically (eg, in their use as hypnotics in over-the-counter sleep aids).

D. TOXICITY AND INTERACTIONS

Sedation is common, especially with diphenhydramine and promethazine. It is much less common with second-generation agents, which do not enter the CNS readily. Antimuscarinic effects such as dry mouth and blurred vision occur with some first-generation drugs in some patients. Alpha-blocking actions, which are significant with phenothiazine derivatives such as promethazine, may cause orthostatic hypotension.

Interactions occur between older antihistamines and other drugs with sedative effects (eg, benzodiazepines and alcohol). Drugs that inhibit hepatic metabolism may result in dangerously high levels of certain antihistaminic drugs that are taken concurrently. For example, azole antifungal drugs and certain other CYP3A4 inhibitors interfere with the metabolism of astemizole and terfenadine, 2 second-generation agents that have been withdrawn from the US market because high plasma concentrations of either antihistamine can precipitate lethal arrhythmias.

HISTAMINE H₂ ANTAGONISTS

A. CLASSIFICATION AND PROTOTYPES

Four H_2 blockers are available; **cimetidine** is the prototype. **Ranitidine, famotidine,** and **nizatidine** differ only in being slightly less toxic than cimetidine. These drugs do not resemble H_1 blockers structurally. They are orally active, with half-lives of 1–3 h. Because they are relatively nontoxic, they can be given in large doses, so that the duration of action of a single dose may be 12–24 h.

B. MECHANISM AND EFFECTS

These drugs produce a surmountable pharmacologic blockade of histamine H_2 receptors. They are relatively selective and have no significant blocking actions at H_1 or autonomic receptors. The only therapeutic effect of clinical importance is the reduction of gastric acid secretion, but this is a very useful action. Blockade of cardiovascular and mast cell H_2 receptor-mediated effects can be demonstrated but has no clinical significance.

C. CLINICAL USE

In acid-peptic disease, especially duodenal ulcer, these drugs reduce symptoms, accelerate healing, and prevent recurrences. Acute ulcer is usually treated with 2 or more doses per day, whereas recurrence of ulcers can often be prevented with a single bedtime dose. H_2 blockers are also effective in accelerating healing and preventing recurrences of gastric peptic ulcers. Intravenous H_2 blockers are useful in preventing gastric erosions and hemorrhage that occur in stressed patients in intensive care units. In Zollinger-Ellison syndrome, which is characterized by acid hypersecretion, severe recurrent peptic ulceration, gastrointestinal bleeding, and diarrhea, these drugs are helpful but large doses are required, and they are not as effective as proton pump inhibitors. Similarly, the H_2 blockers have been used in gastroesophageal reflux disease (GERD), but they are not as effective as proton pump inhibitors (see Chapter 60).

SKILL KEEPER: ANTIHISTAMINE
ADVERSE EFFECTS
(SEE CHAPTERS 8 AND 10)

An elderly dental patient was given promethazine intravenously to reduce anxiety before undergoing an extraction in the dental office. Promethazine is an older first-generation antihistamine. Predict the CNS and autonomic effects of this drug when given intravenously. The Skill Keeper Answer appears at the end of the chapter.

D. TOXICITY

Cimetidine is a potent inhibitor of hepatic drug-metabolizing enzymes and may also reduce hepatic blood flow. Cimetidine also has significant antiandrogen effects in patients receiving high doses. Ranitidine has a weaker inhibitory effect on hepatic drug metabolism; neither it nor the other H_2 blockers appear to have any endocrine effects.

SEROTONIN (5-HYDROXYTRYPTAMINE; 5-HT) & RELATED AGONISTS

Serotonin is produced from tryptophan and stored in vesicles in the enterochromaffin cells of the gut and neurons of the CNS and ENS. After release, it is metabolized by monoamine oxidase. Excess production in the body (eg, in carcinoid syndrome) can be detected by measuring its major metabolite, 5-hydroxyindoleacetic acid (5-HIAA), in the urine. Serotonin plays a physiologic role as a neurotransmitter in both the CNS and the enteric nervous system and may have a role as a local hormone that modulates gastrointestinal activity. Serotonin is also stored (but synthesized to only a minimal extent) in platelets. In spite of the very large number of serotonin receptors (14 identified to date), most of the serotonin *agonists* in clinical use act at $5-HT_{1D}$ receptors. Recently, a partial agonist that acts at $5-HT_4$ receptors was approved for use for gastrointestinal disease, but withdrawn from general use shortly thereafter. Serotonin antagonists in use or under investigation act at $5-HT_2$ and $5-HT_3$ receptors (see drug classification at the beginning of the chapter).

A. RECEPTORS AND EFFECTS

1. 5-HT₁ receptors—$5-HT_1$ receptors are most important in the brain and mediate synaptic inhibition via increased potassium conductance (Table 16–1). Peripheral $5-HT_1$ receptors mediate both excitatory and inhibitory effects in various smooth muscle tissues. $5-HT_1$ receptors are G_i protein-coupled receptors.

2. 5-HT₂ receptors—$5-HT_2$ receptors are important in both brain and peripheral tissues. These receptors mediate synaptic excitation in the CNS and smooth muscle contraction (gut, bronchi, uterus, vessels) or relaxation (other vessels). The mechanisms involve (in different tissues) increased IP_3, decreased potassium conductance, and decreased cAMP. This receptor class probably mediates some of the vasodilation, diarrhea, and bronchoconstriction that occur as symptoms of carcinoid tumor, a neoplasm that releases serotonin and other substances.

3. 5-HT₃ receptors—$5-HT_3$ receptors are found in the CNS, especially in the chemoreceptive area and vomiting center, and in peripheral sensory and enteric nerves. These receptors mediate excitation via a

5-HT-gated cation channel. Antagonists acting at this receptor have proved to be extremely useful antiemetic drugs.

4. 5-HT$_4$ receptors—5-HT$_4$ receptors are found in the gastrointestinal tract and play a role in intestinal motility.

B. Clinical Use

Serotonin has no clinical applications.

C. Other Serotonin Agonists

1. 5-HT$_{1D}$ agonists—**Sumatriptan,** a substituted indole compound, is the prototype. **Naratriptan** and other "-triptans" are similar to sumatriptan. They are effective in the treatment of acute migraine and cluster headache attacks, an observation that strengthens the association of serotonin abnormalities with these headache syndromes. These drugs are active orally; sumatriptan is also available for parenteral administration. Ergot alkaloids, discussed later, are partial agonists at some 5-HT receptors.

2. 5-HT$_4$ Partial agonist—**Tegaserod** is a newer drug that acts as an agonist in the colon. It was approved and briefly marketed for use in chronic constipation, but because of cardiovascular toxicity, its use is now restricted.

3. Serotonin reuptake inhibitors—A number of important antidepressant drugs act to increase activity at central serotonergic synapses by inhibiting the reuptake carrier for 5-HT. These drugs are discussed in Chapter 30. **Dexfenfluramine** (now withdrawn because of cardiotoxicity) was a reuptake inhibitor used exclusively for its appetite-reducing effect. Dexfenfluramine was combined with phentermine, an amphetamine-like anorexiant, in a weight-loss product known as "fen-phen."

SEROTONIN ANTAGONISTS

A. Classification and Prototypes

Ketanserin, phenoxybenzamine, and **cyproheptadine** are effective 5-HT$_2$ blockers. **Ondansetron, granisetron, dolasetron,** and **alosetron** are 5-HT$_3$ blockers. The **ergot alkaloids** are partial agonists (and therefore have some antagonist effects) at 5-HT and other receptors (see later discussion).

B. Mechanisms and Effects

Ketanserin and cyproheptadine are competitive pharmacologic 5-HT$_2$ antagonists. Phenoxybenzamine is an irreversible blocker at this receptor.

Ketanserin, cyproheptadine, and phenoxybenzamine are poorly selective agents. In addition to inhibition of serotonin effects, they also have α-blocking effects (ketanserin, phenoxybenzamine) or H$_1$ blocking effects (cyproheptadine).

Ondansetron, granisetron, and dolasetron are selective 5-HT$_3$ receptor blockers and have a central antiemetic action in the area postrema of the medulla and also on peripheral sensory and enteric nerves.

C. Clinical Uses

Ketanserin has been studied as an antihypertensive drug. Ketanserin, cyproheptadine, and phenoxybenzamine may be of value (separately or in combination) in the treatment of carcinoid tumor, a neoplasm that secretes large amounts of serotonin (and peptides) and causes diarrhea, bronchoconstriction, and flushing.

Ondansetron and its congeners are extremely useful in the control of vomiting associated with cancer chemotherapy and postoperative vomiting. **Alosetron,** another 5-HT$_3$ antagonist, is used in the treatment of women with irritable bowel syndrome associated with diarrhea.

D. Toxicity

Adverse effects of ketanserin are those of α blockade and H$_1$ blockade. The toxicities of ondansetron, granisetron, and dolasetron include diarrhea and headache. Dolasetron has been associated with QRS and QT$_c$ prolongation in the ECG and should not be used in patients with heart disease. Alosetron causes significant constipation in some patients and has been associated with fatal bowel complications.

ERGOT ALKALOIDS

These complex molecules are produced by a fungus found in wet or spoiled grain. They are responsible for the epidemics of "St. Anthony's fire" (ergotism) described during the Middle Ages and up to the present time. There are at least 20 naturally occurring members of the family, but only a few of these and a handful of semisynthetic derivatives are used as therapeutic agents. The ergot alkaloids are partial agonists at α adrenoceptors and 5-HT receptors. The balance of α adrenoceptor versus 5-HT affinity and agonist versus antagonist effect varies from compound to compound and even differs among tissues. Some ergot alkaloids are also agonists at the dopamine receptor.

A. Classification and Effects

The ergot alkaloids may be divided into 3 major subgroups on the basis of the organ or tissue in which they have their primary effects. The receptor effects of the ergot alkaloids are summarized in Table 16–2 and are most marked in the following tissues:

1. Vessels—Ergot alkaloids can produce marked and prolonged α-receptor-mediated vasoconstriction. **Ergotamine** is the prototype. An overdose can cause ischemia and gangrene of the limbs. Because they are partial agonists, the drugs may also block the α-agonist effects of sympathomimetics.

Table 16–2. Effects of some ergot alkaloids at several receptors.

Ergot Alkaloid	Alpha Receptor (α_1)	Dopamine Receptor (D_2)	Serotonin Receptor (5-HT$_2$)	Uterine Smooth Muscle Stimulation
Bromocriptine	−	+++	−	0
Ergonovine	+	+	− (PA)	+++
Ergotamine	− (PA)	0	+ (PA)	+++
Lysergic acid diethylamide (LSD)	+/0	+++	− −/++ in CNS	+

Reproduced, with permission, from Katzung BG, editor: *Basic & Clinical Pharmacology*, 10th ed. McGraw-Hill, 2007.

Agonist effects are indicated by +, antagonist by −, no effect by 0. Relative affinity for the receptor is indicated by the number of + or − signs. PA, partial agonist.

2. Uterus—Ergot alkaloids produce powerful contraction in this tissue, especially near term. **Ergonovine** is the prototype. In pregnancy, the uterine contraction is sufficient to cause abortion or miscarriage. Earlier in pregnancy (and in the nonpregnant uterus) much higher doses of ergot alkaloids are needed to produce this effect. After delivery of the placenta, ergonovine or ergotamine can produce a useful contraction of the uterus that reduces blood loss.

3. Brain—Hallucinations may be prominent with the naturally occurring ergots and with **LSD,** a semisynthetic prototypical hallucinogenic ergot derivative, but are uncommon with the therapeutic ergot derivatives. Although LSD is a potent 5-HT$_2$ blocker in peripheral tissues, its actions in the CNS are thought to be due to agonist actions at dopamine receptors. In the pituitary, some ergot alkaloids are potent dopamine-like agonists and inhibit prolactin secretion. **Bromocriptine** and **pergolide** are among the most potent of the semisynthetic ergot derivatives at these dopamine D_2 receptors in the pituitary and in the basal ganglia (see Chapter 28).

C. CLINICAL USES

1. Migraine—**Ergotamine** has been a mainstay of treatment of acute attacks. Methysergide and ergonovine have

been used for prophylaxis, but methysergide is no longer available in the United States.

2. Obstetric bleeding—**Ergonovine** and ergotamine are effective agents for the reduction of postpartum bleeding.

3. Hyperprolactinemia and parkinsonism—**Bromocriptine** and pergolide are used to reduce prolactin secretion (dopamine is the physiologic prolactin release inhibitor). Bromocriptine also appears to reduce the size of pituitary tumors of the prolactin-secreting cells. Both drugs are used in the treatment of Parkinson's disease.

D. TOXICITY

The toxic effects of ergot alkaloids are quite important, both from a public health standpoint (epidemics of ergotism from spoiled grain) and from the toxicity resulting from overdose or abuse by individuals. Intoxication of grazing animals is sometimes reported by farmers and veterinarians.

1. Vascular effects—Severe prolonged vasoconstriction can result in ischemia and gangrene. The most consistently effective antagonist is nitroprusside. When used for long periods, ergot derivatives may produce an

---

KEY DRUGS

Subclass	Prototype	Other Significant Agents
H$_1$ blockers	Diphenhydramine, loratadine	Chlorpheniramine, fexofenadine
H$_2$ blockers	Cimetidine	Ranitidine, famotidine, nizatidine
5-HT agonists	Sumatriptan, other triptans	
5-HT antagonists	Ketanserin, ondansetron	Alosetron, ergot alkaloids
Ergot alkaloids	Bromocriptine, ergonovine, ergotamine	LSD, pergolide

unusual hyperplasia of connective tissue. This fibroplasia may be retroperitoneal, retropleural, or subendocardial and can cause hydronephrosis or cardiac valvular and conduction system malfunction. Similar lesions are found in some patients with carcinoid, suggesting that this action is probably mediated by agonist effects at serotonin receptors.

2. Gastrointestinal effects—Ergot alkaloids cause gastrointestinal upset (nausea, vomiting, diarrhea) in many individuals.

3. Uterine effects—Marked uterine contractions may be produced. The uterus becomes progressively more sensitive to ergot alkaloids during pregnancy. Although abortion resulting from the use of ergot for migraine is rare, most obstetricians recommend avoidance or very conservative use of these drugs as pregnancy progresses.

4. CNS effects—Hallucinations resembling psychosis are common with LSD but less so with the other ergot alkaloids. Methysergide was occasionally used in the past as an LSD substitute by users of "recreational" drugs.

QUESTIONS

1–2. Your patient has been diagnosed with a rare metastatic carcinoid tumor. This neoplasm is releasing serotonin, bradykinin, and several unknown peptides.

1. The effects of serotonin in this patient are MOST likely to include which one of the following?
   (A) Constipation
   (B) Episodes of bronchospasm
   (C) Hypersecretion of gastric acid
   (D) Hypotension
   (E) Urinary retention

2. In recommending treatment for your carcinoid patient, the one least likely to be helpful is
   (A) Cyproheptadine
   (B) Ketanserin
   (C) Phenoxybenzamine
   (D) Sumatriptan

3. Which of the following drugs can reverse 1 or more smooth muscle effects of circulating histamine in humans?
   (A) Dolasetron
   (B) Epinephrine
   (C) Granisetron
   (D) Ranitidine
   (E) Sumatriptan

4. Many antihistamines (H_1 blockers) have additional nonhistamine-related effects; these are likely to include which one of the following?
   (A) Muscarinic increase in bladder tone
   (B) General anesthetic effects if the drug is injected

   (C) Anti-motion sickness effect
   (D) Increase in total peripheral resistance
   (E) Insomnia

5. Which of the following will result from blockade of H_2 receptors?
   (A) Decreased cAMP in cardiac muscle
   (B) Decreased channel opening in enteric nerves
   (C) Decreased IP_3 in gastric mucosa
   (D) Increased IP_3 in gastric mucosa
   (E) Increased IP_3 in smooth muscle

6. Toxicities of certain H_2 antihistamines include which one of the following?
   (A) Blurred vision
   (B) Diarrhea
   (C) Orthostatic hypotension
   (D) P450 enzyme inhibition
   (E) Sleepiness

7. All of the following statements about possible pharmacologic explanations of 16th and 17th century accounts of witchcraft are reasonable EXCEPT
   (A) Ingestion of bread made with flour from spoiled grain could cause painful burning sensations in the limbs, leading naive individuals to suspect supernatural evil forces
   (B) Similar ingestion could cause "epidemics" of abortions, with similar interpretations
   (C) Similar ingestion by elderly women might cause them to have hallucinations and exhibit behaviors interpretable by others as "casting spells"
   (D) The major substance now known to occur in spoiled grain is LSD, a substance similar to PCP

8. A patient undergoing cancer chemotherapy is vomiting frequently. A drug that might help in this situation is
   (A) Bromocriptine
   (B) Cimetidine
   (C) Ketanserin
   (D) Loratadine
   (E) Ondansetron

9. Which of the following descriptions of H_2 histamine blockers is MOST correct?
   (A) All have long half-lives of 12–24 h
   (B) All available H_2 blockers have approximately equal efficacy
   (C) Famotidine is associated with more drug interactions than other H_2 blockers as a result of inhibition of hepatic P450 systems
   (D) Ranitidine is associated with antiandrogenic effects in some patients

10. Which of the following is a correct application of the drug mentioned?

(A) Alosetron: for obstetric bleeding
(B) Cetirizine: for hay fever
(C) Ergonovine: for Alzheimer's disease
(D) Ondansetron: for acute migraine headache
(E) Ranitidine: for Parkinson's disease

11. Which of the following is most useful in the treatment of hyperprolactinemia?
(A) Bromocriptine
(B) Cimetidine
(C) Ergotamine
(D) Ketanserin
(E) LSD
(F) Ondansetron
(G) Sumatriptan

12. Which of the following is most effective in the treatment of peptic ulcer disease?
(A) Bromocriptine
(B) Cimetidine
(C) Ergotamine
(D) Ketanserin
(E) LSD
(F) Ondansetron
(G) Sumatriptan

13. Which of the following is a serotonin agonist useful for aborting an acute migraine headache and is not derived from a fungus?
(A) Bromocriptine
(B) Cimetidine
(C) Ergotamine
(D) Ketanserin
(E) LSD
(F) Ondansetron
(G) Sumatriptan

14. Which of the following is the most useful for reversing severe ergot-induced vasospasm?
(A) Bromocriptine
(B) Cimetidine
(C) Ergotamine
(D) Ketanserin
(E) LSD
(F) Nitroprusside
(G) Sumatriptan
(H) Ondansetron

ANSWERS

1. Serotonin causes bronchospasm, but the other effects listed are not observed. The answer is **B**.

2. All of the drugs listed have significant blocking effects on 5-HT receptors except sumatriptan, which is an *agonist* at 5-HT_{1D} receptors. The answer is **D**.

3. Dolasetron and granisetron are 5-HT_3 antagonists. Sumatriptan is a 5-HT_{1D} agonist. Ranitidine is a histamine antagonist but blocks the H_2 receptor in the stomach and the heart, not H_1 receptors in smooth muscle. Epinephrine has a *physiologic* antagonist action that reverses histamine's effects on smooth muscle. The answer is **B**.

4. H_1 blockers do not activate muscarinic receptors or mediate vasoconstriction, they cause local but not general anesthesia. They do not cause insomnia. The answer is **C**.

5. H_2 receptors are G_s protein-coupled receptors, like β adrenoceptors. Blockade of this system will cause a *decrease* in cAMP. The answer is **A**.

6. The older H_1 blockers, not H_2 blockers, cause blurred vision, orthostatic hypotension, and sleepiness. Neither group typically causes diarrhea. Cimetidine (unlike other H_2 blockers) is a potent CYP3A4 inhibitor. The answer is **D**.

7. Historians have noted that many of the behaviors described for accused "witches" and their purported victims during the Salem witch trials period of American history resemble signs of ergotism.

SKILL KEEPER ANSWER: ANTIHISTAMINE ADVERSE EFFECTS (SEE CHAPTERS 8 AND 10)

Promethazine very effectively alleviated the anxiety of this elderly woman. However, when she attempted to get out of the dental chair following the procedure, she experienced severe orthostatic hypotension and fainted. In the horizontal position on the floor and later on a couch, she rapidly regained consciousness. Supine blood pressure was low normal, and heart rate was elevated. When she sat up, blood pressure dropped and heart rate increased. Promethazine and several other first-generation H_1 antihistamines are effective α (and M_3) blockers (Chapters 8 and 10). After 30 min supine, the patient was able to stand without fainting and experienced only a slight tachycardia. Older antihistaminic agents readily enter the CNS, causing sedation. This patient felt somewhat sleepy for 2 h but had no further signs or symptoms. If she had glaucoma, she might be at risk for an acute angle closure episode, with markedly increased intraocular pressure as a result of the antimuscarinic action. An elderly man with prostatic hyperplasia might experience urinary retention.

Ergotism is caused by a mixture of naturally occurring ergot alkaloids, not LSD, a semisynthetic ergot derivative. LSD is not similar to PCP (phencyclidine, Chapter 32). The answer is **D.**

8. Ondansetron has significant antiemetic effects. The answer is **E.**

9. H$_2$ blockers have equal efficacies, though their potencies vary. Cimetidine has significant antiandrogenic and CYP3A4-inhibiting effects. The answer is **B.**

10. Alosetron is indicated in irritable bowel syndrome. Ergonovine is used in uterine bleeding. Ondansetron is useful for chemotherapy-induced emesis. Cetirizine is used in the treatment of hay fever. The answer is **B.**

11. Bromocriptine is an effective dopamine agonist in the CNS with the advantage of oral activity. The drug inhibits prolactin secretion by activating pituitary dopamine receptors. The answer is **A.**

12. An H$_2$ blocker is appropriate treatment for peptic ulcer; cimetidine is such a drug. The answer is **B.**

13. Sumatriptan, an agonist at 5-HT$_{1D}$ receptors, is indicated for parenteral treatment of migraine. Ergotamine is also effective for acute migraine but is produced by the fungus *Claviceps purpurea*. The answer is **G.**

14. A very powerful vasodilator is necessary to reverse ergot-induced vasospasm; nitroprusside is such a drug. The answer is **F.**

CHECKLIST

When you complete this chapter, you should be able to:

☐ List the major organ system effects of histamine and serotonin.

☐ Describe the pharmacology of the 2 generations and 3 subgroups of H$_1$ antihistamines; list prototypical agents for each subgroup.

☐ Describe the pharmacology of the H$_2$ antihistamines; name the 4 members of this group.

☐ Describe the action, indication, and toxicity of sumatriptan.

☐ Describe one 5-HT$_2$ and one 5-HT$_3$ antagonist and their major applications.

☐ List the major organ system effects of the ergot alkaloids.

☐ Describe the major clinical applications and toxicities of the ergot drugs.

Vasoactive Peptides

17

Vasoactive peptides are autacoids with significant actions on vascular smooth muscle as well as other tissues. They include vasoconstrictors, vasodilators, and peptides with mixed effects.

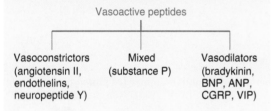

Vasoactive peptides comprise a large class of endogenous substances that function as neurotransmitters as well as local and systemic hormones. The better-known peptides include angiotensin, bradykinin, natriuretic peptides, calcitonin gene-related peptide (CGRP), endothelin, neuropeptide Y (NPY), substance P, and vasoactive intestinal peptide (VIP) (discussed in this chapter) and vasopressin (Chapters 15 and 37), glucagon (Chapter 41), and several opioid peptides (Chapter 31).

Vasoactive peptides probably all act on cell surface receptors. Most act via G protein-coupled receptors and cause the production of well-known second messengers (Table 17–1); a few may open ion channels.

ANGIOTENSIN & ITS ANTAGONISTS

A. Source and Disposition

Angiotensin I is produced from circulating angiotensinogen by **renin,** an enzyme released from the juxtaglomerular apparatus of the kidney. An inactive decapeptide, angiotensin I is converted into **angiotensin II (AII),** an active octapeptide, by **angiotensin-converting enzyme (ACE),** also known as peptidyl dipeptidase or kininase II (see Figure 11–3). Angiotensin II, the active form of the peptide, is rapidly degraded by peptidases (angiotensinases).

B. Effects

AII is a potent arteriolar vasoconstrictor and stimulant of aldosterone release. AII directly increases peripheral vascular resistance and, through aldosterone, causes renal sodium retention. AII also facilitates the release of norepinephrine from adrenergic nerve endings via presynaptic heteroreceptor action (see Chapter 6). All of these effects are mediated by the angiotensin AT_1 receptor, a G_q-coupled receptor. The AT_2 receptor appears to mediate vasodilation via nitric oxide and may be most important during fetal development.

C. Clinical Role

AII was used in the past by intra-arterial infusion to control bleeding in difficult-to-access sites. The peptide is no longer used for this indication. Its major clinical significance is as a pathophysiologic mediator in some cases of hypertension (high-renin hypertension) and in heart failure. Even in normal- and low-renin hypertension, AII *antagonists* have demonstrated clinical benefits. Therefore, AII antagonists are of considerable clinical importance.

D. Angiotensin Antagonists

As noted in Chapter 11, 2 types of antagonists are available. **ACE inhibitors** (eg, **captopril, enalapril**, others) are important agents for the treatment of hypertension and heart failure. AII receptor blockers (eg, **losartan, valsartan**, others) are orally active nonpeptide inhibitors at the AII AT_1 receptor. Block of angiotensin's effects by either of these drug types is often accompanied by a compensatory increase in renin and angiotensin I. Aliskiren, a new orally active renin inhibitor, reduces angiotensin I as well as angiotensin II and has recently been approved for use in hypertension.

VASOPEPTIDASE INHIBITORS

The vasopeptidase enzymes include neutral endopeptidase 24.11 and ACE. A new class of drugs that block both enzymes is in clinical trials, and these drugs (eg, omapatrilat) show considerable efficacy in hypertension and heart failure. Unfortunately, these drugs also cause angioedema in a significant number of patients and have not been approved for clinical use.

	HIGH-YIELD TERMS TO LEARN

Kinins	Family of vasoactive peptides associated with tissue injury and inflammation, eg, bradykinin
Natriuretic peptides	Family of peptides synthesized in brain, heart, and other tissues; have vasodilator as well as natriuretic effects
Neuropeptides	Peptides with prominent roles as neurotransmitters or modulators; many also have potent smooth muscle effects
Peptidase	Family of enzymes that activate or inactivate peptides by hydrolysis, eg, angiotensin-converting enzyme (dipeptidyl peptidase), neutral endopeptidase
Tachykinins	Group of 3 potent neuropeptides: substance P, neurokinin A, and neurokinin B
Vasoactive peptides	Peptides with prominent effects on vascular smooth muscle; many are neuro-peptides as well

BRADYKININ

A. SOURCE AND DISPOSITION

Bradykinin is one of several vasodilator **kinins** produced from kininogen by a family of enzymes, the kallikreins. Bradykinin is rapidly degraded by various peptidases, including ACE.

B. EFFECTS

Bradykinin acts through at least 2 receptors (B_1 and B_2) and causes the production of inositol 1,4,5-trisphosphate, diacylglycerol, cyclic adenosine monophosphate, nitric oxide, and prostaglandins in tissues. It is one of the most potent vasodilators known. The peptide is involved in inflammation and causes edema and pain when released or injected into tissue. Bradykinin can be found in saliva and may play a role in stimulating its secretion.

C. CLINICAL ROLE

Although it has no therapeutic application, bradykinin may play a role in the antihypertensive action of ACE inhibitors, as previously noted (see Chapter 11;

Table 17–1. Some vasoactive peptides and their properties.

Peptide	Properties
Angiotensin II (AII)	↑IP_3, DAG via AT_1 G protein-coupled receptors. Constricts arterioles, increases aldosterone secretion
Bradykinin	↑IP_3, DAG, cAMP, NO. Dilates arterioles, increases capillary permeability, stimulates sensory nerve endings
Brain natriuretic peptide (BNP)	↑cGMP via ANP_A receptors. Dilates vessels, inhibits aldosterone secretion and effects, increases glomerular filtration
Calcitonin gene-related peptide (CGRP)	An extremely potent vasodilator; causes hypotension and reflex tachycardia
Endothelins	↑IP_3, DAG via G protein-coupled ET_A and ET_B receptors. Synthesized in vascular endothelium. Constrict most vessels and contract other smooth muscle
Neuropeptide Y	Causes vasoconstriction and stimulates the heart. Effects mediated in part by IP_3
Substance P, neurokinins	Act on NK_1, NK_2, and NK_3 receptors. Dilate arterioles, contract veins, intestinal, and bronchial smooth muscle, cause diuresis; substance P is a transmitter in sensory pain neurons
Vasoactive intestinal peptide (VIP)	↑cAMP via G protein-coupled receptors VPAC1 and VPAC2. Dilates vessels, relaxes bronchi and intestinal smooth muscle

Figure 11–3). Icatibant, an orally active bradykinin B_2 receptor antagonist, is under intense study in various conditions, but at present there are no FDA-approved bradykinin antagonists.

NATRIURETIC PEPTIDES

A. Source and Disposition

Natriuretic peptides (**atrial natriuretic peptide [ANP]** and **brain natriuretic peptide [BNP]**) are synthesized and stored in the cardiac atria of mammals. BNP has also been isolated from brain tissue. They are released from the atria in response to distension of the chambers. A similar peptide, C-type natriuretic peptide, has been isolated from other tissues. BNP appears to be the most important of these peptides.

B. Effects

Natriuretic peptides activate guanylyl cyclase in many tissues. They act as vasodilators as well as natriuretic (sodium excretion-enhancing) agents. Their renal action includes increased glomerular filtration, decreased proximal tubular sodium reabsorption, and inhibitory effects on renin secretion. The peptides also inhibit the actions of AII and aldosterone. Although they lack positive inotropic action, endogenous natriuretic peptides may play an important compensatory role in congestive heart failure by limiting sodium retention. Blood levels of endogenous BNP have been shown to correlate with the severity of heart failure and can be used as a diagnostic tool.

C. Clinical Role

BNP has showed some benefit in the treatment of acute severe heart failure and is currently available for clinical use as **nesiritide.** This drug is approved for intravenous administration in acute severe heart failure (see Chapter 13) but has significant renal toxicity.

ENDOTHELINS

Endothelins are peptide vasoconstrictors formed in and released by endothelial cells in blood vessels. Endothelins are believed to function as autocrine and paracrine hormones in the vasculature. Three different endothelin peptides (ET-1, ET-2, and ET-3) with minor variations in amino acid sequence have been identified in humans. Two receptors, ET_A and ET_B, have been identified, both of which are coupled to their effectors with G proteins. The ET_A receptor appears to be responsible for the vasoconstriction produced by endothelins.

Endothelins are much more potent than norepinephrine as vasoconstrictors and have a relatively long-lasting effect. The peptides also stimulate the heart, increase natriuretic peptide release, and activate smooth muscle proliferation. The peptides may be involved in some forms of hypertension and other cardiovascular

disorders. The first antagonists to become available are **bosentan** and aprisentan**,** which are approved for use in pulmonary hypertension.

VIP, SUBSTANCE P, CGRP, & NPY

VIP is an extremely potent vasodilator but is probably more important as a neurotransmitter. It is found in the central and peripheral nervous systems and in the gastrointestinal tract. No clinical application has been found for this peptide.

The **neurokinins** (**substance P, neurokinin A,** and **neurokinin B**) act at NK_1 and NK_2 receptors in the CNS and the periphery. Substance P has mixed vascular effects. It is a potent arteriolar vasodilator and a potent *stimulant* of veins and intestinal and airway smooth muscle. The peptide may also function as a local hormone in the gastrointestinal tract. Highest concentrations of substance P are found in those parts of the nervous system that contain neurons subserving pain. **Capsaicin,** the "hot" component of chili peppers, releases substance P from its stores in nerve endings and depletes the peptide. Capsaicin has been approved for topical use on arthritic joints and for postherpetic neuralgia.

Neurokinins appear to be involved in certain CNS conditions, including depression and nausea and vomiting. **Aprepitant** is an oral antagonist at NK_1 receptors and is approved for use in chemotherapy-induced nausea and vomiting.

CGRP is found (along with calcitonin) in high concentrations in the thyroid but is also present in most smooth muscle tissues. The presence of CGRP in smooth muscle suggests a function as a cotransmitter in autonomic nerve endings. CGRP is the most potent hypotensive agent discovered to date and causes reflex tachycardia. Some evidence suggests that CGRP is involved in migraine headache. Currently, there is no clinical application for this peptide.

NPY is a potent vasoconstrictor peptide that also stimulates the heart. NPY is found in both the CNS and peripheral nerves. In the periphery, NPY is most commonly localized as a cotransmitter in adrenergic nerve endings. Several receptor subtypes have been identified.

SKILL KEEPER: ANGIOTENSIN ANTAGONISTS (SEE CHAPTER 11)

Discuss the differences between ACE inhibitors and AT_1-receptor blockers in the context of the peptides described in this chapter. The Skill Keeper Answer appears at the end of the chapter.

QUESTIONS

1. The most correct statement regarding autacoid peptides is,
   (A) Angiotensin I is the most potent of the series that includes angiotensinogen and angiotensin II
   (B) Bradykinin is a potent vasodilator with pain- and edema-inducing effects
   (C) Atrial and brain natriuretic peptides increase cardiac contractility in heart failure
   (D) Because they cannot cross the blood-brain barrier, peptides are not found in the brain
   (E) Bradykinin is inactivated by the enzyme kallikrein

2. Which of the following, if given intravenously, will cause increased gastrointestinal motility and diarrhea?
   (A) Angiotensin II
   (B) Bethanechol
   (C) Bradykinin
   (D) Renin
   (E) Vasoactive intestinal peptide

3. A peptide that causes increased capillary permeability and edema is
   (A) Angiotensin II
   (B) Bradykinin
   (C) Captopril
   (D) Histamine
   (E) Losartan

4. Which of the following causes arteriolar vasoconstriction and venodilation?
   (A) Angiotensin II
   (B) Bradykinin
   (C) Endothelin-1
   (D) Substance P
   (E) Vasoactive intestinal peptide

5. A vasodilator that can be inactivated by proteolytic enzymes is
   (A) Angiotensin I
   (B) Isoproterenol
   (C) Histamine
   (D) Neuropeptide Y
   (E) Vasoactive intestinal peptide

6. Which of the following is released in traumatized tissue, causes pain and edema, and is inactivated by angiotensin-converting enzyme?
   (A) Angiotensin I
   (B) Angiotensin II
   (C) Atrial natriuretic peptide
   (D) Bradykinin
   (E) Calcitonin gene-related peptide
   (F) Endothelin
   (G) Neuropeptide Y
   (H) Renin
   (I) Substance P
   (J) Vasoactive intestinal peptide

7. Which of the following is a decapeptide precursor of a vasoconstrictor substance?
   (A) Angiotensin I
   (B) Angiotensin II
   (C) Atrial natriuretic peptide
   (D) Bradykinin
   (E) Calcitonin gene-related peptide
   (F) Endothelin
   (G) Neuropeptide Y
   (H) Renin
   (I) Substance P
   (J) Vasoactive intestinal peptide

8. Which of the following is an arterial vasodilator found in peripheral and CNS nerves, causes contraction of veins and airway smooth muscle, and is found in afferent pain fibers?
   (A) Angiotensin I
   (B) Angiotensin II
   (C) Atrial natriuretic peptide
   (D) Bradykinin
   (E) Calcitonin gene-related peptide
   (F) Endothelin
   (G) Neuropeptide Y
   (H) Renin
   (I) Substance P
   (J) Vasoactive intestinal peptide

9. Which of the following is an octapeptide vasoconstrictor that increases in the blood of hypertensive patients treated with large doses of diuretics?
   (A) Angiotensin I
   (B) Angiotensin II
   (C) Atrial natriuretic peptide
   (D) Bradykinin
   (E) Calcitonin gene-related peptide
   (F) Endothelin
   (G) Neuropeptide Y
   (H) Renin
   (I) Substance P
   (J) Vasoactive intestinal peptide

10. Which of the following is a vasodilator that increases in the blood or tissues of patients treated with captopril?
    (A) Angiotensin II
    (B) Bradykinin
    (C) Brain natriuretic peptide
    (D) Calcitonin gene-related peptide
    (E) Endothelin
    (F) Neuropeptide Y
    (G) Renin

11. Which of the following is used to treat severe pulmonary hypertension?
    (A) Angiotensin I
    (B) Aprepitant
    (C) Atrial natriuretic peptide
    (D) Bosentan
    (E) Bradykinin
    (F) Enalapril
    (G) Endothelin

12. Which of the following is an antagonist at NK_1 receptors and can be used to prevent or reduce chemotherapy-induced nausea and vomiting?
    (A) Angiotensin I
    (B) Aprepitant
    (C) Atrial natriuretic peptide
    (D) Bosentan
    (E) Bradykinin
    (F) Enalapril
    (G) Endothelin

ANSWERS

1. Angiotensin I is an inactive precursor. Natriuretic peptides have no effect on cardiac contractility. Peptides are found in high concentrations in parts of the brain because they are synthesized there. The answer is **B.**

2. The peptides listed here are not associated with marked increases in gastrointestinal motility; VIP reduces it. Bethanechol, a muscarinic cholinoceptor agonist, is an effective stimulant of the gut. The answer is **B.**

3. Histamine and bradykinin both cause a marked increase in capillary permeability that is often associated with edema, but histamine is not a peptide. The answer is **B.**

4. Substance P is a potent arterial vasodilator and venoconstrictor. The answer is **D.**

5. A peptide, but not an amine, would be altered by proteolytic enzymes. Vasoactive intestinal peptide is the only peptide in the list that is an arteriolar vasodilator. The answer is **E.**

6. Bradykinin is a mediator of pain and edema caused by tissue damage. The answer is **D.**

7. Angiotensin I is a decapeptide. The answer is **A.**

8. Substance P is an arteriolar vasodilator that is also a pain-mediating neurotransmitter. The answer is **I.**

9. Angiotensin II, an octapeptide, increases when blood volume decreases because the compensatory response causes an increase in renin secretion. The answer is **B.**

10. Bradykinin increases because the enzyme inhibited by captopril, converting enzyme, normally degrades kinins in addition to synthesizing angiotensin II (see Figure 11–3). The answer is **B.**

11. Bosentan is an endothelin antagonist approved for use in pulmonary hypertension. The answer is **D.**

12. Aprepitant is used to reduce or prevent chemotherapy-induced nausea and vomiting. The answer is **B.**

SKILL KEEPER ANSWER: ANGIOTENSIN ANTAGONISTS (SEE CHAPTER 11)

Both ACE inhibitors (eg, captopril) and AT_1-receptor blockers (eg, losartan) reduce the effects of the renin-angiotensin-aldosterone system and thereby reduce blood pressure. Both result in a compensatory increase in the release of renin and angiotensin I. The major difference between the 2 types of drugs results from the fact that ACE inhibitors increase the circulating levels of bradykinin because bradykinin is normally inactivated by ACE. The increase in bradykinin contributes to the hypotensive action of ACE inhibitors but is probably also responsible for the high incidence of cough associated with ACE inhibitor use. The cough is believed to result from prostaglandins synthesized as a result of the increased bradykinin. AT_1-receptor blockers have a lower incidence of cough.

CHECKLIST

When you complete this chapter, you should be able to:

☐ Name an antagonist of angiotensin at its receptor and at least 2 drugs that reduce the formation of angiotensin II.

☐ Outline the major effects of bradykinin and brain natriuretic peptide.

☐ Describe the functions of converting enzyme (peptidyl dipeptidase, kininase II).

☐ List 2 potent vasoconstrictor peptides.

☐ Describe the effects of vasoactive intestinal peptide and substance P.

☐ Describe the clinical applications of bosentan and aprepitant.

Prostaglandins & Other Eicosanoids

The eicosanoids are an important group of endogenous fatty acid derivatives that are produced from arachidonic acid. Arachidonic acid is derived from cell membrane lipids. Two major families of eicosanoids are generated by the enzymes cyclooxygenase (producing prostaglandins) and lipoxygenase (producing leukotrienes).

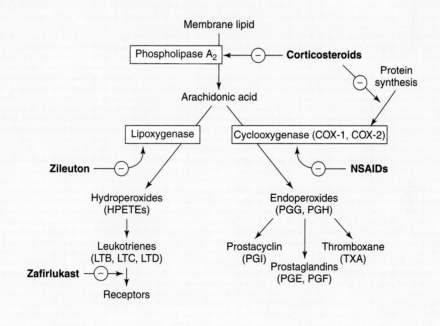

EICOSANOID AGONISTS

A. CLASSIFICATION

The principal eicosanoid subgroups are the cyclic molecules, including prostaglandins, prostacyclin, thromboxanes and the straight-chain leukotrienes. Prostacyclin, thromboxane, and other members of the prostaglandin group are cyclized derivatives of arachidonic acid. The leukotrienes retain the straight-chain configuration of arachidonic acid. There are several series for most of the principal subgroups, based on different substituents (indicated by letters A, B, etc) and different numbers of double bonds (indicated by a subscript number) in the molecule.

HIGH-YIELD TERMS TO LEARN

Abortifacient	A drug used to cause an abortion. Example: Prostaglandin $F_{2\alpha}$
Cyclooxygenase	Enzyme that converts arachidonic acid to PGG and PGH, the precursors of the prostaglandins
Dysmenorrhea	Painful uterine cramping activated by prostaglandins released during menstruation
Endoperoxide	General term for prostaglandin precursors, eg, PGG, PGH
Great vessel transposition	Congenital anomaly in which the pulmonary artery exits from the left ventricle and the aorta from the right ventricle. Incompatible with life after birth unless a large patent ductus or ventricular septal defect is present
Lipoxygenase	Enzyme that converts arachidonic acid to leukotriene precursors (HPETEs)
NSAID	Nonsteroidal anti-inflammatory drug, eg, aspirin, ibuprofen, celecoxib. Inhibitor of cyclooxygenase
Patent ductus arteriosus	Persistence after birth of the fetal connection between the pulmonary artery and the aorta
Phospholipase A_2	Enzyme in the cell membrane that generates arachidonic acid from membrane lipid constituents
Slow-reacting substance of anaphylaxis (SRS-A)	Material originally identified by bioassay from tissues of animals undergoing anaphylactic shock; now recognized as a mixture of leukotrienes, especially LTC_4, and LTD_4

B. Synthesis

Active eicosanoids are synthesized in response to a wide variety of stimuli (eg, physical injury, immune reactions). These stimuli activate phospholipases in the cell membrane or cytoplasm, and arachidonic acid (a tetraenoic fatty acid) is released from membrane phospholipids. Arachidonic acid is then metabolized by several mechanisms, 2 of which are most important. First, metabolism to straight-chain products is performed by **lipoxygenase,** ultimately producing leukotrienes. Alternatively, cyclization by the enzyme **cyclooxygenase** (COX) may occur, resulting in the production of prostacyclin, prostaglandins, or thromboxane. COX exists in at least 2 forms. **COX-1** is found in many tissues; the prostaglandins produced in these tissues by COX-1 appear to be important for a variety of normal physiologic processes (see later discussion). In contrast, **COX-2** is found primarily in inflammatory cells; the products of its actions play a major role in tissue injury (eg, inflammation). COX-2 is also responsible for synthesis of prostacyclin in the vascular endothelium and of prostaglandins important in renal function. Thromboxane is preferentially synthesized in platelets, whereas prostacyclin is synthesized in the endothelial cells of vessels. Naturally occurring eicosanoids have very short half-lives (seconds to minutes) and are inactive when given orally.

Replacement of tetraenoic (4 double bonds) fatty acids in the diet with trienoic (3 double bonds) or pentaenoic (5 double bonds) precursors results in the synthesis of much less active prostaglandin and leukotriene products. Thus dietary therapy with fatty oils from plant or cold-water fish sources can be useful in conditions involving eicosanoids.

C. Mechanism of Action

Most eicosanoid effects appear to be brought about by activation of cell surface receptors (Table 18–1) that are coupled by the G_s protein to adenylyl cyclase (producing cyclic adenosine monophosphate [cAMP]) or by the G_q protein to the phosphatidylinositol cascade (producing inositol 1,4,5-trisphosphate [IP_3] and diacylglycerol [DAG] second messengers).

D. Effects

A vast array of effects are produced in smooth muscle, platelets, the CNS, and other tissues. Some of the most important effects are summarized in Table 18–1. Eicosanoids most directly involved in pathologic processes include prostaglandin (PG) $F_{2\alpha}$, thromboxane A_2 (TXA$_2$), and the leukotrienes LTC_4 and LTD_4. LTC_4 and LTD_4 comprise the important mediator of bronchoconstriction, **slow-reacting substance of anaphylaxis (SRS-A).** Leukotriene LTB_4 is a chemotactic factor important in inflammation. PGE_2 and prostacyclin may play important roles as endogenous vasodilators. PGE_1 and its derivatives have significant protective effects on

Table 18–1. Effects of some important eicosanoids.

Effect	PGE_2	$PGF_{2\alpha}$	PGI_2	TXA_2	LTB_4	LTC_4	LTD_4
Major receptors	EP_{1-4}	$FP_{A,B}$	IP	$TP_{\alpha,\beta}$	$BLT_{1,2}$	$CysLT_2$	$CysLT_1$
Vascular tone	↓	↑ or ↓	↓↓	↑↑↑	?	↑ or ↓	↑ or ↓
Bronchial tone	↓↓	↑↑	↓	↑↑↑	?	↑↑↑↑	↑↑↑↑
Uterine tone	↑↑	↑↑↑	↓	↑↑	?	?	?
Platelet aggregation	↑ or ↓		↓↓↓	↑↑↑	?	?	?
Leukocyte chemotaxis	?	?	?	?	↑↑↑↑	↑↑	↑↑

? = unknown effect

the gastric mucosa. The mechanism may involve increased secretion of bicarbonate and mucus, decreased acid secretion, or both. PGE_1 and PGE_2 relax vascular and other smooth muscle. PGE_2 appears to be the natural vasodilator that maintains patency of the ductus arteriosus during fetal development. PGE_2 and $PGF_{2\alpha}$ are released in large amounts from the endometrium during menstruation and may play a physiologic role in labor. PGE_2 appears to be involved in the physiologic ripening of the cervix at term. Dysmenorrhea is associated with uterine contractions induced by prostaglandins, especially $PGF_{2\alpha}$. Platelet aggregation is strongly activated by thromboxane. $PGF_{2\alpha}$ reduces intraocular pressure (see later discussion), but it is not known whether this is a physiologic effect of endogenous $PGF_{2\alpha}$. Therapeutic effects of prostaglandins are described below.

E. CLINICAL USES

1. Obstetrics—PGE_2 and $PGF_{2\alpha}$ are involved in contraction of the uterus. PGE_2 (as **dinoprostone**) is approved for use to ripen the cervix at term before induction of labor with oxytocin. Both PGE_2 and $PGF_{2\alpha}$ have been used as abortifacients in the second trimester of pregnancy. Although effective in inducing labor at term, they produce more adverse effects (nausea, vomiting, diarrhea) than do other oxytocics (eg, oxytocin) used for this application. In Europe, the PGE_1 analog **misoprostol** has been used extensively with the progesterone antagonist mifepristone (RU 486) as an extremely effective and safe abortifacient combination. Misoprostol has been used for this purpose in combination with either methotrexate or mifepristone in the United States.

2. Pediatrics—PGE_1 is given as an infusion to maintain patency of the ductus arteriosus in infants with transposition of the great vessels until surgical correction can be undertaken.

3. Pulmonary hypertension and dialysis—Prostacyclin (PGI_2) is approved for use (as **epoprostenol**)

in severe pulmonary hypertension and to prevent platelet aggregation in dialysis machines.

4. Peptic ulcer associated with NSAID use—Misoprostol is approved in the United States for the prevention of peptic ulcers in patients who must take high doses of NSAIDs for arthritis and who have a history of ulcer associated with this use.

5. Urology—PGE_1 (as **alprostadil**) is used in the treatment of impotence. Preparations are available for injection as well as for insertion into the urethra.

6. Ophthalmology—**Latanoprost,** a $PGF_{2\alpha}$ derivative, is used extensively for the treatment of glaucoma. **Bimatoprost, travoprost,** and **unoprostone** are newer, related drugs. These agents apparently increase the outflow of aqueous humor, thus reducing intraocular pressure.

EICOSANOID ANTAGONISTS

Phospholipase A_2 and cyclooxygenase can be inhibited by drugs; some of these inhibitors are mainstays in the treatment of inflammation (see the drug classification figure, page 157 as well as Chapter 36). **Zileuton** is a selective inhibitor of lipoxygenase; some cyclooxygenase inhibitors exert a mild inhibitory effect on leukotriene synthesis. Inhibitors of the receptors for the prostaglandins and the leukotrienes are being actively sought. **Zafirlukast** and **montelukast,** inhibitors at the LTD_4 receptor, are currently available for the treatment of asthma (Chapter 20).

A. CORTICOSTEROIDS

As indicated in the drug classification, corticosteroids inhibit the production of arachidonic acid by phospholipases in the membrane. This effect is mediated by intracellular steroid receptors that, when activated by an appropriate steroid, increase expression of specific proteins capable of inhibiting phospholipase. Steroids also inhibit the synthesis of COX-2. These actions are

KEY DRUGS		
Subclass	**Prototype**	**Other Significant Agents**
Prostaglandins	PGE_2, $PGF_{2\alpha}$	PGE_1
Prostacyclin	PGI_2	
Thromboxane	TXA_2	
Leukotrienes	LTB_4, LTC_4	LTD_4
Leukotriene inhibitors	Zafirlukast, zileuton	
Phospholipase inhibitors	Prednisone, hydrocortisone	See Chapter 39
Cyclooxygenase inhibitors	Aspirin, ibuprofen	See Chapter 36

thought to be the major mechanisms of the important anti-inflammatory action of corticosteroids.

B. NSAIDS

Aspirin and other nonsteroidal (ie, noncorticosteroid) anti-inflammatory drugs inhibit cyclooxygenase and the production of the thromboxane, prostaglandin, and prostacyclin branches of the synthetic path (see drug classification figure). Most of the currently available NSAIDs nonselectively inhibit both COX-1 and COX-2. In fact, many inhibit COX-1 somewhat more effectively than COX-2, the isoform thought to be responsible for synthesis of inflammatory eicosanoids. Selective COX-2 inhibitors include **celecoxib**; **rofecoxib** and **valdecoxib** were withdrawn from the market because of reports of cardiovascular toxicity (see Chapter 36).

Inhibition of cyclooxygenase by aspirin, unlike that by other NSAIDs, is irreversible. It is thought that some cases of aspirin allergy result from diversion of arachidonic acid to the leukotriene pathway when the cyclooxygenase-catalyzed prostaglandin pathway is blocked. The resulting increase in leukotriene synthesis causes the bronchoconstriction that is typical of aspirin allergy. For unknown reasons, this form of aspirin allergy is more common in individuals with nasal polyps.

The antiplatelet action of aspirin results from the fact that inhibition of thromboxane synthesis is essentially permanent in platelets; they lack the machinery for new protein synthesis. In contrast, inhibition of prostacyclin synthesis in the vascular endothelium is temporary because these cells can synthesize new enzyme. Inhibition of prostaglandin synthesis also results in important anti-inflammatory effects. Inhibition of synthesis of fever-inducing prostaglandins in the brain produces the antipyretic action of NSAIDs. Closure of a patent ductus arteriosus in an otherwise normal infant can be accelerated with an NSAID such as indomethacin or ibuprofen.

C. LEUKOTRIENE ANTAGONISTS

As noted, an inhibitor of lipoxygenase (zileuton) and LTD_4 (and LTE_4) receptor antagonists (zafirlukast, montelukast) are available for clinical use. Currently, these agents are approved only for use in asthma (see Chapter 20).

QUESTIONS

1. Your patient calls the office complaining that your last prescription has caused severe diarrhea. Which of the following is frequently associated with increased gastrointestinal motility and diarrhea?
   (A) Corticosteroids
   (B) Leukotriene LTB_4
   (C) Misoprostol
   (D) Timolol
   (E) Zileuton

2. Which of the following drugs inhibits cyclooxygenase irreversibly?
   (A) Aspirin
   (B) Hydrocortisone
   (C) Ibuprofen
   (D) Indomethacin
   (E) Zileuton

3. Which of the following drugs causes vasodilation?
   (A) Angiotensin II
   (B) Ergotamine
   (C) Prostaglandin $PGF_{2\alpha}$
   (D) Prostacyclin
   (E) Thromboxane

4. A patient complains of severe dysmenorrhea. A uterine stimulant derived from membrane lipid in the endometrium is
   (A) Angiotensin II
   (B) Histamine

(C) Prostacyclin (PGI$_2$)
(D) Prostaglandin PGE$_2$
(E) Serotonin

5. Inflammation is a complex tissue reaction that includes the release of cytokines, leukotrienes, prostaglandins, and peptides. Prostaglandins involved in inflammatory processes are typically produced from arachidonic acid by
(A) Cyclooxygenase -1
(B) Cyclooxygenase -2
(C) Glutathione-S-transferase
(D) Lipoxygenase
(E) Phospholipase A$_2$

6. Which of the following is a recognized clinical indication for eicosanoids or their inhibitors?
(A) Angina pectoris
(B) Essential hypertension
(C) Patent ductus arteriosus
(D) Supraventricular reentry arrhythmia
(E) Type 2 diabetes mellitus

7. A 60-year-old woman has glaucoma after cataract surgery. Which of the following can be used to reduce intraocular pressure?
(A) Leukotriene LTD$_4$ or its analogs
(B) Prostaglandin PGE$_2$ or its analogs
(C) Prostaglandin PGF$_{2\alpha}$ or its analogs
(D) Slow-reacting substance of anaphylaxis (SRS-A)
(E) Thromboxane TXA$_2$ or its analogs

8. Which of the following is a reversible inhibitor of platelet cyclooxygenase?
(A) Alprostadil
(B) Aspirin
(C) Ibuprofen
(D) Leukotriene LTC$_4$
(E) Misoprostol
(F) Prednisone
(G) Prostacyclin
(H) Zafirlukast
(I) Zileuton

9. Which of the following is a component of slow-reacting substance of anaphylaxis (SRS-A)?
(A) Alprostadil
(B) Aspirin
(C) Ibuprofen
(D) Leukotriene LTC$_4$
(E) Misoprostol
(F) Prednisone
(G) Prostacyclin
(H) Zafirlukast
(I) Zileuton

10. Which of the following reduces the activity of phospholipase A$_2$?

(A) Alprostadil
(B) Aspirin
(C) Ibuprofen
(D) Leukotriene LTC$_4$
(E) Misoprostol
(F) Prednisone
(G) Prostacyclin
(H) Zafirlukast
(I) Zileuton

11. A 17-year-old patient complains that he gets severe shortness of breath whenever he takes aspirin for headache. Increased levels of which of the following may be responsible, in part, for some cases of aspirin hypersensitivity?
(A) Alprostadil
(B) Aspirin
(C) Ibuprofen
(D) Leukotriene LTC$_4$
(E) Misoprostol
(F) Prednisone
(G) Prostacyclin
(H) Zafirlukast
(I) Zileuton

12. Which of the following is a leukotriene receptor blocker?
(A) Alprostadil
(B) Aspirin
(C) Ibuprofen
(D) Leukotriene LTC$_4$
(E) Misoprostol
(F) Prednisone
(G) Prostacyclin
(H) Zafirlukast
(I) Zileuton

ANSWERS

1. Beta-blockers (eg, timolol), corticosteroids, and zileuton do not cause diarrhea. LTB$_4$ is a chemotactic factor. The answer is **C**.

2. Hydrocortisone and other corticosteroids inhibit phospholipase. Ibuprofen and indomethacin inhibit cyclooxygenase reversibly, whereas zileuton inhibits lipoxygenase. The answer is **A**.

3. Prostacyclin (PGI$_2$) is a very potent vasodilator. The answer is **D**.

4. Although serotonin and, in some species, histamine may cause uterine stimulation, these substances are not derived from membrane lipid. Prostacyclin relaxes the uterus (see Table 18–1). The answer is **D**.

5. Phospholipase A$_2$ converts membrane phospholipid to arachidonic acid. Cyclooxygenases convert arachidonic acid to prostaglandins. COX-2 is the

enzyme believed to be responsible for this reaction in inflammatory cells. The answer is **B.**

6. A persistent patent ductus arteriosus can often be induced to close by inhibiting the production of the endogenous vasodilator PGE_2 by means of an NSAID such as indomethacin or ibuprofen. Conversely, in transposition of the great vessels, it is important to maintain the ductus patent until the anomaly can be surgically corrected. Patency of the ductus is maintained by means of a constant infusion of PGE_2. The answer is **C.**

7. $PGF_{2\alpha}$ and several of its analogs reduce intraocular pressure. The answer is **C.**

8. NSAIDs other than aspirin are reversible inhibitors of cyclooxygenase. The answer is **C.**

9. The leukotriene C and D series are major components of SRS-A. The answer is **D.**

10. Corticosteroids cause inhibition of phospholipase A_2, the enzyme that releases arachidonic acid from membrane lipids. The answer is **F.**

11. It is thought that the leukotrienes may be produced in increased amounts when cyclooxygenase is blocked; in patients with aspirin hypersensitivity, this might precipitate the bronchoconstriction often observed in this condition. The answer is **D.**

12. Zafirlukast is a blocker of LTD_4 receptors. The answer is **H.**

CHECKLIST

When you complete this chapter, you should be able to:

☐ List the major effects of PGE_2, $PGF_{2\alpha}$, PGI_2, LTB_4, LTC_4, and LTD_4.

☐ List important sites of synthesis and the effects of thromboxane and prostacyclin in the vascular system.

☐ List the currently available therapeutic antagonists of leukotrienes and prostaglandins and their targets (receptors or enzymes).

☐ Explain the different effects of aspirin on prostaglandin synthesis and on leukotriene synthesis.

Nitric Oxide, Donors, & Inhibitors

Nitric oxide (NO) is a common product of the metabolism of arginine in many tissues. It is thought to be an important paracrine vasodilator, and it may also play a role in cell death and in neurotransmission; it therefore qualifies as an autacoid. NO is also released from several important vasodilator drug molecules.

ENDOGENOUS NO

Endogenous NO is synthesized by a family of enzymes collectively called **NO synthase (NOS)**. These intracellular enzymes are activated by calcium influx or by cytokines. Arginine, the primary substrate, is converted by NOS to citrulline and NO. Three forms of NO synthase are known: isoform 1 (bNOS, cNOS, or nNOS, a constitutive form found in epithelial and neuronal cells); isoform 2 (iNOS or mNOS, an inducible form found in macrophages and smooth muscle cells); and isoform 3 (eNOS, a constitutive form found in endothelial cells). Nitric oxide synthase can be inhibited by arginine analogs such as N^{G}-monomethyl-L-arginine (L-NMMA). Under some circumstances (eg, ischemia), NO may be formed from endogenous nitrate ion. NO is not stored in cells. Because it is a gas at body temperature, NO very rapidly diffuses from its site of synthesis to surrounding tissues. Drugs that cause endogenous NO release do so by stimulating its synthesis by NOS. Such drugs include acetylcholine, other muscarinic agonists, and histamine.

EXOGENOUS NO DONORS

NO is released from several important drugs, including **nitroprusside** (Chapter 11), **nitrates,** (Chapter 12), and **nitrites.** Release from nitroprusside occurs spontaneously in the blood in the presence of oxygen, whereas release from nitrates and nitrites is enzymatic and intracellular and requires the presence of thiol compounds such as cysteine. Tolerance may develop to nitrates and nitrites if endogenous thiol compounds are depleted.

EFFECTS OF NO

A. SMOOTH MUSCLE

NO is a powerful vasodilator in all vascular beds and a potent relaxant in most other smooth muscle tissues.

> **SKILL KEEPER:**
> **NONINNERVATED RECEPTORS**
> **(SEE CHAPTER 6)**
>
> *List the noninnervated receptors found in blood vessels and describe their second-messenger mechanisms of action.* The Skill Keeper Answer appears at the end of the chapter.

The mechanism of this effect involves activation of guanylyl cyclase and the synthesis of cyclic guanosine monophosphate (cGMP). This cGMP, in turn, facilitates the dephosphorylation and inactivation of myosin light chains, which results in relaxation of smooth muscle. NO plays a physiologic role in erectile tissue function, in which smooth muscle relaxation is required to bring about the influx of blood that causes erection.

B. CELL ADHESION

NO has effects on cell adhesion that result in reduced platelet aggregation and reduced neutrophil adhesion to vascular endothelium. The latter effect is probably due to reduced expression of adhesion molecules by endothelial cells.

C. INFLAMMATION

NO appears to *facilitate* inflammation both directly and through the stimulation of prostaglandin synthesis by cyclooxygenase 2.

CLINICAL APPLICATIONS OF NO INHIBITORS AND DONORS

Although *inhibitors* of NO synthesis are of great research interest, none are currently in clinical use. NO can be *inactivated* by heme, but application of this approach is in preclinical research.

In contrast, drugs that *release* endogenous NO and *donors* of the molecule were in use long before NO was

---

HIGH-YIELD TERMS TO LEARN

Endothelium-derived relaxing factor, EDRF	A mixture of nitric oxide and other vasodilator substances synthesized in vascular endothelium
Nitric oxide donor	A molecule from which nitric oxide can be released (eg, arginine, nitroprusside, nitroglycerin)
cNOS, iNOS, eNOS	Naturally occurring isoforms of nitric oxide synthase: respectively, constitutive (NOS-1), inducible (NOS-2), and endothelial (NOS-3) isoforms

---

discovered and continue to be very important in clinical medicine. The cardiovascular applications of nitroprusside (Chapter 11) and the nitrates and nitrites (Chapter 12) have been discussed. The treatments of preeclampsia and of pulmonary hypertension and acute respiratory distress syndrome are currently under clinical investigation. Early results from the pulmonary disease studies appear promising, and one preparation of NO gas (INOmax) has been approved for use in neonates with hypoxic respiratory failure.

Preclinical studies suggest that NO donor drugs or dietary supplementation with arginine may assist in slowing atherosclerosis, especially in grafted organs. In contrast, *acute rejection* of grafts may involve up-regulation of NOS enzymes, and inhibition of these enzymes may prolong graft survival.

QUESTIONS

1. Which one of the following does not *contain* nitric oxide, but causes it to be released from endogenous precursors, resulting in vasodilation?
   (A) Amyl nitrite
   (B) Arginine
   (C) Histamine
   (D) Isosorbide dinitrate
   (E) Nitroprusside

2. A molecule that stimulates nitric oxide synthase (NOS), especially the eNOS (NOS 3) isoform, is
   (A) Acetylcholine
   (B) Citrulline
   (C) Isoproterenol
   (D) Nitroglycerin
   (E) Nitroprusside

3. The inducible isoform of nitric oxide synthase (iNOS, isoform 2) is found primarily in
   (A) Cartilage
   (B) Eosinophils

   (C) Macrophages
   (D) Platelets
   (E) Vascular endothelial cells

4. The primary endogenous substrate for nitric oxide synthase (NOS) is
   (A) Acetylcholine
   (B) Angiotensinogen
   (C) Arginine
   (D) Citrulline
   (E) Heme

5. Which of the following is a recognized effect of nitric oxide (NO)?
   (A) Arrhythmia
   (B) Bronchoconstriction
   (C) Constipation
   (D) Inhibition of acute graft rejection
   (E) Pulmonary vasodilation

6. Which of the following is an approved application for NO administered as a gas?
   (A) Asthma
   (B) Dysmenorrhea
   (C) Patent ductus arteriosus
   (D) Pulmonary hypertension
   (E) Rejection after renal transplant

ANSWERS

1. Nitroprusside and organic nitrites (eg, amyl nitrite) and nitrates (eg, isosorbide dinitrate) contain NO groups that can be released as NO. Arginine is the normal source of endogenous NO. Histamine stimulates the production of NO from arginine. The answer is **C.**

2. Acetylcholine is the only molecule in this list that stimulates the endogenous production of NO by NOS. The answer is **A.**

3. The inducible form of NOS is associated with inflammation and the enzyme is found in macrophages. The answer is **C**.

4. Arginine is the substrate and citrulline (along with NO) is the product of NOS. The answer is **C**.

5. NO does not cause arrhythmias or constipation. It causes bronchodilation and may hasten graft rejection. NO does cause pulmonary vasodilation. The answer is **E**.

6. Thus far, NO gas has been approved for use by inhalation in neonatal hypoxic respiratory failure and adult pulmonary hypertension. The answer is **D**.

SKILL KEEPER ANSWER: NONINNERVATED RECEPTORS (SEE CHAPTER 6)

Endothelial cells lining blood vessels have noninnervated muscarinic receptors. These M_3 receptors use the G_q-coupling protein to activate phospholipase C, which releases inositol 1,4,5-trisphosphate and diacylglycerol from membrane lipids. eNOS is activated and NO is released, causing vasodilation. Histamine H_1 receptors are also found in the vascular endothelium and similarly cause vasodilation through the synthesis and release of NO. Other noninnervated (or poorly innervated) receptors found in blood vessels include α_2 and β_2 receptors. The α_2 receptors use G_i to inhibit adenylyl cyclase, reducing cyclic adenosine monophosphate (cAMP) and causing contraction in the vessel. (Recall that the blood pressure-lowering action of α_2 agonists is mediated by actions in the CNS, not in the vessels.) Conversely, β_2 receptors activate adenylyl cyclase via G_s and increase cAMP, resulting in relaxation.

CHECKLIST

When you complete this chapter, you should be able to:

☐ Name the enzyme responsible for the synthesis of NO in tissues.

☐ List the major beneficial and toxic effects of endogenous NO.

☐ List 2 drugs that cause release of endogenous NO.

☐ List 2 drugs that spontaneously or enzymatically break down in the body to release NO.

Bronchodilators & Other Drugs Used in Asthma

Asthma is a disease characterized by airway inflammation and episodic, reversible bronchospasm. Drugs useful in asthma include bronchodilators (smooth muscle relaxants) and anti-inflammatory drugs. Bronchodilators include sympathomimetics, especially β_2-selective agonists, muscarinic antagonists, methylxanthines, and leukotriene receptor blockers. Anti-inflammatory drugs include corticosteroids, mast cell stabilizers, and an anti-IgE antibody. Leukotriene antagonists play a dual role.

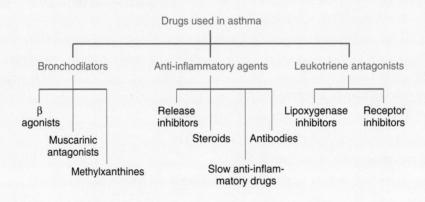

PATHOPHYSIOLOGY OF ASTHMA

The immediate cause of asthmatic bronchoconstriction is the release of several mediators from IgE-sensitized mast cells and other cells involved in immunologic responses (Figure 20–1). These mediators include the leukotrienes LTC_4 and LTD_4. In addition, chemoattractant mediators such as LTB_4 attract inflammatory cells to the airways. Finally, several cytokines and some enzymes are released, leading to chronic inflammation. Chronic inflammation leads to marked bronchial hyperreactivity to various inhaled substances, including antigens, histamine, muscarinic agonists, and irritants such as SO_2 and cold air. This reactivity is partially mediated by vagal reflexes.

STRATEGIES OF ASTHMA THERAPY

Acute asthmatic bronchospasm must be treated promptly and effectively with bronchodilators. Beta$_2$ agonists, muscarinic antagonists, and theophylline and its derivatives are available for this indication. Long-term preventive treatment requires control of the inflammatory process in the airways. The most important anti-inflammatory drugs in the treatment of chronic asthma are the corticosteroids and drugs (such as cromolyn and nedocromil) that inhibit release of mediators from mast cells and other inflammatory cells. In early results, anti-IgE antibodies also appear promising for chronic therapy. The leukotriene antagonists may have effects on both bronchoconstriction and inflammation.

HIGH-YIELD TERMS TO LEARN

Bronchial hyperreactivity	Pathologic increase in the bronchoconstrictor response to antigens and irritants; caused by bronchial inflammation
IgE-mediated disease	Disease caused by excessive or misdirected immune response mediated by IgE antibodies. Example: asthma
Mast cell degranulation	Exocytosis of granules from mast cells with release of mediators of inflammation and bronchoconstriction
Phosphodiesterase (PDE)	Family of enzymes that degrade cyclic nucleotides to nucleotides, eg, cAMP (active) to AMP (inactive); various isoforms, some degrade cGMP to GMP
Tachyphylaxis	Rapid loss of responsiveness to a stimulus (eg, a drug)

BETA-ADRENOCEPTOR AGONISTS

A. PROTOTYPES AND PHARMACOKINETICS

The most important sympathomimetics used to reverse asthmatic bronchoconstriction are the β_2-selective agonists, although epinephrine and isoproterenol are still available and used occasionally (see Chapter 9). Of the selective agents, **albuterol, terbutaline,** and **metaproterenol**[*] are the most important in the United States. **Salmeterol** and **formoterol** are long-acting β_2-selective agonists. Beta agonists are given almost exclusively by inhalation, usually from pressurized aerosol canisters but occasionally by nebulizer. The inhalational route decreases the systemic dose (and adverse effects) while delivering an effective dose locally to the airway smooth muscle. The older drugs have durations of action of 6 h or less; salmeterol and formoterol act for 12 h or more.

B. MECHANISM AND EFFECTS

These agents act by stimulating adenylyl cyclase and increasing cyclic adenosine monophosphate (cAMP) in smooth muscle cells (Figure 20–2). The increase in cAMP results in a powerful bronchodilator response.

C. CLINICAL USE

Sympathomimetics are used very extensively in asthma. Shorter acting sympathomimetics (albuterol, metaproterenol, terbutaline) should be used only for acute episodes of bronchospasm (not for prophylaxis), whereas the long-acting agents (salmeterol, formoterol) should be used for prophylaxis, and not for acute episodes. In almost all patients, the shorter acting β agonists are the most effective bronchodilators available and therefore the drugs of choice for acute asthma. Many patients with chronic obstructive pulmonary disease (COPD) also benefit, although the incidence of toxicity is increased in this condition.

D. TOXICITY

Skeletal muscle tremor is a common adverse β_2 effect. Beta$_2$ selectivity is relative. At high clinical dosage, these agents have significant β_1 effects. Even when they are given by inhalation, some cardiac effect (tachycardia) is common. Other adverse effects are rare. When the agents are used excessively, arrhythmias may occur. Loss of responsiveness (tolerance, tachyphylaxis) is an unwanted effect of excessive use of the short-acting sympathomimetics. Patients with COPD often have concurrent cardiac disease and may have arrhythmias even at normal dosage.

SKILL KEEPER: SYMPATHOMIMETICS IN ASTHMA (SEE CHAPTER 9)

The sympathomimetic bronchodilators are drugs of choice in acute asthma. Compare the properties of direct- and indirect-acting sympathomimetics relative to the therapeutic goals in asthma. Which type is superior and why? The Skill Keeper Answer appears at the end of the chapter.

METHYLXANTHINES

A. PROTOTYPES AND PHARMACOKINETICS

The methylxanthines are purine derivatives. Three major methylxanthines are found in plants and provide the stimulant effects of 3 common beverages: **caffeine**

---

[*]Do not confuse metaproterenol, a β_2 agonist, with metoprolol, a β-blocker.

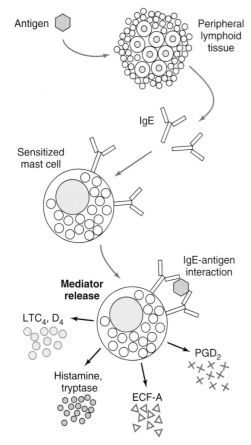

Figure 20–1. Immunologic model for the pathogenesis of asthma. Exposure to antigen causes synthesis of IgE, which binds to and sensitizes mast cells and other inflammatory cells. When such sensitized cells are challenged with antigen, a variety of mediators are released that can account for most of the signs of the early bronchoconstrictor response in asthma. LTC_4, D_4, leukotrienes C_4 and D_4; ECF-A, eosinophil chemotactic factor-A; PGD_2, prostaglandin D_2. (Modified and reproduced, with permission, from Gold WW: Cholinergic pharmacology in asthma. In: *Asthma Physiology, Immunopharmacology, and Treatment.* Austen KF, Lichtenstein LM, editors. Academic Press, 1974.)

(in coffee), **theophylline** (tea), and **theobromine** (cocoa). Theophylline is the only member of this group important in the treatment of asthma. The drug and several analogs are orally active and available as various salts and as the base. Theophylline is available in both prompt-release and slow-release forms. Theophylline is eliminated by P450 drug-metabolizing enzymes in the liver. Clearance varies with age (highest in young

adolescents), smoking status (higher in smokers), and concurrent use of other drugs that inhibit or induce hepatic enzymes.

B. MECHANISM OF ACTION

The methylxanthines inhibit phosphodiesterase (PDE), the enzyme that degrades cAMP to AMP (see Figure 20–2), and thus increase cAMP. This anti-PDE effect, however, requires high concentrations of the drug. Methylxanthines also block adenosine receptors in the CNS and elsewhere, but a relationship between this action and the bronchodilating effect has not been clearly established. It is possible that bronchodilation is caused by a third as yet unrecognized action.

C. EFFECTS

In asthma, bronchodilation is the most important therapeutic action of theophylline. Increased strength of contraction of the diaphragm has been demonstrated in some patients. Other effects of therapeutic doses include CNS stimulation, cardiac stimulation, vasodilation, a slight increase in blood pressure (probably caused by the release of norepinephrine from adrenergic nerves), and increased gastrointestinal motility.

D. CLINICAL USE

The major clinical indication for the use of methylxanthines is asthma, but none of this class of compounds is as safe or effective as the β agonists. Slow-release theophylline (for control of nocturnal asthma) is the most important methylxanthine in clinical use. Another methylxanthine derivative, **pentoxifylline,** is promoted as a remedy for intermittent claudication; this effect is said to result from decreased viscosity of the blood. Of course, the nonmedical use of the methylxanthines in coffee, tea, and cocoa is far greater, in total quantities consumed, than the medical uses of the drugs.

E. TOXICITY

The common adverse effects include gastrointestinal distress, tremor, and insomnia. Severe nausea and vomiting, hypotension, cardiac arrhythmias, and convulsions may result from overdosage. Very large overdoses (eg, in suicide attempts) are potentially lethal because of the arrhythmias and convulsions. Beta-blockers are useful in reversing severe cardiovascular toxicity from theophylline.

MUSCARINIC ANTAGONISTS

A. PROTOTYPES AND PHARMACOKINETICS

Atropine and other naturally occurring belladonna alkaloids were used for many years in the treatment of asthma but have been replaced by **ipratropium,** a quaternary antimuscarinic agent designed for aerosol use. This drug is delivered to the airways by pressurized

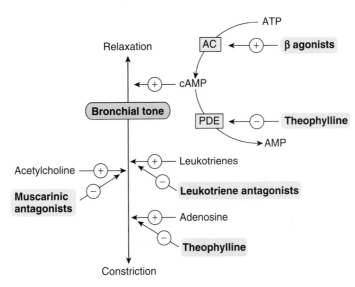

Figure 20–2. Possible mechanisms of β agonists, muscarinic antagonists, theophylline, and leukotriene antagonists in altering bronchial tone in asthma. AC, adenylyl cyclase; PDE, phosphodiesterase.

aerosol and has little systemic action. **Tiotropium** is a longer-acting analog.

B. MECHANISM OF ACTION

When given as an aerosol, ipratropium competitively blocks muscarinic receptors in the airways and effectively prevents bronchoconstriction mediated by vagal discharge. If given systemically (not an approved use), the drug is indistinguishable from other short-acting muscarinic blockers.

C. EFFECTS

Muscarinic antagonists reverse bronchoconstriction in some asthma patients (especially children) and in many patients with COPD. They have no effect on the inflammatory aspects of asthma.

D. CLINICAL USE

Ipratropium is useful in one third to two thirds of asthmatic patients; β₂ agonists are effective in almost all. For acute bronchospasm, therefore, the β agonists are usually preferred. However, in COPD, which is often associated with acute episodes of bronchospasm, the antimuscarinic agents may be more effective and less toxic than β agonists.

E. TOXICITY

Because these agents are delivered directly to the airway and are minimally absorbed, systemic effects are small. When given in excessive dosage, minor atropine-like toxic effects may occur (Chapter 8). In contrast to the β₂ agonists, muscarinic antagonists do not cause tremor or arrhythmias.

CROMOLYN & NEDOCROMIL

A. PROTOTYPES AND PHARMACOKINETICS

Cromolyn (disodium cromoglycate) and nedocromil are unusual chemicals: They are extremely insoluble, so that even massive doses given orally or by aerosol result in minimal systemic blood levels. They are given by aerosol for asthma. **Cromolyn** is the prototype of this group.

B. MECHANISM OF ACTION

The mechanism of action of these drugs is poorly understood but appears to involve a decrease in the release of mediators (such as leukotrienes and histamine) from mast cells. The drugs have no bronchodilator action but can prevent bronchoconstriction caused by a challenge with antigen to which the patient is allergic. Cromolyn and nedocromil are capable of preventing both early and late responses to challenge (Figure 20–3).

C. EFFECTS

Because they are not absorbed from the site of administration, cromolyn and nedocromil have only local effects. When administered orally, cromolyn has some efficacy in preventing food allergy. Similar actions have been demonstrated after local application in the conjunctiva and the nasopharyngeal tract for allergic reactions in these tissues.

D. CLINICAL USES

Asthma (especially in children) is the most important use for cromolyn and nedocromil. Nasal and eyedrop

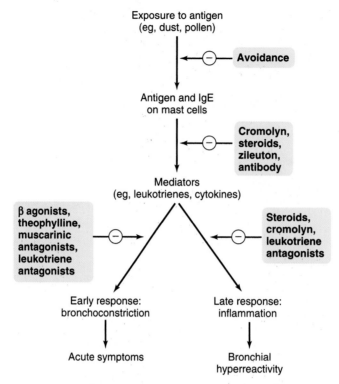

Figure 20–3. Summary of treatment strategies in asthma. (Modified and redrawn from Cockcroft DW: The bronchial late response in the pathogenesis of asthma and its modulation by therapy. *Allergy Asthma Immunol* 1985;55:857.)

formulations of cromolyn are available for hay fever, and an oral formulation is used for food allergy.

E. TOXICITY

These drugs may cause cough and irritation of the airway when given by aerosol. Rare instances of drug allergy have been reported.

CORTICOSTEROIDS

A. PROTOTYPES AND PHARMACOKINETICS

All of the corticosteroids are potentially beneficial in severe asthma (see Chapter 39). However, because of their toxicity, systemic (oral) corticosteroids are used chronically only if other therapies are unsuccessful. In contrast, local aerosol administration of surface-active corticosteroids (eg, **beclomethasone, budesonide, dexamethasone, flunisolide, fluticasone, mometasone**) is relatively safe; inhaled corticosteroids have become common first-line therapy for individuals with moderate to severe asthma. Important intravenous corticosteroids for status asthmaticus include prednisolone (the active metabolite of prednisone) and hydrocortisone.

B. MECHANISM OF ACTION

Corticosteroids reduce the synthesis of arachidonic acid by phospholipase A_2 and inhibit the expression of COX-2, the inducible form of cyclooxygenase (see Chapter 18). It has also been suggested that corticosteroids increase the responsiveness of β adrenoceptors in the airway.

C. EFFECTS

See Chapter 39 for details. Glucocorticoids bind to intracellular receptors and activate glucocorticoid response elements (GREs) in the nucleus, resulting in synthesis of substances that prevent the full expression of inflammation and allergy. Reduced activity of phospholipase A_2 is thought to be particularly important in asthma because the leukotrienes that result from eicosanoid synthesis are extremely potent bronchoconstrictors and may also participate in the late inflammatory response (Figure 20–3).

D. CLINICAL USE

Inhaled glucocorticoids are now considered appropriate (even for children) in most cases of moderate asthma that are not fully responsive to aerosol β agonists. It is believed that such early use may prevent the severe, progressive

---

KEY DRUGS

Subclass	Prototypes	Other Significant Agents
Beta agonists	Albuterol, salmeterol	Metaproterenol, terbutaline, formoterol
Methylxanthines	Theophylline	Aminophylline (a theophylline salt), caffeine, theobromine
Muscarinic antagonists	Ipratropium	Tiotropium
Release inhibitors	Cromolyn	Nedocromil
Glucocorticoids	Beclomethasone	Prednisone
Leukotriene antagonists	Zafirlukast, zileuton	Montelukast

---

inflammatory changes characteristic of long-standing asthma. This is a shift from earlier beliefs that steroids should be used only in severe refractory asthma. In such cases of severe asthma, patients are usually hospitalized and stabilized on daily systemic prednisone and then switched to inhaled or alternate-day oral therapy before discharge. In status asthmaticus, parenteral steroids are lifesaving and apparently act more promptly than in ordinary asthma. Their mechanism of action in this condition is not fully understood. (See Chapter 39 for other uses.)

E. Toxicity

Local aerosol administration can occasionally result in a very small degree of adrenal suppression, but this is rarely significant. More commonly, changes in oropharyngeal flora result in candidiasis. If oral therapy is required, adrenal suppression can be reduced by using alternate-day therapy (ie, giving the drug in slightly higher dosage every other day rather than smaller doses every day). The major systemic toxicities of the glucocorticoids described in Chapter 39 are much more likely to occur if systemic treatment is required for more than 2 weeks, as in severe refractory asthma. Regular use of inhaled steroids *does* cause mild growth retardation in children, but these children eventually reach full predicted adult stature.

LEUKOTRIENE ANTAGONISTS

These drugs interfere with the synthesis or the action of the leukotrienes (see also Chapter 18). Although their value has been established, they are not as effective as corticosteroids in severe asthma.

A. Leukotriene Receptor Blockers

Zafirlukast and **montelukast** are antagonists at the LTD_4 leukotriene receptor (see Table 18–1). The LTE_4 receptor is also blocked. These drugs are orally active and have been shown to be effective in preventing exercise-, antigen-, and aspirin-induced bronchospasm. They are not recommended for acute episodes of asthma. Toxicity is generally low. Rare reports of Churg-Strauss syndrome, allergic granulomatous angiitis, have appeared, but an association with these drugs has not been established.

B. Zileuton

Zileuton is an orally active drug that selectively inhibits 5-lipoxygenase, a key enzyme in the conversion of arachidonic acid to leukotrienes. The drug is effective in preventing both exercise- and antigen-induced bronchospasm. It is also effective against "aspirin allergy," the bronchospasm that results from ingestion of aspirin by individuals who apparently divert all eicosanoid production to leukotrienes when the cyclooxygenase pathway is blocked (Chapter 18). The toxicity of zileuton includes occasional elevation of liver enzymes, and this drug is therefore less popular than the receptor blockers.

ANTI-IGE ANTIBODY

Omalizumab is a humanized murine monoclonal antibody to human IgE. It binds to the IgE on sensitized mast cells and prevents activation by asthma triggers and subsequent release of inflammatory mediators. It was approved in 2003 for the prophylactic management of asthma, and initial reports have been positive. It is very expensive and must be administered parenterally.

QUESTIONS

1. One effect that theophylline, nitroglycerin, isoproterenol, and histamine have in common is
   (A) Direct stimulation of cardiac contractile force
   (B) Tachycardia

(C) Increased gastric acid secretion
(D) Postural hypotension
(E) Throbbing headache

2. A 23-year-old woman is using an albuterol inhaler for frequent acute episodes of asthma and describes symptoms that she ascribes to the albuterol. Which of the following is NOT a recognized action of albuterol?
(A) Diuretic effect
(B) Positive inotropic effect
(C) Skeletal muscle tremor
(D) Smooth muscle relaxation
(E) Tachycardia

3. A 10-year-old child has severe asthma and was hospitalized 5 times between the ages of 7 and 9. He is now receiving outpatient medications that have greatly reduced the frequency of severe attacks. Which of the following is most likely to have adverse effects when used daily over long periods for severe asthma?
(A) Albuterol by aerosol
(B) Beclomethasone by aerosol
(C) Cromolyn by inhaler
(D) Prednisone by mouth
(E) Theophylline in long-acting oral form

4. Nedocromil has as its major action
(A) Block of calcium channels in lymphocytes
(B) Block of mediator release from mast cells
(C) Block of phosphodiesterase in mast cells and basophils
(D) Smooth muscle relaxation in the bronchi
(E) Stimulation of cortisol release by the adrenals

5–6. A 16-year-old patient is in the emergency room receiving nasal oxygen. She has a heart rate of 135/min, a respiratory rate of 40/min, and a peak expiratory flow less than 50% of the predicted value. Wheezing and rales are audible without a stethoscope.

5. Which of the following drugs does NOT have a direct bronchodilator effect?
(A) Epinephrine
(B) Terbutaline
(C) Nedocromil
(D) Theophylline
(E) Ipratropium

6. After successful treatment of the acute attack, the patient was referred to the outpatient clinic for follow-up treatment of her asthma. Which of the following is NOT an established prophylactic strategy for asthma?
(A) Avoidance of antigen exposure
(B) Blockade of histamine receptors
(C) Blockade of leukotriene receptors

(D) Inhibition of phospholipase A_2
(E) Inhibition of release of mediators from mast cells and leukocytes

7. Mr Green is a 60-year-old former smoker with severe COPD and cardiac disease associated with frequent episodes of bronchospasm. Which of the following is a bronchodilator useful in chronic obstructive pulmonary disease (COPD) and least likely to cause cardiac arrhythmia?
(A) Aminophylline
(B) Cromolyn
(C) Epinephrine
(D) Ipratropium
(E) Metaproterenol
(F) Metoprolol
(G) Prednisone
(H) Salmeterol
(I) Zafirlukast
(J) Zileuton

8. Which of the following is a nonselective but very potent and efficacious bronchodilator that is not active by the oral route?
(A) Aminophylline
(B) Cromolyn
(C) Epinephrine
(D) Ipratropium
(E) Metaproterenol
(F) Metoprolol
(G) Prednisone
(H) Salmeterol
(I) Zafirlukast
(J) Zileuton

9. Which of the following is a prophylactic agent that appears to stabilize mast cells?
(A) Aminophylline
(B) Cromolyn
(C) Epinephrine
(D) Ipratropium
(E) Metaproterenol
(F) Metoprolol
(G) Prednisone
(H) Terbutaline
(I) Zafirlukast
(J) Zileuton

10. Which of the following is a direct bronchodilator that is most often used in asthma by the oral route?
(A) Cromolyn
(B) Epinephrine
(C) Ipratropium
(D) Metaproterenol
(E) Metoprolol
(F) Prednisone
(G) Salmeterol

(H) Theophylline
(I) Zileuton

11. Which of the following in its parenteral form is life-saving in severe status asthmaticus and acts, at least in part, by inhibiting phospholipase A_2?
(A) Aminophylline
(B) Cromolyn
(C) Epinephrine
(D) Ipratropium
(E) Metaproterenol
(F) Metoprolol
(G) Prednisone/prednisolone
(H) Salmeterol
(I) Zafirlukast
(J) Zileuton

12. Which of the following has overdose toxicity that includes insomnia, arrhythmias, and convulsions?
(A) Aminophylline
(B) Cromolyn
(C) Epinephrine
(D) Ipratropium
(E) Metaproterenol
(F) Metoprolol
(G) Prednisone/prednisolone
(H) Salmeterol
(I) Zafirlukast
(J) Zileuton

ANSWERS

1. Theophylline does not ordinarily cause headache. Nitroglycerin does not increase gastric acid secretion. Isoproterenol does not cause either. Histamine may cause all of the effects listed. The answer is **B**.

2. Albuterol is a β_2-selective receptor agonist, but in moderate to high doses it induces β_1 cardiac effects as well as β_2-mediated smooth and skeletal muscle effects. The answer is **A**.

3. If oral corticosteroids must be used, alternate-day therapy is preferred because it interferes less with normal growth in children. The answer is **D**.

4. The answer is **B**, inhibition of mediator release from mast cells. The mechanism for this effect is not known.

5. Neither nedocromil nor cromolyn is capable of reversing bronchospasm; their action is prophylactic. The answer is **C**.

6. Histamine does not appear to play a significant role in asthma, and antihistaminic drugs, even in high doses, are of little or no value. The answer is **B**.

7. Ipratropium is the bronchodilator that is most likely to be useful in COPD without causing arrhythmias. The answer is **D**.

8. Epinephrine is still one of the most potent and efficacious agents available for asthma. However, because it is nonselective, β_2-selective agents are preferred. The answer is **C**.

9. Cromolyn is useful only for prophylaxis. Like nedocromil, the drug stabilizes mast cells (ie, prevents mediator release). The answer is **B**.

10. Theophylline is a bronchodilator that is active by the oral route. The answer is **H**.

11. Parenteral corticosteroids such as prednisolone (the active metabolite of prednisone) are lifesaving in status asthmaticus. They probably act by reducing production of leukotrienes (see Chapter 18). The answer is **G**.

12. Aminophylline, a salt form of the base theophylline, can cause severe and potentially lethal overdose toxicity. The answer is **A**.

SKILL KEEPER ANSWER: SYMPATHOMIMETICS IN ASTHMA (SEE CHAPTER 9)

Direct-acting sympathomimetics are usually rapid in onset and short acting (eg, epinephrine, albuterol; exceptions: salmeterol, formoterol). Most direct-acting sympathomimetics have poor oral bioavailability. Indirect-acting sympathomimetics are usually longer acting and have good bioavailability (eg, ephedrine). An important disadvantage of the indirect-acting group is their CNS activity: most enter the CNS and produce undesirable stimulation. Even more important in asthma is the lack of receptor selectivity of the indirect-acting group. Because they release norepinephrine and epinephrine from stores, they produce all the α- and β_1-adrenoceptor-mediated effects of these catecholamines, most of which are undesirable in asthma. In contrast, the direct-acting agents can be tailored for selective β_2 activity. Furthermore, local application by aerosol administration is convenient and greatly reduces the systemic toxicity associated with oral or other systemic routes.

CHECKLIST

When you complete this chapter, you should be able to:

☐ Describe the strategies of drug treatment of asthma.

☐ List the major classes of drugs used in asthma.

☐ Describe the mechanisms of action of these drug groups.

☐ List the major adverse effects of the prototype asthma drugs.

PART V

Drugs That Act in the Central Nervous System

Introduction to CNS Pharmacology

21

TARGETS OF CNS DRUG ACTION

Most drugs that act on the CNS appear to do so by changing ion flow through transmembrane channels of nerve cells.

A. TYPES OF ION CHANNELS

Ion channels of neuronal membranes are of 2 major types: voltage gated and ligand gated (Figure 21–1). Voltage-gated ion channels respond to changes in membrane potential. They are concentrated on the axons of nerve cells and include the sodium channels responsible for action potential propagation. Cell bodies and dendrites also have voltage-sensitive ion channels for potassium and calcium. Ligand-gated ion channels, also called ionotropic receptors, respond to chemical neurotransmitters that bind to receptor subunits present in their macromolecular structure. Neurotransmitters also bind to G protein-coupled receptors (metabotropic receptors) that can modulate voltage-gated ion channels. Neurotransmitter-coupled ion channels are found on cell bodies and on both the presynaptic and the postsynaptic sides of synapses.

B. TYPES OF RECEPTOR-CHANNEL COUPLING

In the case of ligand-gated ion channels, activation (or inactivation) is initiated by the interaction between chemical neurotransmitters and their receptors (see

Figure 21–1). Coupling may be (1) through a receptor that acts directly on the channel protein (**B**), (2) through a receptor that is coupled to the ion channel through a G protein (**C**), or (3) through a receptor coupled to a G protein that modulates the formation of diffusible second messengers, including cyclic adenosine monophosphate (cAMP), inositol trisphosphate (IP_3), and diacylglycerol (DAG), which secondarily modulate ion channels (**D**).

C. ROLE OF THE ION CURRENT CARRIED BY THE CHANNEL

Excitatory postsynaptic potentials (EPSPs) are usually generated by the opening of sodium or calcium channels. In some synapses, similar depolarizing potentials result from the *closing* of potassium channels. Inhibitory postsynaptic potentials (IPSPs) are usually generated by the opening of potassium or chloride channels. For example, activation of postsynaptic metabotropic receptors increases the efflux of potassium. Presynaptic inhibition can occur via a decrease in calcium influx elicited by activation of metabotropic receptors.

SITES & MECHANISMS OF DRUG ACTION

A small number of neuropharmacologic agents exert their effects through direct interactions with molecular

---

HIGH-YIELD TERMS TO LEARN

Voltage-gated ion channels	Transmembrane ion channels regulated by changes in membrane potential
Ligand-gated ion channels	Transmembrane ion channels that are regulated by interactions between neurotransmitters and their receptors (also called ionotropic receptors)
Metabotropic receptors	G protein-coupled receptors that respond to neurotransmitters either by a direct action of G proteins on ion channels or by G protein enzyme activation that leads to formation of diffusible second messengers
EPSP	Excitatory postsynaptic potential; a depolarizing potential change
IPSP	Inhibitory postsynaptic potential; a hyperpolarizinq potential change
Synaptic mimicry	Ability of an administered chemical to mimic the actions of the natural neurotransmitter: a criterion for identification of a putative neurotransmitter

---

components of ion channels on axons. Examples include certain anticonvulsants (eg, carbamazepine, phenytoin), local anesthetics, and some drugs used in general anesthesia. However, the effects of most therapeutically important CNS drugs are exerted mainly at synapses. Possible mechanisms are indicated in Figure 21–2. Thus, drugs may act presynaptically to alter the synthesis, storage, release, reuptake, or metabolism of transmitter chemicals. Other drugs can activate or block both pre- and postsynaptic receptors for specific transmitters or can interfere with the actions of second messengers. The selectivity of CNS drug action is largely based on the fact that different groups of neurons use different neurotransmitters and that they are segregated into networks that subserve different CNS functions. A few neurotoxic substances damage or kill nerve cells. For example, 1-methyl-4-phenyl-1, 2, 3, 6-tetrahydropyridine (MPTP) is cytotoxic to neurons of the nigrostriatal dopaminergic pathway.

ROLE OF CNS ORGANIZATION

The CNS contains 2 types of neuronal systems: hierarchical and diffuse.

A. HIERARCHICAL SYSTEMS

These systems are delimited in their anatomic distribution and generally contain large myelinated, rapidly conducting fibers. Hierarchical systems control major sensory and motor functions. The major excitatory transmitters in these systems are aspartate and glutamate. These systems also include numerous small inhibitory interneurons, which use γ-aminobutyric acid (GABA) or glycine as transmitters. Drugs that affect hierarchical systems often have profound effects on the overall excitability of the CNS.

B. DIFFUSE SYSTEMS

Diffuse systems are broadly distributed, with single cells frequently sending processes to many different areas. The axons are fine and branch repeatedly to form synapses with many cells. Axons commonly have periodic enlargements (varicosities) that contain transmitter vesicles. The transmitters in diffuse systems are often amines (norepinephrine, dopamine, serotonin) or peptides that commonly exert actions on metabotropic receptors. Drugs that affect these systems will often have marked effects on such CNS functions as attention, appetite, and emotional states.

TRANSMITTERS AT CENTRAL SYNAPSES

A. CRITERIA FOR TRANSMITTER STATUS

To be accepted as a neurotransmitter, a candidate chemical must (1) be present in higher concentration in the synaptic area than in other areas (ie, must be localized in appropriate areas), (2) be released by electrical or chemical stimulation via a calcium-dependent mechanism, and (3) produce the same sort of postsynaptic response that is seen with physiologic activation of the synapse (ie, must exhibit synaptic mimicry). Table 21–1 lists the most important chemicals currently accepted as neurotransmitters in the CNS.

B. ACETYLCHOLINE

Approximately 5% of brain neurons have receptors for acetylcholine (ACh). Most CNS responses to ACh are mediated by a large family of G protein-coupled muscarinic M_1 receptors that lead to slow excitation when activated. The ionic mechanism of slow excitation involves a *decrease* in membrane permeability to potassium. Of the nicotinic receptors present in the CNS

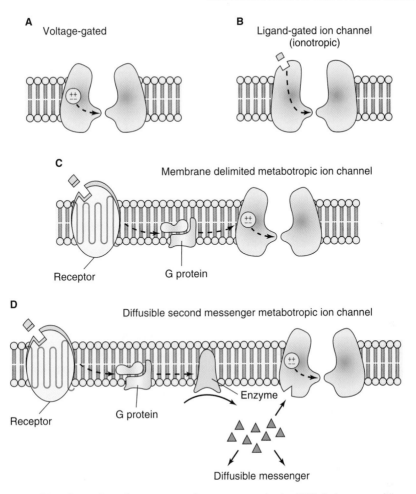

Figure 21–1. Types of ion channels and neurotransmitter receptors in the CNS: **A** shows a voltage-gated ion channel in which the voltage sensor controls the gating (broken arrow). **B** shows a ligand-gated ion channel in which binding of the neurotransmitter to the ionotropic channel receptor controls the gating. **C** shows a metabotropic receptor coupled to a G protein that can interact directly with an ion channel. **D** shows a receptor coupled to a G protein that activates an enzyme; the activated enzyme generates a diffusible second messenger that can interact with an ion channel. (Reproduced, with permission, from Katzung BG, editor: *Basic & Clinical Pharmacology*, 10th ed. McGraw-Hill, 2007.)

(they are less common than muscarinic receptors), those on the Renshaw cells activated by motor axon collaterals in the spinal cord are the best characterized. Drugs affecting the activity of cholinergic systems in the brain include the acetylcholinesterase inhibitors used in Alzheimer's disease (eg, tacrine) and the muscarinic blocking agents used in parkinsonism (eg, benztropine).

C. DOPAMINE

Dopamine exerts slow inhibitory actions at synapses in specific neuronal systems commonly via G protein-coupled activation of potassium channels (postsynaptic)or inactivation of calcium channels (presynaptic). The D_2 receptor is the main dopamine subtype in basal ganglia neurons, and it is widely distributed at the supraspinal level. Dopaminergic pathways include the nigrostriatal, mesolimbic, and tuberoinfundibular tracts. In addition to the 2 receptors listed in Table 21–1, 3 other dopamine receptor subtypes have been identified (D_3, D_4, and D_5). Drugs that block the activity of dopaminergic pathways include older antipsychotics (eg, chlorpromazine, haloperidol). Drugs that increase brain dopaminergic activity include CNS stimulants (eg, amphetamines) and antiparkinsonism drugs (eg, levodopa).

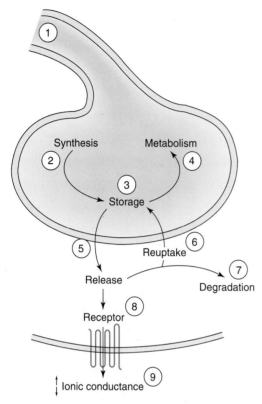

Figure 21–2. Sites of CNS drug action. Drugs may alter (1) the action potential in the presynaptic fiber; (2) the synthesis of transmitter; (3) the storage of transmitter; (4) the metabolism of transmitter within the nerve ending; (5) the release of transmitter; (6) the reuptake or (7) extracellular disposition of transmitter; (8) the postsynaptic receptor; or (9) the postsynaptic effects that follow receptor activation. (Reproduced, with permission, from Katzung BG, editor: *Basic & Clinical Pharmacology,* 10th ed. McGraw-Hill, 2007.)

D. NOREPINEPHRINE

Noradrenergic neuron cell bodies are mainly located in the brain stem and the lateral tegmental area of the pons. These neurons fan out broadly to provide most regions of the CNS with diffuse noradrenergic input. Excitatory effects are produced by activation of α_1 and β_1 receptors. Inhibitory effects are caused by activation of α_2 and β_2 receptors. CNS stimulants (eg, amphetamines, cocaine), monoamine oxidase inhibitors (eg, phenelzine), and tricyclic antidepressants (eg, amitriptyline) are examples of drugs that enhance the activity of noradrenergic pathways.

E. SEROTONIN

Most serotonin (5-hydroxytryptamine; 5-HT) pathways originate from cell bodies in the raphe or midline regions of the pons and upper brain stem; these pathways innervate most regions of the CNS. Multiple 5-HT receptor subtypes have been identified and, with the exception of the 5-HT_3 subtype, all are metabotropic. 5-HT_{1A} receptors and GABA_B receptors share the same potassium channel. Serotonin can cause excitation or inhibition of CNS neurons depending on the receptor subtype activated. Both excitatory and inhibitory actions can occur on the same neuron if appropriate receptors are present. Most of the agents used in the treatment of major depressive disorders affect serotonergic pathways (eg, tricyclic antidepressants, selective serotonin reuptake inhibitors). The actions of some CNS stimulants and newer antipsychotic drugs (eg, olanzapine) also appear to be mediated via effects on serotonergic transmission. Reserpine, which may cause severe depression of mood, depletes vesicular stores of both serotonin and norepinephrine in CNS neurons.

F. GLUTAMIC ACID

Most neurons in the brain are excited by glutamic acid. High concentrations of glutamic acid in synaptic vesicles are achieved by the vesicular glutamate transporter (VGLUT). Both ionotropic and metabotropic receptors have been characterized. Subtypes of glutamate receptors include the *N*-methyl-D-aspartate (NMDA) receptor, which is blocked by phencyclidine (PCP) and ketamine. NMDA receptors appear to play a role in synaptic plasticity related to learning and memory. Memantine is an NMDA antagonist introduced for treatment of Alzheimer's dementia. Excessive activation of NMDA receptors after neuronal injury may be responsible for cell death. Glutamate metabotropic receptor activation can result in G protein-coupled activation of phospholipase C or inhibition of adenylyl cyclase.

G. GABA AND GLYCINE

GABA is the primary neurotransmitter mediating IPSPs in neurons in the brain; it is also important in the spinal cord. GABA_A receptor activation opens chloride ion channels. GABA_B receptors (activated by baclofen, a centrally-acting muscle relaxant) are coupled to G proteins that either open potassium channels or close calcium channels. Fast IPSPs are blocked by GABA_A receptor antagonists, and slow IPSPs are blocked by GABA_B receptor antagonists. Drugs that influence GABA_A receptor systems include sedative-hypnotics (eg, barbiturates, benzodiazepines, zolpidem) and some anticonvulsants (eg, gabapentin, tiagabine, vigabatrin). Glycine receptors, which are more numerous in the cord than in the brain, are blocked by strychnine, a spinal convulsant.

Table 21–1. Neurotransmitter pharmacology in the CNS.

Transmitter	Anatomical Distribution	Receptor Subtypes	Receptor Mechanisms
Acetylcholine	Cell bodies at all levels, short and long axons	Muscarinic, M_1; blocked by pirenzepine and atropine	Excitatory; ↓ K^+ conductance; ↑ IP_3 and DAG
		Muscarinic, M_2; blocked by atropine	Inhibitory; ↑ K^+ conductance; ↓ cAMP
	Motoneuron–Renshaw cell synapse	Nicotinic, N	Excitatory; ↑ cation conductance
Dopamine	Cell bodies at all levels, short, medium, and long axons	D_1; blocked by phenothiazines	Inhibitory; ↑cAMP
		D_2; blocked by phenothiazines and haloperidol	Inhibitory (presynaptic); ↓ Ca^{2+} conductance;
			Inhibitory (postsynaptic); ↑ K^+ conductance; ↓ cAMP
Norepinephrine	Cell bodies in pons and brain stem project to all levels	$Alpha_1$; blocked by prazosin	Excitatory; ↓ K^+ conductance; ↑ IP_3 and DAG
		$Alpha_2$; activated by clonidine	Inhibitory (presynaptic); ↓ Ca^{2+} conductance
			Inhibitory (postsynaptic); ↑ K^+ conductance; ↓ cAMP
		$Beta_1$; blocked by propranolol	Excitatory; ↓ K^+ conductance; ↑ cAMP
		$Beta_2$; blocked by propranolol	Inhibitory; ? increase in electrogenic sodium pump
Serotonin (5-hydroxy-tryptamine)	Cell bodies in midbrain and pons project to all levels	5-HT_{1A}; buspirone is a partial agonist	Inhibitory; ↑ K^+ conductance
		5-HT_{2A}; blocked by clozapine, risperidone, and olanzapine	Excitatory; ↓ K^+ conductance; ↑ IP_3 and DAG
		5-HT_3; blocked by ondansetron	Excitatory; ↑ cation conductance
		5-HT_4	Excitatory; ↓ K^+ conductance; ↑ cAMP
GABA	Supraspinal interneurons; spinal interneurons involved in presynaptic inhibition	$GABA_A$; facilitated by benzodiazepines and zolpidem	Inhibitory; ↑ Cl^- conductance
		$GABA_B$; activated by baclofen	Inhibitory (presynaptic); ↓ Ca^{2+} conductance
			Inhibitory (postsynaptic); ↑ K^+ conductance
Glutamate, aspartate	Relay neurons at all levels	Four subtypes; NMDA subtype blocked by phencyclidine, ketamine and memantine	Excitatory; ↑ Ca^{2+} or cation conductance
		Metabotropic subtypes	Inhibitory (presynaptic); ↓ Ca^{2+} conductance ↓ cAMP
			Excitatory (postsynaptic); ↓ K^+ conductance, ↑ IP_3 and DAG

(continued)

Table 21–1. Neurotransmitter pharmacology in the CNS. (*continued*)

Transmitter	Anatomical Distribution	Receptor Subtypes	Receptor Mechanisms
Glycine	Interneurons in spinal cord and brain stem	Single subtype; blocked by strychnine	Inhibitory; ↑ Cl⁻ conductance
Opioid peptides	Cell bodies at all levels	Three major subtypes: mu, delta, kappa	Inhibitory (presynaptic); $\downarrow Ca^{2+}$ conductance; ↓ cAMP
			Inhibitory (postsynaptic); ↑ K⁺ conductance; ↓ cAMP

Adapted, with permission, from Katzung BG, editor: *Basic & Clinical Pharmacology,* 9th ed. Appleton & Lange, 2004.

H. Peptide Transmitters

Many peptides have been identified in the CNS, and some meet most or all of the criteria for acceptance as neurotransmitters. The best defined peptides are the opioid peptides (beta-endorphin, met- and leu-enkephalin, and dynorphin), which are distributed at all levels of the neuraxis. Some of the important therapeutic actions of opioid analgesics (eg, morphine)are mediated via activation of receptors for these endogenous peptides. Substance P is a mediator of slow EPSPs in neurons involved in nociceptive sensory pathways in the spinal cord and brain stem. Peptide transmitters differ from nonpeptide transmitters in that (1) the peptides are synthesized in the cell body and transported to the nerve ending via axonal transport, and (2) no reuptake or specific enzyme mechanisms have been identified for terminating their actions.

I. Endocannabinoids

These are brain lipid derivatives (eg, 2-arachidonyl-glycerol) that bind to receptors for cannabinoids found in marijuana. They are synthesized and released postsynaptically after membrane depolarization but travel backward acting presynaptically (retrograde) to decrease transmitter release.

SKILL KEEPER:
BIODISPOSITION OF CNS
DRUGS (SEE CHAPTER 1)

1. *What characteristics of drug molecules afford access to the CNS?*

2. *What concerns do you have regarding CNS drug use in the pregnant patient?*

3. *How are CNS drugs eliminated from the body?*

The Skill Keeper Answers appear at the end of the chapter.

QUESTIONS

1. Which of the following chemicals does NOT satisfy the criteria for a neurotransmitter role in the CNS?
   (A) Acetylcholine
   (B) Dopamine
   (C) Glycine
   (D) Nitric oxide
   (E) Substance P

2. Many therapeutically useful drugs act via brain dopaminergic systems. Which mechanism underlying their actions is NOT likely to be useful in the management of Parkinson's disease?
   (A) Inhibition of dopamine reuptake
   (B) Increase in dopamine synthesis
   (C) Activation of dopamine receptors
   (D) Inhibition of dopamine metabolism
   (E) Blockade of dopamine receptors

3. Neurotransmitters may
   (A) Increase chloride conductance to cause inhibition
   (B) Increase potassium conductance to cause excitation
   (C) Increase sodium conductance to cause inhibition
   (D) Increase calcium conductance to cause inhibition
   (E) Exert all of the above actions

4. Which neurotransmitter does NOT change membrane excitability by decreasing K⁺ conductance?
   (A) Acetylcholine
   (B) Dopamine
   (C) Glutamic acid
   (D) Norepinephrine
   (E) Serotonin

5. Which receptor shares the same potassium channel as the 5-HT$_{1A}$ receptor?
   (A) Delta opioid receptor
   (B) Dopamine D$_2$ receptor
   (C) GABA$_B$ receptor

(D) Muscarinic M_1 receptor
(E) Substance P receptor

6. Which compound is most likely to function as a neurotransmitter in hierarchical systems?
(A) Dopamine
(B) Glutamate
(C) Met-enkephalin
(D) Norepinephrine
(E) Serotonin

7. Which statement about beta-endorphin is accurate?
(A) It is exclusively located in the spinal cord
(B) Enzymes for its synthesis are located in nerve endings
(C) It selectively activates delta opioid receptors
(D) Its postsynaptic effects are terminated by active reuptake
(E) Its actions are mainly inhibitory

8. Activation of metabotropic receptors located presynaptically causes inhibition by decreasing the inward flux of
(A) Calcium
(B) Chloride
(C) Potassium
(D) Sodium
(E) None of the above

9. This compound is found in diffuse neuronal systems in the CNS, particularly in the raphe nuclei; it appears to play a major role in the expression of mood because many antidepressant drugs are thought to increase its functional activity.
(A) Acetylcholine
(B) Dopamine
(C) Histamine
(D) Serotonin
(E) Substance P

10. In strychnine poisoning, convulsions occur because of antagonistic effects at receptors for
(A) Aspartate
(B) GABA
(C) Glutamate
(D) Glycine
(E) Norepinephrine

11. Cyclic adenosine monophosphate (cAMP) functions as a diffusible second messenger that can modify voltage-gated ion channels after activation of which of the following receptors?
(A) Acetylcholine M_1 receptors
(B) Beta adrenoceptors
(C) 5-HT$_3$ receptors
(D) GABA$_A$ receptors
(E) Glycine receptors

12. One of the first neurotransmitter receptors to be identified in the CNS is located on the Renshaw cell in the spinal cord. Activation of this receptor results in excitation via an increase in cation conductance independently of G proteins. Which compound is most likely to activate this receptor?
(A) Aspartate
(B) Baclofen
(C) Glutamate
(D) Nicotine
(E) Serotonin

13. This compound decreases the functional activities of several CNS neurotransmitters, including dopamine, norepinephrine, and serotonin. At high doses it may cause parkinsonism-like extrapyramidal system dysfunction.
(A) Amphetamine
(B) Baclofen
(C) Diazepam
(D) Ketamine
(E) Reserpine

14. This amine neurotransmitter is found in high concentrations in cell bodies in the pons and brain stem; at some sites, release of transmitter is autoregulated via presynaptic inhibition.
(A) Acetylcholine
(B) Dopamine
(C) Glutamate
(D) Norepinephrine
(E) Substance P

ANSWERS

1. Nitric oxide synthase (NOS), the enzyme that generates nitric oxide (NO), is found in some neurons in the CNS. However, a role for NO in synaptic transmission in the CNS has not been established. The answer is **D.**

2. The neuropathology of Parkinson's disease involves degeneration of dopaminergic neurons in the nigrostriatal pathway. Drugs that facilitate dopaminergic transmission have value in the management of parkinsonism. Levodopa increases dopamine synthesis; bromocriptine activates dopamine receptors; and selegiline inhibits dopamine metabolism. Drugs that act as inhibitors of brain dopamine *transporters* could have important therapeutic applications in Parkinson's disease and in the treatment of hyperprolactinemia. Antagonists of brain dopamine receptors are associated with extrapyramidal dysfunction, and such drugs are likely to exacerbate parkinsonism. The answer is **E.**

3. Activation of chloride or potassium ion channels often generates inhibitory postsynaptic potentials

(IPSPs). Activation of sodium and *inhibition* of potassium ion channels generate excitatory postsynaptic potentials (EPSPs). The answer is **A.**

4. A decrease in K^+ conductance is associated with neuronal excitation. With the exception of dopamine, all of the neurotransmitters listed are able to cause excitation by this mechanism via their activation of specific receptors: acetylcholine (M_1), glutamate (metabotropic), norepinephrine (α_1 and β_1), and serotonin (5-HT$_{2A}$). The answer is **B.**

5. GABA$_B$ receptors and 5-HT$_{1A}$ receptors share the same potassium ion channel, with a G protein involved in the coupling mechanism. The spasmolytic drug baclofen is an activator of GABA$_B$ receptors in the spinal cord. The anxiolytic drug buspirone may act as a partial agonist at brain 5-HT$_{1A}$ receptors. The answer is **C.**

6. Catecholamines (dopamine, norepinephrine), opioid peptides, and serotonin act as neurotransmitters in nonspecific or diffuse neuronal systems. Glutamate is the primary excitatory transmitter in hierarchical neuronal systems. The answer is **B.**

7. The opioid peptides are widely distributed in the CNS at all levels of the neuraxis and are synthesized in the cell bodies. They activate several receptor subtypes and cause inhibition. No mechanism has been described for termination of the synaptic actions of endogenous peptides. The answer is **E.**

8. Activation of metabotropic receptors located presynaptically results in the inhibition of calcium influx with a resultant decrease in the release of neurotransmitter from nerve endings. This type of presynaptic inhibition occurs after activation of dopamine D_2, norepinephrine α_2, glutamate, and mu opioid peptide receptors. The answer is **A.**

9. Several amine transmitters may be involved in the control of mood states, especially norepinephrine and serotonin. Many of the cell bodies of serotonergic neurons are found in the raphe nuclei. Most of the drugs used for the treatment of major depressive disorders increase serotonergic activity in the CNS. The answer is **D.**

10. Activation of both GABA$_A$ and glycine receptors present on neurons in the spinal cord leads to membrane hyperpolarization via increases in chloride ion conductance. In the case of glycine, its inhibitory action at the level of the spinal cord is opposed by strychnine. The answer is **D.**

11. Metabotropic receptors can modulate voltage-gated ion channels directly (membrane-delimited action) and also by the formation of diffusible second messengers through G protein-mediated effects on enzymes involved in their synthesis. A classic example of the latter type of action is provided by the β adrenoceptor, which generates cAMP via the activation of adenylyl cyclase. The answer is **B.**

SKILL KEEPER ANSWERS: BIODISPOSITION OF CNS DRUGS (SEE CHAPTER 1)

1. *Lipid solubility is an important characteristic of most CNS drugs in terms of their ability to cross the blood-brain barrier. Access to the CNS of water-soluble (polar) molecules is limited to those of low molecular weight such as lithium ion and ethanol.*

2. *CNS drugs readily cross the placental barrier and enter the fetal circulation. Concerns during pregnancy include possible effects on fetal development and the potential for drug effects on the neonate if CNS drugs are used near the time of delivery.*

3. *With the exception of lithium, almost all CNS drugs require metabolism to more water-soluble (polar) metabolites for their elimination. Thus, drugs that modify the activities of drug-metabolizing enzymes may impact on the clearance of CNS drugs, perhaps affecting the intensity or duration of their effects.*

12. Nicotinic receptors on the Renshaw cell are activated by the release of ACh from motoneuron collaterals. This results in the release of glycine, which, via interaction with its receptors on the motoneuron, causes membrane hyperpolarization, an example of feedback inhibition. The receptors were so named because of their activation by nicotine. The answer is **D.**

13. In addition to depleting vesicular stores of norepinephrine in sympathetic nerve endings, reserpine depletes brain dopamine and causes parkinsonism-like adverse effects. Reserpine also decreases vesicular stores of norepinephrine and serotonin in CNS neurons, which can result in depression of mood. The answer is **E.**

14. Cell bodies of noradrenergic neurons located in the pons and brain stem project to all levels of the CNS. Agents that activate presynaptic α_2 receptors on such neurons (eg, clonidine, methyldopa) decrease central noradrenergic activity, an action thought to result in decreased vasomotor outflow. The answer is **D.**

CHECKLIST

When you complete this chapter, you should be able to:

☐ Explain the difference between voltage-gated and ligand-gated ion channels.

☐ List the criteria for accepting a chemical as a neurotransmitter.

☐ Identify the major excitatory and inhibitory CNS neurotransmitters in the CNS.

☐ Identify the sites of drug action at synapses and the mechanisms by which drugs modulate synaptic transmission.

☐ Give an example of a CNS drug that influences neurotransmitter functions at the level of (a) synthesis, (b) metabolism, (c) release, (d) reuptake, and (e) receptor.

Sedative-Hypnotic Drugs

The sedative-hypnotics belong to a chemically heterogeneous class of drugs, almost all of which produce dose-dependent CNS depressant effects. A major subgroup is the benzodiazepines, but representatives of other subgroups, including barbiturates, and miscellaneous agents (carbamates, alcohols, and cyclic ethers) are still in use. Newer drugs with distinctive characteristics include the anxiolytic buspirone, several widely used hypnotics (zolpidem, zaleplon, eszopiclone), and ramelteon, a novel drug used in sleep disorders.

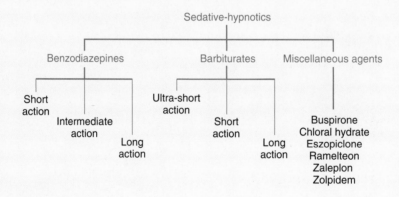

PHARMACOKINETICS

A. ABSORPTION AND DISTRIBUTION

Most of the sedative-hypnotic drugs are lipid soluble and are absorbed well from the gastrointestinal tract, with good distribution to the brain. Drugs with the highest lipid solubility (eg, **thiopental**) enter the CNS rapidly and can be used as induction agents in anesthesia. The CNS effects of thiopental are terminated by rapid **redistribution** of the drug from brain to other highly perfused tissues, including skeletal muscle. Other drugs with a rapid onset of CNS action include eszopiclone, zaleplon, and zolpidem.

B. METABOLISM AND EXCRETION

Sedative-hypnotics are metabolized before elimination from the body, mainly by hepatic enzymes. Metabolic rates and pathways vary among different drugs. Many benzodiazepines are converted initially to **active metabolites** with long half-lives. After several days of therapy with some drugs (eg, diazepam, flurazepam), accumulation of active metabolites can lead to excessive sedation. Lorazepam and oxazepam undergo extrahepatic conjugation and do not form active metabolites. With the exception of phenobarbital, which is excreted partly unchanged in the urine, the barbiturates are extensively metabolized. Chloral hydrate is oxidized to trichloroethanol, an active metabolite. Rapid metabolism by liver enzymes is responsible for the short duration of action of zolpidem. Zaleplon undergoes even more rapid hepatic metabolism by aldehyde oxidase and cytochrome P450. Eszopiclone is also metabolized by cytochrome P450, with a half-life of 6 h. The duration of CNS actions of sedative-hypnotic drugs ranges from

HIGH-YIELD TERMS TO LEARN

Sedation	Reduction of anxiety
Anxiolytic	A drug that reduces anxiety, a sedative
Hypnosis	Induction of sleep
REM Sleep	Phase of sleep associated with rapid eye movements; most dreaming takes place during REM sleep
Tolerance	Reduction in drug effect requiring an increase in dosage to maintain the same response
Physiologic Dependence	The state of response to a drug whereby removal of the drug evokes unpleasant symptoms, usually the opposite of the drug's effects
Psychological Dependence	The state of response to a drug whereby the drug taker feels compelled to use the drug and suffers anxiety when separated from the drug
Anesthesia	Loss of consciousness associated with absence of response to pain
Coma	Extremely deep anesthesia or depression of brain activity; precursor to respiratory and circulatory failure

just a few hours (eg, zaleplon < zolpidem = triazolam = eszopiclone < chloral hydrate) to more than 30 h (eg, chlordiazepoxide, clorazepate, diazepam, phenobarbital).

MECHANISMS OF ACTION

No single mechanism of action for sedative-hypnotics has been identified, and the different chemical subgroups may have different actions. Certain drugs (eg, benzodiazepines) facilitate neuronal membrane inhibition by actions at specific receptors.

A. Benzodiazepines

Receptors for benzodiazepines (BZ receptors) are present in many brain regions, including the thalamus, limbic structures, and the cerebral cortex. The BZ receptors form part of a $GABA_A$ receptor-chloride ion channel macromolecular complex, a pentameric structure assembled from 5 subunits each with 4 transmembrane domains. A major isoform of the $GABA_A$ receptor consists of two $alpha_1$, two $beta_2$, and one $gamma_2$ subunits. In this isoform, the binding site for benzodiazepines is between an $alpha_1$ and the $gamma_2$ subunit. However, benzodiazepines also bind to other $GABA_A$ receptor isoforms that contain $alpha_2$, $alpha_3$, and $alpha_5$ subunits. Binding of benzodiazepines facilitates the inhibitory actions of GABA, which are exerted through increased chloride ion conductance (Figure 22–1). Benzodiazepines increase the *frequency* of GABA-mediated chloride ion channel opening. **Flumazenil** reverses the CNS effects of benzodiazepines and is classified as an **antagonist** at BZ

receptors. Certain beta-carbolines have a high affinity for BZ receptors and can elicit anxiogenic and convulsant effects. These drugs are classified as **inverse agonists.**

B. Barbiturates

Barbiturates depress neuronal activity in the midbrain reticular formation, facilitating and prolonging the inhibitory effects of GABA and glycine. Barbiturates also bind to multiple isoforms of the $GABA_A$ receptor but at different sites from those with which benzodiazepines interact. Their actions are not antagonized by flumazenil. Barbiturates increase the *duration* of GABA-mediated chloride ion channel opening. They may also block the excitatory transmitter glutamic acid, and, at high concentration, sodium channels.

C. Other Drugs

The hypnotics **zolpidem, zaleplon,** and **eszopiclone** are not benzodiazepines but appear to exert their CNS effects via interaction with certain benzodiazepine receptors, classified as BZ_1 or omega$_1$ subtypes. In contrast to benzodiazepines, these drugs bind more selectively, interacting only with $GABA_A$ receptor isoforms that contain $alpha_1$ subunits. Their CNS depressant effects can be antagonized by flumazenil.

PHARMACODYNAMICS

The CNS effects of most sedative-hypnotics depend on dose, as shown in Figure 22–2. These effects range from sedation and relief of anxiety (anxiolysis), through

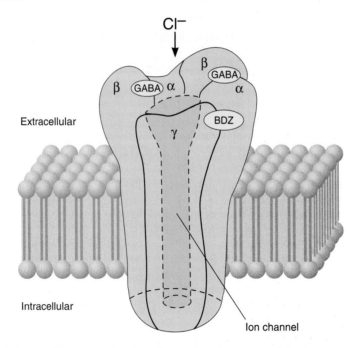

Figure 22–1. A model of the GABA$_A$ receptor-chloride ion channel macromolecular complex consisting of 5 membrane-spanning subunits. Multiple forms of α, β and γ subunits are arranged in different pentameric combinations (receptor heterogeneity). GABA interacts with α or β subunits triggering chloride channel opening with resulting membrane hyperpolarization. Binding of benzodiazepines facilitates channel opening but does not directly initiate choride current. (Modified and reproduced with permission, from Zorumski CF, Isenberg KE: Insights into the structure and function of GABA receptors: Ion channels and psychiatry. Am J Psychiatry 1991;148:162.)

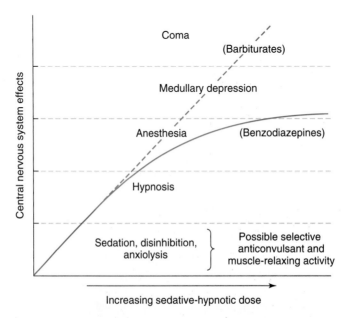

Figure 22–2. Relationships between dose of benzodiazepines and barbiturates and their CNS effects.

hypnosis (facilitation of sleep), to anesthesia and coma. Depressant effects are additive when 2 or more drugs are given together. The steepness of the dose–response curve varies among drug groups; those with flatter curves, such as benzodiazepines and the newer hypnotics (eg, zolpidem), are safer for clinical use.

A. SEDATION

Sedative actions, with relief of anxiety, occur with all drugs in this class. Anxiolysis is usually accompanied by some impairment of psychomotor functions, and behavioral disinhibition may also occur. In animals, most conventional sedative-hypnotics release punishment-suppressed behavior.

B. HYPNOSIS

Sedative-hypnotics can promote sleep onset and increase the duration of the sleep state. Rapid eye movement (REM) sleep duration is usually decreased at high doses; a rebound increase in REM sleep may occur on withdrawal from chronic drug use. Effects on sleep patterns occur infrequently with newer hypnotics such as zaleplon and zolpidem.

C. ANESTHESIA

At high doses of most older sedative-hypnotics loss of consciousness may occur, with amnesia and suppression of reflexes. Anterograde amnesia is more likely with benzodiazepines than with other sedative-hypnotics. Anesthesia can be produced by most barbiturates (eg, thiopental) and certain benzodiazepines (eg, midazolam).

D. ANTICONVULSANT ACTIONS

Suppression of seizure activity occurs with high doses of most of the barbiturates and some of the benzodiazepines, but this is usually at the cost of marked sedation. Selective anticonvulsant action (ie, suppression of convulsions at doses that do not cause severe sedation) occurs with only a few of these drugs (eg, phenobarbital, clonazepam). High doses of intravenous diazepam, lorazepam, or phenobarbital are used in status epilepticus. In this condition, heavy sedation is desirable.

E. MUSCLE RELAXATION

Relaxation of skeletal muscle only occurs with high doses of most sedative-hypnotics. However, diazepam is effective at sedative dose levels for specific spasticity states, including cerebral palsy. Meprobamate also has some selectivity as a muscle relaxant.

F. MEDULLARY DEPRESSION

High doses of conventional sedative-hypnotics, especially alcohols and barbiturates, can cause depression of medullary neurons, leading to respiratory arrest, hypotension, and cardiovascular collapse. These effects are the cause of death in suicidal overdose.

SKILL KEEPER: LOADING DOSE (SEE CHAPTER 3)

Four hours after ingestion of an unknown quantity of phenobarbital, a patient was hospitalized and the drug concentration in the plasma was found to be 50 mg/L. Assume that in this patient pharmacokinetic parameters for phenobarbital are as follows: oral bioavailability, 100%; V_d, 40 L; CL, 6 L/day; half-life, 4 days. Estimate the dose of phenobarbital ingested. The Skill Keeper Answer appears at the end of the chapter.

G. TOLERANCE AND DEPENDENCE

Tolerance—a decrease in responsiveness—occurs when sedative-hypnotics are used chronically or in high dosage. Cross-tolerance may occur among different chemical subgroups. Psychological dependence occurs frequently with most sedative-hypnotics and is manifested by the compulsive use of these drugs to reduce anxiety. Physiologic dependence constitutes an altered state that leads to an abstinence syndrome (withdrawal state) when the drug is discontinued. Withdrawal signs, which may include anxiety, tremors, hyperreflexia, and seizures, occur more commonly with shorter acting drugs. The dependence liability of zolpidem, zaleplon, and eszopiclone may be less than that of the benzodiazepines since withdrawal symptoms are minimal following their abrupt discontinuance.

CLINICAL USES

Most of these uses can be predicted from the pharmacodynamic effects outlined previously.

A. ANXIETY STATES

Benzodiazepines are favored in the drug treatment of acute anxiety states and for rapid control of panic attacks. Although it is difficult to demonstrate the superiority of one drug over another, alprazolam and clonazepam have greater efficacy than other benzodiazepines in the longer term treatment of panic and phobic disorders. *Note the increasing use of newer antidepressants in the treatment of chronic anxiety states (see Chapter 30).*

B. SLEEP DISORDERS

Benzodiazepines, including estazolam, flurazepam, and triazolam, have been widely used in primary insomnia and for the management of certain other sleep disorders. Lower doses should be used in elderly patients who are more sensitive to their CNS depressant effects. More recently, in insomnia there has been increasing use of zolpidem, zaleplon, and eszopiclone. These newer hypnotics appear to

KEY DRUGS		
Subclass	**Prototypes**	**Other Significant Agents**
Benzodiazepines	Diazepam	Alprazolam, chlordiazepoxide, clonazepam, flurazepam, lorazepam, oxazepam, triazolam
Benzodiazepine antagonist	Flumazenil	
Barbiturates	Phenobarbital	Amobarbital, pentobarbital, secobarbital, thiopental
Alcohols	Ethanol	Chloral hydrate
Carbamates	Meprobamate	
Other hypnotics	Zolpidem	Eszopiclone, zaleplon
Atypicals	Buspirone, ramelteon	

cause less daytime cognitive impairment than most benzodiazepines and have minimal effects on sleep patterns. Note that sedative-hypnotics including benzodiazepines are not recommended for breathing-related sleep disorders.

C. Other Uses

Thiopental is commonly used for the induction of anesthesia, and certain benzodiazepines (eg, diazepam, midazolam) are used as components of anesthesia protocols, including those used in day surgery. Special uses include the management of seizure disorders (eg, clonazepam, phenobarbital) and bipolar disorder (eg, clonazepam) and treatment of muscle spasticity (eg, diazepam). Longer acting benzodiazepines (eg, chlordiazepoxide, diazepam) are used in the management of withdrawal states in persons physiologically dependent on ethanol and other sedative-hypnotics.

TOXICITY

A. Psychomotor Dysfunction

This includes cognitive impairment, decreased psychomotor skills, and unwanted daytime sedation. These adverse effects are more common with benzodiazepines that have active metabolites with long half-lives (eg, diazepam, flurazepam), but can also occur following a single dose of a short-acting benzodiazepine like triazolam. The dosage of a sedative-hypnotic should be reduced in elderly patients, who are more susceptible to drugs that cause psychomotor dysfunction. In such patients excessive daytime sedation has been shown to increase the risk of falls and fractures. Anterograde amnesia may also occur with benzodiazepines, especially when used at high dosage, an action that forms the basis for their criminal use in cases of "date rape." Zolpidem and the newer hypnotics cause modest

day-after psychomotor depression with few amnestic effects. However, all prescription drugs used as sleep aids may cause functional impairment, including "sleep driving," defined as "driving while not fully awake after ingestion of a sedative-hypnotic product, with no memory of the event."

B. Additive CNS Depression

This occurs when sedative-hypnotics are used with other drugs in the class as well as with alcoholic beverages, antihistamines, antipsychotic drugs, opioid analgesics, and tricyclic antidepressants. This is the most common type of drug interaction involving sedative-hypnotics.

C. Overdosage

Overdosage causes severe respiratory and cardiovascular depression; these potentially lethal effects are more likely to occur with alcohols, barbiturates, and carbamates than with benzodiazepines or the newer hypnotics such as zolpidem. Management of intoxication requires maintenance of a patent airway and ventilatory support. Flumazenil may reverse CNS depressant effects of benzodiazepines, eszopiclone, zolpidem, and zaleplon but has no beneficial actions in overdosage with other sedative-hypnotics.

D. Other Adverse Effects

Barbiturates and carbamates (but not benzodiazepines, eszopiclone, zolpidem, or zaleplon) induce the formation of liver microsomal enzymes that metabolize drugs. This enzyme induction may lead to multiple drug interactions. Barbiturates may also precipitate acute intermittent porphyria in susceptible patients. Chloral hydrate may displace coumarins from plasma protein binding sites and increase anticoagulant effects.

ATYPICAL SEDATIVE-HYPNOTICS

A. BUSPIRONE

Buspirone is a selective anxiolytic, with minimal CNS depressant effects (it does not affect driving skills) and has no anticonvulsant or muscle relaxant properties. The drug interacts with the 5-HT$_{1A}$ subclass of brain serotonin receptors as a partial agonist, but the precise mechanism of its anxiolytic effect is unknown. Buspirone has a slow onset of action (>1 week) and is used in generalized anxiety disorder (GAD). Tolerance development is minimal with chronic use. Side effects of buspirone include tachycardia, paresthesias, pupillary constriction, and gastrointestinal distress. Buspirone has minimal abuse liability and is not a schedule-controlled drug.

B. RAMELTEON

This novel hypnotic drug, which activates melatonin receptors located in the suprachiasmatic nuclei of the CNS, is reported to decrease the latency of sleep onset, with minimal rebound insomnia or withdrawal symptoms. Unlike conventional hypnotics, ramelteon appears to have minimal abuse liability and is not a controlled substance. The drug is metabolized by hepatic cytochrome P450, forming an active metabolite. Its adverse effects include dizziness, fatigue, and endocrine changes, including decreased testosterone and increased prolactin.

QUESTIONS

1. Which of the following is most likely to result from treatment with moderate-high doses of diazepam?
   (A) Alleviation of the symptoms of major depressive disorder
   (B) Agitation and possible hyperreflexia with abrupt discontinuance after chronic use
   (C) Increased porphyrin synthesis
   (D) Improved performance on tests of psychomotor function
   (E) Retrograde amnesia

2. A 56-year-old very overweight man complains of not sleeping well and feeling tired during the day. He tells his physician that his wife is the cause of the problem because she wakes him up several times during the night because of his loud snores. This appears to be a breathing-related sleep disorder, so you should probably write a prescription for
   (A) Clorazepate
   (B) Flurazepam
   (C) Secobarbital
   (D) Triazolam
   (E) None of the above

3. Which statement concerning the barbiturates is accurate?

(A) Symptoms of the abstinence syndrome are more severe during withdrawal from phenobarbital than from secobarbital
(B) Compared with barbiturates, the benzodiazepines exhibit a steeper dose–response relationship
(C) Barbiturates may increase the half-lives of drugs metabolized by the liver
(D) Alkalinization of the urine will accelerate the elimination of phenobarbital
(E) Respiratory depression caused by barbiturate overdosage can be reversed by flumazenil

4. Which statement is accurate?
   (A) Alprazolam is effective in the management of obsessive–compulsive disorders
   (B) Clonazepam is effective in certain seizure disorders
   (C) Diazepam is the drug of choice for chronic management of bipolar affective disorder
   (D) Ramelteon is useful in status epilepticus
   (E) Symptoms of the alcohol withdrawal state may be alleviated by treatment with buspirone

5–6. A 24-year-old computer programmer has a "nervous disposition," according to his wife. He is easily startled, worries about inconsequential matters, and sometimes complains of stomach cramps. At night he grinds his teeth in his sleep. There is no current history of drug abuse.

5. Assuming that the symptoms experienced by this young man are those indicative of generalized anxiety disorder (GAD), the most appropriate drug for treatment would be
   (A) Buspirone
   (B) Midazolam
   (C) Phenobarbital
   (D) Triazolam
   (E) Zolpidem

6. Regarding the characteristic properties of the drug most likely to be of value, the physician should inform the patient to anticipate
   (A) A need to continually increase drug dosage because of tolerance
   (B) A significant effect of the drug on memory
   (C) Additive CNS depression with alcoholic beverages
   (D) That the drug will take a week or so to begin working
   (E) That if he stops taking the drug abruptly he will experience withdrawal signs

7. Which of the following best describes the mechanism of action of benzodiazepines?
   (A) Activate GABA$_B$ receptors in the spinal cord
   (B) Block glutamate receptors in hierarchical neuronal pathways in the brain

(C) Increase the frequency of opening of chloride ion channels that are coupled to GABA$_A$ receptors

(D) Inhibit GABA transaminase to increase brain levels of GABA

(E) Stimulate the release of GABA from nerve endings in the brain

8. An 82-year-old woman, otherwise healthy for her age, has difficulty sleeping. Triazolam is prescribed for her at one half of the conventional adult dose.

8. Which statement about the use of triazolam in this elderly patient is accurate?
(A) Ambulatory dysfunction does not occur in elderly patients taking one half of the conventional adult dose
(B) Hypertension is a common adverse effect of benzodiazepines in patients older than 70 years
(C) Over-the-counter cold medications may antagonize the hypnotic effects of the drug
(D) She may experience amnesia, especially if she also drinks alcoholic beverages
(E) Triazolam is distinctive in that it does not cause rebound insomnia on abrupt discontinuance

9. The most likely explanation for the increased sensitivity of elderly patients following administration of a single dose of a benzodiazepine is
(A) Changes in brain function that accompany the aging process
(B) Decreased renal function
(C) Increased cerebral blood flow
(D) Decreased hepatic metabolism of lipid-soluble drugs
(E) Changes in plasma protein binding

10. A 28-year-old woman has sporadic attacks of intense anxiety with marked physical symptoms, including hyperventilation, tachycardia, and sweating. If she is diagnosed as suffering from a panic disorder, the most appropriate drug to use is
(A) Alprazolam
(B) Chloral hydrate
(C) Flurazepam
(D) Propranolol
(E) Ramelteon

11. Which of the following drugs may increase anticoagulant effects by displacement of warfarin from plasma protein binding sites and is inactive until converted in the body to an active metabolite?
(A) Buspirone
(B) Chloral hydrate
(C) Clorazepate
(D) Secobarbital
(E) Zaleplon

12. Which drug used chronically in maintenance treatment of patients with tonic-clonic or partial seizure states increases hepatic metabolism of warfarin and phenytoin?
(A) Chlordiazepoxide
(B) Meprobamate
(C) Phenobarbital
(D) Triazolam
(E) Zolpidem

13. A 40-year-old patient with liver dysfunction is scheduled for a surgical procedure. Lorazepam can be used for preanesthetic sedation in this patient without concern for excessive CNS depression because the drug is
(A) A selective anxiolytic like buspirone
(B) Actively secreted in the renal proximal tubule
(C) Conjugated extrahepatically
(D) Eliminated via the lungs
(E) Reversible by administration of naloxone

14. This hypnotic drug facilitates the inhibitory actions of GABA, but it lacks anticonvulsant or muscle relaxing properties and has minimal effect on sleep architecture.
(A) Buspirone
(B) Diazepam
(C) Flurazepam
(D) Phenobarbital
(E) Zaleplon

15. The most frequent type of drug interaction that occurs in patients using benzodiazepines is
(A) Additive CNS depression
(B) Antagonism of sedative or hypnotic actions
(C) Competition for plasma protein binding
(D) Induction of liver drug-metabolizing enzymes
(E) Inhibition of liver drug-metabolizing enzymes

ANSWERS

1. Diazepam has no more effectiveness than placebo in the treatment of major depressions. Benzodiazepines do not increase activity of drug-metabolizing enzymes or enzymes involved in porphyrin synthesis. At high doses, benzodiazepines may cause anterograde, not retrograde, amnesia. With abrupt discontinuance after chronic use, anxiety and agitation may occur, sometimes with hyperreflexia and, rarely, seizures. The answer is **B.**

2. Benzodiazepines and barbiturates are contraindicated in breathing-related sleep disorders because they further compromise ventilation. In obstructive sleep apnea (pickwickian syndrome), obesity is a major risk factor. The best prescription you can give this patient is to lose weight. The answer is **E.**

3. Withdrawal symptoms from use of the shorter acting barbiturate secobarbital are more severe than with phenobarbital. The dose–response curve for benzodiazepines is flatter than that for barbiturates. Induction of liver drug-metabolizing enzymes occurs with barbiturates and may lead to decreases in half-life of other drugs. Flumazenil is an antagonist at BZ receptors and is used to reverse CNS depressant effects of benzodiazepines. As a weak acid (pK_a, 7), phenobarbital will be more ionized (nonprotonated) in the urine at alkaline pH and less reabsorbed in the renal tubule. The answer is **D.**

4. Benzodiazepines have no significant therapeutic benefit in the management of obsessive–compulsive disorders. Clonazepam has been used commonly as an anticonvulsant and also has efficacy in certain anxiety states, including agoraphobia. Clonazepam (not diazepam) has also been used as a backup drug in bipolar affective disorder. The answer is **B.**

5. Buspirone, longer acting benzodiazepines, and newer antidepressants (see Chapter 30) are effective in the management of GAD. Midazolam and triazolam are short-acting benzodiazepines used in anesthesia protocols and for sleep disorders, respectively. The answer is **A.**

6. Buspirone is a selective anxiolytic with pharmacologic characteristics quite different from sedative-hypnotics. Buspirone has minimal effects on cognition or memory; it is not additive with ethanol in terms of CNS depression; tolerance is minimal; and it has no dependence liability. Buspirone is not effective in *acute* anxiety because it has a slow onset of action. The answer is **D.**

7. Benzodiazepines exert most of their CNS effects by increasing the inhibitory effects of GABA, interacting with components of the $GABA_A$ receptor-chloride ion channel macromolecular complex to increase the frequency of chloride ion channel opening. Benzodiazepines do not affect GABA metabolism or release, and they are not GABA receptor agonists because they do not interact directly with the binding site for GABA. The answer is **C.**

8. In elderly patients taking benzodiazepines, hypotension is far more likely than an increase in blood pressure. The elderly are more prone to CNS depressant effects of hypnotics; even a dose reduction of 50% may still cause excessive sedation with possible ambulatory impairment. Additive CNS depression occurs commonly with drugs used in OTC cold medications, and rebound insomnia can occur with abrupt discontinuance of benzodiazepines used as sleeping pills. Alcohol enhances psychomotor depression and the amnestic effects of the benzodiazepines. The answer is **D.**

9. Decreased blood flow to vital organs, including the liver and kidney, occurs during the aging process. These changes may contribute to cumulative effects of sedative-hypnotic drugs. However, this does not explain the enhanced sensitivity of the elderly patient to a **single** dose of a central depressant, which appears to be due to changes in brain function that accompany aging. The answer is **A.**

10. Alprazolam and clonazepam are the most effective of the benzodiazepines for the treatment of panic disorders. Propranolol is commonly used to attenuate excessive sympathomimetic activity in persons who suffer from performance anxiety ("stage fright"). The answer is **A.**

11. Chloral hydrate, a prodrug is metabolized to trichloroethanol, the active moiety. It can displace drugs from plasma protein binding sites and may cause bleeding when administered to patients given warfarin. Clorazepate is also a prodrug forming nordiazepam, the active metabolite. Benzodiazepines do not displace other drugs from plasma protein binding sites. The answer is **B.**

12. Chronic administration of phenobarbital increases the activity of hepatic drug-metabolizing enzymes, including cytochrome P450 isozymes. This can increase the rate of metabolism of drugs administered concomitantly, with decreases in the intensity and duration of their effects. The answer is **C.**

13. The elimination of most benzodiazepines involves their metabolism by liver enzymes, including cytochrome P450 isozymes. In a patient with liver dysfunction, lorazepam, which is metabolized extrahepatically, is less likely to cause excessive CNS depression. Benzodiazepines are not eliminated via the kidneys or lungs. Flumazenil is used to reverse excessive CNS depression caused by benzodiazepines. The answer is **C.**

**SKILL KEEPER ANSWER:
LOADING DOSE
(SEE CHAPTER 3)**

Because the half-life of phenobarbital is 4 days, one may assume that the plasma concentration 4 h after drug ingestion is of an order of magnitude similar to that of the peak plasma level. If so, and assuming 100% bioavailability, then

$$Dose\ ingested = Plasma\ concentration \times V_d$$
$$= 50\ mg/L \times 40\ L$$
$$= 2000\ mg$$

14. Eszopiclone, zaleplon, and zolpidem are related hypnotics that, although structurally different from benzodiazepines, appear to have a similar mechanism of action. However, these drugs are not effective in seizures or in muscle spasticity states. Compared with benzodiazepines, the newer hypnotics are less likely to alter sleep patterns. Buspirone is not a hypnotic! The answer is **E**.

15. The most common drug interaction involving sedative-hypnotics is additive CNS depression. Additive effects can be predicted with concomitant use of alcoholic beverages, anticonvulsants, opioid analgesics, and phenothiazines. Less obvious but equally important is enhanced CNS depression with many antihistamines, and tricyclic antidepressants. The answer is **A**.

CHECKLIST

When you complete this chapter, you should be able to:

☐ Identify major drugs in each sedative-hypnotic subgroup.

☐ Recall the significant pharmacokinetic features of the sedative-hypnotic drugs commonly used for treatment of anxiety and sleep disorders.

☐ Describe the proposed mechanisms of action of benzodiazepines, barbiturates, and zolpidem.

☐ List the pharmacodynamic actions of major sedative-hypnotics in terms of their clinical uses and their adverse effects.

☐ Identify the distinctive properties of buspirone, eszopiclone, ramelteon, zaleplon, and zolpidem.

☐ Describe the symptoms and management of overdose of sedative-hypnotics and withdrawal from physiological dependence.

Alcohols

23

Ethanol, a sedative-hypnotic drug, is the most important alcohol of pharmacologic interest. It has few medical applications but its abuse causes major medical and socioeconomic problems. Other alcohols of toxicologic importance are methanol and ethylene glycol. Several important drugs discussed in this chapter are used to prevent the potentially life-threatening ethanol withdrawal syndrome, to treat chronic alcoholism or to treat acute methanol and ethylene glycol poisoning.

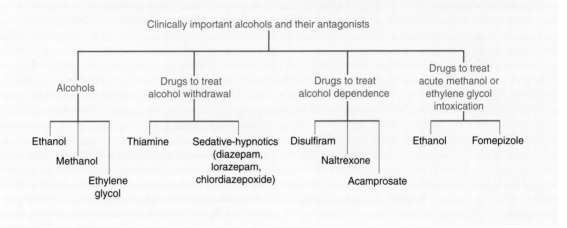

ETHANOL

A. PHARMACOKINETICS

After ingestion, ethanol is rapidly and completely absorbed; the drug is then distributed to most body tissues, and its volume of distribution is equivalent to that of total body water (0.5–0.7 L/kg). Two enzyme systems metabolize ethanol to acetaldehyde (Figure 23–1).

1. Alcohol dehydrogenase (ADH)—This cytosolic, NAD-dependent enzyme, found mainly in the liver and gut, accounts for the metabolism of low to moderate doses of ethanol. Because of the limited supply of the coenzyme NAD, the reaction has *zero-order kinetics,* resulting in a fixed capacity for ethanol metabolism of 7–10 g/h. Gastrointestinal metabolism of ethanol is lower in women than in men.

2. Microsomal ethanol oxidizing system (MEOS)—At blood ethanol levels above 100 mg/dL, the liver microsomal mixed function oxidase system that catalyzes most phase I drug metabolizing reactions (see Chapter 2) contributes significantly to ethanol metabolism (Figure 23-1). Chronic ethanol consumption induces cytochrome P450 enzyme synthesis and MEOS activity; this increase may be partially responsible for the development of tolerance to ethanol. The primary isoform of cytochrome P450 induced by ethanol—2E1 (see Table 4-3)—converts acetaminophen to a hepatotoxic metabolite.

Acetaldehyde formed from the oxidation of ethanol by either ADH or MEOS is rapidly metabolized to acetate by aldehyde dehydrogenase, a mitochondrial enzyme found in the liver and many other tissues. Aldehyde dehydrogenase is inhibited by **disulfiram** and other drugs,

---

HIGH-YIELD TERMS TO LEARN

Alcoholism	Compulsive use of ethanol
Psychologic and physiologic dependence	States wherein deprivation of a drug results in severe anxiety and craving (psychologic) and/or physical symptoms (physiologic dependence)
Tolerance, cross-tolerance	State of adaptation to a drug that results in reduced effects at a given dosage; cross-tolerance is tolerance to a second drug developed as a result of chronic exposure to a first drug
Alcohol withdrawal syndrome	The characteristic syndrome of insomnia, tremor, agitation, seizures, and autonomic instability engendered by deprivation in an individual who is physically dependent on ethanol
Delirium tremens (DTs)	Severe form of alcohol withdrawal whose main symptoms are sweating, tremor, confusion and hallucinations
Fetal alcohol syndrome	A syndrome of craniofacial dysmorphia, heart defects and mental retardation caused by the teratogenic effects of ethanol consumption during pregnancy
Wernicke-Korsakoff syndrome	A syndrome of ataxia, confusion and paralysis of the extraocular muscles that is associated with chronic alcoholism and thiamine deficiency

---

including **metronidazole, oral hypoglycemics,** and some **cephalosporins.** Some individuals, primarily of Asian descent, have genetic deficiency of aldehyde dehydrogenase. After consumption of even small quantities of ethanol, these individuals experience nausea and a flushing reaction from accumulation of acetaldehyde.

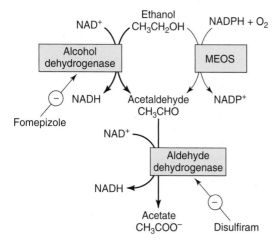

Figure 23–1. Metabolism of ethanol by alcohol dehydrogenase (ADH) and the microsomal ethanol-oxidizing system (MEOS). Alcohol dehydrogenase and aldehyde dehydrogenase are inhibited by fomepizole and disulfiram, respectively. (Reproduced, with permission, from Katzung BG, editor: *Basic & Clinical Pharmacology*, 10th ed. McGraw-Hill, 2007).

B. ACUTE EFFECTS

1. CNS—The major acute effects of ethanol on the CNS include sedation, loss of inhibition, impaired judgment, slurred speech, and ataxia. In nontolerant individuals, impairment of driving ability is thought to occur at ethanol blood levels between 60 mg/dL and 80 mg/dL. Blood levels of 120 to 160 mg/dL are usually associated with gross drunkenness. Levels greater than 300 mg/dL may lead to loss of consciousness, anesthesia, and coma with sometimes fatal respiratory and cardiovascular depression. Blood levels >500 mg/dL are usually lethal. Chronic alcoholics who are tolerant to the effects of ethanol can function almost normally at much higher blood concentrations than occasional drinkers. Additive CNS depression occurs with concomitant ingestion of ethanol and a wide variety of CNS depressants, including sedative-hypnotics, opioid agonists, and many drugs that block muscarinic and H_1 histamine receptors.

The molecular mechanisms underlying the complex CNS effects of ethanol are not fully understood. Specific receptors for ethanol have not been identified. Instead, ethanol appears to modulate the function of a number of signaling proteins. It facilitates the action of GABA at $GABA_A$ receptors, inhibits the ability of glutamate to activate NMDA (N-methyl-D-aspartate) receptors, and modifies the activities of adenyl cyclase, phospholipase C, and ion channels. It has been suggested that alcohol "blackouts" may result from interference with NMDA receptors.

2. Other organ systems—Ethanol, even at relatively low blood concentrations, significantly depresses the heart. Vascular smooth muscle is relaxed, which leads to vasodilation, sometimes with marked hypothermia. Ethanol relaxes uterine smooth muscle.

C. CHRONIC EFFECTS

1. Tolerance and dependence—Tolerance occurs mainly as a result of CNS adaptation and to a lesser extent by an increased rate of ethanol metabolism. There is cross-tolerance to sedative-hypnotic drugs that facilitate GABA activity (eg, benzodiazepines and barbiturates). Both psychological and physical dependence are marked.

2. Liver—Liver disease is the most common medical complication of chronic alcohol abuse. Reduced gluconeogenesis can lead to hypoglycemia. Progressive loss of liver function occurs with reversible fatty liver progressing to irreversible hepatitis, cirrhosis, and liver failure. Hepatic dysfunction is often more severe in women than in men and in both men and women infected with hepatitis B or C virus.

3. Gastrointestinal system—Irritation, inflammation, bleeding, and scarring of the gut wall occur after chronic heavy use of ethanol and may cause absorption defects and exacerbate nutritional deficiencies. Chronic alcohol abuse greatly increases the risk of pancreatitis.

4. CNS—Peripheral neuropathy is the most common neurologic abnormality in chronic alcoholics. More rarely, thiamine deficiency, along with ethanol abuse, leads to the **Wernicke-Korsakoff** syndrome, which is characterized by ataxia, confusion, and paralysis of the extraocular muscles. Prompt treatment with parenteral thiamine is essential to prevent a permanent memory disorder known as Korsakoff's psychosis.

5. Endocrine system—Gynecomastia, testicular atrophy, and salt retention occur, partly because of altered steroid metabolism in the cirrhotic liver.

6. Cardiovascular system—Excessive chronic ethanol use is associated with an increased incidence of hypertension, anemia, and dilated cardiomyopathy. Acute drinking for several days ("binge" drinking) can cause arrhythmias. However, the ingestion of modest quantities of ethanol (10–15 g/day) raises serum levels of high-density lipoprotein (HDL) cholesterol and may *protect* against coronary heart disease.

7. Fetal alcohol syndrome—Ethanol use in pregnancy is associated with teratogenic effects that include mental retardation (most common), growth deficiencies, microcephaly, and a characteristic underdevelopment of the midface region. Facial abnormalities are particularly associated with heavy consumption of alcohol during the first trimester of pregnancy.

8. Neoplasia—Ethanol is not a primary carcinogen, but its chronic use is associated with an increased incidence of neoplastic diseases in the gastrointestinal tract and a small increase in the risk of breast cancer.

9. Immune system—Chronic alcohol abuse has complex effects on immune functions because it enhances inflammation in the liver and pancreas and inhibits immune function in other tissues. Heavy use predisposes to infectious pneumonia.

SKILL KEEPER: ELIMINATION HALF-LIFE (SEE CHAPTER 1)

Search "high and low" through drug information resources and you will not find data on the elimination half-life of ethanol! Can you explain why this is the case? The Skill Keeper Answer appears at the end of the chapter.

D. TREATMENT OF ACUTE AND CHRONIC ALCOHOLISM

1. Excessive CNS depression—Intoxication resulting from acute ingestion of ethanol is managed by maintenance of vital signs and prevention of aspiration after vomiting. Intravenous dextrose is standard. Thiamine administration is used to protect against the Wernicke-Korsakoff syndrome, and correction of electrolyte imbalance may also be required.

2. Alcohol withdrawal syndrome—In individuals physically dependent on ethanol, discontinuance can lead to a withdrawal syndrome characterized by insomnia, tremor, anxiety, and, in severe cases, life-threatening seizures and delirium tremens (DTs). Peripheral effects include nausea, vomiting, diarrhea, and arrhythmias. The abstinence syndrome is managed by correction of electrolyte imbalance and administration of thiamine and a sedative-hypnotic. A long-acting benzodiazepine (eg, diazepam, chlordiazepoxide) is preferred unless the patient has compromised liver function, in which case a short-acting benzodiazepine with less complex metabolism (eg, lorazepam) is preferred.

3. Treatment of alcoholism—Alcoholism is a complex sociomedical problem, characterized by a high relapse rate. Several CNS neurotransmitter systems appear to be targets for drugs that reduce the craving for alcohol. The opioid receptor antagonist naltrexone has proved to be useful in some patients, presumably through its ability to decrease the effects of endogenous opioid peptides in the brain. Acamprosate, an NMDA glutamate receptor antagonist, is also FDA approved for treatment of alcoholism, and agents under investigation include ondansetron (a 5-HT$_3$ serotonin receptor antagonist; Chapters 16 and 60) and topiramate (an antiepileptic drug; Chapter 24). The aldehyde dehydrogenase inhibitor disulfiram is used adjunctively in some treatment programs. If ethanol is consumed by a patient who has taken disulfiram, acetaldehyde accumulation leads to nausea, headache, flushing, and hypotension (Figure 23–1).

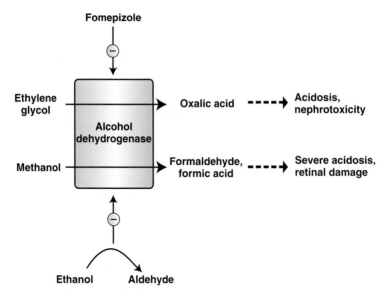

Figure 23–2. The oxidation of ethylene glycol and methanol by alcohol dehydrogenase creates metabolites that cause serious toxicity. Ethanol, a substrate preferred by ADH, is used in methanol or ethylene glycol poisoning to slow the rate of formation of toxic metabolites. Fomepizole, an inhibitor of alcohol dehydrogenase, is an alternative to ethanol.

OTHER ALCOHOLS

A. METHANOL

Methanol (wood alcohol), a constituent of windshield cleaners and "canned heat," is sometimes ingested intentionally. Intoxication causes visual dysfunction, gastrointestinal distress, shortness of breath, loss of consciousness, and coma. Methanol is metabolized to formaldehyde and formic acid, which can cause severe acidosis, retinal damage, and blindness. The formation of formaldehyde is retarded by prompt intravenous administration of ethanol, which acts as a preferred substrate for alcohol dehydrogenase and competitively inhibits the oxidation of methanol, and by **fomepizole,** an inhibitor of alcohol dehydrogenase (Figure 23–2).

B. ETHYLENE GLYCOL

Industrial exposure to ethylene glycol (by inhalation or skin absorption) or self-administration (eg, by drinking antifreeze products) leads to severe acidosis and renal damage from the metabolism of ethylene glycol to oxalic acid. Prompt treatment with ethanol, which competes for oxidation by alcohol dehydrogenase, or fomepizole may slow or prevent formation of this toxic metabolite (Figure 23–2).

KEY DRUGS

Subclass	Prototypes	Other Significant Agents
Alcohols	Ethanol	Methanol, ethylene glycol
Drugs for alcohol withdrawal syndrome	Diazepam	Lorazepam, chlordiazepoxide
Drugs for alcoholism	Naltrexone, acamprosate	Disulfiram
Antidotes for methanol or ethylene glycol poisoning	Ethanol, fomepizole	

QUESTIONS

1. A 45-year-old moderately obese man has been drinking heavily for 72 h. This level of drinking is much higher than his regular habit of drinking 1 alcoholic drink per day. His only significant medical problem is mild hypertension, which is adequately controlled by metoprolol. With this history, this man is at significant risk for
   (A) Arrhythmia
   (B) Bacterial pneumonia
   (C) Hyperthermia
   (D) Tonic-clonic seizures
   (E) Wernicke-Korsakoff syndrome

2. A 42-year-old man with a history of alcoholism is brought to the emergency department in a confused and delirious state. He has truncal ataxia and ophthalmoplegia. The most appropriate immediate course of action is to administer diazepam plus
   (A) Chlordiazepoxide
   (B) Disulfiram
   (C) Folic acid
   (D) Fomepizole
   (E) Thiamine

3. The cytochrome P450-dependent microsomal ethanol oxidizing system (MEOS) pathway of ethanol metabolism is MOST likely to be maximally activated under the condition of low concentrations of:
   (A) Acetaldehyde
   (B) Ethanol
   (C) NAD^+
   (D) NADPH
   (E) Oxygen

4. A freshman student (weight, 70 kg) attends a college party where he rapidly consumes a quantity of an alcoholic beverage that results in a blood level of 500 mg/dL. Assuming that this young man has not had an opportunity to develop tolerance to ethanol, his present condition is BEST characterized as
   (A) Able to walk, but not in a straight line
   (B) Alert and competent to drive a car
   (C) Comatose and near death
   (D) Sedated with increased reaction times
   (E) Slightly inebriated

5. The regular consumption of a glass or 2 of wine each day with meals may decrease the risk of
   (A) Cancer
   (B) Coronary heart disease
   (C) Gastritis
   (D) Psychological dependence
   (E) Viral hepatitis

6–7. A homeless middle-aged male patient presents in the emergency department in a state of intoxication. You note that he is behaviorally disinhibited and rowdy. He tells you that he has recently consumed about a pint of a red-colored liquid that his friends were using to "get high." He complains that his vision is blurred and that it is "like being in a snowstorm." His breath smells a bit like formaldehyde. He is acidotic.

6. The most likely cause of this patient's intoxicated state is the ingestion of
   (A) Ethanol
   (B) Ethylene glycol
   (C) Isopropanol
   (D) Hexane
   (E) Methanol

7. After assessing and stabilizing the patient's airway, respiration, and circulatory status, ethanol was administered intravenously. The purpose of the ethanol was to
   (A) Accelerate the rate of elimination of the toxic liquid that he consumed
   (B) Combat his acidosis
   (C) Inhibit the metabolic production of a toxic metabolite of the poison
   (D) Prevent alcohol withdrawal seizures
   (E) Sedate the patient

8. The regular ingestion of moderate or heavy amounts of alcohol predisposes to hepatic damage after overdose of acetaminophen because ethanol
   (A) Blocks acetaminophen metabolism
   (B) Causes thiamine deficiency
   (C) Displaces acetaminophen from plasma proteins
   (D) Induces liver drug-metabolizing enzymes
   (E) Inhibits renal clearance of acetaminophen

9. In addition to an increased risk of severe liver disease, people with alcoholism are at increased risk for
   (A) Angina
   (B) Heart failure
   (C) Pulmonary hypertension
   (D) Renal insufficiency
   (E) CNS tumors

10. A 23-year-old pregnant woman with alcoholism presented to the emergency department in the early stages of labor. She had drunk large amounts of alcohol throughout her pregnancy. This patient's infant is at high risk of a syndrome that includes
    (A) Ambiguous genitalia in a male fetus and normal genitalia in a female fetus
    (B) Failure of closure of the atrial septum or ventricular septum
    (C) Limb or digit malformation
    (D) Mental retardation and craniofacial abnormalities
    (E) Underdevelopment of the lungs

11. The combination of ethanol and disulfiram results in nausea and hypotension as a result of the accumulation of
    (A) Acetaldehyde
    (B) Acetate
    (C) Methanol
    (D) NADH
    (E) Pyruvate

12. The intense craving experienced by individuals who are trying to recover from chronic alcohol abuse can be ameliorated by a drug that is an
    (A) Agonist of α_1 adrenoceptors
    (B) Agonist of serotonin receptors
    (C) Antagonist of β_2 adrenoceptors
    (D) Antagonist of opioid receptors
    (E) Inhibitor of cyclooxygenase

ANSWERS

1. This man's regular rate of alcohol consumption is not high enough to put him at risk of long-term consequences such as Wernicke-Korsakoff syndrome, increased susceptibility to bacterial pneumonia, or alcohol withdrawal seizures. This pattern of "binge drinking" does put him at increased risk of cardiac arrhythmia. The answer is **A**.

2. This patient has the symptoms of Wernicke's encephalopathy, including delirium, gait disturbances, and paralysis of the external eye muscles. The condition results from thiamine deficiency but is rarely seen in the absence of alcoholism. The diazepam is administered to prevent the alcohol withdrawal syndrome. The answer is **E**.

3. The microsomal ethanol oxidizing system (MEOS) contributes most to ethanol metabolism at relatively high blood alcohol concentrations (>100 mg/dL), when the alcohol dehydrogenase pathway is saturated due to depletion of NAD^+. So, the MEOS system contributes most when the NAD^+ concentration is low. NADPH and oxygen are cofactors for MEOS reactions. The concentration of acetaldehyde does not appear to affect the rate of either the ADH or the MEOS reactions. The answer is **C**.

4. The blood level of ethanol achieved in this person almost certainly was estimated postmortem. The quantity of ethanol ingested can be calculated from the product of plasma level and volume of distribution (0.5–0.7 L/kg). In this case, the young man ingested 200 g of ethanol, the equivalent of more than 20 fluid ounces (550 mL) of distilled 80 proof spirits. The answer is **C**.

5. Compared with those who abstain, individuals who regularly ingest modest quantities of ethanol (1 or 2 drinks daily) are reported to have a *decreased* risk of coronary heart disease. The chronic use of ethanol is a risk factor for the other items listed. The answer is **B**.

6. Behavioral disinhibition is a feature of early intoxication from ethanol and most other alcohols but not the solvent, hexane. Ocular dysfunction, including horizontal nystagmus and diplopia, is also a common finding in poisoning with alcohols, but the complaint of "flickering white spots before the eyes" or "being in a snowstorm" is highly suggestive of methanol intoxication. In some cases, the odor of formaldehyde may be present on the breath. In this patient, blood methanol levels should be determined as soon as possible. The answer is **E**.

7. In patients with suspected methanol intoxication, ethanol (10% solution) is often given intravenously before laboratory diagnosis is confirmed to inhibit the ADH-catalyzed formation of toxic metabolites. The answer is **C**.

8. Chronic use of ethanol causes induction of a cytochrome P450 2E1 isozyme that converts acetaminophen to a cytotoxic metabolite. This appears to be the explanation for the increased susceptibility to acetaminophen-induced hepatotoxicity found in individuals who regularly ingest alcohol. The answer is **D**.

9. Chronic use of ethanol damages the heart and causes a dilated cardiomyopathy with ventricular hypertrophy and fibrosis. Heart failure can ensue. The answer is **B**.

SKILL KEEPER ANSWER: ELIMINATION HALF-LIFE (SEE CHAPTER 1)

Drug information resources do not provide data on the elimination half-life of ethanol because, in the case of this drug, it is not constant. The elimination of ethanol follows **zero-order kinetics** *because the drug is metabolized at a constant rate irrespective of its concentration in the blood (see Chapter 3). The pharmacokinetic relationship between elimination half-life, volume of distribution, and clearance, given by*

$$t_{1/2} = \frac{0.693 \times V_d}{CL}$$

is not applicable to ethanol. Its rate of metabolism is constant, but its clearance decreases with an increase in blood level. The arithmetic plot of ethanol blood level versus time follows a straight line (not exponential decay).

10. This woman's infant is at risk for fetal alcohol syndrome, a syndrome associated with mental retardation, abnormalities of the head and face, and growth deficiency. This syndrome is a leading cause of mental retardation. The answer is **D.**

11. The nausea, hypotension, and ill feeling that result from drinking ethanol while also taking disulfiram stems from acetaldehyde accumulation. Disulfiram inhibits acetaldehyde dehydrogenase, the enzyme that converts acetaldehyde to acetate. The answer is **A.**

12. Naltrexone, a competitive inhibitor of opioid receptors, decreases the craving for alcohol in patients who are recovering from alcoholism. The answer is **D.**

CHECKLIST

When you complete this chapter, you should be able to:

☐ Sketch the biochemical pathways for ethanol metabolism and indicate where fomepizole and disulfiram act.

☐ Summarize characteristic pharmacodynamic and pharmacokinetic properties of ethanol.

☐ Relate blood alcohol levels in a nontolerant individual to CNS depressant effects of acute alcohol ingestion.

☐ Identify the toxic effects of chronic ethanol ingestion.

☐ Describe the fetal alcohol syndrome.

☐ Describe the treatment of ethanol overdosage.

☐ Outline the pharmacotherapy of (1) the alcohol withdrawal syndrome and (2) alcoholism.

☐ Describe the toxicity and treatment of acute poisoning with (1) methanol and (2) ethylene glycol.

Antiseizure Drugs

Epilepsy comprises a group of chronic syndromes that involve the recurrence of seizures (ie, limited periods of abnormal discharge of cerebral neurons). Effective antiseizure drugs have, to varying degrees, selective depressant actions on such abnormal neuronal activity. However, they vary in terms of their mechanisms of action and in their effectiveness in specific seizure disorders.

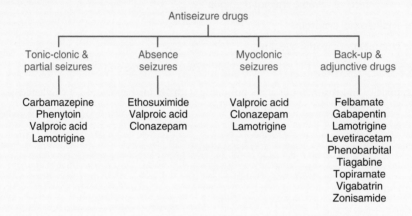

PHARMACOKINETICS

Antiseizure drugs are commonly used for long periods of time, and consideration of their pharmacokinetic properties is important for avoiding toxicity and drug interactions. For some of these drugs (eg, phenytoin), determination of plasma levels and clearance in individual patients may be necessary for optimum therapy. In general, antiseizure drugs are well absorbed orally and have good bioavailability. Most antiseizure drugs are metabolized by hepatic enzymes, and in some cases active metabolites are formed. Resistance to antiseizure drugs may involve increased expression of drug transporters at the level of the blood-brain barrier.

Pharmacokinetic drug interactions are common in this drug group. In the presence of drugs that inhibit antiseizure drug metabolism or displace anticonvulsants from plasma protein binding sites, plasma concentrations of the antiseizure agents may reach toxic levels.

On the other hand, drugs that induce hepatic drug-metabolizing enzymes (eg, rifampin) may result in plasma levels of the antiseizure agents that are inadequate for seizure control. Several antiseizure drugs are themselves capable of inducing hepatic drug metabolism, especially carbamazepine and phenytoin.

A. PHENYTOIN

The oral bioavailability of phenytoin is variable because of individual differences in first-pass metabolism. Phenytoin metabolism is nonlinear; elimination kinetics shift from first-order to zero-order at moderate to high dose levels. The drug binds extensively to plasma proteins (97–98%), and free (unbound) phenytoin levels in plasma are increased transiently by drugs that compete for binding (eg, carbamazepine, sulfonamides, valproic acid). The metabolism of phenytoin is enhanced in the presence of inducers of liver metabolism (eg, phenobarbital, rifampin) and inhibited by other drugs

HIGH-YIELD TERMS TO LEARN	
Seizures	Finite episodes of brain dysfunction resulting from abnormal discharge of cerebral neurons
Partial seizures, simple	Consciousness preserved; manifested variously as convulsive jerking, paresthesias, psychic symptoms (altered sensory perception, illusions, hallucinations, affect changes), and autonomic dysfunction
Partial seizures, complex	Impaired consciousness that is preceded, accompanied, or followed by psychological symptoms
Tonic-clonic seizures, generalized	Tonic phase (less than 1 min) involves abrupt loss of consciousness, muscle rigidity, and respiration arrest; clonic phase (2–3 min) involves jerking of body muscles, with lip or tongue biting, and fecal and urinary incontinence; formerly called grand mal
Absence seizures, generalized	Impaired consciousness (often abrupt onset and brief), sometimes with automatisms, loss of postural tone, or enuresis; begin in childhood (formerly, petit mal) and usually cease by age 20 years
Myoclonic seizures	Single or multiple myoclonic muscle jerks
Status epilepticus	A series of seizures (usually tonic-clonic) without recovery of consciousness between attacks; it is a life-threatening emergency

(eg, cimetidine, isoniazid). Phenytoin induces hepatic drug metabolism, decreasing the effects of other antiepileptic drugs including carbamazepine, clonazepam, and lamotrigine. **Fosphenytoin** is a water-soluble prodrug form of phenytoin that is used parenterally.

B. CARBAMAZEPINE

Carbamazepine induces formation of liver drug-metabolizing enzymes that increase metabolism of the drug itself and may increase the clearance of many other anticonvulsant drugs including clonazepam, lamotrigine and valproic acid. Carbamazepine metabolism can be inhibited by other drugs (eg, propoxyphene, valproic acid). A related drug, oxcarbazepine, is less likely to be involved in drug interactions.

C. VALPROIC ACID

In addition to competing for phenytoin plasma protein binding sites, valproic acid inhibits the metabolism of carbamazepine, ethosuximide, phenytoin, phenobarbital, and lamotrigine. Hepatic biotransformation of valproic acid leads to formation of a toxic metabolite that has been implicated in the hepatotoxicity of the drug.

D. NEWER DRUGS

Gabapentin, levetiracetam, and vigabatrin are unusual in that they are eliminated by the kidney, largely in unchanged form. These agents have virtually no drug-drug pharmacokinetic interactions. Felbamate and topiramate undergo both hepatic metabolism and renal

elimination of intact drug. Lamotrigine is eliminated via hepatic glucuronidation.

MECHANISMS OF ACTION

The general effect of antiseizure drugs is to suppress repetitive action potentials in epileptic foci in the brain. Different mechanisms are involved in achieving this effect. In the case of some drugs, multiple mechanisms may contribute to their antiseizure activities. Some of the recognized mechanisms are described next.

A. SODIUM CHANNEL BLOCKADE

At therapeutic concentrations, phenytoin, carbamazepine, and lamotrigine block voltage-gated sodium channels in neuronal membranes. This action is rate dependent (ie, dependent on the frequency of neuronal discharge) and results in prolongation of the inactivated state of the Na^+ channel and the refractory period of the neuron. Phenobarbital, valproic acid, and zonisamide may exert similar effects at high doses.

B. GABA-RELATED TARGETS

As described in Chapter 22, benzodiazepines interact with specific receptors on the $GABA_A$ receptor-chloride ion channel macromolecular complex. In the presence of benzodiazepines, the *frequency* of chloride ion channel opening is increased; these drugs facilitate the inhibitory effects of GABA. Phenobarbital and other barbiturates also enhance the inhibitory actions of

GABA but interact with a different receptor site on chloride ion channels that results in an increased *duration* of chloride ion channel opening.

GABA aminotransaminase (GABA-T) is an important enzyme in the termination of action of GABA. The enzyme is irreversibly inactivated by vigabatrin at therapeutic plasma levels and can also be inhibited by valproic acid at very high concentrations. Tiagabine inhibits a GABA transporter (GAT-1) in neurons and glia, prolonging the action of the neurotransmitter. Gabapentin is a structural analog of GABA, but it does not activate GABA receptors directly and its mechanism of antiseizure action is unclear. Other drugs that may facilitate the inhibitory actions of GABA include felbamate, topiramate, and valproic acid.

C. CALCIUM CHANNEL BLOCKADE

Ethosuximide inhibits low-threshold (T type) Ca^{2+} currents, especially in thalamic neurons that act as pacemakers to generate rhythmic cortical discharge. A similar action is reported for valproic acid.

D. OTHER MECHANISMS

In addition to its action on calcium channels, valproic acid causes neuronal membrane hyperpolarization, possibly by enhancing K^+ channel permeability. In addition to its actions on sodium channels and GABA-chloride channels, phenobarbital also acts as an antagonist at some glutamate receptors. Felbamate blocks glutamate NMDA receptors. Topiramate blocks sodium channels and potentiates the actions of GABA and may also block glutamate receptors.

SKILL KEEPER:
ANTIARRHYTHMIC DRUG
ACTIONS (SEE CHAPTER 14)

1. *Which of the mechanisms of action of antiseizure drugs have theoretical implications regarding their activity in cardiac arrhythmias?*

2. *Can you recall any clinical uses of antiseizure drugs in the management of cardiac arrhythmias?*

The Skill Keeper Answers appear at the end of the chapter.

CLINICAL USES

Diagnosis of a specific seizure type is important for prescribing the most appropriate antiseizure drug (or combination of drugs). Drug choice is usually made on the basis of established efficacy in the specific seizure state that has been diagnosed, the prior responsiveness of the patient, and the anticipated toxicity of the drug. Treatment may involve combinations of drugs, following the principle of adding known effective agents if the preceding drugs are not sufficient.

A. GENERALIZED TONIC-CLONIC SEIZURES

Valproic acid, or carbamazepine, or phenytoin are the drugs of choice for generalized tonic-clonic (grand mal) seizures. Phenobarbital (or primidone) is now considered to be an alternative agent in adults but continues to be a primary drug in infants. Lamotrigine and topiramate are also approved drugs for this indication, and several others may be used adjunctively in refractory cases.

B. PARTIAL SEIZURES

The drugs of first choice are carbamazepine (or oxcarbazepine), or lamotrigine, or phenytoin. Alternatives include felbamate, phenobarbital, topiramate, and valproic acid. Many of the newer anticonvulsants can be used adjunctively, including gabapentin and pregabalin, a structural congener.

C. ABSENCE SEIZURES

Ethosuximide or valproic acid are the preferred drugs because they cause minimal sedation. Ethosuximide is often used in uncomplicated absence seizures if patients can tolerate its gastrointestinal side effects. Valproic acid is particularly useful in patients who have concomitant generalized tonic-clonic or myoclonic seizures. Clonazepam, is effective as an alternative drug but has the disadvantages of causing sedation and tolerance. Lamotrigine, levetiracetam, and zonisamide are also effective in absence seizures.

D. MYOCLONIC & ATYPICAL ABSENCE SYNDROMES

Myoclonic seizure syndromes are usually treated with valproic acid; lamotrigine is approved for adjunctive use, but is commonly used as monotherapy. Clonazepam can be effective, but the high doses required cause drowsiness. Levetiracetam, topiramate, and zonisamide are also used as backup drugs in myoclonic syndromes. Felbamate has been used adjunctively with the primary drugs but has hematotoxic and hepatotoxic potential.

E. STATUS EPILEPTICUS

Intravenous diazepam or lorazepam is usually effective in terminating attacks and providing short-term control. For prolonged therapy, intravenous phenytoin is usually used because it is highly effective and less sedating than benzodiazepines or barbiturates. However, phenytoin may cause cardiotoxicity (perhaps because of its solvent propylene glycol), and fosphenytoin (water soluble) may prove to be safer. Phenobarbital has also been used in status epilepticus, especially in children. In very severe status epilepticus that does not respond to these measures, general anesthesia may be used.

F. OTHER CLINICAL USES

Several antiseizure drugs are effective in the management of bipolar affective disorders, especially valproic acid, which now is often used as a first-line drug in the treatment of mania. Carbamazepine and lamotrigine have also been used successfully in bipolar disorder. Carbamazepine is the drug of choice for trigeminal neuralgia, and its congener oxcarbazine may provide similar analgesia with fewer adverse effects. Gabapentin has efficacy in pain of neuropathic origin, including postherpetic neuralgia, and, like phenytoin, may have some value in migraine.Pregabalin is also approved for neuropathic pain.

TOXICITY

Chronic therapy with antiseizure drugs is associated with specific toxic effects, the most important of which are listed in Table 24–1.

A. TERATOGENICITY

Children born of mothers taking anticonvulsant drugs have an increased risk of congenital malformations. Neural tube defects (eg, spina bifida) are associated with the use of valproic acid; carbamazepine has been implicated as a cause of craniofacial anomalies and spina bifida; and a fetal hydantoin syndrome has been described after phenytoin use by pregnant women.

B. OVERDOSAGE TOXICITY

Most of the commonly used anticonvulsants are CNS depressants, and respiratory depression may occur with overdosage. Management is primarily supportive (airway management, mechanical ventilation), and flumazenil may be used in benzodiazepine overdose.

C. LIFE-THREATENING TOXICITY

Fatal hepatotoxicity has occurred with valproic acid, with greatest risk to children younger than 2 years and

Table 24–1. Adverse effects and complications of the use of antiepileptic drugs.

Antiepileptic Drug	Adverse Effects
Benzodiazepines	Sedation, tolerance, dependence
Carbamazepine	Diplopia, cognitive dysfunction, drowsiness, ataxia; rare occurrence of severe blood dyscrasias and Stevens-Johnson syndrome; teratogenic potential; induction of drug metabolism
Ethosuximide	Gastrointestinal distress, lethargy, headache, behavioral changes
Felbamate	Aplastic anemia, hepatic failure
Gabapentin	Dizziness, sedation, ataxia, nystagmus
Lamotrigine	Dizziness, ataxia, nausea, rash, rare Stevens-Johnson syndrome
Levetiracetam	Dizziness, sedation, weakness, irritability; hallucinations and psychosis have occurred
Oxcarbazepine	Similar to carbamazepine, but hyponatremia is more common; unlike carbamazepine, does not induce drug metabolism
Phenobarbital	Sedation, cognitive dysfunction, tolerance, dependence, induction of hepatic drug metabolism; primidone is similar
Phenytoin	Nystagmus, diplopia, sedation, gingival hyperplasia, hirsutism, anemias, peripheral neuropathy, osteoporosis, induction of hepatic drug metabolism
Tiagabine	Abdominal pain, nausea, dizziness, tremor, asthenia; drug metabolism is not induced
Topiramate	Drowsiness, dizziness, ataxia, psychomotor slowing and memory impairment, paresthesias, weight loss, acute myopia
Valproic acid	Drowsiness, nausea, tremor, hair loss, weight gain, hepatotoxicity; inhibition of hepatic drug metabolism
Vigabatrin	Sedation, dizziness, weight gain; visual field defects with long-term use, which may not be reversible
Zonisamide	Dizziness, confusion, agitation, diarrhea, weight loss, rash, Stevens-Johnson syndrome

---

KEY DRUGS

Subclass	Prototype	Other Significant Agents
Barbiturates	Phenobarbital	Primidone
Benzodiazepines	Diazepam	Clonazepam, clorazepate, lorazepam, nitrazepam
Carboxylic acids	Valproic acid	Sodium valproate
Hydantoins	Phenytoin	Fosphenytoin
Succinimides	Ethosuximide	Phensuximide
Tricyclics	Carbamazepine	Oxcarbazepine
Newer agents	Felbamate, gabapentin, lamotrigine, levetiracetam, pregabalin, tiagabine, topiramate, vigabatrin, zonisamide	

---

patients taking multiple anticonvulsant drugs. Lamotrigine has caused skin rashes and life-threatening Stevens-Johnson syndrome or toxic epidermal necrolysis. Children are at higher risk (1–2% incidence), especially if they are also taking valproic acid. Zonisamide may also cause severe skin reactions. Reports of aplastic anemia and acute hepatic failure have limited the use of felbamate to severe, refractory seizure states.

D. WITHDRAWAL

Withdrawal from antiseizure drugs should be accomplished gradually to avoid increased seizure frequency and severity. In general, withdrawal from anti-absence drugs is more easily accomplished than withdrawal from drugs used in partial or generalized tonic-clonic seizure states.

QUESTIONS

1. A 26-year-old woman develops a seizure disorder characterized by recurrent contractions of the muscles in the right hand, which then spread to the right arm and to the right side of the face ("jacksonian march"). Consciousness is not impaired, and the attacks usually last for only 1 or 2 min. Which drug is NOT likely to be useful in the treatment of this patient?
   (A) Carbamazepine
   (B) Ethosuximide
   (C) Lamotrigine
   (D) Phenytoin
   (E) Primidone

2. A 9-year-old child is having learning difficulties at school. He has brief lapses of awareness with eyelid fluttering that occur every 5–10 min. EEG studies reveal brief 3-Hz spike and wave discharges appearing synchronously in all leads. Which drug would be effective in this child without the disadvantages of excessive sedation or tolerance development?
   (A) Clonazepam
   (B) Diazepam
   (C) Ethosuximide
   (D) Felbamate
   (E) Phenobarbital

3. Which statement concerning proposed mechanisms of action of anticonvulsant drugs is false?
   (A) Diazepam facilitates GABA-mediated inhibitory actions
   (B) Ethosuximide selectively blocks K^+ ion channels in thalamic neurons
   (C) Phenobarbital has multiple actions, including enhancement of the effects of GABA, antagonism of glutamate receptors, and blockade of Na^+ ion channels
   (D) Phenytoin prolongs the inactivated state of the Na^+ ion channel
   (E) Vigabatrin elevates brain GABA levels

4. Which antiseizure drug is most likely to elevate the plasma concentration of other drugs administered concomitantly?
   (A) Carbamazepine
   (B) Diazepam
   (C) Phenobarbital
   (D) Phenytoin
   (E) Valproic acid

5. The most appropriate drug for treatment of a young woman who suffers from myoclonic jerking with no

overt signs of neurologic deficit or history of generalized tonic-clonic seizures is
(A) Carbamazepine
(B) Ethosuximide
(C) Phenobarbital
(D) Valproic acid
(E) Vigabatrin

6. Which of the following is NOT important when treating a young female patient with valproic acid?
   (A) She should be advised that gastrointestinal distress is a likely side effects
   (B) Her liver enzymes should be monitored
   (C) She should be examined every 2 or 3 mo for deep tendon reflex activity
   (D) She should contact her physician immediately if she becomes pregnant
   (E) She should be made aware that weight gain is common

7. Which statement concerning the pharmacokinetics of antiseizure drugs is accurate?
   (A) At high doses, phenytoin elimination follows first-order kinetics
   (B) Valproic acid may increase the activity of hepatic ALA synthase and the synthesis of porphyrins
   (C) The administration of phenytoin to patients in methadone maintenance programs has led to symptoms of opioid overdose, including respiratory depression
   (D) Although ethosuximide has a half-life of approximately 40 h, the drug is usually taken twice a day
   (E) Treatment with vigabatrin may reduce the effectiveness of oral contraceptives

8. With chronic use in seizure states, the adverse effects of this drug include coarsening of facial features, hirsutism, gingival hyperplasia, and osteomalacia.
   (A) Carbamazepine
   (B) Ethosuximide
   (C) Gabapentin
   (D) Phenytoin
   (E) Valproic acid

9. Which statement about vigabatrin is accurate?
   (A) Blocks neuronal reuptake of GABA
   (B) Drug of choice in absence seizures
   (C) Is established to be teratogenic in humans
   (D) Life-threatening skin disorders may occur
   (E) Visual field defects occur in up to one third of patients

10. Withdrawal of antiseizure drugs can cause increased seizure frequency and severity. Withdrawal is least likely to be a problem with
    (A) Clonazepam
    (B) Diazepam
    (C) Ethosuximide
    (D) Phenobarbital
    (E) Phenytoin

11. A young patient who suffers from bipolar disorder has failed to respond adequately to lithium. Which drug is most likely to be effective in this patient?
    (A) Diazepam
    (B) Gabapentin
    (C) Phenytoin
    (D) Valproic acid
    (E) Zonisamide

12. The mechanism of antiseizure activity of carbamazepine is
    (A) Block of sodium ion channels
    (B) Block of calcium ion channels
    (C) Facilitation of GABA actions on chloride ion channels
    (D) Glutamate receptor antagonism
    (E) Inhibition of GABA transaminase

13. Which statement about phenytoin is accurate?
    (A) Displaces sulfonamides from plasma proteins
    (B) Drug of choice in myoclonic seizures
    (C) Half-life is increased if used with phenobarbital
    (D) Isoniazid (INH) decreases steady-state blood levels of phenytoin
    (E) Toxicity may occur with only small increments in dose

14. A young male patient suffers from a seizure disorder characterized by tonic rigidity of the extremities followed in 15–30 s by tremor progressing to massive jerking of the body. This clonic phase lasts for 1 or 2 minutes, leaving the patient in a stuporous state. The antiseizure drug of choice for long-term management of this patient is
    (A) Carbamazepine
    (B) Clonazepam
    (C) Ethosuximide
    (D) Felbamate
    (E) Tiagabine

ANSWERS

1. Simple partial seizures can have the characteristics described in this patient. The jacksonian march is due to progression of epileptiform discharges in the contralateral motor cortex. Phenytoin, carbamazepine, primidone, and lamotrigine are effective in partial seizures. The succinimides (ethosuximide, phensuximide) are not effective in partial seizures or in generalized tonic-clonic seizure states. The answer is **B.**

2. Two of the drugs listed are effective in absence seizures. Ethosuximide is not excessively sedating, and tolerance does not develop to its antiseizure activity. Clonazepam is effective but exerts troublesome CNS depressant effects, and tolerance develops with chronic use. The answer is **C**.

3. The mechanism of action of ethosuximide is thought to involve blockade of T-type Ca^{2+} ion channels in thalamic neurons. The drug does not block K^+ ion channels, which in any case would be likely to result in an increase (rather than a decrease) in neuronal excitability. The answer is **B**.

4. With chronic use, barbiturates, carbamazepine, and phenytoin all induce the formation of hepatic drug-metabolizing enzymes. This action may lead to a *decrease* in the plasma concentration of other drugs used concomitantly. Valproic acid, an inhibitor of drug metabolism, can increase the plasma levels of many drugs, including carbamazepine, lamotrigine, phenobarbital, and phenytoin. Benzodiazepines have no major effects on the metabolism of other drugs. The answer is **E**.

5. Valproic acid is highly effective in specific myoclonic syndromes and is the drug of choice. Clonazepam and lamotrigine (not listed) are backup drugs. None of the other drugs listed are effective. The answer is **D**.

6. Valproic acid causes gastrointestinal distress and is potentially hepatotoxic. Its use in pregnancy has been associated with teratogenicity (neural tube defects). Weight gain is common in patients taking valproic acid. Peripheral neuropathy, including diminished deep tendon reflexes in the lower extremities, occurs with the chronic use of phenytoin, not valproic acid. The answer is **C**.

7. Monitoring of plasma concentration of phenytoin may be critical in establishing an effective dosage because of nonlinear elimination kinetics at high doses. Valproic acid has no effect on porphyrin synthesis. The enzyme-inducing activity of phenytoin has led to symptoms of opioid *withdrawal*, presumably because of an increase in the rate of metabolism of methadone. Vigabatrin does not affect the metabolism of oral contraceptives. Twice-daily dosage of ethosuximide reduces the severity of adverse gastrointestinal effects. The answer is **D**.

8. Common adverse effects of phenytoin include nystagmus, diplopia, and ataxia. With chronic use, abnormalities of vitamin D metabolism and coarsening of facial features may occur. Gingival overgrowth and hirsutism also occur. The answer is **D**.

9. Vigabatrin inhibits the enzyme GABA transaminase and does not block transporter mechanisms for GABA reuptake. Long-term use for partial seizures is associated with visual field defects that may not be reversible. Because of its toxic potential the drug is relegated to use for partial seizures in patients refractory to the standard drugs. The answer is **E**.

10. Dose tapering is an important principle in antiseizure drug withdrawal. As a rule, withdrawal from drugs used in absence seizures is easier than withdrawal from drugs used for partial and tonic-clonic seizures. Withdrawal is most difficult in patients who have been treated with barbiturates and benzodiazepines. The answer is **C**.

11. Several antiseizure drugs have some effectiveness in bipolar disorder. Valproic acid is recognized to be an appropriate first-line treatment for mania and is also used together with lithium in maintenance treatment. Carbamazepine and lamotrigine may also be of value. The answer is **D**.

12. Carbamazepine's mechanism of action is similar to that of phenytoin, blocking sodium ion channels. Ethosuximide blocks calcium channels; benzodiazepines and barbiturates facilitate the inhibitory actions of GABA; topiramate may block glutamate receptors; and vigabatrin inhibits GABA metabolism. The answer is **A**.

SKILL KEEPER ANSWERS: ANTIARRHYTHMIC DRUG ACTIONS (SEE CHAPTER 14)

1. *Close similarities of structure and function exist between voltage-gated sodium channels in neurons and in cardiac cells. Drugs that exert antiseizure actions via their blockade of sodium channels in the CNS have the potential for a similar action in the heart. Delayed recovery of sodium channels from their inactivated state subsequently slows the rising phase of the action potential in Na^+-dependent fibers and is characteristic of group I antiarrhythmic drugs. In theory, antiseizure drugs that block calcium ion channels might also have properties akin to those of group IV antiarrhythmic drugs.*

2. *In practice, the only antiseizure drug that has been used in cardiac arrhythmias is phenytoin, which has characteristics similar to group IB antiarrhythmic drugs. Phenytoin has been used for arrhythmias resulting from cardiac glycoside overdose and for ventricular arrhythmias unresponsive to lidocaine.*

13. Sulfonamides can displace phenytoin from its binding sites, increasing the plasma free fraction of the drug. Induction of liver drug-metabolizing enzymes by phenobarbital results in a *decreased* half-life of phenytoin, and isoniazid *increases* plasma levels of phenytoin by inhibiting its metabolism. Because of the dose-dependent elimination kinetics of phenytoin, some toxicity may occur with only small increments in dose. The answer is **E.**

14. This patient is suffering from generalized tonic-clonic seizures. The drugs of choice are carbamazepine, phenytoin, or valproic acid. Clonazepam and ethosuximide are not effective in this type of seizure disorder. Fosphenytoin is available for parenteral use in the management of status epilepticus. Tiagabine is approved for adjunctive use only in partial seizures. The answer is **A.**

CHECKLIST

When you complete this chapter, you should be able to:

☐ List the drugs of choice for partial seizures, generalized tonic-clonic seizures, absence and myoclonic seizures, and status epilepticus.

☐ Identify the mechanisms of antiseizure drug action at the levels of specific ion channels and/or neurotransmitter systems.

☐ Describe the main pharmacokinetic features and list the adverse effects of carbamazepine, phenytoin, and valproic acid.

☐ Identify the distinctive toxicities of new antiseizure drugs.

☐ Describe the important pharmacokinetic and pharmacodynamic considerations relevant to the long-term use of antiseizure drugs.

General Anesthetics

25

General anesthesia is a state characterized by unconsciousness, analgesia, amnesia, skeletal muscle relaxation, and loss of reflexes. Drugs used as general anesthetics are CNS depressants with actions that can be induced and terminated more rapidly than those of conventional sedative-hypnotics.

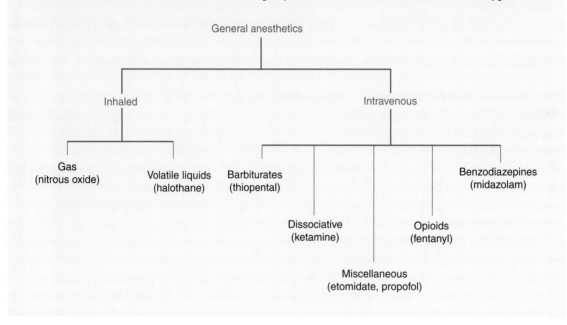

STAGES OF ANESTHESIA

Modern anesthetics act very rapidly and achieve deep anesthesia quickly. With older and more slowly acting anesthetics, the progressively greater depth of central depression associated with increasing dose or time of exposure is traditionally described as **stages of anesthesia.**

A. STAGE 1: ANALGESIA

In this stage the patient has decreased awareness of pain, sometimes with amnesia. Consciousness may be impaired but is not lost.

B. STAGE 2: DISINHIBITION

The patient appears to be delirious and excited. Amnesia occurs, reflexes are enhanced, and respiration is typically irregular; retching and incontinence may occur.

C. STAGE 3: SURGICAL ANESTHESIA

In this stage the patient is unconscious and has no pain reflexes; respiration is very regular, and blood pressure is maintained.

HIGH-YIELD TERMS TO LEARN	
Balanced anesthesia	Anesthesia produced by a combination of drugs, often including both inhaled and intravenous agents
Inhalation anesthesia	Anesthesia induced by inhalation of drug
Minimal alveolar anesthetic concentration (MAC)	The alveolar concentration of an anesthetic that is required to prevent a response to a standardized painful stimulus in 50% of patients
Analgesia	A state of decreased awareness of pain, sometimes with amnesia
General anesthesia	A state of unconsciousness, analgesia, and amnesia, with skeletal muscle relaxation and loss of reflexes

D. STAGE 4: MEDULLARY DEPRESSION

The patient develops severe respiratory and cardiovascular depression that requires mechanical and pharmacologic support.

ANESTHESIA PROTOCOLS

Anesthesia protocols vary depending on the proposed type of diagnostic, therapeutic, or surgical intervention. For minor procedures, **conscious sedation** techniques that combine intravenous agents with local anesthetics (see Chapter 26) are often used. These can provide profound analgesia, with retention of the patient's ability to maintain a patent airway and respond to verbal commands. For more extensive surgical procedures, anesthesia protocols commonly include the use of intravenous drugs to induce the anesthetic state, inhaled anesthetics (with or without intravenous agents) to maintain an anesthetic state, and neuromuscular blocking agents to effect muscle relaxation (see Chapter 27). Vital sign monitoring remains the standard method of assessing "depth of anesthesia" during surgery. Cerebral monitoring, automated techniques based on quantification of anesthetic effects on the electroencephalograph (EEG), is also useful.

MECHANISMS OF ACTION

The mechanisms of action of general anesthetics are varied. As CNS depressants, these drugs usually increase the threshold for firing of CNS neurons. The potency of inhaled anesthetics is roughly proportionate to their lipid solubility. Mechanisms of action include effects on ion channels by interactions of anesthetic drugs with membrane lipids or proteins with subsequent effects on central neurotransmitter mechanisms. Inhaled anesthetics, barbiturates, benzodiazepines, etomidate, and propofol facilitate γ-aminobutyric acid (GABA)-mediated inhibition at GABA$_A$ receptors. These receptors are sensitive to clinically relevant concentrations of the anesthetic agents and exhibit the appropriate stereospecific effects in the case of enantiomeric drugs. Ketamine does not produce its effects via facilitation of GABA$_A$ receptor functions, but possibly via its antagonism of the action of the excitatory neurotransmitter glutamic acid on the N-methyl-D-aspartate (NMDA) receptor. Most inhaled anesthetics also inhibit nicotinic ACh receptor isoforms at moderate to high concentrations. The strychnine-sensitive glycine receptor is another ligand-gated ion channel that may function as a "target" for certain inhaled anesthetics. CNS neurons in different regions of the brain have different sensitivities to general anesthetics; inhibition of neurons involved in pain pathways occurs before inhibition of neurons in the midbrain reticular formation.

INHALED ANESTHETICS

A. CLASSIFICATION AND PHARMACOKINETICS

The agents currently used in inhalation anesthesia are nitrous oxide (a gas) and several easily vaporized liquid halogenated hydrocarbons, including halothane, desflurane, enflurane, isoflurane, sevoflurane, and methoxyflurane. They are administered as gases; their partial pressure, or "tension," in the inhaled air or in blood or other tissue is a measure of their concentration. Because the standard pressure of the total inhaled mixture is atmospheric pressure (760 mm Hg at sea level), the partial pressure may also be expressed as a percentage. Thus, 50% nitrous oxide in the inhaled air would have a partial pressure of 380 mm Hg. The speed of induction of anesthetic effects depends on several factors, discussed next.

1. Solubility—The more rapidly a drug equilibrates with the blood, the more quickly the drug passes into the brain to produce anesthetic effects. Drugs with a low

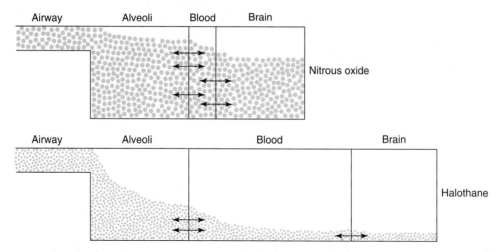

Figure 25–1. Why induction of anesthesia is slower with more soluble anesthetic gases and faster with less soluble ones. In this schematic diagram, solubility is represented by the size of the blood compartment (the more soluble the gas, the larger is the compartment). For a given concentration or partial pressure of the 2 anesthetic gases in the inspired air, it will take much longer with halothane than with nitrous oxide for the blood partial pressure to rise to the same partial pressure as in the alveoli. Because the concentration in the brain can rise no faster than the concentration in the blood, the onset of anesthesia will be much slower with halothane than with nitrous oxide. (Reproduced, with permission, from Katzung BG, editor: *Basic & Clinical Pharmacology*, 10th ed. McGraw-Hill, 2007.)

blood:gas partition coefficient (eg, nitrous oxide) equilibrate more rapidly than those with a higher blood solubility (eg, halothane), as illustrated in Figure 25–1. Partition coefficients for inhalation anesthetics are shown in Table 25–1.

2. Inspired gas partial pressure—A high partial pressure of the gas in the lungs results in more rapid

achievement of anesthetic levels in the blood. This effect can be taken advantage of by the initial administration of gas concentrations higher than those required for maintenance of anesthesia.

3. Ventilation rate—The greater the ventilation, the more rapid is the rise in alveolar and blood partial pressure of the agent and the onset of anesthesia

Table 25–1. Properties of inhalation anesthetics.

Anesthetic	Blood: Gas Partition Coefficient	Minimum Alveolar Concentration (%)[a]	Metabolism
Nitrous oxide	0.47	>100	None
Desflurane	0.42	6.5	<0.1%
Sevoflurane	0.69	2.0	2–5% (fluoride)
Isoflurane	1.40	1.4	<2%
Enflurane	1.80	1.7	8%
Halothane	2.30	0.75	>40%
Methoxyflurane	12	0.16	>70% (fluoride)

[a]Minimum alveolar concentration (MAC) is the anesthetic concentration that eliminates the response in 50% of patients exposed to a standardized painful stimulus. In this table, MAC is expressed as a percentage of the inspired gas mixture.
Modified and reproduced, with permission, from Katzung BG, editor: *Basic & Clinical Pharmacology*, 10th ed. Appleton & Lange, 2007.

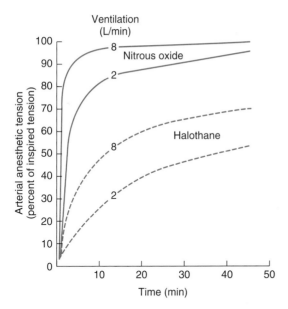

Figure 25–2. Ventilation rate and arterial anesthetic tensions. Increased ventilation (8 versus 2 L/min) has a much greater effect on equilibration of halothane than nitrous oxide. (Reproduced, with permission, from Katzung BG, editor: *Basic & Clinical Pharmacology*, 10th ed. McGraw-Hill, 2007.)

(Figure 25–2). This effect is taken advantage of in the induction of the anesthetic state.

4. Pulmonary blood flow—At high pulmonary blood flows, the gas partial pressure rises at a slower rate; thus, the speed of onset of anesthesia is reduced. At low flow rates, onset is faster. In circulatory shock, this effect may accelerate the rate of onset of anesthesia with agents of high blood solubility.

5. Arteriovenous concentration gradient—Uptake of soluble anesthetics into highly perfused tissues may decrease gas tension in mixed venous blood. This can influence the rate of onset of anesthesia because achievement of equilibrium is dependent on the difference in anesthetic tension between arterial and venous blood.

B. ELIMINATION

Anesthesia is terminated by redistribution of the drug from the brain to the blood and elimination of the drug through the lungs. The rate of recovery from anesthesia using agents with low blood:gas partition coefficients is faster than that of anesthetics with high blood solubility. This important property has led to the introduction of several newer inhaled anesthetics (eg, desflurane, sevoflurane), which, because of their low blood solubility, are characterized by recovery times that are considerably

shorter than is the case with older agents. Halothane and methoxyflurane are metabolized by liver enzymes to a significant extent (see Table 25–1). Metabolism of halothane and methoxyflurane has only a minor influence on the speed of recovery from their anesthetic effect but does play a role in potential toxicity of these anesthetics.

C. MINIMUM ALVEOLAR ANESTHETIC CONCENTRATION

The potency of inhaled anesthetics is best measured by the minimum alveolar anesthetic concentration (MAC), defined as the alveolar concentration required to eliminate the response to a standardized painful stimulus in 50% of patients. Each anesthetic has a defined MAC (see Table 25–1), but this value may vary among different patients depending on age, cardiovascular status, and use of adjuvant drugs. Estimations of MAC value suggest a relatively "steep" dose–response relationship for inhaled anesthetics. MACs for infants and elderly patients are lower than those for adolescents and young adults. When several anesthetic agents are used simultaneously, their MAC values are additive.

D. EFFECTS OF INHALED ANESTHETICS

1. CNS effects—Inhaled anesthetics decrease brain metabolic rate. They reduce vascular resistance and thus increase cerebral blood flow. This may lead to an increase in intracranial pressure. High concentrations of enflurane may cause spike-and-wave activity and muscle twitching, but this effect is unique to this drug. Although nitrous oxide has low anesthetic potency (ie, a high MAC), it exerts marked analgesic and amnestic actions.

2. Cardiovascular effects—Most inhaled anesthetics decrease arterial blood pressure moderately. Enflurane and halothane are myocardial depressants that decrease cardiac output, whereas isoflurane, desflurane, and sevoflurane cause peripheral vasodilation. Nitrous oxide is less likely to lower blood pressure than are other inhaled anesthetics. Blood flow to the liver and kidney is decreased by most inhaled agents. Inhaled anesthetics depress myocardial function—nitrous oxide least. Halothane, and to a lesser degree isoflurane, may sensitize the myocardium to the arrhythmogenic effects of catecholamines.

3. Respiratory effects—Although rate of respiration may be increased, all inhaled anesthetics cause a dose-dependent decrease in tidal volume and minute ventilation, leading to an increase in arterial CO_2 tension. Inhaled anesthetics decrease ventilatory response to hypoxia even at subanesthetic concentrations (eg, during recovery). Nitrous oxide has the smallest effect on respiration. Most inhaled anesthetics are bronchodilators, but desflurane is a pulmonary irritant and may cause bronchospasm. The pungency of enflurane causing breath-holding limits its use in anesthesia induction.

4. Toxicity—Postoperative hepatitis has occurred (rarely) after halothane anesthesia in patients experiencing hypovolemic shock or other severe stress. The mechanism of hepatotoxicity is unclear but may involve formation of reactive metabolites that cause direct toxicity or initiate immune-mediated responses. Fluoride released by metabolism of methoxyflurane (and possibly both enflurane and sevoflurane) may cause renal insufficiency after prolonged anesthesia. Prolonged exposure to nitrous oxide decreases methionine synthase activity and may lead to megaloblastic anemia. Susceptible patients may develop **malignant hyperthermia** when anesthetics are used together with neuromuscular blockers (especially succinylcholine). This rare condition is thought in some cases to be due to mutations in the gene loci corresponding to the ryanodine receptor (RyR1). Other chromosomal loci for malignant hyperthermia include mutant alleles of the gene encoding skeletal muscle L-type calcium channels. The uncontrolled release of calcium by the sarcoplasmic reticulum of skeletal muscle leads to muscle spasm, hyperthermia, and autonomic lability. Dantrolene is indicated for the treatment of this life-threatening condition, with supportive management.

> ## SKILL KEEPER: SIGNALING MECHANISMS (SEE CHAPTER 2)
>
> *Like most drugs, the general anesthetics appear to act via interactions with specific receptor molecules involved in cell signaling. For review purposes, try to recall the major types of **signaling mechanisms** relevant to the actions of drugs that act via receptors. The Skill Keeper Answers appear at the end of the chapter.*

INTRAVENOUS ANESTHETICS

A. BARBITURATES

Thiopental and **methohexital** have high lipid solubility, which promotes rapid entry into the brain and results in surgical anesthesia in one circulation time (< 1 min). These drugs are used for induction of anesthesia and for short surgical procedures. The anesthetic effects of thiopental are terminated by redistribution from the brain to other highly perfused tissues (Figure 25–3), but hepatic metabolism is required for elimination from the body. Barbiturates are respiratory and circulatory depressants; because they depress cerebral blood flow, they can also decrease intracranial pressure.

B. BENZODIAZEPINES

Midazolam is widely used adjunctively with inhaled anesthetics and intravenous opioids. The onset of its

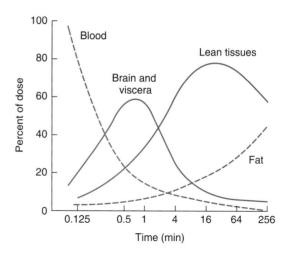

Figure 25–3. Redistribution of thiopental after intravenous bolus administration. (Reproduced, with permission, from Katzung BG, editor: *Basic & Clinical Pharmacology,* 10th ed. McGraw-Hill, 2007.)

CNS effects is slower than that of thiopental, and it has a longer duration of action. Cases of severe postoperative respiratory depression have occurred. The benzodiazepine receptor antagonist, flumazenil, accelerates recovery from midazolam and other benzodiazepines.

C. KETAMINE

This drug produces a state of "dissociative anesthesia" in which the patient remains conscious but has marked catatonia, analgesia, and amnesia. Ketamine is a chemical congener of the psychotomimetic agent, phencyclidine (PCP). The drug is a cardiovascular stimulant, and this action may lead to an increase in intracranial pressure. Emergence reactions, including disorientation, excitation, and hallucinations, which occur during recovery from ketamine anesthesia, can be reduced by the preoperative use of benzodiazepines.

D. OPIOIDS

Morphine and **fentanyl** are used with other CNS depressants (nitrous oxide, benzodiazepines) in anesthesia regimens and are especially valuable in high-risk patients who might not survive a full general anesthetic. Intravenous opioids may cause chest wall rigidity that can impair ventilation. Respiratory depression with these drugs may be reversed postoperatively with naloxone. **Neuroleptanesthesia** is a state of analgesia and amnesia produced when fentanyl is used with droperidol and nitrous oxide. Newer opioids related to fentanyl have been introduced for intravenous anesthesia. Alfentanil and remifentanil have been used for induction of anesthesia. Recovery from the actions of remifentanil is faster than recovery from other opioids

KEY DRUGS		
Subclass	**Prototypes**	**Other Significant Agents**
Inhaled anesthetics		
Volatile liquids	Halothane	Enflurane, desflurane, isoflurane, sevoflurane
Gas	Nitrous oxide	
Intravenous anesthetics		
Barbiturates	Thiopental	Thiamylal, methohexital
Opioids	Morphine	Fentanyl, alfentanil, remifentanil
Phenols	Propofol	
Benzodiazepines	Midazolam	
Dissociative agent	Ketamine	
Imidazole	Etomidate	

used in anesthesia because of its rapid metabolism by blood and tissue esterases.

E. PROPOFOL

Propofol produces anesthesia as rapidly as the intravenous barbiturates, and recovery is more rapid. Propofol has antiemetic actions, and recovery is not delayed after prolonged infusion. The drug is commonly used as a component of balanced anesthesia and as an anesthetic in outpatient surgery. Propofol is also effective in producing prolonged sedation in patients in critical care settings. Propofol may cause marked hypotension during induction of anesthesia, primarily through decreased peripheral resistance. Total body clearance of propofol is greater than hepatic blood flow, suggesting that its elimination includes other mechanisms in addition to metabolism by liver enzymes.

F. ETOMIDATE

This imidazole derivative affords rapid induction with minimal change in cardiac function or respiratory rate and has a short duration of action. The drug is not analgesic, and its primary advantage is in anesthesia for patients with limited cardiac or respiratory reserve. Etomidate may cause pain and myoclonus on injection and nausea postoperatively. Prolonged administration may cause adrenal suppression.

QUESTIONS

1. A new halogenated gas anesthetic has a blood:gas partition coefficient of 0.5 and a MAC value of 1%. Which prediction about this agent is most accurate? (Refer to Table 25–1 for comparison of agents.)
    (A) The new agent will be more potent than halothane
    (B) It will be metabolized by the liver to release fluoride ions
    (C) It will be more soluble in the blood than isoflurane
    (D) Its speed of onset of action will be similar to that of nitrous oxide
    (E) Equilibrium between arterial and venous gas tensions will be achieved very slowly with this agent

2. Which statement concerning the effects of anesthetic agents is false?
    (A) Relaxation of bronchiolar smooth muscle occurs during halothane anesthesia
    (B) Mild generalized muscle twitching occurs at high doses of enflurane
    (C) Chest muscle rigidity often follows the administration of fentanyl
    (D) Intraoperative use of midazolam with inhalation anesthetics may prolong the postanesthesia recovery period
    (E) Severe hepatitis has been reported after the use of desflurane

3. A 23-year-old man has a pheochromocytoma, blood pressure of 190/120 mm Hg, and hematocrit of 50%. Pulmonary function and renal function are normal. His catecholamines are elevated, and he has a well-defined abdominal tumor on MRI. He has been scheduled for surgery. Of the following agents, which one should NOT be included in the anesthesia protocol?
    (A) Desflurane
    (B) Fentanyl
    (C) Halothane
    (D) Midazolam
    (E) Thiopental

4. Which statement concerning nitrous oxide is accurate?

(A) It is a useful component of anesthesia protocols because of its lack of cardiovascular depression

(B) Anemia is a common adverse effect in patients exposed to nitrous oxide for periods longer than 2 h

(C) It is the most potent of the inhaled anesthetics

(D) There is a direct association between the use of nitrous oxide and malignant hyperthermia

(E) 30–50% of nitrous oxide is eliminated via hepatic metabolism

5. Which statement concerning anesthetic MAC value is accurate?
(A) Anesthetics with low MAC value have low potency
(B) MACs give information about the slope of the dose–response curve
(C) Nitrous oxide has an extremely low MAC value
(D) MAC values decrease in elderly patients
(E) Simultaneous use of opioid analgesics increases the MAC for inhaled anesthetics

6. Total intravenous anesthesia with fentanyl has been selected for a frail 72-year-old woman about to undergo cardiac surgery. Which statement about this anesthesia protocol is accurate?
(A) Intravenous opioids will provide useful cardiostimulatory effects
(B) Opioids control the hypertensive response to surgical stimulation
(C) Marked relaxation of skeletal muscles is anticipated
(D) Patient awareness may occur during surgery, with recall after recovery
(E) The patient is likely to experience pain during surgery

7. Which anesthetic has a low blood:gas partition coefficient but is not used for induction of anesthesia because of airway irritation?
(A) Desflurane
(B) Enflurane
(C) Halothane
(D) Isoflurane
(E) Sevoflurane

8–9. A 20-year-old male patient scheduled for hernia surgery was anesthetized with halothane and nitrous oxide; tubocurarine was provided for skeletal muscle relaxation. The patient rapidly developed tachycardia and became hypertensive. Generalized skeletal muscle rigidity was accompanied by marked hyperthermia. Laboratory values revealed hyperkalemia and acidosis.

8. This unusual complication of anesthesia is most likely caused by

(A) Activation of brain dopamine receptors by halothane
(B) Block of automic ganglia by tubocurarine
(C) Excessive release of calcium from the sarcoplasmic reticulum
(D) Pheochromocytoma
(E) Release of acetylcholine from somatic nerve endings at skeletal muscle

9. The patient should be treated immediately with
(A) Atropine
(B) Baclofen
(C) Dantrolene
(D) Edrophonium
(E) Succinylcholine

10. The inhalation anesthetic with the fastest onset of action is
(A) Enflurane
(B) Isoflurane
(C) Nitric oxide
(D) Nitrogen dioxide
(E) Nitrous oxide

11. If ketamine is used as the sole anesthetic in the attempted reduction of a dislocated shoulder joint, its actions will include
(A) Analgesia
(B) Bradycardia
(C) Hypotension
(D) Muscle rigidity
(E) Respiratory depression

12. An intravenous bolus dose of thiopental usually leads to loss of consciousness within 10–15 s. If no further drugs are administered, the patient will regain consciousness in just a few minutes. This is because thiopental is
(A) A good substrate for renal tubular secretion
(B) Exhaled rapidly
(C) Rapidly metabolized by hepatic enzymes
(D) Redistributed from brain to other body tissues
(E) Secreted in the bile

13. Respiratory depression after use of which of the following agents may be reversed by administration of flumazenil?
(A) Desflurane
(B) Fentanyl
(C) Ketamine
(D) Midazolam
(E) Propofol

14. Which of the following agents is associated with a high incidence of disorientation, sensory and perceptual illusions, and vivid dreams during recovery from anesthesia?

(A) Diazepam
(B) Fentanyl
(C) Ketamine
(D) Midazolam
(E) Thiopental

15. For which of these drugs is the following true? Postoperative vomiting is uncommon with this intravenous agent, and patients are able to ambulate sooner than those who receive other anesthetics.
(A) Enflurane
(B) Ketamine
(C) Morphine
(D) Propofol
(E) Remifentanil

ANSWERS

1. Inhaled anesthetics with low blood:gas solubility have a fast onset of action and a short duration of recovery. The new agent described here resembles nitrous oxide but is more potent, as indicated by its low MAC value. Not all halogenated anesthetics undergo significant hepatic metabolism or release fluoride ions. The answer is **D.**

2. Hepatitis after general anesthesia has been linked to use of *halothane,* although the incidence is very low (1 in 20,000–35,000). The results of animal experiments suggest that halothane hepatotoxicity may be due to formation of a toxic metabolite produced under anoxic conditions. Hepatotoxicity has not been reported after administration of desflurane or other inhaled anesthetics. The answer is **E.**

3. Halothane, and to a lesser extent isoflurane (not listed),sensitizes the myocardium to catecholamines. Arrhythmias may occur in patients with cardiac disease who have high circulating levels of epinephrine and norepinephrine (eg, patients with pheochromocytoma). Newer inhaled anesthetics are considerably less arrhythmogenic. The answer is **C.**

4. Anemia has **not** been reported in patients exposed to nitrous oxide anesthesia for periods as long as 6 h. Nitrous oxide is the least potent of the inhaled anesthetics, and the compound has not been implicated in malignant hyperthermia. More than 98% of the gas is eliminated via exhalation. The answer is **A.**

5. MAC value is inversely related to potency; a low MAC means high potency. MAC gives no information about the slope of the dose–response curve. Desflurane has the lowest blood:gas partition coefficient of the inhaled anesthetics. Use of opioid analgesics with inhaled anesthetics lowers the MAC value. As with most CNS depressants, the elderly patient is more sensitive, so MAC values are lower. The answer is **D.**

6. Intravenous opioids (eg, fentanyl) are widely used in anesthesia for cardiac surgery because they provide full analgesia and cause less cardiac depression than inhalation anesthetic agents. They are not cardiac stimulants, and fentanyl is more likely to cause skeletal muscle rigidity than relaxation. Disadvantages of this technique are patient recall (decreased by use of a benzodiazepine)and the occurrence of hypertensive responses to surgical stimulation. The addition of vasodilators (eg, nitroprusside) or a β-blocker (eg, esmolol) may be needed to prevent intraoperative hypertension. The answer is **D.**

7. Desflurane is rarely used for induction of anesthesia because of a high incidence of coughing and sometimes bronchospasm. Despite its low blood:gas partition coefficient, anesthesia with desflurane does not always lead to faster rates of recovery. The answer is **A.**

8. Malignant hyperthermia is a rare but life-threatening reaction that may occur during general anesthesia with halogenated anesthetics and skeletal muscle relaxants, particularly succinylcholine and tubocurarine. Predisposing genetic factors include clinical myopathy associated with mutations in the gene loci for the skeletal muscle ryanodine receptor or L-type calcium channels. The answer is **C.**

9. The drug of choice in malignant hyperthermia is dantrolene, which prevents release of calcium from the sarcoplasmic reticulum of skeletal muscle cells. Appropriate measures must be taken to lower body temperature, control hypertension, and restore acid-base and electrolyte balance. The answer is **C.**

10. The purpose of this question is to point out that there are 3 medically important oxides of nitrogen. Nitric oxide (NO) is a powerful vasodilator (see Chapter 19). Nitrogen dioxide (NO_2) is a pulmonary irritant generated in fermenting silage; it may cause lethal pulmonary damage in farm workers. Nitrous oxide (N_2O) is the inhalation anesthetic agent discussed in this chapter. The answer is **E.**

11. Ketamine is a cardiovascular stimulant, increasing heart rate and blood pressure. This results in part from central sympathetic stimulation and from inhibition of norepinephrine reuptake at sympathetic nerve endings. Analgesia and amnesia occur, with preservation of muscle tone and minimal depression of respiration. The answer is **A.**

12. The high lipophilicity of thiopental ensures rapid entry to the CNS after an intravenous bolus dose. As the blood level falls, thiopental exits the brain and is redistributed to other highly perfused tissues such as the liver and skeletal muscles. Thus, the brain level of thiopental rapidly declines to the

point that consciousness is regained within a few minutes. Ultimately, the elimination of thiopental from the body depends on its metabolism by the liver. The answer is **D.**

13. Flumazenil is a benzodiazepine receptor antagonist (see Chapter 22). It accelerates recovery from post-operative depression of the CNS caused by midazolam and other benzodiazepines used in anesthesia. The short duration of action of flumazenil may necessitate multiple doses. The sedative actions of benzodiazepines are more reliably reversed by flumazenil than is respiratory depression. Use of flumazenil does not obviate the need for adequate monitoring of respiration and provision of ventilatory support when needed. The answer is **D.**

14. The emergence phenomena described are adverse effects of ketamine. Administration of diazepam immediately before ketamine anesthesia reduces the incidence of these effects. The answer is **C.**

15. Propofol is used extensively in anesthesia protocols, including those for day surgery. The favorable properties of the drug include an antiemetic effect and recovery more rapid than that after use of other intravenous drugs. Propofol does not cause cumulative effects, possibly because of its short half-life (2–8 min) in the body. The drug is also used for prolonged sedation in critical care settings. The answer is **D.**

SKILL KEEPER ANSWER: SIGNALING MECHANISMS (SEE CHAPTER 2)

1. *Receptors that modify gene transcription: adrenal and gonadal steroids*

2. *Receptors on membrane-spanning enzymes: insulin*

3. *Receptors activating Janus kinases that modulate STAT molecules: cytokines*

4. *Receptors directly coupled to ion channels: nicotinic (ACh), GABA, glycine*

5. *Receptors coupled to enzymes via G proteins: many endogenous compounds (eg, ACh, NE, serotonin) and drugs*

6. *Receptors that are enzymes or transporters: acetylcholinesterase, angiotensin-converting enzyme, carbonic anhydrase, H^+/K^+ antiporter, and so on*

CHECKLIST

When you complete this chapter, you should be able to:

☐ Name the inhalation anesthetic agents and identify their pharmacodynamic and pharmacokinetic properties.

☐ Describe what is meant by the terms (1) blood:gas partition coefficient and (2) minimum alveolar anesthetic concentration.

☐ Identify proposed molecular targets for the actions of anesthetic drugs.

☐ Describe how the blood:gas partition coefficient of an inhalation anesthetic influences its speed of onset of anesthesia and its recovery time.

☐ Identify the commonly used intravenous anesthetics and point out their main pharmacokinetic and pharmacodynamic characteristics.

Local Anesthetics

Local anesthesia is the condition that results when sensory transmission from a local area of the body to the CNS is blocked. The local anesthetics constitute a group of chemically similar agents (esters and amides) that block the sodium channels of excitable membranes. Because these drugs can be administered by injection in the target area, or by topical application in some cases, the anesthetic effect can be restricted to a localized area (eg, the cornea or an arm). When given intravenously, local anesthetics have effects on other tissues.

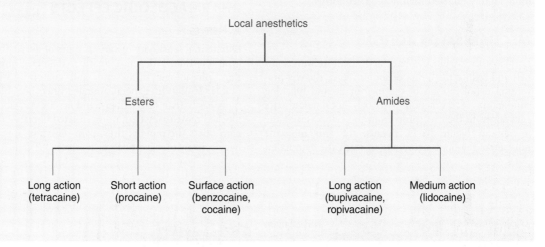

CHEMISTRY

Most local anesthetic drugs are esters or amides of simple benzene derivatives. Subgroups within the local anesthetics are based on this chemical characteristic and on duration of action. The commonly used local anesthetics are weak bases with at least 1 ionizable amine function that can become charged through the gain of a proton (H^+). As discussed in Chapter 1, the degree of ionization is a function of the pK_a of the drug and the pH of the medium. Because the pH of tissue may differ from the physiologic 7.4 (eg, it may be as low as 6.4 in infected tissue), the degree of ionization of the drug will vary. Because the pK_a of most local anesthetics is between 8.0 and 9.0 (benzocaine is an exception), variations in

pH associated with infection can have significant effects on the proportion of ionized to nonionized drug. The question of the active form of the drug (ionized vs. nonionized) is discussed later.

PHARMACOKINETICS

Many shorter acting local anesthetics are readily absorbed into the blood from the injection site after administration. The duration of local action is, therefore, limited unless blood flow to the area is reduced. This can be accomplished by administration of a vasoconstrictor (usually an α agonist sympathomimetic) with the local anesthetic agent. Cocaine is an important exception because it has intrinsic sympathomimetic action due to its inhibition of norepinephrine reuptake into nerve terminals. The longer acting agents (eg, bupivicaine, ropivicaine, tetracaine) are also less dependent on the coadministration of vasoconstrictors. Surface activity (ability to reach superficial nerves when applied to the surface of mucous membranes) is a property of certain local anesthetics, including cocaine and benzocaine.

Metabolism of ester local anesthetics is carried out by plasma cholinesterases (pseudocholinesterases) and is very rapid for procaine (half-life, 1–2 min), slower for cocaine and very slow for tetracaine. The amides are metabolized in the liver, in part by cytochrome P450 isozymes. The half-lives of lidocaine and prilocaine are approximately 1.5 h. Bupivacaine and ropivacaine are the longest acting amide local anesthetics, with half-lives of 3.5 and 4.2 h, respectively. Liver dysfunction may increase the elimination half-life of amide local anesthetics. Acidification of the urine promotes ionization of local anesthetics; the charged forms of such drugs are more rapidly excreted than nonionized forms.

MECHANISM OF ACTION

Local anesthetics block voltage-dependent sodium channels and reduce the influx of sodium ions, thereby preventing depolarization of the membrane and blocking conduction of the action potential. Local anesthetics gain access to their receptors from the cytoplasm or the membrane (Figure 26–1). Because the drug molecule must cross the lipid membrane to reach the cytoplasm,

the more lipid-soluble (nonionized, uncharged) form reaches effective intracellular concentrations more rapidly than does the ionized form. On the other hand, once inside the axon, the ionized (charged) form of the drug is the more effective blocking entity. Thus, both the nonionized and the ionized forms of the drug play important roles, the first in reaching the receptor site and the second in causing the effect. The affinity of the receptor site within the sodium channel for the local anesthetic is a function of the state of the channel, whether it is resting, open, or inactivated, and therefore follows the same rules of use dependence and voltage dependence that were described for the sodium channel-blocking antiarrhythmic drugs (see Chapter 14). In particular, if other factors are equal, rapidly firing fibers are usually blocked before slowly firing fibers. High concentrations of extracellular K^+ may enhance local anesthetic activity, whereas elevated extracellular Ca^{2+} may antagonize it.

PHARMACOLOGIC EFFECTS

A. NERVES

Differential sensitivity of various types of nerve fibers to local anesthetics depends on fiber diameter, myelination, physiologic firing rate, and anatomic location (Table 26–1). In general, smaller fibers are blocked more easily than larger fibers, and myelinated fibers are blocked more easily than unmyelinated fibers. Activated pain fibers fire rapidly; thus, pain sensation appears to be selectively blocked by local anesthetics. Fibers located

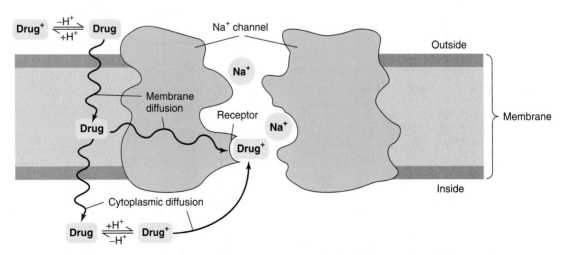

Figure 26–1. Schematic diagram of the sodium channel in an excitable membrane (eg, an axon) and the pathways by which a local anesthetic molecule (*Drug*) may reach its receptor. Sodium ions are not able to pass through the channel when the drug is bound to the receptor. The local anesthetic diffuses within the membrane in its uncharged form. In the aqueous extracellular and intracellular spaces, the charged form (*Drug*) is also present.

Table 26–1. Susceptibility to block of types of nerve fibers.

Fiber Type	Function	Diameter (μm)	Myelination	Conduction Velocity (m/s)	Sensitivity to Block
Type A					
Alpha	Proprioception, motor	12–20	Heavy	70–120	+
Beta	Touch, pressure	5–12	Heavy	30–70	++
Gamma	Muscle spindles	3–6	Heavy	15–30	++
Delta	Pain, temperature	2–5	Heavy	12–30	+++
Type B	Preganglionic, autonomic	<3	Light	3–15	++++
Type C					
Dorsal root	Pain	0.4–1.2	None	0.5–2.3	++++
Sympathetic	Postganglionic	0.3–1.3	None	0.7–2.3	++++

Reproduced, with permission, from Katzung BG, editor: *Basic & Clinical Pharmacology,* 10th ed. McGraw-Hill, 2007.

in the periphery of a thick nerve bundle are blocked sooner than those in the core because they are exposed earlier to higher concentrations of the anesthetic.

B. OTHER TISSUES

The effects of these drugs on the heart are discussed in Chapter 14 (see class I antiarrhythmic agents). Most local anesthetics also have weak blocking effects on skeletal muscle neuromuscular transmission, but these actions have no clinical application. The mood elevation induced by cocaine reflects actions on dopamine or other amine-mediated synaptic transmission in the CNS rather than a local anesthetic action on membranes.

CLINICAL USE

The local anesthetics are commonly used for minor surgical procedures, often in combination with vasoconstrictors such as epinephrine. Onset of action may be accelerated by the addition of sodium bicarbonate, which enhances intracellular access of these weakly basic compounds. Local anesthetics are also used in spinal anesthesia and to produce autonomic blockade in ischemic conditions. Slow epidural infusion at low concentrations has been used successfully for postoperative analgesia (in the same way as epidural opioid infusion; Chapter 31). Repeated epidural injection in anesthetic doses may lead to tachyphylaxis, however.

TOXICITY

A. CNS EFFECTS

The important toxic effects of most local anesthetics are in the CNS. All local anesthetics are capable of producing a spectrum of central effects, including light-headedness

or sedation, restlessness, nystagmus, and tonic-clonic convulsions. Severe convulsions may be followed by coma with respiratory and cardiovascular depression.

B. CARDIOVASCULAR EFFECTS

With the exception of cocaine, all local anesthetics are vasodilators. Patients with preexisting cardiovascular disease may develop heart block and other disturbances of cardiac electrical function at high plasma levels of local anesthetics. Bupivacaine, a racemic mixture of 2 isomers, may produce severe cardiovascular toxicity, including arrhythmias and hypotension. The (S)-isomer, levobupivicaine, appears to be less cardiotoxic. Cardiotoxicity has also been reported for ropivicaine when used for peripheral nerve block. The ability of cocaine to block norepinephrine reuptake at sympathetic neuroeffector junctions and the drug's vasoconstricting actions contribute to cardiovascular toxicity. When used as a drug of abuse, cocaine's cardiovascular toxicity includes severe hypertension with cerebral hemorrhage, cardiac arrhythmias, and myocardial infarction.

C. OTHER TOXIC EFFECTS

Prilocaine is metabolized to products that include *O*-toluidine, an agent capable of converting hemoglobin to methemoglobin. Although it is tolerated in healthy individuals, even moderate methemoglobinemia can cause decompensation in patients with cardiac or pulmonary disease. The ester-type local anesthetics are metabolized to products that can cause antibody formation in some patients. Allergic responses to local anesthetics are rare and can usually be avoided by using an agent from the amide subclass. In high concentrations, local anesthetics may cause a local neurotoxic action that includes histologic damage and permanent impairment of function.

KEY DRUGS		
Subclass	**Prototypes**	**Other Significant Agents**
Esters	Procaine	Benzocaine, cocaine, tetracaine
Amides	Lidocaine	Bupivacaine, etidocaine, prilocaine

SKILL KEEPER: CARDIAC TOXICITY OF LOCAL ANESTHETICS (SEE CHAPTER 14)

Explain how hyperkalemia facilitates the cardiac toxicity of local anesthetics. The Skill Keeper Answer appears at the end of the chapter.

D. TREATMENT OF TOXICITY

Severe toxicity is treated symptomatically; there are no antidotes. Convulsions are usually managed with intravenous diazepam or a short-acting barbiturate such as thiopental. Hyperventilation with oxygen is helpful. Occasionally, a neuromuscular blocking drug may be used to control violent convulsive activity. The cardiovascular toxicity of bupivacaine overdose is difficult to treat and has caused fatalities in healthy young adults.

QUESTIONS

1. Properties of local anesthetics do NOT include
   (A) Blockade of voltage-dependent sodium channels
   (B) Preferential binding to resting channels
   (C) Slowing of axonal impulse conduction
   (D) An increase in membrane refractory period
   (E) Effects on vascular tone

2. The pK$_a$ of bupivicaine is 8.3. In infected tissue at pH 6.3, the fraction of the drug in the ionized form will be
   (A) 1%
   (B) 10%
   (C) 50%
   (D) 90%
   (E) 99%

3. Which statement about the speed of onset of nerve blockade with local anesthetics is correct?
   (A) Faster in onset in infected tissues
   (B) Faster in onset in myelinated fibers
   (C) Faster in onset in hypocalcemia
   (D) Slower in onset in hyperkalemia
   (E) Slower in onset in the periphery of a nerve bundle than in the center of a bundle

4. The most important effect of inadvertent intravenous administration of a large dose of an amide local anesthetic is
   (A) Bronchoconstriction
   (B) Hepatic damage
   (C) Nerve damage
   (D) Renal failure
   (E) Seizures

5. Factors that influence the action of local anesthetics do NOT include
   (A) Acetylcholinesterase activity in the area
   (B) Amount of local anesthetic injected
   (C) Blood flow through the tissue in which the injection is made
   (D) Tissue pH
   (E) Use of vasoconstrictors

6. You have a vial containing 4 mL of a 2% solution of lidocaine. How much lidocaine is present in 1 mL?
   (A) 2 mg
   (B) 8 mg
   (C) 20 mg
   (D) 80 mg
   (E) 200 mg

7. Which statement about the toxicity of local anesthetics is correct?
   (A) Serious cardiovascular reactions are more likely to occur with tetracaine than with bupivacaine
   (B) Cyanosis may occur after injection of large doses of lidocaine, especially in patients with pulmonary disease
   (C) Intravenous injection of local anesthetics may stimulate ectopic cardiac pacemaker activity
   (D) In overdosage, hyperventilation (with oxygen) is helpful to correct acidosis and lower extracellular potassium
   (E) Most local anesthetics cause vasoconstriction

8. Epinephrine added to a solution of lidocaine for a peripheral nerve block will

(A) Increase the risk of convulsions
(B) Increase the duration of anesthetic action of the local anesthetic
(C) Both **A** and **B**
(D) Neither **A** nor **B**

9. A child requires multiple minor surgical procedures in the nasopharynx. Which drug has high surface local anesthetic activity and intrinsic vasoconstrictor actions that reduce bleeding in mucous membranes?
(A) Benzocaine
(B) Bupivacaine
(C) Cocaine
(D) Lidocaine
(E) Procaine

10. A 24-year-old woman was given an epidural anesthetic for pain relief during labor. The drug selected had a slow onset, but a longer duration of action than most of the other local anesthetics. Unfortunately, some of the drug was inadvertently injected intravenously and caused a marked drop in blood pressure and an arrhythmia. The drug used was most likely
(A) Benzocaine
(B) Bupivacaine
(C) Cocaine
(D) Lidocaine
(E) Procaine

11. Prilocaine is relatively contraindicated in patients with cardiovascular or pulmonary disease because the drug
(A) Acts as an antagonist at beta adrenoceptors in the heart and the lung
(B) Can cause decompensation through formation of *O*-toluidine
(C) Inhibits cyclooxygenases in cardiac and pulmonary cells
(D) Is a potent bronchoconstrictor
(E) None of the above

ANSWERS

1. Local anesthetics bind preferentially to sodium channels in the open and inactivated states. Recovery from drug-induced block is 10–1000 times slower than recovery of channels from normal inactivation. Resting channels have a lower affinity for local anesthetics. The answer is **B**.

2. Because the drug is a weak base, it will be more ionized (protonated) at pH values lower than its pK_a. Because the pH given is 2 log units lower (more acid) than the pK_a, the ratio of ionized to nonionized drug will be approximately 99:1. The answer is **E**.

(Recall from Chapter 1 that at a pH equal to pK_a, the ratio is 1:1; at 1 log unit difference, the ratio is approximately 90:10; at 2 units difference, 99:1; and so on).

3. Myelinated nerve fibers are blocked by local anesthetics more readily than unmyelinated ones. See the Skill Keeper answer for an explanation of the effects of hypocalcemia and hyperkalemia on nerve blockade by local anesthetics. The answer is **B**.

4. Of the effects listed, the most important in local anesthetic overdose (of both amide and ester types) concern the CNS. Such effects can include sedation or restlessness, nystagmus, convulsions, coma, and respiratory depression. Intravenous diazepam is commonly used for seizures caused by local anesthetics. The answer is **E**.

5. Local anesthetics are poor substrates for acetylcholinesterase, and the activity of this enzyme does not play a part in terminating the actions of local anesthetics. Ester-type local anesthetics are hydrolyzed by plasma (and tissue) pseudocholinesterases. Individuals with genetically based defects in pseudocholinesterase activity are unusually sensitive to procaine and other esters. The answer is **A**.

6. The fact that you have 4 mL of the solution of lidocaine is irrelevant. A 2% solution of any drug contains 2 g per 100 mL. The amount of lidocaine in 1 mL of a 2% solution is thus 0.02 g, or 20 mg. The answer is **C**.

7. Acidosis resulting from tissue hypoxia favors local anesthetic toxicity because these drugs bind more avidly (or dissociate more slowly) from the sodium channel binding site when they are in the charged state. (Note that *onset* of therapeutic effect may be slower because charged local anesthetics penetrate the membrane less rapidly; see text.) Hyperkalemia depolarizes the membrane, which also favors local anesthetic binding. Oxygenation reduces both acidosis and hyperkalemia. The answer is **D**.

8. Epinephrine will increase the duration of a nerve block when it is administered with short- and medium-duration local anesthetics. As a result of the vasoconstriction that prolongs the duration of this block, less local anesthetic is required, so the risk of toxicity (eg, a convulsion) is reduced. The answer is **B**.

9. Cocaine is the only local anesthetic with intrinsic vasoconstrictor activity due to its action to block the reuptake of norepinephrine released from sympathetic nerve endings (Chapter 9). Cocaine also has significant surface local anesthetic activity and is favored for head, neck, and pharyngeal surgery. The answer is **C**.

10. Bupivacaine appears to be more cardiotoxic than other local anesthetics. Accidental intravenous administration of bupivacaine may lead to arrhythmias and cardiovascular collapse. Cardiotoxicity has also been reported for ropivicaine when used for peripheral nerve block. The answer is **B.**

11. Large doses of prilocaine may cause accumulation of a metabolite (*O*-toluidine) that converts hemoglobin to methemoglobin. Patients may appear cyanotic and the blood "chocolate-colored." High plasma levels of methemoglobin have resulted in decompensation in patients with cardiac or pulmonary disease. The answer is **B.**

 SKILL KEEPER ANSWER: CARDIAC TOXICITY OF LOCAL ANESTHETICS (SEE CHAPTER 14)

Sodium channel blockers (eg, local anesthetics) bind more readily to open (activated) or inactivated sodium channels. Hyperkalemia depolarizes the resting membrane potential, so more sodium channels are in the inactivated state. Conversely, hypercalcemia tends to hyperpolarize the resting potential and reduces the block of sodium channels.

CHECKLIST

When you complete this chapter, you should be able to:

☐ Describe the mechanism of action of local anesthetics.

☐ Know what is meant by the terms "use-dependent blockade" and "state-dependent blockade."

☐ Explain the relationship among tissue pH, drug pK_a, and the rate of onset of local anesthetic action.

☐ List 4 factors that determine the susceptibility of nerve fibers to local anesthetic blockade.

☐ Describe the major toxic effects of the local anesthetics.

Skeletal Muscle Relaxants

27

The drugs in this chapter are divided into 2 dissimilar groups. The neuromuscular blocking drugs, which act at the skeletal myoneural junction, are used to produce muscle paralysis to facilitate surgery or assisted ventilation. The spasmolytic drugs, most of which act in the CNS, are used to reduce abnormally elevated tone caused by neurologic or muscle end plate disease.

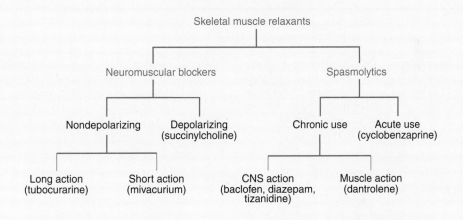

NEUROMUSCULAR BLOCKING DRUGS

A. CLASSIFICATION AND PROTOTYPES

Skeletal muscle contraction is evoked by a nicotinic cholinergic transmission process. Blockade of transmission at the end plate (the postsynaptic structure bearing the nicotinic receptors) is clinically useful in producing muscle relaxation, a requirement for surgical relaxation and control of ventilation. The neuromuscular blockers are quaternary amines structurally related to acetylcholine (ACh). Most are antagonists (nondepolarizing type), and the prototype is **tubocurarine.** One neuromuscular blocker used clinically, **succinylcholine,** is an agonist at the nicotinic end plate receptor (depolarizing type).

B. NONDEPOLARIZING NEUROMUSCULAR BLOCKING DRUGS

1. Pharmacokinetics—All agents are given parenterally. They are highly polar drugs and do not cross the blood:brain barrier. Drugs that are metabolized (eg, mivacurium, by plasma cholinesterase) or eliminated in the bile (eg, vecuronium) usually have shorter durations of action than those eliminated by the kidney (eg, pancuronium, tubocurarine), which usually have durations of action > 35 min. In addition to hepatic metabolism, atracurium clearance involves rapid spontaneous breakdown (Hofmann elimination) to form laudanosine and other products. At high blood levels laudanosine may cause seizures; cisatracurium, a stereoisomer of atracurium, forms less laudanosine.

HIGH-YIELD TERMS TO LEARN

Depolarizing blockade	Neuromuscular paralysis that results from persistent depolarization of the endplate (eg, by succinylcholine)
Desensitization	A phase of blockade by a depolarizing blocker during which the endplate repolarizes but is less than normally responsive to agonists (acetylcholine or succinylcholine)
Malignant hyperthermia	Hyperthermia that results from massive release of calcium from the sarcoplasmic reticulum, leading to uncontrolled contraction and stimulation of metabolism in skeletal muscle
Nondepolarizing blockade	Neuromuscular paralyis that results from pharmacologic antagonism at the acetylcholine receptor of the end plate (eg, by tubocurarine)
Spasmolytic	A drug that reduces abnormally elevated muscle tone (spasm) without paralysis (eg, baclofen, dantrolene)
Stabilizing blockade	Synonym for nondepolarizing blockade

---

2. Mechanism of action—Nondepolarizing drugs prevent the action of ACh at the skeletal muscle end plate (Figure 27–1). They act as surmountable blockers (ie, the blockade can be overcome by increasing the amount of agonist [ACh] in the synaptic cleft). They behave as though they compete with ACh at the receptor, and their effect is reversed by cholinesterase inhibitors. Some drugs in this group may also act directly to plug the ion channel operated by the ACh receptor. Posttetanic potentiation is preserved in the presence of these agents, but tension during the tetanus fades rapidly. See Table 27–1 for additional details.

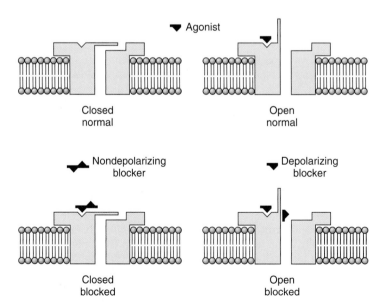

Figure 27–1. Drug interactions with the acetylcholine (ACh) receptor on the skeletal muscle end plate. **Top:** ACh, the normal agonist, opens the sodium channel. **Bottom left:** Nondepolarizing blockers bind to the receptor to prevent opening of the channel. **Bottom right:** Succinylcholine causes initial depolarization (fasciculation) and then persistent depolarization of the channel, which leads to muscle relaxation. (Reproduced, with permission, from Katzung BG, editor: *Basic & Clinical Pharmacology*, 9th ed. McGraw-Hill, 2004.

Table 27–1. Comparison of a typical nondepolarizing neuromuscular blocker (tubocurarine) and a depolarizing blocker (succinylcholine).

Process	Tubocurarine	Succinylcholine Phase I	Succinylcholine Phase II
Administration of tubocurarine	Additive	Antagonistic	Augmented[a]
Administration of succinylcholine	Antagonistic	Additive	Augmented[a]
Effect of neostigmine	Antagonistic	Augmented[a]	Antagonistic
Initial excitatory effect on skeletal muscle	None	Fasciculations	None
Response to tetanic stimulus	Unsustained ("fade")	Sustained[b]	Unsustained
Posttetanic facilitation	Yes	No	Yes

[a]It is not known whether this interaction is additive or synergistic (superadditive).
[b]The amplitude is decreased, but the response is sustained.
Reproduced, with permission, from Katzung BG, editor: *Basic & Clinical Pharmacology,* 9th ed. McGraw-Hill, 2007.

C. Depolarizing Neuromuscular Blocking Drugs

1. Pharmacokinetics—Succinylcholine is composed of 2 ACh molecules linked end to end. Succinylcholine is metabolized by cholinesterase (butyrylcholinesterase or pseudocholinesterase) in the liver and plasma. It has a duration of action of only a few minutes if given as a single dose. Blockade may be prolonged in patients with genetic variants of plasma cholinesterase that metabolize succinylcholine very slowly. Such variant cholinesterases are resistant to the inhibitory action of dibucaine. Succinylcholine is not rapidly hydrolyzed by acetylcholinesterase.

2. Mechanism of action—Succinylcholine acts like a nicotinic agonist and depolarizes the neuromuscular end plate (see Figure 27–1). The initial depolarization is often accompanied by twitching and fasciculations (antagonized by pretreatment with small doses of a nondepolarizing blocker). Because tension cannot be maintained in skeletal muscle without periodic repolarization and depolarization of the end plate, continuous depolarization results in muscle relaxation and paralysis. As with the nondepolarizing blockers, some evidence suggests that succinylcholine can also plug the end plate channels.

When given by continuous infusion, the effect of succinylcholine changes from continuous depolarization (phase I) to gradual repolarization with resistance to depolarization (phase II) (ie, a curare-like block; see Table 27–1).

D. Reversal of Blockade

The action of nondepolarizing blockers is readily reversed by increasing the concentration of normal transmitter at the receptors. This is best accomplished by administration of cholinesterase inhibitors such as neostigmine or pyridostigmine. In contrast, the paralysis produced by depolarizing blockers is *increased* by cholinesterase inhibitors during phase I. During phase II, the block produced by succinylcholine is usually reversible by cholinesterase inhibitors.

E. Toxicity

1. Respiratory paralysis—The action of full doses of neuromuscular blockers leads directly to respiratory paralysis. If mechanical ventilation is not provided, the patient will asphyxiate.

2. Autonomic effects and histamine release—Autonomic ganglia are stimulated by succinylcholine and blocked by tubocurarine. Succinylcholine activates cardiac muscarinic receptors, whereas pancuronium is a moderate blocking agent and causes tachycardia. Tubocurarine and mivacurium are the most likely of these agents to cause histamine release, but it may also occur to a slight extent with atracurium and succinylcholine. Vecuronium and 3 newer nondepolarizing drugs (cisatracurium, doxacurium, pipecuronium) have no significant effects on autonomic functions or histamine release. A summary of these autonomic effects is shown in Table 27–2.

3. Specific effects of succinylcholine—Muscle pain is a common postoperative complaint, and muscle damage may occur. Succinylcholine may cause hyperkalemia, especially in patients with burn or spinal cord injury, peripheral nerve dysfunction, or muscular dystrophy. Increases in intragastric pressure caused by fasciculations may promote regurgitation, with possible aspiration of gastric contents.

4. Interactions—Inhaled anesthetics, especially isoflurane, strongly potentiate and prolong neuromuscular

Table 27–2. Autonomic effects of neuromuscular drugs.

Drug	Effect on Autonomic Ganglia	Effect on Cardiac Muscarinic Receptors	Ability to Release Histamine
Nondepolarizing			
Atracurium	None	None	Slight
Cisatracurium	None	None	None
Doxacurium	None	None	None
Mivacurium	None	None	Moderate
Pancuronium	None	Moderate block	None
Pipecuronium	None	None	None
Tubocurarine	Weak block	None	Moderate
Vecuronium	None	None	None
Depolarizing			
Succinylcholine	Stimulation	Stimulation	Slight

Modified and reproduced with permission from Katzung BG, editor: *Basic & Clinical Pharmacology*, 10th ed. McGraw-Hill, 2007.

blockade. A rare interaction of succinylcholine (and possibly tubocurarine) with inhaled anesthetics can result in malignant hyperthermia. A very early sign of this potentially life-threatening condition following administration of the neuromuscular blocker is contraction of the jaw muscles (trismus). Aminoglycoside antibiotics and antiarrhythmic drugs may potentiate and prolong the relaxant action of neuromuscular blockers to a lesser degree.

SKILL KEEPER: AUTONOMIC CONTROL OF HEART RATE (SEE CHAPTER 6)

Tubocurarine can block bradycardia caused by phenylephrine but has no effect on bradycardia caused by neostigmine. Explain! The Skill Keeper Answer appears at the end of the chapter.

SPASMOLYTIC DRUGS

Certain chronic diseases of the CNS (eg, cerebral palsy, multiple sclerosis, stroke) are associated with abnormally high reflex activity in the neuronal pathways that control skeletal muscle; the result is painful spasm. Bladder and anal sphincter control are also affected in most cases and may require autonomic drugs for management. In other circumstances, acute injury or inflammation of muscle leads to spasm and pain. Such temporary spasm can sometimes be reduced with appropriate drug therapy.

The goal of spasmolytic therapy in both chronic and acute conditions is reduction of excessive skeletal muscle tone without reduction of strength. Reduced spasm results in reduction of pain and improved mobility.

A. DRUGS FOR CHRONIC SPASM

1. Classification—The spasmolytic drugs do not resemble ACh in structure or effect. They act in the CNS or in the skeletal muscle cell rather than at the neuromuscular end plate. The spasmolytic drugs used in treatment of the chronic conditions mentioned previously include **diazepam,** a benzodiazepine (see Chapter 22); **baclofen,** a γ-aminobutyric acid (GABA) agonist; **tizanidine,** a congener of clonidine; and **dantrolene,** an agent that acts on the sarcoplasmic reticulum of skeletal muscle. These agents are usually administered by the oral route. Refractory cases may respond to chronic intrathecal administration of baclofen. **Botulinum toxin** injected into selected muscles can reduce pain caused by severe spasm (see Chapter 6) and also has application in more generalized spastic disorders (eg, cerebral palsy). **Gabapentin,** an antiseizure drug, has been shown to be an effective spasmolytic in patients with multiple sclerosis.

2. Mechanism of action—The spasmolytic drugs act by several mechanisms. Three of the drugs act in the spinal cord. Diazepam facilitates GABA-mediated presynaptic inhibition (see Chapter 22). Baclofen acts as a $GABA_B$ agonist causing membrane hyperpolarization via increased K^+ conductance, an action that decreases

KEY DRUGS

Subclass	Prototypes	Other Significant Agents
Nondepolarizing neuromuscular blockers		
Renal elimination, long duration	Tubocurarine	Pancuronium
Hepatic elimination, intermediate duration	Vecuronium	Rocuronium
Spontaneous or plasma ChE,[a] intermediate-short duration	Atracurium	Mivacurium
Depolarizing blockers	Succinylcholine	
Spasmolytic drugs	Diazepam, baclofen, cyclobenzaprine, dantrolene, tizanidine, botulinum toxin	

[a]ChE: cholinesterase. (Atracurium breaks down spontaneously; mivacurium is metabolized by plasma ChE.)

the release of excitatory neurotransmitters, including substance P. Tizanidine, an imidazoline related to clonidine with significant α_2 agonist activity, reinforces both presynaptic and postsynaptic inhibition in the cord. All 3 drugs reduce the tonic output of the primary spinal motoneurons.

Dantrolene acts in the skeletal muscle cell to reduce the release of activator calcium from the sarcoplasmic reticulum via interaction with the ryanodine receptor (RyR) channel. Cardiac and smooth muscle are minimally depressed. Dantrolene is also effective in the treatment of malignant hyperthermia, a disorder characterized by massive calcium release from the sarcoplasmic reticulum of skeletal muscle. Although rare, malignant hyperthermia can be triggered by general anesthesia protocols that include succinylcholine or tubocurarine (see Chapter 25). In this emergency condition, dantrolene is given intravenously to block calcium release.

3. Toxicity—The sedation produced by diazepam is significant but milder than that produced by other sedative-hypnotic drugs at doses that induce equivalent muscle relaxation. Baclofen produces less sedation than diazepam. Dantrolene causes significant muscle weakness but less sedation than either diazepam or baclofen. Tizanidine may cause drowsiness and hypotension.

B. DRUGS FOR ACUTE MUSCLE SPASM

Many drugs (eg, cyclobenzaprine, methocarbamol, orphenadrine) are promoted for the treatment of acute spasm resulting from muscle injury. Most of these drugs are sedatives or act in the brain stem. **Cyclobenzaprine,** a typical member of this group, is believed to act in the brain stem, possibly by interfering with polysynaptic reflexes that maintain skeletal muscle tone. The drug is active by the oral route and has marked sedative and antimuscarinic actions. Cyclobenzaprine may cause confusion and visual

hallucinations in some patients. None of these drugs used for acute spasm are effective in muscle spasm resulting from cerebral palsy or spinal cord injury.

QUESTIONS

1. Characteristics of phase I depolarizing neuromuscular blockade include
   (A) Easy reversibility with pharmacologic antagonists
   (B) Marked muscarinic blockade
   (C) Muscle fasciculations in the later stages of block
   (D) Reversibility by pyridostigmine
   (E) Well-sustained tension during a period of tetanic stimulation

2–3. A patient underwent a surgical procedure of 2 h. Anesthesia was provided by isoflurane, supplemented by intravenous midazolam and a nondepolarizing muscle relaxant. At the end of the procedure, a low dose of atropine was administered followed by pyridostigmine.

2. The main reason for administering atropine was to
   (A) Prevent spasm of gastrointestinal smooth muscle
   (B) Reverse the effects of the muscle relaxant
   (C) Provide postoperative analgesia
   (D) Prevent activation of cardiac muscarinic receptors
   (E) Enhance the action of pyridostigmine

3. Atropine would probably not be needed to offset effects on the heart during reversal of the effects of a nondepolarizing relaxant if the agent used was
   (A) Atracurium
   (B) Mivacurium
   (C) Pancuronium
   (D) Tubocurarine
   (E) Vecuronium

4. Characteristics of nondepolarizing neuromuscular blockade include which of the following?
   (A) Block of posttetanic potentiation
   (B) Histamine blocking action
   (C) Poorly sustained tetanic tension
   (D) Significant muscle fasciculations during onset of block
   (E) Stimulation of autonomic ganglia

5. Which drug is most effective in the management of malignant hyperthermia?
   (A) Baclofen
   (B) Dantrolene
   (C) Haloperidol
   (D) Succinylcholine
   (E) Vecuronium

6. Succinylcholine is associated with
   (A) Antagonism by pyridostigmine during the early phase of blockade
   (B) Blockade of autonomic ganglia
   (C) Elevated intragastric pressure
   (D) Histamine release in a genetically determined population
   (E) Metabolism at the neuromuscular junction by acetylcholinesterase

7. A 22-year-old anesthesia patient with normal hepatic and renal function was given a bolus intravenous dose of a neuromuscular blocker that should have lasted only 5–10 min. Instead, the patient required mechanical ventilation for over 8 h. Which statement about this problem is accurate?
   (A) The agent administered was atracurium
   (B) This is an example of genetic variation in drug metabolism
   (C) The agent used was tubocurarine
   (D) The problem is due to inadequate activity of acetylcholinesterase
   (E) Neostigmine should be administered to establish the nature of the problem

8. Which drug is most often associated with hypotension caused by histamine release?
   (A) Diazepam
   (B) Pancuronium
   (C) Tizanidine
   (D) Tubocurarine
   (E) Vecuronium

9. Regarding the spasmolytic drugs, which statement is NOT accurate?
   (A) Baclofen acts on neurons in the spinal cord to increase chloride ion conductance
   (B) Cyclobenzaprine is likely to dry oropharyngeal secretions and decrease gut motility
   (C) Dantrolene has little effect on calcium release in cardiac muscle

   (D) Diazepam causes sedation at most doses required to reduce muscle spasms
   (E) Intrathecal use of baclofen is effective in some refractory cases of muscle spasticity

10. Which drug has caused hyperkalemia leading to cardiac arrest in patients with spinal cord injury or muscular dystrophy?
    (A) Baclofen
    (B) Dantrolene
    (C) Succinylcholine
    (D) Tubocurarine
    (E) Vecuronium

11. Atracurium is
    (A) A depolarizing blocker
    (B) An activator of cardiac muscarinic receptors
    (C) Commonly used in the ICU for long-term immobilization
    (D) Inactivated by spontaneous breakdown
    (E) Slowly eliminated in pseudocholinesterase deficiency

12. Which drug has spasmolytic activity and could also be used in the management of seizures caused by overdose of a local anesthetic?
    (A) Baclofen
    (B) Cyclobenzaprine
    (C) Dantrolene
    (D) Diazepam
    (E) Tizanidine

13. Which drug administered in the operating room is used to prevent postoperative pain caused by succinylcholine?
    (A) Baclofen
    (B) Dantrolene
    (C) Diazepam
    (D) Lidocaine
    (E) Vecuronium

14. In anesthesia protocols that include succinylcholine, which of the following is a premonitory sign of malignant hyperthermia?
    (A) Acidosis
    (B) Bradycardia
    (C) Hypotension
    (D) Transient hypothermia
    (E) Trismus

ANSWERS

1. Phase I depolarizing blockade is not associated with muscarinic blockade, nor is it reversible with cholinesterase inhibitors. Muscle fasciculations occur at the start of the action of succinylcholine. The answer is **E**.

2. Acetylcholinesterase inhibitors used for reversing the effects of nondepolarizing muscle relaxants cause increases in ACh at all sites where it acts as a neurotransmitter. To offset the resulting side effects, including bradycardia, a muscarinic blocking agent is used concomitantly. Although atropine is effective, glycopyrrolate is usually preferred since it lacks CNS effects. The answer is **D**.

3. One of the distinctive characteristics of pancuronium is that it can block muscarinic receptors, especially those in the heart. It has sometimes caused tachycardia and hypertension and may cause dysrhythmias in predisposed individuals. The answer is **C**.

4. Nondepolarizing blockers result in poorly sustained tetanic tension. They do not cause ganglionic stimulation or fasciculations at any time during their action. The answer is **C**.

5. Prompt treatment is essential in malignant hyperthermia to control body temperature, correct acidosis, and prevent calcium release. Dantrolene interacts with the RyR channel to block the release of activator calcium from the sarcoplasmic reticulum, preventing the tension-generating interaction of actin with myosin. The answer is **B**.

6. Fasciculations associated with succinylcholine may increase intragastric pressure, with possible complications of regurgitation and aspiration of gastric contents. This complication is more likely in patients with delayed gastric emptying, such as those with esophageal dysfunction or diabetes. Histamine release resulting from succinylcholine is not genetically determined. The answer is **C**.

7. The drug administered was the depolarizing agent succinylcholine. This drug is metabolized by pseudocholinesterase and has a duration of action of just a few minutes in most patients. However, about 1 in 500 persons have a single abnormal gene for pseudocholinesterase. Fewer than 1 in 3000 persons have 2 abnormal genes (homozygous atypical) that produce an enzyme with only 1% of the normal affinity for succinylcholine. In such patients the action of succinylcholine may persist for hours. The answer is **B**.

8. Hypotension may occur with tubocurarine and with the spasmolytic drug tizanidine. In the case of tubocurarine, the decrease in blood pressure may be due partly to histamine release and to ganglionic blockade. Tizanidine causes hypotension via α_2 adrenoceptor activation like its congener clonidine. The answer is **D**.

9. Baclofen activates $GABA_B$ receptors in the spinal cord. However, these receptors are coupled to K^+ channels (see Chapter 21). $GABA_A$ receptors in the CNS modulate chloride ion channels. The answer is **A**.

10. Muscle depolarization by succinylcholine releases potassium, and the ensuing hyperkalemia can be life threatening in terms of cardiac arrest. Patients most susceptible include those with extensive burns, spinal cord injuries, neurologic dysfunction, or intra-abdominal infection. The answer is **C**.

11. Atracurium (nondepolarizing) breaks down spontaneously in the plasma (Hofmann elimination) to form laudanosine, which has a long half-life. Because laudanosine enters the CNS and may cause seizures, prolonged administration of atracurium is usually avoided. The drug has no action on autonomic ganglia or muscarinic receptors. The answer is **D**.

12. Diazepam is both an effective antiseizure drug and a spasmolytic. The spasmolytic action of diazepam is thought to be exerted partly in the spinal cord because it reduces spasm of skeletal muscle in patients with cord transection. Cyclobenzaprine is used for acute local spasm and has no antiseizure activity. The answer is **D**.

SKILL KEEPER ANSWER: AUTONOMIC CONTROL OF HEART RATE (SEE CHAPTER 6)

Reflex changes in heart rate involve ganglionic transmission. Activation of α_1 receptors on blood vessels by phenylephrine elicits a reflex bradycardia because mean blood pressure is increased. One of the characteristic effects of tubocurarine is its block of autonomic ganglia; this action can interfere with reflex changes in heart rate. Tubocurarine would not prevent bradycardia resulting from neostigmine (an inhibitor of acetylcholinesterase) because this occurs via stimulation by ACh of cardiac muscarinic receptors.

13. The action of succinylcholine is antagonized by depolarizing blockers. To prevent skeletal muscle fasciculations and the resulting postoperative pain caused by succinylcholine, a small nonparalyzing dose of a nondepolarizing drug is often given immediately before succinylcholine. The answer is **E**.

14. Bradycardia from activation of muscarinic receptors is characteristic of succinylcholine, and hypotension can result from histamine release. There is no transient phase of hypothermia, but severe contraction of the jaw muscles (trismus) is considered to be a premonitory sign of malignant hyperthermia. Acidosis is a delayed consequence of malignant hyperthermia. The answer is **E**.

CHECKLIST

When you complete this chapter you should be able to:

☐ Describe the transmission process at the skeletal neuromuscular end plate and the points at which drugs can modify this process.

☐ Identify the major nondepolarizing neuromuscular blockers and 1 depolarizing neuromuscular blocker; compare their pharmacokinetics.

☐ Describe the differences between depolarizing and nondepolarizing blockers from the standpoint of tetanic and posttetanic twitch strength.

☐ Describe the method of reversal of nondepolarizing blockade.

☐ List drugs for treatment of skeletal muscle spasticity and identify their sites of action and their adverse effects.

Drugs Used in Parkinsonism & Other Movement Disorders

28

Movement disorders constitute a number of heterogeneous neurologic conditions with very different therapies. They include parkinsonism, Huntington's disease, Wilson's disease, and Gilles de la Tourette's syndrome. Movement disorders, including athetosis, chorea, dyskinesia, dystonia, tics, and tremor, can be caused by a variety of general medical conditions, neurologic dysfunction, and drugs.

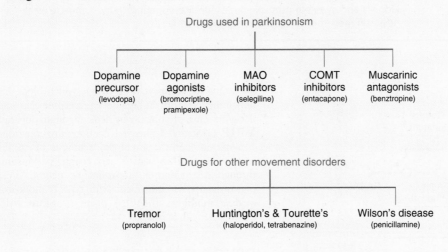

PARKINSONISM

A. PATHOPHYSIOLOGY

Parkinsonism (paralysis agitans) is a common movement disorder that involves dysfunction in the basal ganglia and associated brain structures. Signs include rigidity of skeletal muscles, akinesia (or bradykinesia), flat facies, and tremor at rest (mnemonic **RAFT**).

1. Naturally occurring parkinsonism—The naturally occurring disease is of uncertain origin and occurs with increasing frequency during aging from the fifth or sixth decade of life onward. Pathologic characteristics include a decrease in the levels of striatal dopamine and

the degeneration of dopaminergic neurons in the nigrostriatal tract that normally *inhibit* the activity of striatal GABAergic neurons (Figure 28–1). Most of the postsynaptic dopamine receptors on GABAergic neurons are of the D_2 subclass (negatively coupled to adenylyl cyclase). The reduction of normal dopaminergic neurotransmission leads to excessive *excitatory* actions of cholinergic neurons on striatal GABAergic neurons; thus, dopamine and acetylcholine activities are out of balance in parkinsonism (see Figure 28–1).

2. Drug-induced parkinsonism—Many drugs can cause parkinsonian symptoms; these effects are usually reversible. The most important drugs are the butyrophenone and

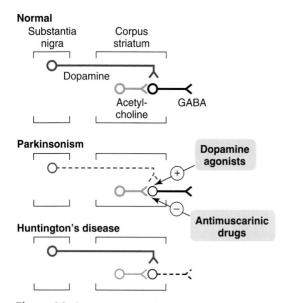

Figure 28–1. Schematic representation of the sequence of neurons involved in parkinsonism and Huntington's chorea. **Top:** Neurons in the normal brain. **Middle:** Neurons in parkinsonism. The dopaminergic neuron is lost. **Bottom:** Neurons in Huntington's disease. The GABAergic neuron is lost. (Reproduced, with permission, from Katzung BG, editor: *Basic & Clinical Pharmacology*, 9th ed. McGraw-Hill, 2004.)

phenothiazine **antipsychotic drugs,** which block brain dopamine receptors. At high doses, **reserpine** causes similar symptoms, presumably by depleting brain dopamine. **MPTP** (1-methyl-4-phenyl-1,2,3,6-tetrahydropyridine), a by-product of the attempted synthesis of an illicit meperidine analog, causes irreversible parkinsonism through destruction of dopaminergic neurons in the nigrostriatal tract. Treatment with type B monoamine oxidase inhibitors (MAOIs) protects against MPTP neurotoxicity in animals.

DRUG THERAPY OF PARKINSONISM

Strategies of drug treatment of parkinsonism involve increasing dopamine activity in the brain, decreasing muscarinic cholinergic activity in the brain, or both. Although several dopamine receptors subtypes are present in the substantia nigra, the benefits of most dopaminergic antiparkinson drugs appear to depend on activation of the D_2 receptor subtype.

A. LEVODOPA

1. **Mechanisms**—Because dopamine has low bioavailability and does not readily cross the blood-brain barrier, its precursor, L-dopa (levodopa), is used. This amino acid enters the brain via an L-amino acid transporter (LAT) and is converted to dopamine by the enzyme aromatic L-amino acid decarboxylase (DOPA decarboxylase), which is present in many body tissues, including the brain.

Levodopa is usually given with **carbidopa,** a drug that does not cross the blood-brain barrier but inhibits DOPA decarboxylase in peripheral tissues. With this combination, the plasma half-life is prolonged, lower doses of levodopa are effective, and there are fewer peripheral side effects.

2. Pharmacologic effects—Levodopa ameliorates the signs of parkinsonism, particularly bradykinesia; moreover, the mortality rate is decreased. However, the drug does not cure parkinsonism, and responsiveness fluctuates and gradually decreases with time, which may reflect progression of the disease. Clinical response fluctuations may, in some cases, be related to the timing of levodopa dosing. In other cases, unrelated to dosing, off-periods of akinesia may alternate over a few hours with on-periods of improved mobility but often with dyskinesias (**on-off phenomena**). In some cases off-periods may respond to apomorphine (see below). Although drug holidays sometimes reduce toxic effects, they rarely affect response fluctuations. However, catechol-*O*-methyltransferase (COMT) inhibitors used adjunctively may improve fluctuations in levodopa responses in some patients (see below).

3. Toxicity—Most adverse effects are dose dependent. Gastrointestinal effects include anorexia, nausea, and emesis and can be reduced by taking the drug in divided doses. Tolerance to the emetic action of levodopa usually occurs after several months.

Postural hypotension is common, especially in the early stage of treatment. Other cardiac effects include tachycardia, asystole, and cardiac arrhythmias (rare).

Dyskinesias occur in up to 80% of patients, with choreoathetosis of the face and distal extremities occurring most often. Some patients may exhibit chorea, ballismus, myoclonus, tics, and tremor.

Behavioral effects may include anxiety, agitation, confusion, delusions, hallucinations, and depression. Levodopa is contraindicated in patients with a history of psychosis.

B. BROMOCRIPTINE AND OTHER DOPAMINE AGONISTS

1. Mechanism of action—Bromocriptine and pergolide (the latter recently withdrawn, see below) are ergot alkaloids that act as partial agonists at dopamine D_2 receptors in the brain; the drugs increase the functional activity of dopamine neurotransmitter pathways, including those involved in extrapyramidal functions.

2. Clinical use—Bromocriptine and pergolide have been used as individual drugs, in combinations with levodopa (and with anticholinergic drugs), and in patients who are refractory to or cannot tolerate levodopa.

3. Toxicity—**Gastrointestinal effects** include anorexia, nausea, and vomiting. **Cardiovascular effects** commonly include postural hypotension, and cardiac

arrhythmias may also occur. Because of its implication in cardiac valvular disease, pergolide was recently withdrawn in the United States. **Dyskinesias** may occur with abnormal movements similar to those caused by levodopa. **Behavioral effects** include confusion, hallucinations, and delusions; these occur more commonly with bromocriptine and pergolide than with levodopa. Like levodopa, these dopamine agonists are contraindicated in patients with a history of psychosis. **Ergot-related effects** include pulmonary infiltrates and erythromelalgia.

4. Pramipexole and ropinirole—Pramipexole and ropinirole are more recently introduced nonergot dopamine receptor agonists. Ropinirole is a relatively pure D_2 receptor agonist, but pramipexole is unusual in that the drug has greater affinity for D_3 receptors. Both are often considered to be first-line drugs in early management of Parkinson's disease. Anorexia, nausea, and vomiting may occur and can be minimized by taking the drugs with meals. Dyskinesias, postural hypotension, lassitude, sleepiness, and fatigue have been reported. Pramipexole may be neuroprotective because it is reported to act as a scavenger for hydrogen peroxide. The dose of pramipexole should be reduced in renal dysfunction. Ropinirole is metabolized in the liver by the CYP1A2 isoform, which also metabolizes caffeine and **warfarin.**

5. Apomorphine—A potent DA receptor agonist, apomorphine injected subcutaneously may provide temporary relief (1-2 h) of "off-periods" of akinesia in patients on dopaminergic therapy. Because of severe nausea, pretreatment with antiemetics (eg, trimethobenzamide) is necessary. Other side effects of apomorphine include dyskinesias, hypotension, drowsiness, and sweating.

C. AMANTADINE

1. Mechanism of action—Amantadine enhances dopaminergic neurotransmission by unknown mechanisms that may involve increasing synthesis or release of dopamine or inhibition of dopamine reuptake. The drug also has muscarinic blocking actions.

2. Pharmacologic effects—Amantadine may improve bradykinesia, rigidity, and tremor but is usually effective for only a few weeks. Amantadine also has antiviral effects.

3. Toxicity—**Behavioral effects** include restlessness, agitation, insomnia, confusion, hallucinations, and acute toxic psychosis. **Dermatologic reactions** include livedo reticularis. **Miscellaneous effects** may include gastrointestinal disturbances, urinary retention, and postural hypotension. Amantadine also causes peripheral edema, which responds to diuretics.

D. SELEGILINE

1. Mechanism of action—Selegiline is a selective inhibitor of MAO type B, the enzyme isoform that metabolizes dopamine in preference to norepinephrine and serotonin. Selegiline may increase brain dopamine levels. Rasagiline, another MAO type B inhibitor, is also available. Both drugs inhibit MAO type A at high doses.

2. Pharmacologic effects—Selegiline is used as an adjunct to levodopa in parkinsonism and has also been used as the sole agent in newly diagnosed patients. Hepatic metabolism of selegiline results in the formation of desmethylselegiline (possibly neuroprotective) and amphetamine.

3. Toxicity—Adverse effects include insomnia, mood changes, dyskinesias, gastrointestinal distress, and hypotension. Meperidine in combination with selegiline has caused agitation, delirium, and death. Selegiline has been implicated in the serotonin syndrome when used in patients taking selective serotonin reuptake inhibitors (see Chapter 30).

E. Catechol-*O*-Methyltransferase Inhibitors

1. Mechanism of action—Entacapone and tolcapone are inhibitors of COMT, the enzyme that converts levodopa to 3-*O*-methyldopa (3OMD). Increased plasma levels of 3OMD are associated with poor response to levodopa partly because the compound competes with levodopa for active transport into the CNS.

2. Clinical uses—The drugs are used individually as adjuncts to levodopa-carbidopa, improving response and prolonging "on-time". A formulation combining levodopa, carbidopa, and entacapone is available.

3. Toxicity—Adverse effects related to increased levels of levodopa include dyskinesias, gastrointestinal distress, and postural hypotension. Levodopa dose reductions may be needed for the first few days of COMT inhibitor use. Other side effects include sleep disturbances and orange discoloration of the urine. Tolcapone increases liver enzymes and has caused acute hepatic failure, necessitating routine monitoring of liver function tests.

F. Acetylcholine-Blocking (Antimuscarinic) Drugs

1. Mechanism of action—These drugs decrease the excitatory actions of cholinergic neurons on cells in the striatum by blocking muscarinic receptors.

2. Pharmacologic effects—Drugs such as benztropine or trihexyphenidyl may improve the tremor and rigidity of parkinsonism but have little effect on bradykinesia. They are used adjunctively in parkinsonism and also alleviate the reversible extrapyramidal symptoms caused by antipsychotic drugs.

3. Toxicity—CNS toxicity includes drowsiness, inattention, confusion, delusions, and hallucinations. Peripheral adverse effects are typical of atropine-like drugs. These agents exacerbate tardive dyskinesias that result from prolonged use of antipsychotic drugs.

SKILL KEEPER: AUTONOMIC DRUG SIDE EFFECTS (SEE CHAPTERS 8 AND 9)

Based on your understanding of the receptors affected by drugs used in Parkinson's disease, what types of autonomic side effects can you anticipate? The Skill Keeper Answers appear at the end of the chapter.

DRUG THERAPY OF OTHER MOVEMENT DISORDERS

A. Tremor

Physiologic and essential tremor are clinically similar conditions characterized by postural tremor. They may be alleviated by β-blocking drugs including **propranolol.** β-Blockers should be used with caution in patients with congestive heart failure, asthma, diabetes, or hypoglycemia. Metoprolol, a β_1-selective antagonist, has been used in patients with concomitant pulmonary disease. Antiepileptic drugs including primidone and topiramate have also been used to treat essential tremor.

B. Huntington's Disease and Tourette's Syndrome

Huntington's disease, an inherited disorder, results from a brain neurotransmitter imbalance such that GABA functions are diminished and dopaminergic functions are enhanced (see Figure 28–1). There may also be a cholinergic deficit because choline acetyltransferase is decreased in the basal ganglia of patients with this disease. Drug therapy involves the use of amine-depleting drugs (eg, **reserpine, tetrabenazine**) or dopamine receptor antagonists (eg, **haloperidol**). Pharmacologic attempts to enhance brain GABA and acetylcholine activities have not been successful in patients with this disease.

Tourette's syndrome is a disorder of unknown cause that responds to haloperidol and other dopamine D_2 receptor blockers, including pimozide. Carbamazepine, clonazepam, and clonidine have also been used.

C. Drug-Induced Dyskinesias

Parkinsonism symptoms caused by antipsychotic agents (see Chapter 29) are usually reversible by lowering drug dosage, changing the therapy to a drug that is less toxic to extrapyramidal function, or treating with a muscarinic blocker. In acute dystonias, parenteral administration of benztropine or diphenhydramine is helpful. Levodopa and bromocriptine are not useful because dopamine

KEY DRUGS

Subgroups	Prototypes	Other Significant Agents
Drugs used in parkinsonism		
Dopamine prodrug	Levodopa	
Dopa decarboxylase inhibitor	Carbidopa	
Dopamine agonist	Bromocriptine	Apomorphine, pramipexole, ropinirole
MAO type B inhibitor	Selegiline	Rasagiline
COMT inhibitor	Entacapone	Tolcapone
Atypical dopamine agonist	Amantadine	
Muscarinic blocker	Benztropine	Biperiden, trihexyphenidyl
Drugs used in tremor	Propranolol	Metoprolol
Drugs used in Huntington's disease and Tourette's syndrome	Haloperidol	Phenothiazines
Drugs used in Wilson's disease	Penicillamine	
Drugs used in restless legs syndrome	Ropinirole	

receptors are blocked by the antipsychotic drugs. **Tardive dyskinesias** that develop from therapy with older antipsychotic drugs are possibly a form of denervation supersensitivity. They are not readily reversed; no specific drug therapy is available.

D. WILSON'S DISEASE

This recessively inherited disorder of copper metabolism results in deposition of copper salts in the liver and other tissues. Hepatic and neurologic damage may be severe or fatal. Treatment involves use of the chelating agent penicillamine (dimethylcysteine), which removes excess copper. Toxic effects of penicillamine include gastrointestinal distress, myasthenia, optic neuropathy, and blood dyscrasias.

E. RESTLESS LEGS SYNDROME

This syndrome, of unknown cause, is characterized by an unpleasant creeping discomfort in the limbs that occurs particularly when the patient is at rest. The disorder is more common in pregnant women and in uremic and diabetic patients. Dopaminergic therapy is the preferred treatment and ropinirole, a long-acting drug, is approved for this condition. Opioid analgesics and benzodiazepines are also used.

QUESTIONS

1–2. Bradykinesia has made drug treatment necessary in a 60-year-old male patient with Parkinson's disease and therapy is to be initiated with levodopa.

1. Regarding the anticipated actions of levodopa, the patient should NOT be informed that

    (A) A netlike reddish to blue discoloration of the skin is a likely side effect of the medication

    (B) He should be careful when he stands up because he may get dizzy

    (C) Taking the drug in divided doses will decrease nausea and vomiting

    (D) The drug will probably improve his symptoms for a period of time but not indefinitely

    (E) Uncontrollable muscle jerks may occur

2. The physician who is prescribing levodopa will (or should) know that the drug

    (A) Causes less severe behavioral side effects if given with carbidopa

    (B) Fluctuates in its effectiveness with increasing frequency as treatment continues

    (C) Prevents extrapyramidal adverse effects of antipsychotic drugs

    (D) Protects against cancer in patients with melanoma

    (E) Toxicity includes pulmonary infiltrates

3. The major reason why carbidopa is of value in parkinsonism is that the compound

    (A) Crosses the blood-brain barrier

    (B) Inhibits monoamine oxidase type A

    (C) Inhibits aromatic L-amino acid decarboxylase

    (D) Inhibits monoamine oxidase type B

    (E) Is converted to the false neurotransmitter carbidopamine

4. Which statement about bromocriptine is accurate?

    (A) It should not be administered to patients taking antimuscarinic drugs

    (B) Its effectiveness in Parkinson's disease requires its metabolic conversion to an active metabolite

(C) The drug is contraindicated in patients with a history of psychosis

(D) The drug should not be administered to patients who have already been treated with levodopa

(E) Mental disturbances occur more commonly with levodopa than with bromocriptine

5. A 72-year-old patient with parkinsonism presents with swollen feet. They are red, tender, and very painful. These symptoms would abate within a few days if the patient stopped taking
(A) Amantadine
(B) Benztropine
(C) Bromocriptine
(D) Levodopa
(E) Selegiline

6. A patient with parkinsonism is being treated with levodopa. He suffers from irregular, involuntary muscle jerks that affect the proximal muscles of the limbs. Which statement about these symptoms is accurate?
(A) The symptoms will usually be reduced if the dose of levodopa is increased
(B) Administration of other drugs that activate dopamine receptors will exacerbate dyskinesias
(C) The symptoms are likely to be alleviated by continued treatment with levodopa
(D) Dyskinesias are less likely to occur if levodopa is administered with carbidopa
(E) Coadministration of muscarinic blockers prevents the occurrence of dyskinesias during treatment with levodopa

7. A 51-year-old patient with parkinsonism is being maintained on levodopa-carbidopa, with adjunctive use of low doses of entacapone, but continues to have off-periods of akinesia. The most appropriate drug to use for immediate (but temporary) relief is
(A) Apomorphine
(B) Benztropine
(C) Carbidopa
(D) Ropinirole
(E) Selegiline

8. Concerning the drugs used in parkinsonism, which statement is accurate?
(A) Levodopa causes mydriasis and can precipitate an attack of acute glaucoma
(B) Useful therapeutic effects of amantadine continue for several years
(C) The primary benefit of antimuscarinic drugs in parkinsonism is their ability to relieve bradykinesia
(D) Dopamine receptor agonists should not be used in Parkinson's disease before a trial of levodopa
(E) The concomitant use of selegiline may increase the peripheral adverse effects of levodopa

9. A previously healthy 50-year-old woman begins to suffer from slowed mentation and develops writhing movements of her tongue and hands. In addition, she has delusions of being persecuted. The woman has no history of psychiatric or neurologic disorders. Although further diagnostic assessment should be made, it is very likely that the most appropriate drug for treatment will be
(A) Amantadine
(B) Bromocriptine
(C) Haloperidol
(D) Levodopa
(E) Trihexyphenidyl

10. In parkinsonian patients who have prostatic hypertrophy or obstructive gastrointestinal disease, great caution must be exercised in the use of this drug (or drugs from the same class)?
(A) Benztropine
(B) Carbidopa
(C) Levodopa
(D) Ropinirole
(E) Selegiline

11. With respect to pramipexole, which of the following is accurate?
(A) Activates brain dopamine receptors
(B) Commonly effective when used as monotherapy in mild parkinsonism
(C) May cause postural hypotension
(D) Not an ergot derivative
(E) All of the above

12. Which drug is protective against the selective neurotoxicity of MPTP, a chemical known to cause the destruction of dopaminergic neurons in the nigrostriatal tract?
(A) Benztropine
(B) Entacapone
(C) Levodopa
(D) Penicillamine
(E) Selegiline

13. Entacapone may be of value in patients being treated with levodopa-carbidopa because it
(A) Activates COMT
(B) Decreases formation of 3OMD
(C) Inhibits monoamine oxidase type B
(D) Inhibits dopamine reuptake
(E) Releases dopamine from nerve endings

14. Which drug is most suitable for management of tremor in a patient who has pulmonary disease?
(A) Diazepam
(B) Levodopa
(C) Metoprolol
(D) Propranolol
(E) Terbutaline

ANSWERS

1. In prescribing levodopa, the patient should be informed about side effects, including gastrointestinal distress, postural hypotension, and dyskinesias. It is reasonable to advise the patient that therapeutic benefits cannot be expected to continue indefinitely. Livedo reticularis (a netlike rash) is an adverse effect of treatment with amantadine. The answer is **A.**

2. Levodopa causes less peripheral toxicity but more behavioral side effects when used with carbidopa. The drug is not effective in antagonizing the akinesia, rigidity, and tremor caused by treatment with antipsychotic agents. Levodopa is a precursor of melanin and may *activate* malignant melanoma. Use of levodopa is not associated with pulmonary dysfunction. The answer is **B.**

3. Carbidopa is an inhibitor of aromatic L-amino acid decarboxylase, the enzyme that converts levodopa to dopamine. Because it does not enter the CNS, the drug acts only on the enzyme present in peripheral tissues (eg, liver). The use of carbidopa in combination with levodopa decreases the dose requirement and reduces peripheral side effects of levodopa. The answer is **C.**

4. The use of dopaminergic agents in combination with antimuscarinic drugs is common in the treatment of parkinsonism. If combined with levodopa, bromocriptine should be used in reduced doses to avoid intolerable adverse effects. Confusion, delusions, and hallucinations occur more frequently with bromocriptine than with levodopa. The answer is **C.**

5. The signs and symptoms described are those of *erythromelalgia,* an adverse effect of bromocriptine. The distal extremities (feet and hands) are usually involved. Arthralgia may occur along with the signs described. The answer is **C.**

6. The form and severity of dyskinesias resulting from levodopa may vary widely in different patients. Dyskinesias occur in up to 80% of patients receiving levodopa for long periods. With continued treatment, dyskinesias may develop at a dose of levodopa that was previously well tolerated. They occur more commonly in patients treated with levodopa in combination with carbidopa or with other dopamine receptor agonists. Muscarinic receptor blockers do not prevent their occurrence. The answer is **B.**

7. Apomorphine, via subcutaneous injection, is used for temporary relief of off-periods of akinesia in patients on dopaminergic therapy. Pretreatment with an antiemetic is essential. The answer is **A.**

8. The mydriatic action of levodopa may increase intraocular pressure; the drug should be used cautiously in open-angle glaucoma and is contraindicated in angle-closure glaucoma. Antimuscarinic drugs may improve the tremor and rigidity of parkinsonism but have little effect on bradykinesia. As a selective inhibitor of MAO type B, selegiline does not exacerbate peripheral adverse effects of levodopa. The answer is **A.**

9. Although further diagnosis is desirable, choreoathetosis with decreased mental abilities and psychosis (paranoia) suggests that this patient has Huntington's disease. Drugs that are partly ameliorative include agents that deplete dopamine (eg, tetrabenazine) or that decrease dopaminergic activity, such as haloperidol. The answer is **C.**

10. Benztropine, a muscarinic receptor antagonist, may cause urinary retention and gastrointestinal effects and should be used with caution in patients with prostatic hypertrophy or obstructive gastrointestinal disease. It is contraindicated in those with angle-closure glaucoma. The answer is **A.**

11. Pramipexole is a nonergot agonist at dopamine receptors and may have greater selectivity for D_3 receptors in the striatum. Pramipexole (or the D_2 receptor antagonist ropinirole) are often chosen for monotherapy of mild parkinsonism, and they sometimes have value in patients who have become refractory to levodopa. Side effects of these drugs include dyskinesias, postural hypotension, and somnolence. The answer is **E.**

12. MPTP causes Parkinson-like extrapyramidal dysfunction by destroying dopaminergic neurons in the nigrostriatal tract. This neurotoxic action

SKILL KEEPER ANSWERS:
AUTONOMIC DRUG SIDE EFFECTS
(SEE CHAPTERS 8 AND 9)

Pharmacologic strategy in Parkinson's disease involves attempts to enhance dopamine functions or antagonize acetylcholine at muscarinic receptors. Thus, peripheral side effects must be anticipated.

1. *Side effects referable to activation of peripheral dopamine (or adrenoceptors in the case of levodopa) include postural hypotension, tachycardia (possible arrhythmias), mydriasis, and emetic responses.*

2. *Side effects referable to antagonism of peripheral muscarinic receptors include dry mouth, mydriasis, urinary retention, and cardiac arrhythmias.*

involves the formation of toxic metabolites from the metabolism of MPTP by monoamine oxidase type B. Toxicity is prevented by selegiline, a selective inhibitor of MAO type B. MPTP is used as an experimental tool in animal models of parkinsonism. The answer is **E**.

13. Entacapone is an inhibitor of COMT used adjunctively in patients treated with levodopa-carbidopa. The drug decreases the formation of 3OMD from levodopa. This improves patient response to levodopa by increasing levodopa levels and by decreasing competition between 3OMD and levodopa for active transport into the brain by L-amino acid carrier mechanism. The answer is **B**.

14. Excessive activation of β adrenoceptors has been implicated in essential tremor, and management commonly involves administration of propranolol. However, the more selective β_1-blocker metoprolol is equally effective and is more suitable in a patient with pulmonary disease. The answer is **C**.

CHECKLIST

When you complete this chapter, you should be able to:

☐ Describe the neurochemical imbalance underlying the symptoms of Parkinson's disease.

☐ Identify the mechanisms by which levodopa, dopamine receptor agonists, selegiline, and muscarinic blocking drugs alleviate parkinsonism.

☐ Describe the therapeutic and toxic effects of the major antiparkinsonism agents.

☐ Identify the compounds that inhibit dopa decarboxylase and COMT and describe their use in parkinsonism.

☐ Identify the chemical agents and drugs that cause parkinsonism symptoms.

☐ Identify the most important drugs used in the management of tremor, Huntington's disease, drug-induced dyskinesias, restless legs syndrome, and Wilson's disease.

Antipsychotic Drugs & Lithium

The antipsychotic drugs (neuroleptics) are used in schizophrenia and are also effective in the treatment of other psychoses and agitated states. Although schizophrenia is not cured by drug therapy, the symptoms, including thought disorder, emotional withdrawal, and hallucinations or delusions, may be ameliorated by antipsychotic drugs. Unfortunately, protracted therapy (years) is often needed and can result in severe toxicity in some patients. In bipolar affective disorder, although lithium has been the mainstay of treatment for many years, the use of newer antipsychotic agents and of several antiseizure drugs is increasing.

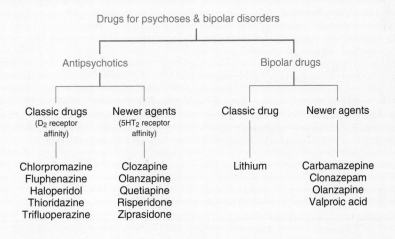

ANTIPSYCHOTIC DRUGS

A. CLASSIFICATION

The major chemical subgroups of older antipsychotic drugs are the **phenothiazines** (eg, chlorpromazine, thioridazine, fluphenazine), the **thioxanthenes** (eg, thiothixene), and the **butyrophenones** (eg, haloperidol).

Newer "second-generation" drugs of varied **heterocyclic** structure are also effective in schizophrenia, including clozapine, loxapine, olanzapine, risperidone, quetiapine, ziprasidone, and aripiprazole. In some cases, these atypical antipsychotic drugs may be somewhat more effective and less toxic than the older drugs.

However, they are much more costly than standard older drugs, most of which are prescribed generically.

B. PHARMACOKINETICS

The antipsychotic drugs are well absorbed when given orally and, because they are lipid soluble, readily enter the CNS and most other body tissues. Many are bound extensively to plasma proteins. These drugs require metabolism by liver enzymes before elimination and have long plasma half-lives that permit once-daily dosing. Parenteral forms of many agents (eg, fluphenazine, haloperidol) are available for both rapid initiation of therapy and depot treatment.

C. Mechanism of Action

1. The dopamine hypothesis—The dopamine hypothesis of schizophrenia proposes that the disorder is caused by a relative excess of functional activity of the neurotransmitter dopamine in specific neuronal tracts in the brain. This hypothesis is based on several observations. First, many antipsychotic drugs block brain dopamine receptors (especially D_2 receptors). Second, dopamine agonist drugs (eg, amphetamine, levodopa) exacerbate schizophrenia. Third, an increased density of dopamine receptors has been detected in certain brain regions of untreated schizophrenics. The dopamine hypothesis of schizophrenia is not fully satisfactory because antipsychotic drugs are only partly effective in most patients and because many effective drugs have a much higher affinity for other receptors than for D_2 receptors.

2. Dopamine receptors—Five different dopamine receptors (D_1–D_5) have been characterized. Each is G protein coupled and contains 7 transmembrane domains. The D_2 receptor, found in the caudate putamen, nucleus accumbens, cerebral cortex, and hypothalamus, is negatively coupled to adenylyl cyclase. The therapeutic efficacy of most of the older antipsychotic drugs correlates with their relative affinity for the D_2 receptor. Unfortunately, there is also a correlation between blockade of D_2 receptors and extrapyramidal dysfunction.

3. Other receptors—Most of the newer atypical antipsychotic agents have higher affinities for other receptors than for the D_2 receptor. For example, α adrenoceptor-blocking action correlates well with antipsychotic effect

for many of the drugs (Table 29–1). Clozapine, a drug with significant D_4 and 5-HT_2 receptor-blocking actions, has very low affinity for D_2 receptors. Most of the newer atypical drugs (eg, olanzapine, quetiapine, and risperidone) have high affinity for 5-HT_{2A} receptors, although they may also interact with D_2 and other receptors. Ziprasidone is an antagonist at the D_2, 5-HT_{2A}, and 5-HT_{1D} receptors and an agonist at the 5-HT_{1A} receptor. The newer antipsychotic agent aripiprazole is a partial agonist at D_2 and 5-HT_{1A} receptors but is a strong antagonist at 5-HT_{2A} receptors. Most of the atypical drugs cause less extrapyramidal dysfunction than standard drugs. With the exception of haloperidol, all antipsychotic drugs block H_1 receptors to some degree.

D. Effects

Dopamine receptor blockade is the major effect that correlates with therapeutic benefit for older antipsychotic drugs. Dopaminergic tracts in the brain include the mesocortical-mesolimbic pathways (regulating mentation and mood), nigrostriatal tract (extrapyramidal function), tuberoinfundibular pathways (control of prolactin release), and chemoreceptor trigger zone (emesis). Mesocortical-mesolimbic dopamine receptor blockade presumably underlies antipsychotic effects, and a similar action on the chemoreceptor trigger zone leads to the useful antiemetic properties of some antipsychotic drugs. Adverse effects resulting from receptor blockade in the other dopaminergic tracts, a major problem with older antipsychotic drugs, include extrapyramidal dysfunction and hyperprolactinemia (see later discussion).

Table 29–1. Relative receptor blocking actions of neuroleptic drugs.

Drug	D_2 Block	D_4 Block	Alpha$_1$ Block	5-HT_2 Block	M Block	H_1 Block
Most phenothiazines and thioxanthines	++	−	++	+	+	+
Thioridazine	++	−	++	+	+++	+
Haloperidol	+++	−	+	−	−	−
Clozapine	−	++	++	++	++	+
Molindone	++	−	+	−	+	+
Olanzapine	+	−	+	++	+	+
Quetiapine	+	−	+	++	+	+
Risperidone	++	−	+	++	+	+
Ziprasidone	++	−	++	++	−	+
Aripiprazole[a]	+	+	+	++	−	+

[a]Partial agonist at D_2 and 5-HT_{1A} receptors and antagonist activity at 5-HT_{2A} receptors.
+, blockade; −, no effect. The number of plus signs indicates the intensity of receptor blockade.

The relative receptor-blocking actions of different antipsychotic drugs are shown in Table 29–1.

E. CLINICAL USE

1. Treatment of schizophrenia—Antipsychotic drugs reduce some of the positive symptoms of schizophrenia, including hyperactivity, bizarre ideation, hallucinations, and delusions. Consequently, they can facilitate functioning in both inpatient and outpatient environments. Beneficial effects may take several weeks to develop. Overall efficacy of the antipsychotic drugs is, for the most part, equivalent in terms of the management of the floridly psychotic forms of the illness, although individual patients may respond best to a specific drug. However, clozapine is effective in some schizophrenic patients resistant to treatment with other antipsychotic drugs. Older drugs are still commonly used in part because of their low cost in comparison with newer agents. However, none of the traditional drugs have much effect on negative symptoms of schizophrenia. Newer atypical drugs are reported to improve some of the negative symptoms of schizophrenia, including emotional blunting, social withdrawal, and lack of motivation.

2. Other psychiatric and neurologic indications—The newer antipsychotic drugs are often used with lithium in the initial treatment of mania. Several second-generation drugs are approved for treatment of acute mania and 2 (olanzapine and aripiprazole) are approved for use in the maintenance treatment of bipolar disorder. The antipsychotic drugs are also used in the management of psychotic symptoms of schizoaffective disorders, in Gilles de la Tourette's syndrome, and for management of toxic psychoses caused by overdosage of certain CNS stimulants. Molindone is used mainly in Tourette's syndrome; it is rarely used in schizophrenia. The newer atypical antipsychotics have also been used to allay psychotic symptoms in patients with Alzheimer's disease and in parkinsonism.

3. Nonpsychiatric indications—With the exception of thioridazine, most phenothiazines have antiemetic actions; prochlorperazine is promoted solely for this indication. H_1 receptor blockade, most often present in short side-chain phenothiazines, provides the basis for their use as antipruritics and sedatives and contributes to their antiemetic effects.

F. TOXICITY

1. Reversible neurologic effects—Dose-dependent extrapyramidal effects include a Parkinson-like syndrome with bradykinesia, rigidity, and tremor. This toxicity may be reversed by a decrease in dose and may be antagonized by concomitant use of muscarinic blocking agents. Extrapyramidal toxicity occurs most frequently with haloperidol and the more potent piperazine side-chain phenothiazines (eg, fluphenazine, trifluoperazine).

Parkinsonism occurs infrequently with clozapine and is much less common with the newer drugs. Other reversible neurologic dysfunctions that occur more frequently with older agents include akathisia and dystonias; these usually respond to treatment with diphenhydramine or muscarinic blocking agents.

2. Tardive dyskinesias—This important toxicity includes choreoathetoid movements of the muscles of the lips and buccal cavity and may be irreversible. Tardive dyskinesias tend to develop after several years of antipsychotic drug therapy but have appeared as early as 6 mo. Antimuscarinic drugs that usually ameliorate other extrapyramidal effects generally *increase* the severity of tardive dyskinesia symptoms. There is no effective drug treatment for tardive dyskinesia. Switching to clozapine does not exacerbate the condition. Tardive dyskinesia may be attenuated *temporarily* by increasing neuroleptic dosage; this suggests that tardive dyskinesia may be caused by dopamine receptor sensitization.

3. Autonomic effects—Autonomic effects result from blockade of peripheral muscarinic receptors and α adrenoceptors and are more difficult to manage in elderly patients. Tolerance to some of the autonomic effects occurs with continued therapy. Thioridazine has the strongest autonomic effects and haloperidol the weakest. Clozapine and most of the atypical drugs have intermediate autonomic effects.

Regarding muscarinic receptor blockade, atropine-like effects (dry mouth, constipation, urinary retention, and visual problems) are often pronounced with the use of thioridazine and phenothiazines with aliphatic side chains (eg, chlorpromazine). These effects also occur with clozapine and most of the atypical drugs but not with ziprasidone or aripiprazole. Antimuscarinic CNS effects may include a toxic confusional state similar to that produced by atropine and the tricyclic antidepressants.

Regarding α receptor blockade, postural hypotension caused by α blockade is a common manifestation of many of the older drugs, especially phenothiazines. In the elderly, measures must be taken to avoid falls resulting from postural fainting. The atypical drugs also block α receptors and can cause orthostatic hypotension. Failure to ejaculate is common in men treated with the phenothiazines.

4. Endocrine and metabolic effects—Endocrine and metabolic effects include hyperprolactinemia, gynecomastia, the amenorrhea-galactorrhea syndrome, and infertility. Most of these side effects are predictable manifestations of dopamine D_2 receptor blockade in the pituitary; dopamine is the normal inhibitory regulator of prolactin secretion. Elevated prolactin is prominent with risperidone. Significant weight gain and hyperglycemia due to a diabetogenic action occur with several of the atypical agents, especially clozapine and olanzapine. These effects may be especially problematic in pregnancy.

Aripiprazole, like ziprasidone, has little or no tendency to cause hyperglycemia, hyperprolactinemia, or weight gain.

5. Neuroleptic malignant syndrome—Patients who are particularly sensitive to the extrapyramidal effects of antipsychotic drugs may develop a malignant hyperthermic syndrome. The symptoms include muscle rigidity, impairment of sweating, hyperpyrexia, and autonomic instability, which may be life threatening. Drug treatment involves the prompt use of dantrolene, diazepam, and dopamine agonists.

6. Sedation—This is more marked with phenothiazines (especially chlorpromazine) than with other antipsychotics; this effect is usually perceived as unpleasant by nonpsychotic individuals. Fluphenazine and haloperidol are the least sedating of the older drugs; aripiprazole appears to be the least sedating of the newer agents.

7. Miscellaneous toxicities—Visual impairment caused by retinal deposits has occurred with **thioridazine**; at high doses, this drug may also cause severe conduction defects in the heart resulting in fatal ventricular arrhythmias. Most of the atypicals, especially **ziprasidone,** prolong the QT interval of the ECG; the underlying myocardial effect may lead to cardiac arrhythmias (eg, torsades). **Clozapine** causes a small but important (1–2%) incidence of agranulocytosis and at high doses has caused seizures.

8. Overdosage toxicity—Poisoning with antipsychotics other than thioridazine is not usually fatal, although the FDA has warned of an increased risk of death in elderly patients with dementia. Hypotension often responds to fluid replacement. Most neuroleptics lower the convulsive threshold and may cause seizures, which are usually managed with diazepam or phenytoin. Thioridazine (and possibly ziprasidone) overdose, because of cardiotoxicity, is more difficult to treat.

LITHIUM & OTHER DRUGS USED IN BIPOLAR (MANIC-DEPRESSIVE) DISORDER

A. Pharmacokinetics

Lithium is absorbed rapidly and completely from the gut. The drug is distributed throughout the body water and cleared by the kidneys at a rate one fifth that of creatinine. The half-life of lithium is about 20 h. Plasma levels should be monitored, especially during the first weeks of therapy, to establish an effective and safe dosage regimen. For acute symptoms the target therapeutic plasma concentration is 0.8–1.2 mEq/L and for maintenance 0.4-0.7 mEq/L Plasma levels of the drug may be altered by changes in body water. Dehydration, or treatment with thiazides, nonsteroidal anti-inflammatory drugs (NSAIDs), angiotensin-converting enzyme inhibitors (ACEIs), and loop diuretics, may result in an increase of lithium in the blood to toxic levels. Caffeine and theophylline increase the renal clearance of lithium.

B. Mechanism of Action

The mechanism of action of lithium is not well defined. The drug inhibits inositol monophosphatase, the rate-limiting enzyme in the recycling of neuronal membrane phosphoinositides involved in the generation of inositol trisphosphate (IP_3) and diacylglycerol (DAG). These second messengers are important in amine neurotransmission, including that mediated by central adrenoceptors and muscarinic receptors (Figure 29–1).Lithium may also act by other mechanisms.

C. Clinical Use

Lithium carbonate continues to be the standard treatment of bipolar disorder (manic-depressive disease), though in acute mania both valproic acid and olanzapine are equally effective. Maintenance therapy with lithium decreases manic behavior and reduces both the frequency and the magnitude of mood swings. Antipsychotics and/or benzodiazepines are commonly required at the initiation of treatment because both lithium and valproic acid have a slow onset of action. Aripiprazole and olanzapine, as well as the anticonvulsants carbamazepine and lamotrigine, are approved for maintenance treatment. Although lithium has protective effects against suicide and self-harm, antidepressant drugs are often used concurrently during maintenance. Note that monotherapy with antidepressants can precipitate mania in bipolar patients.

SKILL KEEPER: RECEPTOR MECHANISMS (SEE CHAPTERS 2, 6, AND 21)

Antipsychotic drugs to varying degrees act as antagonists at several receptor types, including those for acetylcholine, dopamine, norepinephrine, and serotonin. What are the second messenger systems for each of the following receptor subtypes that are blocked by antipsychotic drugs?

1. *D_2*
2. *M_3*
3. *Alpha$_1$*
4. *5-HT$_{2A}$*

The Skill Keeper Answers appear at the end of the chapter.

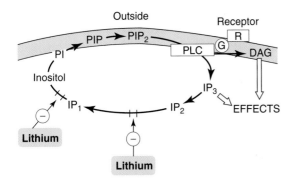

Figure 29–1. Postulated effect of lithium on the inositol trisphosphate (IP$_3$) and diacylglycerol (DAG) second messenger system. The schematic diagram shows the synaptic membrane of a neuron in the brain. PLC, phospholipase C; G, coupling protein; R, receptor; PI, PIP, PIP$_2$, IP$_2$, IP$_1$, intermediates in the production of IP$_3$. By interfering with this cycle, lithium may cause a use-dependent reduction of synaptic transmission. (Modified and reproduced, with permission, from Katzung BG, editor: *Basic & Clinical Pharmacology,* 10th ed. McGraw-Hill, 2007.)

D. TOXICITY

Adverse neurologic effects of lithium include tremor, sedation, ataxia, and aphasia. Thyroid enlargement may occur, but hypothyroidism is rare. Reversible nephrogenic diabetes insipidus occurs commonly at therapeutic drug levels. Edema is a frequent adverse effect of lithium therapy; acneiform skin eruptions occur; and leukocyto-

sis is always present. The issue of dysmorphogenesis is not settled. The use of lithium during pregnancy is thought to increase the incidence of congenital cardiac anomalies (Ebstein's anomaly). Recent analyses suggest that lithium's teratogenic risk is low, but its use during pregnancy appears to contribute to low Apgar scores in the neonate. Consequently, lithium should be withheld 24–48 h before delivery, and its use is contraindicated in nursing mothers.

QUESTIONS

1. Concerning hypotheses for the pathophysiologic basis of schizophrenia, which statement is accurate?
   - (A) All effective antipsychotic drugs have high affinity for dopamine D$_2$ receptors
   - (B) Drugs that block dopamine receptors are used to alleviate psychotic symptoms in parkinsonism
   - (C) Dopamine receptors are decreased in the brains of untreated schizophrenics
   - (D) Drug-induced psychosis can occur without activation of brain dopamine receptors
   - (E) The clinical potency of "second-generation" antipsychotic drugs correlates well with their β adrenoceptor-blocking actions

2. Fluphenazine was prescribed for a young male patient. His schizophrenic symptoms have improved enough for him to register complaints about the side effects of his medication. Which of the following is NOT likely to be on his list?
   - (A) Constipation
   - (B) Disinterest in sex
   - (C) Dizziness if he stands up too quickly

KEY DRUGS		
Subclass	**Prototypes**	**Other Significant Agents**
Phenothiazines Aliphatic Piperidine Piperazine	 Chlorpromazine Thioridazine Trifluoperazine	 Mesoridazine Fluphenazine
Thioxanthines	Thiothixene	
Butyrophenones	Haloperidol	
Heterocyclics ("second generation")	Clozapine	Aripiprazole, olanzapine, quetiapine, risperidone ziprasidone
Drugs for bipolar disorder	Lithium	Aripiprazole, carbamazepine, clonazepam, lamotrigine, olanzapine, valproic acid

(D) Excessive salivation

(E) Small print in the newspaper is hard to see

3. Which statement concerning the adverse effects of antipsychotic drugs is accurate?
   (A) Acute dystonic reactions occur very infrequently with olanzapine
   (B) Blurring of vision and urinary retention are common side effects of haloperidol
   (C) Retinal pigmentation is a dose-dependent toxic effect of clozapine
   (D) The late-occurring choreoathetoid movements caused by conventional antipsychotic drugs are reduced by antimuscarinic agents
   (E) Uncontrollable restlessness in a patient taking antipsychotic medications is alleviated by increasing the drug dose

4. Haloperidol would NOT be an appropriate drug for management of
   (A) Acute mania
   (B) The amenorrhea-galactorrhea syndrome
   (C) Phencyclidine intoxication
   (D) Schizoaffective disorders
   (E) Tourette's syndrome

5. A schizophrenic patient developed bradykinesia, rigidity, and tremor during treatment with haloperidol. His drug therapy was changed to clozapine, which was just as effective in reducing his psychiatric symptoms. However, clozapine did not cause extrapyramidal dysfunction in this patient. The most likely explanation is that clozapine
   (A) Activates GABAergic neurons in the striatum
   (B) Acts presynaptically to block dopamine release
   (C) Has greater blocking actions on brain muscarinic receptors
   (D) Has a low affinity for D_2 receptors
   (E) Is an effective antagonist at α adrenoceptors

6. Which statement concerning the use of lithium in the treatment of bipolar affective disorder is accurate?
   (A) Excessive intake of sodium chloride enhances the toxicity of lithium
   (B) Lithium alleviates the manic phase of bipolar disorder within 24 h
   (C) Lithium does not cross the placental barrier
   (D) Lithium dosage may need to be decreased in patients taking thiazides
   (E) The elimination rate of lithium is equivalent to that of creatinine

7. A 30-year-old male patient is on drug therapy for a psychiatric problem. He complains that he feels "flat" and that he gets confused at times. He has been gaining weight and has lost his sex drive. As he moves his hands, you notice a slight tremor. He tells you that since he has been on medication he is always thirsty and frequently has to urinate. The drug he is most likely to be taking is
   (A) Clozapine
   (B) Haloperidol
   (C) Lithium
   (D) Risperidone
   (E) Trifluoperazine

8. A young male patient recently diagnosed as schizophrenic develops severe muscle cramps with torticollis a short time after drug therapy is initiated with haloperidol. The best course of action would be to
   (A) Add clozapine to the drug regimen
   (B) Discontinue haloperidol and observe the patient
   (C) Give oral diphenhydramine
   (D) Switch the patient to fluphenazine
   (E) Inject benztropine

9. The effective treatment of a bipolar patient has necessitated doses of lithium that result in plasma levels of 1.4 to 1.6 mEq/L. Lately he has begun to suffer from increased motor activity, aphasia, mental confusion, and social withdrawal. The best course of action would be to
   (A) Add amitriptyline to the drug regimen
   (B) Continue lithium and add haloperidol
   (C) Discontinue lithium and start valproic acid
   (D) Discontinue lithium and start clozapine
   (E) Increase the dose of lithium

10. Which of the following drugs is established to be both effective and safe to use in a pregnant patient suffering from bipolar disorder?
    (A) Carbamazepine
    (B) Chlorpromazine
    (C) Lithium
    (D) Olanzapine
    (E) Valproic acid

11. A young patient who has been treated with an antipsychotic drug for a few weeks becomes easily fatigued and experiences periodic fevers. Petechiae are apparent on physical examination, and laboratory studies reveal leukopenia and thrombocytopenia. If a diagnosis is made that the patient is suffering from drug-induced agranulocytosis, he is most likely being treated with
    (A) Chlorpromazine
    (B) Clozapine
    (C) Haloperidol
    (D) Olanzapine
    (E) Risperidone

12. In comparing the characteristics of thioridazine with other older antipsychotic drugs, which of the following statements is accurate?

(A) Most likely to cause extrapyramidal dysfunction
(B) Least likely to cause urinary retention
(C) Most likely to be safe in patients with history of cardiac arrhythmias
(D) Least likely to cause dry mouth
(E) Most likely to cause ocular dysfunction

13. Within days of starting haloperidol treatment for a psychiatric disorder, a young male patient developed severe generalized muscle rigidity and a high temperature. In the emergency department he was incoherent, with increased heart rate, hypotension, and diaphoresis. Laboratory studies indicated acidosis, leukocytosis, and increased creatine kinase. The most likely reason for these symptoms is that the patient was suffering from
(A) Agranulocytosis
(B) A severe bacterial infection
(C) Neuroleptic malignant syndrome
(D) Spastic retrocollis
(E) Tardive dyskinesia

14. Which of the following drugs has a high affinity for 5-HT$_2$ receptors in the brain, does not cause extrapyramidal dysfunction or hematotoxicity, and is reported to increase the risk of significant QT prolongation?
(A) Chlorpromazine
(B) Clozapine
(C) Fluphenazine
(D) Olanzapine
(E) Ziprasidone

ANSWERS

1. Some investigations of the brain of untreated schizophrenics have revealed small *increases* in dopamine receptors. Although most older antipsychotic drugs block D$_2$ receptors, this action is not an absolute requirement for antipsychotic action because clozapine (and several other "second-generation" drugs) has a very low affinity for such receptors. Antipsychotic drugs have no significant actions on beta adrenoceptors. The CNS effects of phencyclidine (PCP) closely parallel an acute schizophrenic episode, but PCP has no actions on brain dopamine receptors. The answer is **D**.

2. Phenothiazines like fluphenazine cause sedation and are antagonists at muscarinic and α adrenoceptors. Postural hypotension, blurring of vision, and constipation are common autonomic side effects, as is dry mouth (not excessive salivation). Effects on the male libido may result from increased prolactin or from increased peripheral conversion of androgens to estrogens. The answer is **D**.

3. Muscarinic blockers exacerbate tardive dyskinesias. Akathisias (uncontrollable restlessness) resulting from antipsychotic drugs may be relieved by a *reduction* in dosage. Retinal pigmentation may occur with thioridazine, not clozapine. Olanzapine has minimal dopamine receptor blocking action and is unlikely to cause acute dystonias. The answer is **A**.

4. Hyperprolactinemia and the amenorrhea-galactorrhea syndrome may occur as an *adverse effect* during treatment with antipsychotic drugs, especially those like haloperidol that strongly antagonize dopamine receptors in the tuberoinfundibular tract. The answer is **B**.

5. Clozapine does have greater muscarinic and α receptor blocking actions than haloperidol, but these are not the primary reasons why the drug is less likely to cause extrapyramidal dysfunction. The main reason is that clozapine has very low affinity for the dopamine D$_2$ receptors in the striatum. The answer is **D**.

6. Clinical effects of lithium are slow in onset and may not be apparent before 1 or 2 weeks of daily treatment. High urinary levels of sodium inhibit renal tubular reabsorption of lithium, thus *decreasing* its plasma levels. Lithium clearance is decreased by distal tubule diuretics (eg, thiazides) because natriuresis stimulates a reflex increase in the proximal tubule reabsorption of both lithium and sodium. Any drug that can cross the blood-brain barrier can cross the placental barrier! The answer is **D**.

7. Confusion, mood changes, decreased sexual interest, and weight gain are symptoms that may be unrelated to drug administration. On the other hand, psychiatric drugs are often responsible for such symptoms. Tremor and symptoms of nephrogenic diabetes insipidus are characteristic adverse effects of lithium that may occur at blood levels within the therapeutic range. The answer is **C**.

8. Acute dystonic reactions are usually very painful and should be treated immediately with parenteral administration of a drug that blocks muscarinic receptors. Adding clozapine will not be protective, and fluphenazine is as likely as haloperidol to cause acute dystonia. Oral administration of diphenhydramine is a possibility, but the patient may find it difficult to swallow and it would take a longer time to act. The answer is **E**.

9. The symptoms described in this patient are toxic effects of lithium. Increasing the dose of lithium will increase blood levels and exacerbate these symptoms. Adding amitriptyline or haloperidol to the regimen would not alleviate the problem. A trial of an alternative drug (eg, olanzapine, carbamazepine, clonazepam, or valproic acid) is appropriate. Unlike

olanzapine, clozapine as a single agent has minimal efficacy in bipolar disorder. The answer is **C.**

10. Carbamazepine and valproic acid are effective in bipolar disorder but are contraindicated in the pregnant patient because of possible effects on fetal development. Although the potential for dysmorphogenesis due to lithium is probably low, the most conservative approach would be to treat the patient with olanzapine. Chlorpromazine has no proven efficacy in bipolar disorder. The answer is **D.**

11. Agranulocytosis occurs in a small percentage of patients taking clozapine. This potentially fatal abnormality can develop rapidly, usually between the sixth and the 18th week of therapy. Hematotoxicity is reversible if clozapine is discontinued immediately after a significant decrease in white blood cell count. The answer is **B.**

12. Atropine-like side effects are more prominent with thioridazine than with other phenothiazines, but the drug is less likely to cause extrapyramidal dysfunction. At high doses, thioridazine causes retinal deposits, which in advanced cases resemble retinitis pigmentosa. The patient may complain of browning of vision. The drug has quinidine-like actions on the heart and, in overdose, may cause arrhythmias and cardiac conduction block. The answer is **E.**

13. The neuroleptic malignant syndrome appears to result from a too-rapid block of dopamine receptors in patients who are highly sensitive to the extrapyramidal effects of antipsychotic drugs. Management involves fever control, use of muscle relaxants (eg, dantrolene or diazepam), and possibly administration of the dopamine receptor agonist bromocriptine. Like most drugs that increase brain dopaminergic activity, bromocriptine may exacerbate psychotic symptoms. The answer is **C.**

14. Many of the newer antipsychotic drugs have a greater affinity for 5-HT$_2$ receptors than dopamine receptors. However, because clozapine is hematotoxic, the choice comes down to olanzapine and ziprasidone, both of which block 5-HT receptors. Of the currently available atypical antipsychotic drugs, ziprasidone carries the greatest risk of QT prolongation. The answer is **E.**

SKILL KEEPER ANSWERS: RECEPTOR MECHANISMS (SEE CHAPTERS 2, 6, AND 21)

1. D_2: G_i linked, ↓cAMP
2. M3: G_q linked, ↑IP$_3$ and DAG
3. Alpha$_1$: G_q linked, ↑IP$_3$ and DAG
4. 5-HT$_{2A}$: G_q linked, ↑IP$_3$ and DAG

CHECKLIST

When you complete this chapter, you should be able to:

☐ Describe the "dopamine hypothesis" of schizophrenia.

☐ Identify 4 receptors blocked by antipsychotic drugs.

☐ Describe the relationship of receptor-blocking actions to the pharmacodynamics of both the older and the newer (atypical) antipsychotics.

☐ Identify the established toxicities of each of the following drugs: chlorpromazine, clozapine, haloperidol, thioridazine, ziprasidone.

☐ Describe tardive dyskinesia and the neuroleptic malignant syndrome.

☐ Identify the distinctive pharmacokinetic features of lithium and list its side effects and toxicities.

☐ List the "alternative" drugs used in bipolar disorder.

Antidepressants

Major depressive disorder, or endogenous depression, is a depression of mood without any obvious medical or situational causes, manifested by an inability to cope with ordinary events or experience pleasure. The drugs used in major depressive disorder are of varied chemical structures; many have effects that enhance the CNS actions of norepinephrine, serotonin, or both.

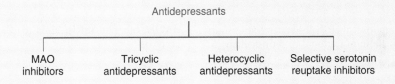

THE AMINE HYPOTHESIS OF MOOD

The **amine hypothesis of mood** postulates that brain amines, particularly norepinephrine (NE) and serotonin (5-HT), are neurotransmitters in pathways that function in the expression of mood. According to the hypothesis, a functional decrease in the activity of such amines is thought to result in depression; a functional increase of activity results in mood elevation. The amine hypothesis is largely based on studies showing that many drugs capable of alleviating symptoms of major depressive disorders enhance the actions of the CNS neurotransmitters 5-HT and NE. Difficulties with this hypothesis include the facts that (1) postmortem studies do not reveal any decreases in the brain levels of NE or 5-HT in patients suffering from depression; (2) although antidepressant drugs may cause changes in brain amine activity within hours, weeks may be required for them to achieve clinical effects; (3) most antidepressants ultimately cause a *down*-regulation of amine receptors; and (4) at least 1 effective antidepressant, bupropion, has minimal effects on brain NE or 5-HT.

DRUG CLASSIFICATION & PHARMACOKINETICS

A. Tricyclic Antidepressants

Tricyclic antidepressants (TCAs; eg, **imipramine, amitriptyline**) are structurally related to the phenothiazine antipsychotics and share certain of their pharmacologic effects. The TCAs are well absorbed orally but may undergo first-pass metabolism. They have high volumes of distribution and are not readily dialyzable. Extensive hepatic metabolism is required before their elimination; plasma half-lives of 8–36 h usually permit once-daily dosing. Both amitriptyline and imipramine form active metabolites, nortriptyline and desipramine, respectively.

B. Heterocyclics

These drugs have varied structures and include second-generation antidepressants (eg, **amoxapine, bupropion, maprotiline, trazodone**) and newer, third-generation drugs (**duloxetine, mirtazapine, nefazodone, venlafaxine**). The pharmacokinetics of most of these agents are similar to those of the TCAs. Nefazodone and

---

HIGH-YIELD TERMS TO LEARN	
Amine hypothesis of mood	The hypothesis that major depressive disorders result from a functional deficiency of norepinephrine or serotonin at synapses in the CNS
Tricyclics	A group of structurally related drugs resembling phenothiazines chemically; block reuptake of both norepinephrine and serotonin
MAO inhibitors	Drugs that inhibit monoamine oxidase type A, which metabolizes norepinephrine and serotonin, or monoamine oxidase B, which metabolizes dopamine
Selective serotonin reuptake inhibitors	A group of drugs that selectively inhibit the serotonin transporters of the nerve-ending membrane
Heterocyclics (second- and third-generation antidepressants)	Drugs of varied chemical structures; several have actions different from those of tricyclic antidepressants or selective serotonin reuptake inhibitors

---

trazodone are exceptions; their half-lives are quite short and usually require administration 2 or 3 times daily.

C. Selective Serotonin Reuptake Inhibitors

Fluoxetine is the prototype of a group of drugs that are selective serotonin reuptake inhibitors (SSRIs). All of them require hepatic metabolism and have half-lives of 18–24 h. However, fluoxetine forms an active metabolite with a half-life of several days (the basis for a once-weekly formulation). Other members of this group (eg, **citalopram, escitalopram, fluvoxamine, paroxetine, sertraline**) do not form long-acting metabolites.

D. Monoamine Oxidase Inhibitors

Monoamine oxidase inhibitors (MAOIs; eg, **phenelzine, tranylcypromine**) are structurally related to amphetamines and are orally active. The older, standard drugs inhibit both MAO-A, which metabolizes NE, 5-HT, and tyramine, and MAO-B, which metabolizes dopamine. Tranylcypromine is the fastest in onset of effect but has a shorter duration of action (about 1 week) than other MAOIs (2–3 weeks). In spite of these prolonged actions, the MAOIs are given daily. They are inhibitors of hepatic drug-metabolizing enzymes and cause drug interactions. Selegiline, a selective inhibitor of MAO type B, was recently approved for treatment of depression.

MECHANISMS OF ANTIDEPRESSANT ACTION

Potential sites of action of antidepressants at CNS synapses are shown in Figure 30–1. By means of several mechanisms, most antidepressants cause potentiation of the neurotransmitter actions of NE, 5-HT, or both. The only exception is bupropion, which has an unknown mechanism of action. Long-term use of tricyclics and

MAOIs, but not SSRIs, leads to *down-regulation* of β receptors.

A. TCAs

The acute effect of tricyclic drugs is to inhibit the reuptake mechanisms (transporters) responsible for the termination of the synaptic actions of both NE and 5-HT in the brain. This presumably results in potentiation of their neurotransmitter actions at postsynaptic receptors.

B. Heterocyclic Antidepressants

The acute actions of heterocyclics are varied. Some second-generation drugs inhibit the reuptake of NE (eg, amoxapine, maprotiline); some have more action on 5-HT reuptake (eg, trazodone; Table 30–1). The third-generation drugs duloxetine and venlafaxine are potent inhibitors of both 5-HT and NE transporters. Mirtazapine has a unique action to increase amine release from nerve endings by antagonism of presynaptic α_2 adrenoceptors involved in feedback inhibition. Antagonism of 5-HT_{2A} and 5-HT_{2c} receptors has been implicated in the antidepressant actions of nefazodone, and possibly both mirtazapine and trazodone. The mechanism of antidepressant action of bupropion is unknown—the drug has no effects on either 5-HT or NE receptors, or on amine transporters.

C. SSRIs

The acute effect of the SSRIs is a highly selective action on the 5-HT transporters.

D. MAOIs

The MAOIs increase brain amine levels by interfering with their metabolism in the nerve endings, resulting in an increase in the vesicular stores of NE and 5-HT. When neuronal activity discharges the vesicles,

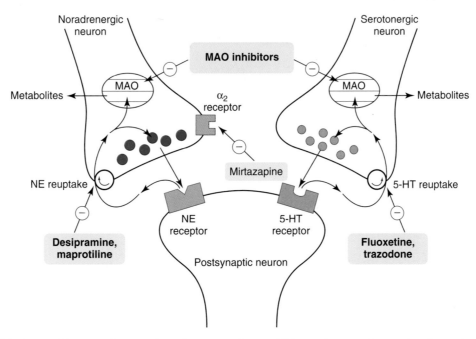

Figure 30–1. Possible sites of action of antidepressant drugs. Inhibition of neuronal reuptake of norepinephrine (NE) and serotonin (5-HT) increases the synaptic activities of these neurotransmitters. Inhibition of monoamine oxidase increases the presynaptic stores of both NE and 5-HT, which leads to increased neurotransmitter effects. Blockade of the presynaptic α_2 autoreceptor prevents feedback inhibition of the release of NE. ***Note:*** These are acute actions of antidepressants.

increased amounts of the amines are released, presumably enhancing the actions of these neurotransmitters.

PHARMACOLOGIC EFFECTS

A. AMINE UPTAKE BLOCKADE

The drugs that block NE transporters in the CNS (eg, tricyclics, maprotiline, venlafaxine) also inhibit the reuptake of NE at nerve endings in the autonomic nervous system. Likewise, MAOIs increase NE in sympathetic nerve terminals. In both cases, this can lead to peripheral autonomic sympathomimetic effects. However, long-term use of MAOIs can decrease blood pressure.

B. SEDATION

Sedation is a common CNS effect of tricyclic drugs and some heterocyclic agents, especially mirtazapine and trazodone (Table 30–1), the latter drug commonly prescribed for this purpose and as a sleeping aid. MAOIs, SSRIs, and bupropion are more likely to cause CNS-stimulating effects.

C. MUSCARINIC RECEPTOR BLOCKADE

Antagonism of muscarinic receptors occurs with all tricyclics and is particularly marked with amitriptyline and

doxepin (see Table 30–1). The newer agents appear to be less potent antimuscarinics with the notable exception of nefazodone, and to a lesser extent amoxapine and maprotiline. Atropine-like effects are minimal with the other heterocyclics, the SSRIs, and bupropion.

D. CARDIOVASCULAR EFFECTS

Cardiovascular effects occur most commonly with tricyclics and include hypotension from α adrenoceptor blockade and depression of cardiac conduction. The latter effect may lead to arrhythmias.

E. SEIZURES

Because the convulsive threshold is lowered by TCAs and MAOIs, seizures may occur with overdoses of these agents. Overdoses of maprotiline and the SSRIs have also caused seizures.

CLINICAL USES

A. MAJOR DEPRESSIVE DISORDERS

Major depression is the primary clinical indication for the antidepressant drugs. Patients typically vary in their responsiveness to individual agents. Because of more tolerable side effects and safety in overdose (see later

Table 30–1. Pharmacodynamic characteristics of antidepressants.[a]

Drug	Sedation	Muscarinic Receptor Block	NE Reuptake Block	5-HT Reuptake Block
Tricyclics				
Amitriptyline, doxepin	+++	+++	++	+++
Desipramine	+	++	+++	0
Imipramine	++	++	++	+++
Nortriptyline	++	++	++	+++
Heterocyclics (second generation)				
Amoxapine	++	++	++	+
Bupropion	0	0	0	0
Maprotiline	++	++	+++	0
Trazodone	+++	0	0	+
Heterocyclics (third generation)				
Duloxetine	0	0	++	+++
Mirtazapine[b]	+++	0	0	0
Nefazodone	++	+++	0	+
Venlafaxine	0	0	++	+++
SSRIs				
(eg, fluoxetine)	0	0	0	+++

[a]0 = none; + = slight; ++ = moderate; +++ = marked.
[b]Significant α_2 adrenoceptor antagonism.

discussion), the newer drugs (SSRIs, certain heterocyclics) are now the most widely prescribed agents. However, none of the newer antidepressants have been shown to be more effective overall than tricyclic drugs. As alternative agents, tricyclic drugs continue to be most useful in patients with psychomotor retardation, sleep disturbances, poor appetite, and weight loss. MAOIs are thought to be most useful in patients with significant anxiety, phobic features, and hypochondriasis. Selegiline, the MAO type B inhibitor used in parkinsonism (see Chapter 28), is now available in a skin-patch formulation for treatment of depression. SSRIs may decrease appetite; overweight patients often lose weight on these drugs, at least during the first 6–12 mo of treatment. Concerns have been expressed that SSRIs and newer heterocyclics may increase suicide risk in children and adolescents. However, most consultants believe that these drugs are more likely to prevent suicide than to cause it.

B. OTHER CLINICAL USES

TCAs are also used in the treatment of bipolar affective disorders, acute panic attacks, phobic disorders (compare with alprazolam; Chapter 22), enuresis, attention deficit hyperkinetic disorder, and chronic pain states. High doses of venlafaxine show efficacy in neuropathic pain. Duloxetine is also approved for pain of diabetic neuropathy. Clomipramine and the SSRIs are effective in obsessive–compulsive disorders. SSRIs are also approved for use in patients who suffer from generalized anxiety disorders, panic attacks, social phobias, bulimia, and premenstrual dysphoric disorder and may also be useful in the treatment of alcohol dependence. Bupropion is used for management of patients attempting to withdraw from nicotine dependence.

TOXICITY & DRUG INTERACTIONS

A. TCAs

The adverse effects of TCAs are largely predictable from their pharmacodynamic actions. These include (1) excessive sedation, lassitude, fatigue, and, occasionally, confusion; (2) sympathomimetic effects, including tachycardia, agitation, sweating, and insomnia; (3) atropine-like effects; (4) orthostatic hypotension, ECG abnormalities, and cardiomyopathies; (5) tremor and paresthesias; and (6) weight gain. Overdosage with tricyclics is extremely

Table 30–2. Drug interactions observed with antidepressant medications.

Antidepressant	Taken With	Consequence
Fluoxetine	Lithium, tricyclics, warfarin	Increased blood levels of the second drug; doses may need to be decreased
Fluvoxamine	Alprazolam, theophylline, tricyclics, warfarin	Increased blood levels of the second drug; doses may need to be decreased
MAO inhibitors	Sympathomimetics, tyramine, SSRIs	Hypertensive crisis, "serotonin syndrome"
Nefazodone	Alprazolam, triazolam	Increased blood levels of the second drug; doses may need to be decreased
Paroxetine	Procyclidine, theophylline, tricyclics, warfarin	Increased blood levels of the second drug; doses may need to be decreased
Sertraline	Tricyclics, warfarin	Increased effects; doses may need to be decreased
Tricyclics	CNS depressants (eg, ethanol, sedative-hypnotics)	Additive CNS depression[a]
	Clonidine, guanethidine, methyldopa	Decreased antihypertensive effects

[a]Includes tricyclics and heterocyclics with sedative actions (eg, mirtazapine, nefazodone, and trazodone).

hazardous, and the ingestion of as little as a 2-week supply has been lethal. Manifestations include (1) agitation, delirium, neuromuscular irritability, convulsions, and coma; (2) respiratory depression and circulatory collapse; (3) hyperpyrexia; and (4) cardiac conduction defects and severe arrhythmias. The "3 Cs"—coma, convulsions, and cardiotoxicity—are characteristic. Tricyclic drug interactions (Table 30–2) include additive depression of the CNS with other central depressants, including ethanol, barbiturates, benzodiazepines, and opioids. Tricyclics may also cause reversal of the antihypertensive action of guanethidine by blocking its transport into sympathetic nerve endings. Less commonly, tricyclics may interfere with the antihypertensive actions of methylnorepinephrine (the active metabolite of methyldopa) and clonidine.

B. HETEROCYCLIC DRUG TOXICITY

Mirtazapine causes weight gain and is markedly sedating, as is trazodone. Amoxapine, maprotiline, mirtazapine, and trazodone cause some autonomic effects. Amoxapine is also a dopamine receptor blocker and may cause akathisia, parkinsonism, and the amenorrhea-galactorrhea syndrome. Adverse effects of bupropion include anxiety, agitation, dizziness, dry mouth, aggravation of psychosis, and, at high doses, seizures. Seizures and cardiotoxicity are prominent features of overdosage with amoxapine and maprotiline. Venlafaxine causes a dose-dependent increase in blood pressure and has CNS stimulant effects similar to those of the SSRIs. Severe withdrawal symptoms can occur, even after missing a single dose of venlafaxine.

Both nefazodone and venlafaxine are inhibitors of cytochrome P450 isozymes. Through this action, nefazodone inhibits the metabolism of alprazolam and triazolam, and venlafaxine inhibits the metabolism of haloperidol (see Table 30–2). Although it rarely happens, nefazodone has caused life-threatening hepatotoxicity requiring liver transplantation. Duloxetine is also reported to cause liver dysfunction.

C. SSRI TOXICITY

Fluoxetine and the other SSRIs may cause nausea, headache, anxiety, agitation, insomnia, and sexual dysfunction. Jitteriness can be alleviated by starting with low doses or by adjunctive use of benzodiazepines. Extrapyramidal effects early in treatment may include akathisia, dyskinesias, and dystonic reactions. Seizures are a consequence of gross overdosage. Cardiac effects of citalopram overdose include QT prolongation. A withdrawal syndrome has been described for SSRIs that includes nausea, dizziness, anxiety, tremor, and palpitations.

The SSRIs are inhibitors of hepatic cytochrome P450 isozymes, an action that has led to increased activity of other drugs, including TCAs and warfarin (see Table 30–2). Citalopram causes fewer drug interactions than other SSRIs.

A **serotonin syndrome** was first described for an interaction between fluoxetine and an MAOI (see later discussion). This life-threatening syndrome includes severe muscle rigidity, myoclonus, hyperthermia, cardiovascular instability, and marked CNS stimulatory effects, including seizures. Drugs implicated include MAOIs,

---

KEY DRUGS

Subclass	Prototypes	Other Significant Agents
Tricyclic drugs	Amitriptyline, imipramine	Clomipramine, desipramine, doxepin, nortriptyline
Heterocyclics (second generation)	Amoxapine, bupropion, maprotiline, trazodone	
Heterocyclics (third generation)	Duloxetine mirtazapine, nefazodone, venlafaxine	
Selective serotonin reuptake inhibitors	Fluoxetine	Citalopram, fluvoxamine, paroxetine, sertraline
MAO inhibitors	Phenelzine	Tranylcypromine, selegiline

TCAs, dextromethorphan, meperidine, St. John's wort, and possibly illicit recreational drugs such as MDMA ("ecstasy"). Antiseizure drugs, muscle relaxants, and blockers of 5-HT receptors (eg, cyproheptadine) have been used in the management of the syndrome.

D. MAOI TOXICITY

Adverse effects of the traditional MAOIs include hypertensive reactions in response to indirectly acting sympathomimetics, hyperthermia, and CNS stimulation leading to agitation and convulsions. Hypertensive crisis may occur in patients taking MAOIs who consume food that contains high concentrations of the indirect sympathomimetic tyramine. In the absence of indirect sympathomimetics, MAOIs typically *lower* blood pressure; overdosage with these drugs may result in shock, hyperthermia, and seizures. MAOIs administered together with SSRIs have resulted in the **serotonin syndrome.**

QUESTIONS

1. A 28-year-old woman presents with symptoms of major depression that are unrelated to a general medical condition, bereavement, or substance abuse. She is not currently taking any prescription or over-the-counter medications. Drug treatment is to be initiated with an SSRI. In your information to the patient, you would tell her that
   (A) Divided doses may help to reduce nausea and gastrointestinal distress
   (B) Muscle cramps and twitches sometimes occur
   (C) She should inform you if she anticipates using other prescription drugs

   (D) The drug may require 2 weeks or more to become effective
   (E) All of the above

2. Concerning the proposed mechanisms of action of antidepressant drugs, which statement is accurate?
   (A) Bupropion inhibits NE and 5-HT transporters
   (B) Chronic treatment with a TCA leads to the up-regulation of adrenoceptors
   (C) Elevation in amine metabolites in cerebrospinal fluid is characteristic of depressed patients before drug therapy
   (D) MAOIs selectively decrease the metabolism of NE
   (E) The acute effect of venlafaxine is to block the neuronal reuptake of both NE and 5-HT in the CNS

3. Which of the following effects is NOT likely to occur during treatment with imipramine?
   (A) Alpha adrenoceptor blockade
   (B) Elevation of the seizure threshold
   (C) Mydriasis
   (D) Sedation
   (E) Urinary retention

4. A 54-year-old male patient who was prescribed fluoxetine for depression has decided he wants to stop taking the drug. When questioned, he said that it affected his sexual performance and that "he wasn't getting any younger." You ascertain that he is also trying to overcome his dependency on tobacco products. If you decide to reinstitute drug therapy in this patient, the best choice would be
   (A) Bupropion
   (B) Citalopram

(C) Imipramine
(D) Sertraline
(E) Venlafaxine

5. Regarding the clinical use of antidepressant drugs, which statement is accurate?
   (A) Chronic use of antidepressants increases the activity of hepatic drug-metabolizing enzymes
   (B) In selecting an appropriate drug for treatment of depression, the history of patient response to specific drugs is a valuable guide
   (C) In the treatment of major depressive disorders, sertraline is usually more effective than fluoxetine
   (D) Tricyclics are highly effective in depressions with attendant anxiety, phobic features, and hypochondriasis
   (E) Weight gain often occurs during the first few months in patients taking SSRIs

6–7. A patient under treatment for a major depressive disorder is brought to the emergency department after ingesting 30 times the normal daily therapeutic dose of amitriptyline.

6. Of the following possible signs and symptoms in this patient, which is likely to be observed?
   (A) Coma and shock
   (B) Decreased body temperature
   (C) Increased bowel sounds
   (D) Hypertension
   (E) Pinpoint pupils

7. In severe TCA overdose, it would be of little value to
   (A) Administer lidocaine (to control cardiac arrhythmias)
   (B) Institute hemodialysis (to hasten drug elimination)
   (C) Administer bicarbonate and potassium chloride (to correct acidosis and hypokalemia)
   (D) Provide intravenous diazepam (to control seizures)
   (E) Maintain the rhythm of the heart by electrical pacing

8. This heterocyclic antidepressant has caused rare but life-threatening hepatotoxicity requiring liver transplantation. It has been withdrawn from the market in Canada and Europe.
   (A) Citalopram
   (B) Desipramine
   (C) Nefazodone
   (D) Selegiline
   (E) Tranylcypromine

9. A recently bereaved 80-year-old female patient was treated with a benzodiazepine for several weeks after the death of her husband, but she did not like the daytime sedation it caused even at low dose. Living independently, she has no major medical problems but appears rather infirm for her age and has poor eyesight. Because her depressive symptoms are not abating, you decide on a trial of an antidepressant medication. Which drug would be the most appropriate choice for this patient?
   (A) Amitriptyline
   (B) Mirtazapine
   (C) Paroxetine
   (D) Phenelzine
   (E) Trazodone

10. SSRIs are much less effective than tricyclic antidepressants in the management of
    (A) Bulimia
    (B) Chronic pain of neuropathic origin
    (C) Generalized anxiety disorder
    (D) Obsessive–compulsive disorder
    (E) Premenstrual dysphoric disorder

11. Which of the following drugs is most likely to be of value in obsessive–compulsive disorders?
    (A) Amitriptyline
    (B) Bupropion
    (C) Clomipramine
    (D) Desipramine
    (E) Venlafaxine

12. Compared with other antidepressant drugs, mirtazapine has the distinctive ability to act as an antagonist of
    (A) Alpha$_2$ adrenoceptors
    (B) Beta adrenoceptors
    (C) D$_2$ receptors
    (D) NE transporters
    (E) 5-HT transporters

13. Of the following drugs, which has established clinical uses that include attention deficit hyperkinetic disorder, enuresis, and chronic pain?
    (A) Bupropion
    (B) Fluvoxamine
    (C) Imipramine
    (D) Phenelzine
    (E) Selegiline

14. Which of the following drugs is most likely to increase plasma levels of alprazolam, theophylline, and warfarin?
    (A) Bupropion
    (B) Clomipramine
    (C) Fluvoxamine
    (D) Imipramine
    (E) Phenelzine

ANSWERS

1. All of the statements are appropriate regarding the initiation of treatment with SSRIs in a depressed patient. In addition, you should tell the patient that the SSRIs have CNS-stimulating effects. They may cause agitation, anxiety, "the jitters," and insomnia. The evening is not the best time to take such drugs. The answer is **E**.

2. The mechanism of action of bupropion is unknown, but the drug does not inhibit NE or 5-HT transporters. Levels of NE and 5-HT metabolites in the cerebrospinal fluid of depressed patients before drug treatment are not higher than normal. *Down-regulation* of adrenoceptors appears to be a common feature of chronic treatment of depression with tricyclic drugs. Older MAOIs used in depression are nonselective. The answer is **E**.

3. Tricyclics modify peripheral sympathetic effects in 2 ways: through blockade of NE reuptake at neuroeffector junctions and through α-adrenoceptor blockade. Sedation and atropine-like side effects are common with tricyclics. In contrast to sedative-hypnotics, tricyclics lower the threshold to seizures. The answer is **B**.

4. SSRIs and venlafaxine can cause sexual dysfunction with decreased libido, erectile dysfunction, and anorgasmia. TCAs may also decrease libido or prevent ejaculation. Of the heterocyclics, bupropion is the least likely to affect sexual performance. The drug is also purportedly useful in withdrawal from nicotine dependence, which could be helpful in this patient. The answer is **A**.

5. No antidepressant has been shown to increase hepatic drug metabolism. MAO inhibitors are most likely to be effective in depression with attendant anxiety, phobic features, and hypochondriasis. SSRIs are usually associated with weight loss, at least during the first 6 mo of treatment. There is no evidence that any SSRI is more effective than another or more effective overall than a tricyclic drug in antidepressant efficacy. However, an individual patient may respond more favorably to a specific drug. The answer is **B**.

6. Anticholinergic effects common in tricyclic drug overdosage include increased body temperature, decreased bowel sounds, tachycardia, and dilated pupils. Hypotension occurs frequently owing to marked blockade at α adrenoceptors. The answer is **A**.

7. TCA overdose is a medical emergency. The "3 Cs"— coma, convulsions, and cardiac problems—are the most common causes of death. Widening of the QRS complex on the ECG is a major diagnostic feature of cardiac toxicity. Arrhythmias resulting from cardiac toxicity require the use of drugs with the least effect on cardiac conductivity (eg, lidocaine). There is no evidence that hemodialysis (or hemoperfusion) increases the rate of elimination of TCAs. The answer is **B**.

8. The drugs listed include two MAO inhibitors, a TCA, a SSRI, and one heterocyclic drug—nefazodone. Hepatotoxicity is a very rare adverse effect of antidepressant drugs. However, in the case of nefazodone, life-threatening hepatic failure has occurred. The answer is **C**.

9. Older patients are more likely to be sensitive to antidepressant drugs that cause sedation, atropine-like side effects, or postural hypotension. Tricyclics and MAO inhibitors cause many autonomic side effects; mirtazapine and trazodone are highly sedating. Paroxetine (or another SSRI) is often the best choice in such patients because it is the least likely of the drugs listed to exert such actions. The answer is **C**.

10. SSRIs are not effective in chronic pain of neuropathic origin. All of the other uses are approved indications with clinical effectiveness equivalent or superior to that of tricyclic drugs. The answer is **B**.

11. Clomipramine, a tricyclic, is a more selective inhibitor of 5-HT reuptake than other drugs in its class. This activity appears to be important in the treatment of obsessive–compulsive disorder. The SSRIs have now become the drugs of choice for this disorder because they are safer in overdose than tricyclics. The answer is **C**.

12. Mirtazapine is an antagonist at presynaptic α_2 receptors, facilitating NE release by opposing feedback inhibition. The drug also blocks histamine H_1 receptors (it is very sedating), $5\text{-}HT_2$ receptors, and $5\text{-}HT_3$ receptors. It has minimal inhibitory activity on amine transporters. The answer is **A**.

13. Enuresis is an established indication for tricyclics, which are also used as back-up drugs to methylphenidate in attention deficit hyperkinetic disorder. Chronic pain states, which may be unresponsive to conventional analgesics, often respond to TCAs. The answer is **C**.

14. Fluvoxamine is an inhibitor of hepatic cytochrome P450 3A4, the major P450 isoform involved in drug metabolism. Dosages of alprazolam, theophylline, and warfarin may need to be reduced if any of these drugs are given concomitantly with fluvoxamine. The answer is **C**.

CHECKLIST

When you complete this chapter, you should be able to:

☐ Describe the probable mechanisms and the major properties of TCAs.

☐ List the toxic effects that occur during chronic therapy and with an acute overdose of TCAs.

☐ Identify the second- and third-generation heterocyclic antidepressants and their distinctive properties.

☐ Identify the SSRIs and list their major characteristics.

☐ Describe the therapeutic use and toxic effects of MAOIs.

☐ Identify the major drug interactions associated with antidepressant drugs.

Opioid Analgesics & Antagonists

31

The opioids include natural opiates and semisynthetic alkaloids derived from the opium poppy, pharmacologically similar synthetic surrogates, and endogenous peptides. On the basis of the nature of their interaction with opioid receptors, the drugs are classified as agonists, mixed agonist-antagonists, and antagonists.

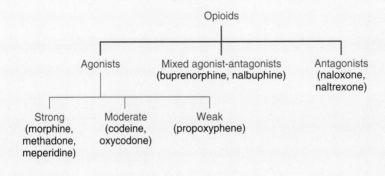

Opioid peptides released from nerve endings modulate transmission in the brain and spinal cord and in primary afferents via their interaction with specific receptors. Many of the pharmacologic actions of opiates and synthetic opioid drugs are effected via their interactions with endogenous opioid peptide receptors.

CLASSIFICATION

The opioid analgesics and related drugs are derived from several chemical subgroups and may be classified in several ways.

A. Spectrum of Clinical Uses

Opioid drugs can be subdivided on the basis of their major therapeutic uses (eg, analgesics, antitussives, and antidiarrheal drugs).

B. Strength of Analgesia

On the basis of their relative abilities to relieve pain, the analgesic opioids may be classified as strong, moderate,

and weak agonists. Partial agonists are opioids that exert less analgesia than morphine, the prototype of a strong analgesic, or full agonist.

C. Ratio of Agonist to Antagonist Effects

Opioid drugs may be classified as agonists (receptor activators [full or partial]), antagonists (receptor blockers), or mixed agonist-antagonists, which are capable of activating one opioid receptor subtype and blocking another subtype.

PHARMACOKINETICS

A. Absorption and Distribution

Most drugs in this class are well absorbed when taken orally, but morphine, hydromorphone, and oxymorphone undergo extensive first-pass metabolism. In most cases, opioids can be given parenterally, and sustained-release forms of some drugs are now available, including morphine and oxycodone. Opioid drugs are widely distributed to body tissues. They cross the placental barrier

---

HIGH-YIELD TERMS TO LEARN

Opiate	A drug derived from alkaloids of the opium poppy
Opioid	The class of drugs that includes opiates, opiopeptins, and all synthetic and semi-synthetic drugs that mimic the actions of the opiates
Opioid peptides	Endogenous peptides that act on opioid receptors
Opioid agonist	A drug that activates some or all opioid receptor subtypes and does not block any
Partial agonist	A drug that can activate an opioid receptor to effect a submaximal response
Opioid antagonist	A drug that blocks some or all opioid receptor subtypes
Mixed agonist-antagonist	A drug that activates some opioid receptor subtypes and blocks other opioid receptor subtypes

---

and exert effects on the fetus that can result in both respiratory depression and, with continuous exposure, physical dependence in neonates.

B. METABOLISM

With few exceptions, the opioids are metabolized by hepatic enzymes, usually to inactive glucuronide conjugates, before their elimination by the kidney. However, morphine-6-glucuronide has analgesic activity equivalent to that of morphine, and morphine-3-glucuronide (the primary metabolite) is neuroexcitatory. Codeine, oxycodone, and hydrocodone are metabolized by cytochrome CYP2D6, an isozyme exhibiting genotypic variability. In the case of codeine this may be responsible for variability in analgesic response because the drug is demethylated by CYP2D6 to form the active metabolite, morphine. The ingestion of alcohol causes major increases in the peak serum levels of several opioids, including hydromorphone and oxymorphone. Meperidine is metabolized to normeperidine, which may cause seizures at high plasma levels. Depending on the specific drug, the duration of their analgesic effects ranges from 1–2 h (eg, fentanyl) to 6–8 h (eg, buprenorphine). However, long-acting formulations of some drugs may provide analgesia for 24 h or more. The elimination half-life of opioids may increase in patients with liver disease. Remifentanil, a congener of fentanyl, is metabolized by plasma and tissue esterases and has a very short half-life.

MECHANISMS OF ACTION

A. RECEPTORS

Many of the effects of opioid analgesics have been interpreted in terms of their interactions with specific receptors for endogenous peptides in the CNS and peripheral tissues. Certain opioid receptors are located on primary afferents and spinal cord pain *transmission* neurons (ascending pathways) and on neurons in the midbrain and medulla (descending pathways) that function in pain *modulation* (Figure 31–1). Other opioid receptors that may be involved in altering *reactivity* to pain are located on neurons in the basal ganglia, the hypothalamus, the limbic structures, and the cerebral cortex. Three major opioid receptor subtypes have been extensively characterized pharmacologically: μ, δ, and κ receptors. All 3 receptor subtypes appear to be involved in antinociceptive and analgesic mechanisms. The μ-receptor activation plays a major role in the respiratory depressant actions of opioids; κ-receptor activation appears to be involved in sedative actions; δ-receptor activation may play a role in the development of tolerance.

B. OPIOID PEPTIDES

Opioid receptors are thought to be activated by endogenous peptides under physiologic conditions. These peptides (eg, enkephalins, dynorphin, beta-endorphin) are synthesized in the soma and transported to the nerve endings where they accumulate in synaptic vesicles. On release from nerve endings, they bind to opioid receptors and can be displaced from binding by opioid antagonists. Although it remains unclear whether these peptides function as classic neurotransmitters, they appear to modulate transmission at many sites in the brain and spinal cord and in primary afferents. Opioid peptides are also found in the adrenal medulla and neural plexus of the gut.

C. IONIC MECHANISMS

Opioid analgesics *inhibit* synaptic activity partly through direct activation of opioid receptors and partly through release of the endogenous opioid peptides, which are themselves inhibitory to neurons. All 3 major opioid receptors are coupled to their effectors by G proteins and

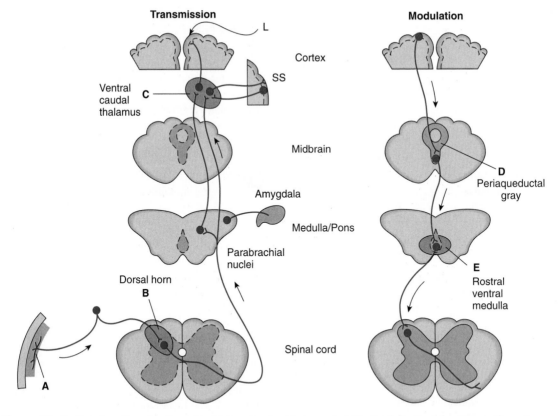

Figure 31–1. Putative sites of action of opioid analgesics (darker color). On the left, sites of action on the pain transmission pathway from the periphery to the higher centers are shown. **A:** Direct action of opioids on inflamed or damaged peripheral tissues. **B:** Inhibition also occurs in the spinal cord. **C:** Possible sites of action in the thalamus. Different thalamic regions project to somatosensory (SS) or limbic (L) cortex. Parabrachial nuclei (medulla/pons) project to the amygdala. On the right, actions of opioids on pain-modulating neurons in the midbrain (**D**), rostral central medulla (**E**), and the locus caeruleus indirectly control pain transmission pathways by enhancing descending inhibition to the dorsal horn. (Reproduced, with permission, from Katzung BG, editor: *Basic & Clinical Pharmacology,* 10th ed. McGraw-Hill, 2007.)

activate phospholipase C or inhibit adenylyl cyclase. At the postsynaptic level, activation of these receptors can open K^+ ion channels to cause membrane hyperpolarization (inhibitory postsynaptic potentials). At the presynaptic level, opioid receptor activation can close voltage-gated Ca^{2+} ion channels to inhibit neurotransmitter release (Figure 31–2). Presynaptic actions result in the inhibition of release of multiple neurotransmitters, including acetylcholine (ACh), norepinephrine, serotonin, glutamate, and substance P.

ACUTE EFFECTS

A. ANALGESIA

The opioids are the most powerful drugs available for the relief of pain. They attenuate both emotional and sensory aspects of the pain experience. Strong agonists (ie, those

with the highest analgesic efficacy, full agonists) include morphine, methadone, meperidine, fentanyl, levorphanol, and heroin. Codeine, hydrocodone, and oxycodone are partial agonists with mild to moderate analgesic efficacy. Propoxyphene is a very weak agonist drug.

B. SEDATION AND EUPHORIA

These effects may occur at doses below those required for maximum analgesia. The sedation is additive with other CNS depressants, but there is little amnesia. Some patients experience dysphoric effects from opioid drugs. At higher doses, the drugs may cause mental clouding and result in a stuporous, or even a comatose, state.

C. RESPIRATORY DEPRESSION

Opioid actions in the medulla lead to inhibition of the respiratory center, with decreased response to carbon

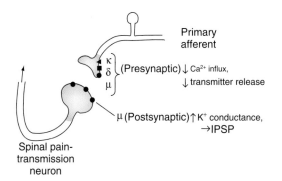

Figure 31–2. Spinal sites of opioid action. The μ, κ, and δ agonists reduce excitatory transmitter release from presynaptic terminals of nociceptive primary afferents. The μ agonists also hyperpolarize second-order pain transmission neurons by increasing K⁺ conductance, evoking an inhibitory postsynaptic potential. (Reproduced, with permission, from Katzung BG, editor: *Basic & Clinical Pharmacology*, 10th ed. McGraw-Hill, 2007.)

dioxide challenge. With full agonists, respiratory depression may be seen at conventional analgesic doses. Increased PCO_2 may cause cerebrovascular dilation, resulting in increased blood flow and increased intracranial pressure. Opioid analgesics are relatively contraindicated in patients with head injuries.

D. ANTITUSSIVE ACTIONS

Suppression of the cough reflex by unknown mechanisms is the basis for the clinical use of opioids as antitussives.

E. NAUSEA AND VOMITING

Nausea and vomiting are caused by activation of the chemoreceptor trigger zone and are increased by ambulation.

F. GASTROINTESTINAL EFFECTS

Constipation occurs through decreased intestinal peristalsis, which is probably mediated by effects on opioid receptors in the enteric nervous system. This powerful action is the basis for the clinical use of these drugs as antidiarrheal agents.

G. SMOOTH MUSCLE

Opioids (with the exception of meperidine) cause contraction of biliary tract smooth muscle, which may cause biliary colic or spasm, increased ureteral and bladder sphincter tone, and a reduction in uterine tone, which may contribute to prolongation of labor.

H. MIOSIS

Pupillary constriction is a characteristic effect of all opioids except meperidine, which has a muscarinic

blocking action. Miosis is blocked by the opioid antagonist naloxone and by atropine.

I. MISCELLANEOUS

Opioid analgesics, especially morphine, can cause flushing and pruritus in part through histamine release. They cause release of ADH and prolactin, but may inhibit the release of LH. Exaggerated responses to opioid analgesics may occur in patients with adrenal insufficiency or hypothyroidism.

SKILL KEEPER: OPIOID PEPTIDES AND SUBSTANCE P (SEE CHAPTERS 6 AND 17)

These peptides are relevant to understanding the analgesic actions of opioid-analgesic drugs in terms of CNS function. What are the roles of these peptides in peripheral tissues? The Skill Keeper Answer appears at the end of the chapter.

CHRONIC EFFECTS

A. TOLERANCE

Marked tolerance can develop to the just-mentioned acute pharmacologic effects, with the exception of miosis and constipation. The mechanism of opioid tolerance development may involve receptor "uncoupling." Antagonists of glutamate NMDA receptors (eg, ketamine), as well as δ-receptor antagonists, are reported to block opioid tolerance. Although there is **cross-tolerance** between different opioid agonists, it is not complete. This provides the basis for "opioid rotation," whereby analgesia is maintained (eg, in cancer patients) by changing from one drug to another.

B. DEPENDENCE

Physical dependence is an anticipated physiologic response to chronic therapy with drugs in this group, particularly the strong agonists. Physical dependence is revealed on abrupt discontinuance as an **abstinence syndrome,** which includes rhinorrhea, lacrimation, chills, gooseflesh, muscle aches, diarrhea, yawning, anxiety, and hostility. A more intense state of **precipitated withdrawal** results when an opioid antagonist is administered to a physically dependent individual.

CLINICAL USES

A. ANALGESIA

Treatment of relatively constant moderate to severe pain is the major indication. Although oral formulations are most commonly used, buccal and suppository forms of some drugs are available. In the acute setting, strong agonists are usually given parenterally. Prolonged analgesia, with some reduction in adverse effects, can be achieved with epidural administration of certain strong agonist drugs (eg, fentanyl and morphine). Fentanyl has also been used by the transdermal route, providing analgesia for up to 72 h. For less severe pain and in the chronic setting, moderate agonists are given by the oral route, sometimes in combinations with acetaminophen or NSAIDs.

B. Cough Suppression

Useful oral antitussive drugs include codeine and dextromethorphan. The latter, an over-the counter drug, has recently been the subject of FDA warnings regarding its abuse potential. Large doses of dextromethorphan may cause hallucinations, confusion, excitation, increased or decreased pupil size, nystagmus, seizures, coma, and decreased breathing.

C. Treatment of Diarrhea

Selective antidiarrheal opioids include diphenoxylate and loperamide. They are given orally.

D. Management of Acute Pulmonary Edema

Morphine (parenteral) may be useful in acute pulmonary edema because of its hemodynamic actions; its calming effects probably also contribute to relief of the pulmonary symptoms.

E. Anesthesia

Opioids are used as preoperative medications and as intraoperative adjunctive agents in balanced anesthesia protocols. High-dose intravenous opioids (eg, morphine, fentanyl) are often the major component of anesthesia for cardiac surgery.

F. Opioid Dependence

Methadone, one of the longer acting opioids, is used in the management of opioid withdrawal states and in maintenance programs for addicts. In withdrawal states, methadone permits a slow tapering of opioid effect that diminishes the intensity of abstinence symptoms. Buprenorphine (see later discussion) has an even longer duration of action and is sometimes used in withdrawal states. In maintenance programs, the prolonged action of methadone blocks the euphoria-inducing effects of doses of shorter acting opioids (eg, heroin, morphine).

TOXICITY

Most of the adverse effects of the opioid analgesics (eg, nausea, constipation, respiratory depression) are predictable extensions of their pharmacologic effects. In addition, overdose and drug interaction toxicities are very important.

A. Overdose

A triad of pupillary constriction, comatose state, and respiratory depression is characteristic; the latter is responsible for most fatalities. Diagnosis of overdosage is confirmed if intravenous injection of naloxone, an antagonist drug, results in prompt signs of recovery. Treatment of overdose involves the use of antagonists such as naloxone and other therapeutic measures, especially ventilatory support.

B. Drug Interactions

The most important drug interactions involving opioid analgesics are additive CNS depression with ethanol, sedative-hypnotics, anesthetics, antipsychotic drugs, tricyclic antidepressants, and antihistamines. Concomitant use of certain opioids (eg, meperidine) with monoamine oxidase inhibitors increases the incidence of hyperpyrexic coma. Meperidine has also been implicated in the serotonin syndrome when used with selective serotonin reuptake inhibitors.

AGONIST-ANTAGONIST DRUGS

A. Analgesic Activity

The analgesic activity of mixed agonist-antagonists varies with the individual drug but is somewhat less than that of strong full agonists like morphine. Buprenorphine, butorphanol, and nalbuphine afford greater analgesia than pentazocine, which is similar to codeine in analgesic efficacy.

B. Receptors

Butorphanol, nalbuphine, and pentazocine are κ agonists, with weak μ-receptor antagonist activity. Butorphanol may act as a partial agonist or antagonist at the μ receptor.

Buprenorphine is a μ-receptor agonist with weak antagonist effects at κ and δ receptors. These characteristics can lead to decreased analgesia or even precipitate withdrawal symptoms, when such drugs are used in patients taking conventional full μ-receptor agonists. Buprenorphine has a long duration of effect because it binds strongly to μ receptors. Although prolonged activity of buprenorphine may be clinically useful (eg, to suppress withdrawal signs in dependency states), this property renders its effects resistant to naloxone reversal. In overdose, respiratory depression caused by nalbuphine is also resistant to naloxone reversal. Naloxone is included in some formulations of these agonist-antagonist drugs to discourage abuse.

C. Effects

The mixed agonist-antagonist drugs often cause sedation at analgesic doses. Dizziness, sweating, and nausea may also occur, and anxiety, hallucinations, and nightmares are possible adverse effects. Respiratory depression

KEY DRUGS

Subclass	Prototypes	Other Significant Agents
Strong agonists	Morphine	Fentanyl, heroin, levorphanol, meperidine, methadone
Moderate agonists	Codeine	Oxycodone, hydrocodone
Weak agonists	Propoxyphene	
Mixed agonist-antagonists	Pentazocine	Buprenorphine, butorphanol, nalbuphine
Antagonists	Naloxone	Nalmefene, naltrexone
Antitussive	Dextromethorphan	Codeine
Antidiarrheal	Diphenoxylate	Loperamide

may be less intense than with pure agonists but is not predictably reversed by naloxone. Tolerance develops with chronic use but is less than the tolerance that develops to the pure agonists, and there is minimal cross-tolerance. Physical dependence occurs, but the abuse liability of mixed agonist-antagonist drugs is less than that of the full agonists.

OPIOID ANTAGONISTS

Naloxone, nalmefene, and naltrexone are pure opioid receptor antagonists that have few other effects at doses that produce marked antagonism of agonist effects. These drugs have greater affinity for μ receptors than for other opioid receptors. The major clinical use of the opioid antagonists is in the management of acute opioid overdose. Naloxone and nalmelfene are given intravenously. Because naloxone has a short duration of action (1–2 h), multiple doses may be required in opioid analgesic overdose. Nalmefene has a duration of action of 8–12 h. Naltrexone has a long elimination half-life, blocking the actions of strong agonists (eg, heroin) for up to 48 h after oral use. Naltrexone decreases the craving for ethanol and is approved for adjunctive use in alcohol dependency programs.

QUESTIONS

1–2. A 63-year-old man is undergoing radiation treatment as an outpatient for metastatic bone cancer. His pain has been managed with a fixed combination of oxycodone plus acetaminophen taken orally. Despite increasing doses of the analgesic combination, the pain is getting worse.

1. The most appropriate oral medication for his increasing pain is
   (A) Buprenorphine
   (B) Codeine plus aspirin
   (C) Levorphanol
   (D) Pentazocine
   (E) Propoxyphene

2. Because of tolerance, it is possible that this patient will have to increase the dose of the analgesic as his condition progresses. Tolerance will not develop to a significant extent with respect to
   (A) Constipation
   (B) Euphoria
   (C) Nausea and vomiting
   (D) Sedation
   (E) Urinary retention

3. Opioid peptides inhibit the release of substance P, an excitatory neurotransmitter, from primary afferent nerve endings in the spinal cord. The ionic mechanism involves
   (A) Activation of chloride ion channels
   (B) Decreased influx of calcium ions
   (C) Facilitation of the efflux of potassium ions
   (D) Prevention of sodium ion influx
   (E) None of the above

4. You are on your way to take an examination and you suddenly get an attack of diarrhea. If you stop at a nearby drugstore for an over-the-counter opioid with antidiarrheal action, you will be asking for
   (A) Codeine
   (B) Dextromethorphan
   (C) Diphenoxylate

(D) Loperamide
(E) Nalbuphine

5. Fentanyl patches used to provide analgesia have caused
   (A) Coughing
   (B) Diarrhea
   (C) Hypertension
   (D) Relaxation of skeletal muscle
   (E) Respiratory depression

6. An emergency department patient with severe pain thought to be of gastrointestinal origin received 80 mg of meperidine. He subsequently developed a severe reaction characterized by tachycardia, hypertension, hyperpyrexia, and seizures. Questioning revealed that the patient had been taking a drug for a psychiatric condition. Which drug is most likely to be responsible for this untoward interaction with meperidine?
   (A) Alprazolam
   (B) Bupropion
   (C) Lithium
   (D) Mirtazapine
   (E) Phenelzine

7. Genetic polymorphism in drug metabolism is established to be responsible for variations in analgesic response to
   (A) Buprenorphine
   (B) Codeine
   (C) Meperidine
   (D) Methadone
   (E) Propoxyphene

8. Opioid analgesics are either contraindicated or must be used with extreme caution in several clinical situations. For morphine, such situations include
   (A) Adrenal insufficiency
   (B) Biliary tract surgery
   (C) Hypothyroidism
   (D) Late stage of labor
   (E) All of the above

9–10. A heroin addict comes to the emergency department in an anxious and agitated state. He complains of chills, muscle aches, and diarrhea; he has also been vomiting. His symptoms include hyperventilation and hyperthermia. He claims to have had an intravenous "fix" approximately 12 h ago. The attending physician notes that pupil size is greater than normal.

9. What is the most likely cause of these signs and symptoms?
   (A) The patient has overdosed with an opioid
   (B) These are early signs of the toxicity of MPTP, a contaminant in "street heroin"

   (C) The signs and symptoms are those of the abstinence syndrome
   (D) In addition to opioids, the patient has been taking barbiturates
   (E) The patient has hepatitis B

10. Which drug will be most effective in alleviating the symptoms experienced by this patient?
    (A) Acetaminophen
    (B) Buprenorphine
    (C) Codeine
    (D) Diazepam
    (E) Naltrexone

11. Which statement about nalbuphine is accurate?
    (A) Activates μ receptors
    (B) Does not cause respiratory depression
    (C) Is nonsedating
    (D) Pain-relieving action is not superior to that of codeine
    (E) Response to naloxone in overdose may be unreliable

12. Which drug does not activate opioid receptors, has been proposed as a maintenance drug in treatment programs for opioid addicts, and, with a single oral dose, will block the effects of injected heroin for up to 48 h?
    (A) Amphetamine
    (B) Buprenorphine
    (C) Methadone
    (D) Naltrexone
    (E) Propoxyphene

13. Which statement about dextromethorphan is accurate?
    (A) Activates κ receptors
    (B) Analgesia equivalent to pentazocine
    (C) Highly effective antiemetic
    (D) Less constipation than codeine
    (E) No abuse potential

14. Which drug is a full agonist at opioid receptors and has excellent oral bioavailability, analgesic activity equivalent to that of morphine, a longer duration of action, and milder withdrawal signs on abrupt discontinuance than morphine?
    (A) Fentanyl
    (B) Hydromorphone
    (C) Methadone
    (D) Nalbuphine
    (E) Oxycodone

15. Which statement about propoxyphene is accurate?
    (A) Analgesia equivalent to oxycodone
    (B) Antagonist at μ receptors
    (C) Causes dose-limiting diarrhea
    (D) Highly effective cough suppressant
    (E) Seizures in overdose

ANSWERS

1. In most situations, pain associated with metastatic carcinoma will ultimately necessitate the use of an opioid analgesic that is equivalent in strength to morphine, so levorphanol would be indicated. Pentazocine or the combination of codeine plus salicylate would not be as effective as the original drug combination. Propoxyphene is even less active than codeine alone. Buprenorphine, a mixed agonist-antagonist, is not usually recommended for cancer-associated pain because of its analgesic "ceiling" and because of possible dysphoric and psychotomimetic effects. The answer is **C.**

2. Chronic use of strong opioid analgesics leads to the development of tolerance to their analgesic, euphoric, and sedative actions. Tolerance also develops to their emetic effects and to effects on some smooth muscle, including the urethral sphincter muscle. However, tolerance does not develop significantly to the constipating or miotic actions of the opioid analgesics. The answer is **A.**

3. Activation of opioid peptide receptors on primary afferent nerve endings (involved in nociception) inhibits the release of excitatory transmitters, including glutamic acid and substance P. The ionic mechanism involves a decrease in the influx of calcium ions. The answer is **B.**

4. Codeine and possibly nalbuphine could decrease gastrointestinal peristalsis, but not without marked side effects (and a prescription). Dextromethorphan is a cough suppressant. The other 2 drugs listed are opioids with antidiarrheal actions. Diphenoxylate is not available over-the-counter because it is a constituent of a proprietary combination that includes atropine sulfate (Lomotil). The answer is **D.**

5. The fentanyl transdermal patch releases the drug over 72 h. The blood levels achieved provide analgesia in pain states but can increase arterial PCO_2 because of depression of the brainstem respiratory center. This effect has contributed to severe respiratory depression with occasional fatalities. The answer is **E.**

6. Concomitant administration of meperidine and monoamine oxidase inhibitors has resulted in life-threatening hyperpyrexic reactions that may culminate in seizures or coma. Note that concomitant use of selective serotonin reuptake inhibitors and meperidine has resulted in the serotonin syndrome, another life-threatening drug interaction (see Chapter 30). The answer is **E.**

7. Codeine, hydrocodone, and oxycodone are metabolized by the cytochrome P450 isoform CYP2D6 and variations in analgesic response to these drugs have been attributed to genotypic polymorphisms in this isozyme. In the case of codeine this may be especially important since the drug is demethylated by CYP2D6 to form the more active metabolite, morphine. The answer is **B.**

8. Morphine and other strong opioid agonists cause exaggerated effects in patients with Addison's disease and in hypothyroidism. These drugs are contraindicated in head injury because they depress respiration, causing cerebral vasodilation, which may increase intracranial pressure. The opioids also contract biliary smooth muscle and may cause spasm or colic. If given during labor, they may cause respiratory depression in the newborn. The answer is **E.**

9. The signs and symptoms are those of withdrawal in a patient physically dependent on an opioid agonist. They usually start within 6–10 h after the last dose; their intensity depends on the degree of physical dependence and peak effects usually occur at 36–48 h. Mydriasis is a prominent feature of the abstinence syndrome; other symptoms include rhinorrhea, lacrimation, piloerection, muscle jerks, and yawning. The answer is **C.**

10. Prevention of signs and symptoms of withdrawal after chronic use of a strong opiate like heroin requires replacement with another strong opioid analgesic drug. Methadone is most commonly used, but buprenorphine is also effective, binding strongly to μ receptors. Acetaminophen and codeine will not be effective. Beneficial effects of diazepam are restricted to relief of anxiety and agitation. The antagonist drug naltrexone may exacerbate withdrawal symptoms. The answer is **B.**

11. Mixed agonist-antagonist drugs like nalbuphine may have analgesic efficacy superior to that of codeine but not equivalent to that of strong agonists. Although mixed agonist-antagonist drugs are less likely to cause respiratory depression than μ activators, if depression does occur reversal with opioid antagonists is unpredictable. Sedation is common. The answer is **E.**

12. The opioid antagonist naltrexone has a much longer half-life than naloxone, and its effects may last 2 days. A high degree of client compliance would be required for naltrexone to be of value in opioid dependence treatment programs. The same reservation is applicable to the use of naltrexone in alcoholism. The answer is **D.**

13. Dextromethorphan, the active component in many over-the-counter cough suppressants, has no appreciable analgesic activity. In comparison with codeine, also an effective antitussive, dextromethorphan causes less constipation. When formulated

properly and used in small amounts, dextromethorphan can be safely used as a cough suppressant. However, overdose toxicity in toddlers has raised concern and abuse of the drug in powdered form has caused disorientation, hallucinations, seizures and death. The answer is **D.**

14. Fentanyl, hydromorphone, and methadone are full agonists with analgesic efficacy similar to that of morphine. Fentanyl, when given intravenously, has a duration of action of just 60–90 min. Hydromorphone has poor oral bioavailability. Methadone has the greatest bioavailability of the drugs used orally, and its effects are more prolonged. Tolerance and physical dependence develop, and dissipate, more slowly with methadone than with morphine. These properties underlie the use of methadone for detoxification and maintenance programs. The answer is **C.**

15. Propoxyphene is chemically related to methadone but has very low analgesic activity. Propoxyphene causes a small additive analgesic effect when used in combination with aspirin or acetaminophen. Overdosage of propoxyphene results in severe toxicity, including respiratory depression, circulatory collapse, pulmonary edema, and seizures. The answer is **E.**

SKILL KEEPER ANSWERS: OPIOPEPTINS AND SUBSTANCE P (SEE CHAPTERS 6 AND 17)

1. *Precursor molecules that release opioid peptides are found at various peripheral sites, including the adrenal medulla and the pituitary gland and in some secretomotor neurons and interneurons in the enteric nervous system. In the gut these peptides appear to inhibit the release of ACh, presumably from parasympathetic nerve endings, and thereby inhibit peristalsis. In other tissues, opioid peptides may stimulate the release of transmitters or act as neurohormones.*

2. *Substance P, an undecapeptide, is a member of the tachykinin peptide group. It is an important sensory neuron transmitter in the enteric nervous system and, of course, in primary afferents involved in nociception. Substance P contracts intestinal and bronchiolar smooth muscle but is an arteriolar vasodilator (possibly via nitric oxide release). It may also play a role in renal and salivary gland functions.*

CHECKLIST

When you complete this chapter, you should be able to:

☐ Identify 3 opioid receptor subtypes and describe 2 ionic mechanisms that result from such activation.

☐ Name the major opioid agonists, rank them in terms of analgesic efficacy, and identify specific dynamic or kinetic characteristics.

☐ Describe the cardinal signs and treatment of opioid drug "overdose" and of the "withdrawal" syndrome.

☐ List acute and chronic adverse effects of opioid analgesics.

☐ Identify an opioid receptor antagonist and a mixed agonist-antagonist.

☐ Identify opioids used for antitussive effects and for antidiarrheal effects.

Drugs of Abuse

Drug abuse is usually taken to mean the use of an illicit drug or the excessive or nonmedical use of a licit drug. It also denotes the deliberate use of chemicals that generally are not considered drugs by the lay public but may be harmful to the user. A primary motivation for drug abuse appears to be the anticipated feeling of pleasure derived from the CNS effects of the drug. If physiologic dependence is present, prevention of an abstinence syndrome acts as a reinforcement to continued drug abuse.

SEDATIVE-HYPNOTICS

The sedative-hypnotic drugs are responsible for many cases of drug abuse. The group includes **ethanol, barbiturates,** and **benzodiazepines.** Benzodiazepines are commonly prescribed drugs for anxiety and, as Schedule IV drugs, are judged by the US government to have low abuse liability (Table 32–1). Short-acting barbiturates (eg, secobarbital) have high addiction potential. Ethanol is not listed in schedules of controlled substances with abuse liability.

A. EFFECTS

Sedative-hypnotics reduce inhibitions, suppress anxiety, and produce relaxation. All of these actions are thought to encourage repetitive use and the development of psychological dependence. The drugs are CNS depressants, and their depressant effects are enhanced by concomitant use of opioid analgesics, antipsychotic agents, marijuana, and any other drug with sedative properties. Acute overdoses commonly result in death through depression of the medullary respiratory and cardiovascular centers (Table 32–2). Management of overdose includes maintenance of a patent airway plus ventilatory support. Flumazenil can be used to reverse the CNS depressant effects of benzodiazepines, but there is no antidote for barbiturates or ethanol.

Flunitrazepam (Rohypnol), a potent rapid-onset benzodiazepine with marked amnestic properties, has been used in "date rape." Added to alcoholic beverages, chloral hydrate or γ-hydroxybutyrate (GHB; sodium oxybate) also render the victim incapable of resisting rape. The latter compound, a minor metabolite of GABA, binds to GABA$_B$ receptors in the CNS. When used as a "club drug," GHB causes euphoria, enhanced sensory perception, and amnesia.

B. WITHDRAWAL

Physiologic dependence occurs with continued use of sedative-hypnotics; the signs and symptoms of the withdrawal (abstinence) syndrome are most pronounced with drugs that have a half-life of less than 24 h (eg, ethanol, secobarbital, methaqualone). However, physiologic dependence may occur with any sedative-hypnotic, including the longer acting benzodiazepines. The most important signs of withdrawal derive from excessive *CNS stimulation* and include anxiety, tremor, nausea and vomiting, delirium, and hallucinations (see Table 32–2). **Seizures** are not uncommon and may be life threatening.

Treatment of sedative-hypnotic withdrawal involves administration of a long-acting sedative-hypnotic (eg, chlordiazepoxide or diazepam) to suppress the acute withdrawal syndrome, followed by gradual dose reduction. Clonidine or propranolol may also be of value to suppress sympathetic overactivity.

A syndrome of **therapeutic withdrawal** has occurred on discontinuance of sedative-hypnotics after long-term therapeutic administration. In addition to the symptoms of classic withdrawal presented in Table 32–2, this syndrome includes weight loss, paresthesias, and headache. (See Chapters 22 and 23 for additional details.)

OPIOID ANALGESICS

A. EFFECTS

The most commonly abused drugs in this group are **heroin, morphine, oxycodone,** and, among health professionals, **meperidine** and **fentanyl.** The effects of intravenous heroin are described by abusers as a "rush" or orgasmic feeling followed by euphoria and then sedation. Intravenous administration of opioids is associated with rapid development of tolerance and psychological and physiologic dependence. Oral administration or smoking of opioids causes milder effects, with a slower onset of tolerance and dependence. Overdose of opioids leads to respiratory depression progressing to coma and

---

HIGH-YIELD TERMS TO LEARN

Tolerance	A decreased response to a drug, necessitating larger doses to achieve the same effect. This can result from increased disposition of the drug (metabolic tolerance), an ability to compensate for the effects of a drug (behavioral tolerance), or changes in receptor or effector systems involved in drug actions (functional tolerance)
Psychological dependence	Compulsive drug-using behavior in which the individual uses the drug for personal satisfaction, often in the face of known risks to health; addiction
Physiologic dependence	A state characterized by signs and symptoms, frequently the opposite of those *caused* by a drug, when it is withdrawn from chronic use or when the dose is abruptly lowered; also called physical dependence
Abstinence syndrome	A term used to describe the signs and symptoms that occur on withdrawal of a drug in a physiologically dependent person
Controlled substance	A drug deemed to have abuse liability that is listed on governmental Schedules of Controlled Substances.[a] Such schedules categorize illicit drugs, control prescribing practices, and mandate penalties for illegal possession, manufacture, and sale of listed drugs. Controlled substance schedules are presumed to reflect current attitudes toward substance abuse; therefore, which drugs are regulated depends on a social judgment
Designer drug	A synthetic derivative of a drug, with slightly modified structure but no major change in pharmacodynamic action. Circumvention of the Schedules of Controlled Drugs is a motivation for the illicit synthesis of designer drugs

[a]An example of such a schedule promulgated by the US Drug Enforcement Agency is shown in Table 32–1. Note that the criteria given by the agency do not always reflect the actual pharmacologic properties of the drugs.

---

death (see Table 32–2). Overdose is managed with intravenous naloxone or nalmefene and ventilatory support.

B. WITHDRAWAL

Deprivation of opioids in physiologically dependent individuals leads to an abstinence syndrome that includes lacrimation, rhinorrhea, yawning, sweating, weakness, gooseflesh ("cold turkey"), nausea and vomiting, tremor, muscle jerks ("kicking the habit"), and hyperpnea (see Table 32–2). Although extremely unpleasant, withdrawal from opioids is rarely fatal (unlike withdrawal from sedative-hypnotics). Treatment involves replacement of the illicit drug with a pharmacologically equivalent agent (eg, methadone), followed by slow dose reduction. Clonidine and buprenorphine, a longer acting opioid, have also been used to suppress withdrawal symptoms. The administration of naloxone to a person who is using strong opioids (but not overdosing) may cause

Table 32–1. Schedules of controlled drugs.

Schedule	Criteria	Examples
I	No medical use; high addiction potential	Flunitrazepam, heroin, LSD, mescaline, PCP, MDA, MDMA, STP
II	Medical use; high addiction potential	Amphetamines, cocaine, methylphenidate, short-acting barbiturates, strong opioids
III	Medical use; moderate abuse potential	Anabolic steroids, barbiturates, dronabinol, ketamine, moderate opioid agonists
IV	Medical use; low abuse potential	Benzodiazepines, chloral hydrate, mild stimulants (eg, phentermine, sibutramine), most hypnotics (eg, zaleplon, zolpidem), weak opioids

Adapted, with permission, from Katzung BG, editor: *Basic & Clinical Pharmacology*, 10th ed. McGraw-Hill, 2007.

Table 32–2. Signs and symptoms of overdose and withdrawal from selected drugs of abuse.

Drug	Overdose Effects	Withdrawal Symptoms
Amphetamines, methylphenidate, cocaine[a]	Agitation, hypertension, tachycardia, delusions, hallucinations, hyperthermia, seizures, death	Apathy, irritability, increased sleep time, disorientation, depression
Barbiturates, benzodiazepines, ethanol[b]	Slurred speech, "drunken" behavior, dilated pupils, weak and rapid pulse, clammy skin, shallow respiration, coma, death	Anxiety, insomnia, delirium, tremors, seizures, death
Heroin; other strong opioids	Constricted pupils, clammy skin, nausea, drowsiness, respiratory depression, coma, death	Nausea, chills, cramps, lacrimation, rhinorrhea, yawning, hyperpnea, tremor

[a]Cardiac arrhythmias, myocardial infarction, and stroke occur more frequently in cocaine overdose.
[b]Ethanol withdrawal includes the excited hallucinatory state of delirium tremens.

more rapid and more intense symptoms of withdrawal (precipitated withdrawal). Neonates born to mothers physiologically dependent on opioids require special management of withdrawal symptoms.

STIMULANTS

A. CAFFEINE AND NICOTINE

1. Effects—Caffeine (in beverages) and nicotine (in tobacco products) are legal in most Western cultures even though they have adverse medical effects. In the United States, cigarette smoking is a major preventable cause of death; tobacco use is associated with a high incidence of cardiovascular, respiratory, and neoplastic disease. Psychological dependence on caffeine and nicotine has been recognized for some time. More recently, demonstration of abstinence signs and symptoms has provided evidence for physiologic dependence.

2. Withdrawal—Withdrawal from caffeine is accompanied by lethargy, irritability, and headache. The anxiety and mental discomfort experienced from discontinuing nicotine are major impediments to quitting the habit.

3. Toxicity—Acute toxicity from overdosage of caffeine or nicotine includes excessive CNS stimulation with tremor, insomnia, and nervousness; cardiac stimulation and arrhythmias; and, in the case of nicotine, respiratory paralysis (Chapters 6 and 7). Severe toxicity has been reported in small children who ingest discarded nicotine gum or nicotine patches, which are used as substitutes for tobacco products.

B. AMPHETAMINES

1. Effects—Amphetamines inhibit transporters of CNS amines including dopamine, norepinephrine, and serotonin. They cause a feeling of euphoria and self-confidence that contributes to the rapid development of

psychological dependence. Drugs in this class include **dextroamphetamine** and **methamphetamine** ("speed"), a crystal form of which ("ice") can be smoked. Chronic high-dose abuse leads to a psychotic state (with delusions and paranoia) that is difficult to differentiate from schizophrenia. Symptoms of overdose include agitation, restlessness, tachycardia, hyperthermia, hyperreflexia, and possibly seizures (see Table 32–2). There is no specific antidote, and supportive measures are directed toward control of body temperature and protection against cardiac arrhythmias and seizures. Chronic abuse of amphetamines is associated with the development of necrotizing arteritis, leading to cerebral hemorrhage and renal failure.

2. Tolerance and withdrawal—Tolerance can be marked, and an abstinence syndrome, characterized by increased appetite, sleepiness, exhaustion, and mental depression, can occur on withdrawal. Antidepressant drugs may be indicated.

3. Congeners of amphetamines—Several chemical congeners of amphetamines have hallucinogenic properties. These include 2,5-dimethoxy-4-methylamphetamine (**DOM, STP**), methylene dioxyamphetamine (**MDA**), and methylenedioxymethamphetamine (**MDMA; "ecstasy"**). MDMA has a more selective action than amphetamine on the serotonin transporter in the CNS. The drug is purported to facilitate interpersonal communication and act as a sexual enhancer. Positron emission tomography studies of the brains of regular users of MDMA show a depletion of neurons in serotonergic tracts. Overdose toxicity includes hyperthermia, symptoms of the serotonin syndrome (see Chapter 30) and seizures. A withdrawal syndrome with protracted depression has been described in chronic users of MDMA.

C. COCAINE

1. Effects—Cocaine, also an inhibitor of the CNS transporters of dopamine, norepinephrine and serotonin, has marked amphetamine-like effects ("super-speed"). Its abuse continues to be widespread in the United States partly because of the availability of a free-base form ("crack") that can be smoked. The euphoria, self-confidence, and mental alertness produced by cocaine are short lasting and positively reinforce its continued use.

Overdoses with cocaine commonly result in fatalities from arrhythmias, seizures, or respiratory depression (see Table 32–2). Cardiac toxicity is partly due to blockade of norepinephrine reuptake by cocaine; its local anesthetic action contributes to the production of seizures. In addition, the powerful vasoconstrictive action of cocaine may lead to severe hypertensive episodes, resulting in myocardial infarcts and strokes. No specific antidote is available. Cocaine abuse during pregnancy is associated with increased fetal morbidity and mortality.

2. Withdrawal—The abstinence syndrome after withdrawal from cocaine is similar to that after amphetamine discontinuance. Severe depression of mood is common and strongly reinforces the compulsion to use the drug. Antidepressant drugs may be indicated. Infants born to mothers who abuse cocaine (or amphetamines) have possible teratogenic abnormalities (cystic cortical lesions) and increased morbidity and mortality and may be cocaine dependent. The signs and symptoms of CNS stimulant overdose and withdrawal are listed in Table 32–2.

HALLUCINOGENS

A. PHENCYCLIDINE

The arylcyclohexylamine drugs include **phencyclidine** (PCP; "angel dust") and ketamine ("special K") and are antagonists at the glutamate NMDA receptor (Chapter 21). Phenyclidine is probably the most dangerous of the currently popular hallucinogenic agents. Psychotic reactions are common with PCP, and impaired judgment often leads to reckless behavior. This drug should be classified as a **psychotomimetic.** Effects of overdosage with PCP include nystagmus, marked hypertension, and seizures, which may be fatal. Parenteral benzodiazepines (eg, diazepam, lorazepam) are used to curb excitation and protect against seizures.

B. MISCELLANEOUS HALLUCINOGENIC AGENTS

Several drugs with hallucinogenic effects have been classified as having abuse liability, including **lysergic acid diethylamide** (LSD), **mescaline,** and **psilocybin.** Hallucinogenic effects may also occur with scopolamine and other antimuscarinic agents. Terms that have been used to describe the CNS effects of such drugs include "psychedelic" and "mind revealing." The perceptual and psychological effects of such drugs are usually accompanied by marked somatic effects, particularly nausea, weakness, and paresthesias. Panic reactions ("bad trips") may also occur. There is little evidence that use of these agents leads to the development of physiologic dependence.

MARIJUANA

A. CLASSIFICATION

Marijuana ("grass") is a collective term for the psychoactive constituents present in crude extracts of the plant *Cannabis sativa* (hemp), the active principles of which include the cannabinoid compounds **tetrahydrocannabinol (THC),** cannabidiol (CBD), and cannabinol (CBN). **Hashish** is a partially purified material that is more potent.

B. CANNABINOIDS

Endogenous cannabinoids in the CNS, which include anadamide and 2-arachidonyl glycerol, are released postsynaptically and act as retrograde messengers to inhibit the presynaptic release of conventional transmitters. The receptors for these compounds are thought to be the "targets" for exogenous cannabinoids present in marijuana.

C. EFFECTS

CNS effects of marijuana include a feeling of being "high," with euphoria, disinhibition, uncontrollable laughter, changes in perception, and achievement of a dreamlike state. Mental concentration may be difficult. Vasodilation occurs, and the pulse rate is characteristically increased. Habitual users show a reddened conjunctiva. A mild withdrawal state has been noted only in long-term heavy users of marijuana. The dangers of marijuana use concern its impairment of judgment and reflexes, effects that are potentiated by concomitant use of sedative-hypnotics, including ethanol. Potential therapeutic effects of marijuana include its ability to decrease intraocular pressure and its antiemetic actions. **Dronabinol** (a controlled-substance formulation of THC) is used to combat severe nausea.

INHALANTS

Certain gases or volatile liquids are abused because they provide a feeling of euphoria or disinhibition.

A. ANESTHETICS

This group includes nitrous oxide, chloroform, and diethylether. These agents are hazardous because they affect judgment and induce loss of consciousness. Inhalation of nitrous oxide as the pure gas (with no oxygen) has caused asphyxia and death. Ether is highly flammable.

B. INDUSTRIAL SOLVENTS

Solvents and a wide range of volatile compounds are present in commercial products such as gasoline, paint thinners, aerosol propellants, glues, rubber cements, and shoe polish. Because of their ready availability, these substances are most frequently abused by children in early adolescence. Active ingredients that have been

KEY DRUGS

Subclass	Prototypes	Other Significant Agents
Sedative-hypnotics	Ethanol, phenobarbital, chlordiazepoxide	Diazepam, methaqualone secobarbital, GHB
Opioids	Heroin	Fentanyl, meperidine, other strong μ receptor activators
Stimulants	Amphetamine, cocaine caffeine, nicotine	Methamphetamine, phenmetrazine, DOM, MDA, MDMA
Hallucinogens	LSD, PCP, ketamine	Mescaline, scopolamine
Marijuana	"Grass"	Dronabinol, hashish
Inhalants	Nitrous oxide, toluene, amyl nitrite	Benzene, chloroform, ether, isobutyl nitrite

identified include benzene, hexane, methylethylketone, toluene, and trichloroethylene. Many of these are toxic to the liver, kidneys, lungs, bone marrow, and peripheral nerves and cause brain damage in animals.

C. ORGANIC NITRITES

Amyl nitrite, isobutyl nitrite, and other organic nitrites are referred to as "poppers" and are mainly used as sexual intercourse "enhancers." Inhalation of the nitrites causes dizziness, tachycardia, hypotension, and flushing. With the exception of methemoglobinemia, few serious adverse effects have been reported.

STEROIDS

In many countries, including the United States, anabolic steroids are controlled substances based on their potential for abuse. Effects sought by abusers are increases in muscle mass and strength rather than euphoria. However, excessive use can have adverse behavioral, cardiovascular, and musculoskeletal effects.

SKILL KEEPER: DRUG OF ABUSE OVERDOSE SIGNS AND SYMPTOMS (SEE CHAPTERS 22 AND 31)

In an emergency situation, behavioral manifestations of the toxicity of drugs of abuse can be of assistance in diagnosis. What other readily detectable markers will also be helpful? The Skill Keeper Answer appears at the end of the chapter.

Acne (sometimes severe), premature closure of the epiphyses, and masculinization in females are anticipated androgenic adverse effects. Hepatic dysfunction has been reported, and the anabolic steroids may pose an increased risk of myocardial infarct. Behavioral manifestations include increases in libido and aggression ("roid rage"). A withdrawal syndrome has been described with fatigue and depression of mood.

QUESTIONS

1–3. A 42-year-old homemaker suffers from anxiety with phobic symptoms and occasional panic attacks. She uses over-the-counter antihistamines for allergic rhinitis and claims that ethanol use is "just 1 or 2 glasses of wine with dinner." Alprazolam is prescribed, and the patient is maintained on the drug for 3 years, with several dose increments over that time period. Her family notices that she does not seem to be improving and that her speech is often slurred in the evenings. She is finally hospitalized with severe withdrawal signs one weekend while attempting to end her dependence on drugs.

1. Which statement about the use of alprazolam is accurate?
   (A) Additive CNS depression occurs with ethanol
   (B) Benzodiazepines are controlled drugs judged to have low abuse liability
   (C) On abrupt discontinuance of alprazolam after 4 weeks of treatment, withdrawal signs may occur
   (D) Tolerance can occur with chronic use of any benzodiazepine
   (E) All of the above statements are accurate

2. The main reason for hospitalization of this patient was to be able to effectively control
   (A) Anxiety
   (B) Cardiac arrhythmias
   (C) Respiratory depression
   (D) Seizures
   (E) Thyroid dysfunction

3. The symptoms experienced by this hospitalized patient can best be managed by the administration of
   (A) Amphetamine
   (B) Diazepam
   (C) Oxycodone
   (D) Propranolol
   (E) Secobarbital

4. Which statement about abuse of the opioid analgesics is false?
   (A) A patient experiencing withdrawal from heroin is free of the symptoms of abstinence in 6–8 days
   (B) In withdrawal from opioids, clonidine may be useful in reducing symptoms caused by sympathetic overactivity
   (C) Lacrimation, rhinorrhea, yawning, and sweating are early signs of withdrawal from opioid analgesics
   (D) Naloxone may precipitate a severe withdrawal state in abusers of opioid analgesics with symptoms starting in less than 15–30 min
   (E) Methadone alleviates most of the symptoms of heroin withdrawal

5. A young male patient is brought to the emergency department of a hospital suffering from an overdose of cocaine after its intravenous administration. His symptoms are NOT likely to include
   (A) Agitation
   (B) Bradycardia
   (C) Hyperthermia
   (D) Myocardial infarct
   (E) Seizures

6. Which drug in overdose is known to cause the potentially fatal "serotonin syndrome"?
   (A) Cocaine
   (B) Fentanyl
   (C) MDMA ("XTC, ecstasy")
   (D) Mescaline
   (E) Phencyclidine

7. Which statement about hallucinogens is accurate?
   (A) Mescaline and related hallucinogens exert their CNS actions through dopaminergic systems in the brain
   (B) Teratogenic effects occur with the use of LSD during pregnancy

   (C) Scopolamine is unique among hallucinogens in that animals will self-administer it
   (D) Dilated pupils, tachycardia, tremor, and increased alertness are characteristic effects of psilocybin
   (E) PCP can be anticipated to cause dry mouth and urinary retention

8. Which statement about inhalants is accurate?
   (A) Solvent inhalation is mainly a drug abuse problem in petroleum industry workers
   (B) Euphoria, numbness, and tingling sensations with visual and auditory disturbances occur in most persons who inhale organic nitrites
   (C) Methemoglobinemia is a common toxicologic problem after repetitive inhalation of industrial solvents
   (D) Nitrous oxide is the most commonly abused drug by medical personnel working in hospitals
   (E) The use of isobutyl nitrite is likely to cause headache

9. Which sign or symptom is likely to occur with marijuana?
   (A) Bradycardia
   (B) Conjunctival reddening
   (C) Hypertension
   (D) Increased psychomotor performance
   (E) Mydriasis

10–11. A college student is brought to the emergency department by friends. The physician is informed that the student had taken a drug and then "went crazy." The patient is agitated and delirious. Several persons are required to hold him down. His skin is warm and sweaty, and his pupils are dilated. Bowel sounds are normal. Signs and symptoms include tachycardia, marked hypertension, hyperthermia, increased muscle tone, and both horizontal and vertical nystagmus.

10. The most likely cause of these signs and symptoms is intoxication from
    (A) Hashish
    (B) LSD
    (C) Mescaline
    (D) PCP
    (E) Scopolamine

11. The management of this patient is likely to include
    (A) Activated charcoal
    (B) Administration of norepinephrine
    (C) Amitriptyline if psychosis ensues
    (D) Atropine to control hyperthermia
    (E) Urinary alkalinization to increase drug elimination

12. This agent has sedative and amnestic properties. Small doses added to alcoholic beverages are not

readily detected by taste and have been used in date rape attacks. The drug is chemically related to a brain inhibitory neurotransmitter. Which agent most closely resembles the description given?

(A) Amyl nitrite
(B) Flunitrazepam
(C) Gamma-hydroxybutyrate
(D) Hashish
(E) Tetrahydrocannabinol

ANSWERS

1. Therapeutic doses of benzodiazepines may lead to physiologic dependence with withdrawal symptoms including anxiety and agitation observable on abrupt discontinuance after a few weeks of treatment. Like most sedative-hypnotics, benzodiazepines are schedule-controlled, exhibiting dependence liability and development of tolerance. Additive depression occurs with ethanol and many other CNS drugs. The answer is **E.**

2. This patient is probably withdrawing from dependence on both alprazolam and alcohol use. In addition to the symptoms described previously, abrupt withdrawal from sedative-hypnotic dependence may include hyperreflexia progressing to seizures, with ensuing coma and possibly death. The risk of a convulsion is increased if the patient abruptly withdraws from ethanol use at the same time. The answer is **D.**

3. Detoxification during withdrawal from physiologic dependence on barbiturates, benzodiazepines, or ethanol involves the use of a long-acting sedative hypnotic with dose tapering. Chlordiazepoxide or diazepam is used frequently. However, depending on the severity of symptoms, initial management may require parenteral diazepam or lorazepam, the latter drug often favored in hepatic dysfunction. The answer is **B.**

4. Symptoms of opioid withdrawal usually begin within 6–8 h, and the acute course may last 6–8 days. However, a secondary phase of heroin withdrawal, characterized by bradycardia, hypotension, hypothermia, and mydriasis, may last 26–30 weeks. Methadone is commonly used in detoxification of the heroin addict because it is a strong agonist, has high oral bioavailability, and has a relatively long half-life. The answer is **A.**

5. Overdoses with amphetamines or cocaine have many signs and symptoms in common. However, the ability of cocaine to block the reuptake of norepinephrine at sympathetic nerve terminals results in greater cardiotoxicity. Tachycardia is the rule, with the possibility of an arrhythmia, infarct, or stroke. The answer is **B.**

6. The serotonin syndrome is associated with drugs that inhibit serotonin transporters in the CNS. MDMA has greater affinity for the serotonin transporter than other CNS stimulants. This sometimes fatal syndrome includes hyperthermia, muscle rigidity, myoclonus, cardiovascular instability, mental status changes, and possibly seizures. The answer is **C.**

7. Psilocybin, mescaline, and LSD have similar central (via serotonergic systems) and peripheral (sympathomimetic) effects. None of these hallucinogenic drugs have been shown to have teratogenic potential. Unlike most hallucinogens, PCP acts as a positive reinforcer of self-administration in animals. Scopolamine blocks muscarinic receptors but is not a positive reinforcer. The answer is **D.**

8. Male preteens are most likely to "experiment" with solvent inhalation. This can result in central and peripheral neurotoxicity, liver and kidney damage, and pulmonary disease. Opioids, including fentanyl and meperidine, are the most widely abused drugs by medical personnel working in hospitals. Industrial solvents rarely cause methemoglobinemia, but this (and headaches) may occur after excessive use of nitrites. The answer is **E.**

9. Two of the most characteristic signs of marijuana use are increased pulse rate and reddening of the conjunctiva. Decreases in blood pressure and in psychomotor performance occur. Pupil size is NOT changed by marijuana. The answer is **B.**

SKILL KEEPER ANSWER: DRUG OF ABUSE OVERDOSE SIGNS AND SYMPTOMS (SEE CHAPTERS 22 AND 31)

Readily detectable markers that may assist in diagnosis of the cause of drug overdose toxicity include changes in heart rate, blood pressure, respiration, body temperature, sweating, bowel signs, and pupillary responses. For example, in the case of drugs of abuse, tachycardia, hypertension, increased body temperature, decreased bowel signs, and mydriasis are common characteristics of overdose of CNS stimulants, including amphetamines, cocaine, and most hallucinogens.

Make a brief list of characteristics that would enable you to identify overdose with opioids and with sedative-hypnotics.

10. The signs and symptoms point to PCP intoxication. The presence of both horizontal and vertical nystagmus is pathognomonic. The answer is **D.**

11. Management of PCP overdose involves ventilatory support and control of seizures (with a benzodiazepine), hypertension, and hyperthermia. Antipsychotic drugs (eg, haloperidol) may also be useful for psychosis. None of the drugs listed are of value. PCP is secreted into the stomach, so removal of the drug may be hastened by activated charcoal or nasogastric suction. PCP is a weak base, and its renal elimination may be accelerated by urinary *acidification.* The answer is **A.**

12. Flunitrazepam fits part of the description of this date rape drug, but it is not chemically related to known neurotransmitters. Gamma-hydroxybutyrate (GHB; "liquid ecstasy"), a popular street drug, is structurally related to γ-aminobutyric acid. GHB causes amnesia and in overdose has resulted in seizures, coma, and death. The answer is **C.**

CHECKLIST

When you complete this chapter, you should be able to:

☐ Identify the major drugs that are commonly abused.

☐ Describe the signs and symptoms of overdose with, and withdrawal from, CNS stimulants, opioid analgesics, and sedative-hypnotics, including ethanol.

☐ Describe the general principles of the management of overdose of commonly abused drugs.

☐ Identify the most likely causes of death from commonly abused agents.

PART VI
Drugs with Important Actions on Blood, Inflammation, & Gout

Agents Used in Anemias & Hematopoietic Growth Factors

33

Blood cells play essential roles in oxygenation of tissues, coagulation, protection against infectious agents, and tissue repair. Blood cell deficiency is a relatively common occurrence that can have profound repercussions. The most common cause of erythrocyte deficiency, or anemia, is insufficient supply of iron, vitamin B_{12}, or folic acid, substances required for normal production of erythrocytes. Pharmacologic treatment of these types of anemia usually involves replacement of the missing substance. An alternative therapy for treatment of certain types of anemia and for treatment of deficiency in other types of blood cells is administration of recombinant hematopoietic growth factors, which stimulate the production of various lineages of blood cells and regulate blood cell function.

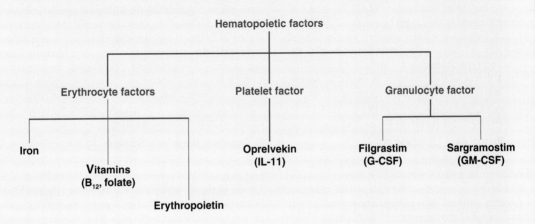

HIGH-YIELD TERMS TO LEARN

Cobalamin	Vitamin B_{12}
dTMP synthesis	A set of biochemical reactions that produce deoxythymidylate (dTMP), an essential constituent of DNA synthesis. The cycle depends on the conversion of dihydrofolate to tetrahydrofolate by the enzyme dihydrofolate reductase (Figure 33–1)
G-CSF	Granulocyte colony-stimulating factor, a hematopoietic growth factor that regulates production and function of neutrophils
GM-CSF	Granulocyte-macrophage colony-stimulating factor, a hematopoietic growth factor that regulates production of granulocytes (basophils, eosinophils, and neutrophils), and other myeloid cells
Hemochromatosis	A condition of chronic excess total body iron that is caused either by an inherited abnormality of iron absorption or by frequent transfusions to treat certain types of hemolytic disorders (eg, thalassemia major)
Megaloblastic anemia	A deficiency in serum hemoglobin and erythrocytes in which the erythrocytes are abnormally large. Results from either folate or vitamin B_{12} deficiency anemia
Microcytic anemia	A deficiency in serum hemoglobin and erythrocytes in which the erythrocytes are abnormally small. Often caused by iron deficiency
Neutropenia	An abnormal decrease in the number of neutrophils in the blood; patients with neutropenia are susceptible to serious infection
Pernicious anemia	A form of megaloblastic anemia that results from a lack of intrinsic factor, a protein that is produced by gastric mucosal cells and is required for intestinal absorption of vitamin B_{12}
Thrombocytopenia	An abnormal decrease in the number of platelets in the blood; patients with thrombocytopenia are susceptible to hemorrhage

BLOOD CELL DEFICIENCIES

A. IRON AND VITAMIN DEFICIENCY ANEMIAS

Microcytic hypochromic anemia, caused by iron deficiency, is the most common type of anemia. Megaloblastic anemias are caused by a deficiency of vitamin B_{12} or folic acid, cofactors required for the normal maturation of red blood cells. Pernicious anemia, the most common type of vitamin B_{12} deficiency anemia, is caused by a defect in the synthesis of **intrinsic factor**, a protein required for efficient absorption of dietary vitamin B_{12}, or by surgical removal of that part of the stomach that secretes intrinsic factor.

B. OTHER BLOOD CELL DEFICIENCIES

Deficiency in the concentration of the various lineages of blood cells can be a manifestation of a disease or a side effect of radiation or cancer chemotherapy. Recombinant DNA-directed synthesis of hematopoietic growth factors now makes possible the treatment of more patients with deficiencies in erythrocytes, neutrophils, and platelets. Some of these growth factors also play an important role in hematopoietic stem cell transplantation.

IRON

A. ROLE OF IRON

Iron is the essential metallic component of heme, the molecule responsible for the bulk of oxygen transport in the blood. Although most of the iron in the body is contained in hemoglobin, an important fraction is bound to **transferrin**, a transport protein, and **ferritin**, a storage protein. Deficiency of iron occurs most often in women because of menstrual blood loss and in vegetarians or malnourished individuals because of inadequate dietary iron intake. Children and pregnant women have increased requirements for iron.

B. REGULATION OF IRON STORES

Although iron is an essential ion, excessive amounts are highly toxic. As a result, a complex system has evolved for the transport and storage of free iron (Figure 33–1). Since there is no mechanism for the efficient excretion of iron, regulation of body iron content occurs through modulation of intestinal absorption. As a result, increased gastrointestinal iron absorption can cause iron overload and organ dysfunction.

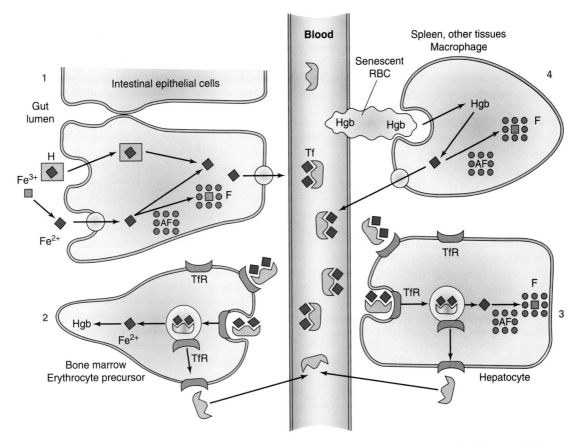

Figure 33–1. Absorption, transport, and storage of iron. Intestinal epithelial cells actively absorb inorganic iron and heme iron. Ferrous iron that is absorbed or released from absorbed heme iron **(1)** is actively transported into the blood or complexed with apoferritin (AF) and stored as ferritin. In the blood, iron is transported by transferrin (Tf) to erythroid precursors in the bone marrow for synthesis of hemoglobin (Hb) **(2)** or to hepatocytes for storage as ferritin **(3)**. The transferrin iron transferrin-iron complex binds to transferrin receptors (TfR) in erythroid precursors and hepatocytes and is internalized. After release of the iron, the TfR-Tf complex is recycled to the plasma membrane and Tf is released. Macrophages that phagocytize senescent erythrocytes (RBC) reclaim the iron from the RBC hemoglobin and either export it or store it as ferritin **(4)**. Hepatocytes employ several mechanisms to take up iron, and store the iron as ferritin. (Reproduced, with permission, from Katzung BG, editor: *Basic & Clinical Pharmacology*, 10th ed. McGraw-Hill, 2007.)

1. Absorption—Dietary iron in the form of heme and the ferrous ion (Fe^{2+}) are taken up by specialized transporters in intestinal epithelials cells and oxidized in the mucosal cell to the ferric (Fe^{3+}) form.

2. Storage—Ferric iron is stored in the mucosa (bound to ferritin) or carried elsewhere in the body (bound to transferrin). Excess iron is stored in the protein-bound form in macrophages and hepatocytes and, in cases of gross overload, in parenchymal cells of the skin, heart, and other organs.

3. Elimination—Minimal amounts of iron are lost from the body with sweat and saliva and in exfoliated skin and intestinal mucosal cells.

C. CLINICAL USE

Iron deficiency anemia is the only indication for the use of iron. Iron deficiency can be diagnosed from red blood cell changes (microcytic cell size, due to diminished hemoglobin content) and from measurements of serum and bone marrow iron stores. The disease is treated by dietary ferrous iron supplementation and, in special cases, by parenteral administration of the metal. Iron should *not* be given in hemolytic anemia because iron stores are elevated, not depressed, in this type of anemia.

D. TOXICITY OF IRON (SEE ALSO CHAPTER 58)

1. Signs and symptoms—Acute iron intoxication is most common in children and usually occurs as a result of accidental ingestion of iron supplementation tablets. Depending on the dose, necrotizing gastroenteritis, shock, metabolic acidosis, coma, and death may result. Chronic iron overload, known as **hemochromatosis,** damages the organs that store excess iron (heart, liver, pancreas). Hemochromatosis occurs most often in individuals with an inherited abnormality of iron absorption and those who receive frequent transfusions for treatment of hemolytic disorders (eg, thalassemia major).

2. Treatment of acute iron intoxication—Immediate treatment is necessary and usually consists of removal of unabsorbed tablets from the gut, correction of acid-base and electrolyte abnormalities, and parenteral administration of **deferoxamine,** which chelates circulating iron.

3. Treatment of chronic iron toxicity—Treatment of the genetic form of hemochromatosis is usually by phlebotomy. Hemochromatosis that is due to frequent transfusions is treated with chronic administration of an iron chelator such as deferoxamine.

VITAMIN B$_{12}$

A. ROLE OF VITAMIN B$_{12}$

Vitamin B$_{12}$ (cobalamin), a cobalt-containing molecule, is, along with folic acid, a cofactor in the transfer of 1-carbon units, a step necessary for the synthesis of DNA. Impairment of DNA synthesis affects all cells, but because red blood cells must be produced continuously, deficiency of either vitamin B$_{12}$ or folic acid usually manifests first as anemia. In addition, vitamin B$_{12}$ deficiency can cause neurologic defects, which may become irreversible if not treated promptly.

B. PHARMACOKINETICS

Vitamin B$_{12}$ is produced only by bacteria; this vitamin cannot be synthesized by multicellular organisms. It is absorbed from the gastrointestinal tract in the presence of **intrinsic factor**, a product of the parietal cells of the stomach. Plasma transport is accomplished by binding to transcobalamin II. Vitamin B$_{12}$ is stored in the liver in large amounts; a normal individual has enough to last 5 years. The 2 available forms of vitamin B$_{12}$, cyanocobalamin and hydroxocobalamin, have similar pharmacokinetics, but hydroxocobalamin has a longer circulating half-life.

C. PHARMACODYNAMICS

Vitamin B$_{12}$ is essential in 2 reactions: conversion of methylmalonyl-coenzyme A (CoA) to succinyl-CoA and conversion of homocysteine to methionine. The second reaction is linked to folic acid metabolism and synthesis of deoxythymidylate (dTMP; Figure 33–1, section 2), a precursor required for DNA synthesis. In vitamin B$_{12}$ deficiency, folates accumulate as N^5-methyltetrahydrofolate; the supply of tetrahydrofolate is depleted; and the production of red blood cells slows. Administration of folic acid to patients with vitamin B$_{12}$ deficiency helps refill the tetrahydrofolate pool (see Figure 33–1, section 3) and partially or fully corrects the anemia. However, the exogenous folic acid does not correct the neurologic defects of vitamin B$_{12}$ deficiency.

D. CLINICAL USE AND TOXICITY

The 2 available forms of vitamin B$_{12}$—hydroxocobalamin and cyanocobalamin—have equivalent effects. The major application is in the treatment of naturally occurring pernicious anemia and anemia caused by gastric resection. Because vitamin B$_{12}$ deficiency anemia is almost always caused by inadequate absorption, therapy should be by replacement of vitamin B$_{12}$, using parenteral therapy. Neither form of vitamin B$_{12}$ has significant toxicity.

FOLIC ACID

A. ROLE OF FOLIC ACID

Like vitamin B$_{12}$, folic acid is required for normal DNA synthesis, and its deficiency usually presents as megaloblastic anemia. In addition, deficiency of folic acid during pregnancy increases the risk of neural tube defects in the fetus.

B. PHARMACOKINETICS

Folic acid is readily absorbed from the gastrointestinal tract. Only modest amounts are stored in the body, so a decrease in dietary intake is followed by anemia within a few months.

C. PHARMACODYNAMICS

Folic acid is converted to tetrahydrofolate by the action of dihydrofolate reductase (see Figure 33–1, section 3). One important set of reactions involving tetrahydrofolate and dihydrofolate constitutes the dTMP cycle (see Figure 33–2, section 2), which supplies the dTMP required for DNA synthesis. Rapidly dividing cells are highly sensitive to folic acid deficiency. For this reason, antifolate drugs are useful in the treatment of various infections and cancers.

D. CLINICAL USE AND TOXICITY

Folic acid deficiency is most often caused by dietary insufficiency or malabsorption. Anemia resulting from

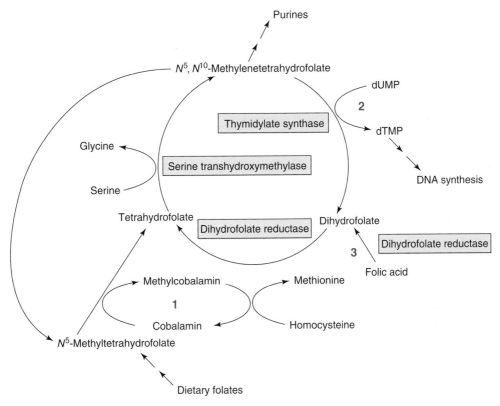

Figure 33–2. Enzymatic reactions that use folates. Section 1 shows the vitamin B_{12}-dependent reaction that allows most dietary folates to enter the tetrahydrofolate cofactor pool and becomes the "folate trap" in vitamin B_{12} deficiency. Section 2 shows the dTMP cycle. Section 3 shows the pathway by which folate enters the tetrahydrofolate cofactor pool. Double arrows indicate pathways with more than 1 intermediate step. (Reproduced, with permission, from Katzung BG, editor: *Basic & Clinical Pharmacology*, 10th ed. McGraw-Hill, 2007.)

folic acid deficiency is readily treated by oral folic acid supplementation. Because maternal folic acid deficiency is associated with increased risk of neural tube defects in the fetus, folic acid supplementation is recommended prior to and during pregnancy. Folic acid supplements will correct the anemia but not the neurologic deficits of vitamin B_{12} deficiency. Therefore, vitamin B_{12} deficiency must be ruled out before one selects folic acid as the sole therapeutic agent in the treatment of a patient with megaloblastic anemia. Folic acid has no recognized toxicity.

HEMATOPOIETIC GROWTH FACTORS

Over a dozen glycoprotein hormones that regulate the differentiation and maturation of stem cells within the bone marrow have been identified. Several growth factors, produced by recombinant DNA technology, have FDA approval for treatment of patients with blood cell deficiencies.

SKILL KEEPER: ROUTES OF ADMINISTRATION (SEE CHAPTER 1)

All of the recombinant hematopoietic growth factors approved for clinical use are administered by injection. Why can these growth factors not be given orally? Which 3 routes of administration require drug injection? How do these 3 routes compare with regard to onset and duration of drug action and risk of adverse effects? The Skill Keeper Answers appear at the end of the chapter.

A. ERYTHROPOIETIN

Erythropoietin is produced by the kidney; reduction in its synthesis is responsible for the anemia of renal failure.

KEY DRUGS

Subclass	Prototypes	Other Significant Agents
Oral iron supplements	Ferrous sulfate	Ferrous gluconate, ferrous fumarate
Parenteral iron	Iron dextran	
Vitamin B$_{12}$	Cyanocobalamin	Hydroxocobalamin
Folic acid	Folic acid	
Red cell colony-stimulating factor	Erythropoietin	Darbepoetin alpha
Myeloid growth factors	Filgrastim (G-CSF)	Sargramostim (GM-CSF)
Megakaryocyte factor	Oprelvekin (IL-11)	

Through activation of receptors on erythroid progenitors in the bone marrow, erythropoietin stimulates the production of red cells and increases their release from the bone marrow.

Erythropoietin is routinely used for the anemia associated with renal failure and is sometimes effective for patients with other forms of anemia (eg, primary bone marrow disorders or anemias secondary to cancer chemotherapy or HIV treatment, bone marrow transplantation, AIDS, or cancer). Erythropoietin's acute toxicity is minimal. However, when it or other erythropoietic agents are allowed to increase hematocrit excessively (ie, hemoglobin level >12 g/dL), there is increased risk of thrombosis and cardiovascular events. **Darbepoetin alpha**, a glycosylated form of erythropoietin, has a much longer half-life.

B. MYELOID GROWTH FACTORS

Filgrastim (granulocyte colony-stimulating factor; **G-CSF**) and **sargramostim** (granulocyte-macrophage colony-stimulating factor; **GM-CSF**) stimulate the production and function of neutrophils. GM-CSF also stimulates the production of other myeloid and megakaryocyte progenitors. G-CSF and, to a lesser degree, GM-CSF mobilize hematopoietic stem cells (ie, increase their concentration in peripheral blood).

Both growth factors are used to accelerate the recovery of neutrophils after cancer chemotherapy and to treat other forms of secondary and primary neutropenia (eg, aplastic anemia, congenital neutropenia). When given to patients soon after autologous stem cell transplantation, G-CSF reduces the time to engraftment and the duration of neutropenia. G-CSF is used to mobilize peripheral blood stem cells in preparation for autologous and allogeneic stem cell transplantation. The toxicity of G-CSF is minimal, although the drug sometimes causes bone pain. GM-CSF can cause more severe effects, including fever, arthralgias, and capillary damage with edema. Allergic reactions are rare. **Pegfilgrastim**, a covalent conjugation product of filgrastim and a form of polyethylene glycol, has a much longer serum half-life than recombinant G-CSF.

C. MEGAKARYOCYTE GROWTH FACTORS

Oprelvekin (interleukin-11 [**IL-11**]) stimulates the growth of primitive megakaryocytic progenitors and increases the number of peripheral platelets. IL-11 is used for the treatment of patients who have had a prior episode of thrombocytopenia after a cycle of cancer chemotherapy. In such patients, it reduces the need for platelet transfusions. The most common side effects of IL-11 are fatigue, headache, dizziness, and fluid retention.

QUESTIONS

1–4. A 23-year-old pregnant woman is referred by her obstetrician for evaluation of anemia. She is in her fourth month of pregnancy and has no history of anemia; her grandfather had pernicious anemia. Her hemoglobin is 10 g/dL (normal, 12–16 g/dL).

1. If this woman has macrocytic anemia, an increased serum concentration of transferrin, and a normal serum concentration of vitamin B$_{12}$, the most likely cause of her anemia is deficiency of
   (A) Cobalamin
   (B) Erythropoietin
   (C) Folic acid
   (D) Intrinsic factor
   (E) Iron

2. If the patient had the deficiency identified in Question 1, her infant would have a higher than normal risk of
   (A) Cardiac abnormality
   (B) Congenital neutropenia

(C) Kidney damage
(D) Limb deformity
(E) Neural tube defect

3. The laboratory data for your pregnant patient indicate that she does not have macrocytic anemia but instead has microcytic anemia. Optimal treatment of normocytic or mild microcytic anemia associated with pregnancy uses
(A) A high-fiber diet
(B) Erythropoietin injections
(C) Ferrous sulfate tablets
(D) Folic acid supplements
(E) Hydroxocobalamin injections

4. If this patient has a young child at home and is taking iron-containing prenatal supplements, she should be warned that they are a common source of accidental poisoning in young children and advised to make a special effort to keep these pills out of her child's reach. Toxicity associated with acute iron poisoning usually includes
(A) Dizziness, hypertension, and cerebral hemorrhage
(B) Hyperthermia, delirium, and coma
(C) Hypotension, cardiac arrhythmias, and seizures
(D) Necrotizing gastroenteritis, shock, and metabolic acidosis
(E) Severe hepatic injury, encephalitis, and coma

5. The iron stored in intestinal mucosal cells is complexed to
(A) Apoferritin
(B) Intrinsic factor
(C) Oprelvekin
(D) Transcobalamin II
(E) Transferrin

6. Which of the following is MOST likely to be required by a 5-year-old boy with chronic renal insufficiency?
(A) Cyanocobalamin
(B) Deferoxamine
(C) Erythropoietin
(D) Filgrastim (G-CSF)
(E) Oprelvekin (IL-11)

7. In a patient who requires filgrastim (G-CSF) after being treated with anticancer drugs, the therapeutic objective is to prevent
(A) Allergic reactions
(B) Cancer recurrence
(C) Excessive bleeding
(D) Hypoxia
(E) Systemic infection

8. The megaloblastic anemia that results from vitamin B_{12} deficiency is due to inadequate supplies of

(A) Cobalamin
(B) dTMP
(C) Folic acid
(D) Homocysteine
(E) N^5-methyltetrahydrofolate

9–10. After undergoing surgery for breast cancer, a 53-year-old woman is scheduled to receive 4 cycles of cancer chemotherapy. The cycles are to be administered every 3–5 weeks. Her first cycle was complicated by severe chemotherapy-induced thrombocytopenia.

9. During the second cycle of chemotherapy, it would be appropriate to consider treating this patient with
(A) Darbepoetin alpha
(B) Filgrastim (G-CSF)
(C) Iron dextran
(D) Oprelvekin (IL-11)
(E) Vitamin B_{12}

10. Twenty months after finishing her chemotherapy, the woman had a relapse of breast cancer. The cancer was now unresponsive to standard doses of chemotherapy. The decision was made to treat the patient with high-dose chemotherapy followed by autologous stem cell transplantation. Which of the following drugs is most likely to be used to mobilize the peripheral blood stem cells needed for the patient's autologous stem cell transplantation?
(A) Erythropoietin
(B) Filgrastim (G-CSF)
(C) Folic acid
(D) Intrinsic factor
(E) Oprelvekin (interleukin-11)

ANSWERS

1. Deficiencies of folic acid or vitamin B_{12} are the most common causes of megaloblastic anemia. If a patient with this type of anemia has a normal serum vitamin B_{12} concentration, folate deficiency is the most likely cause of the anemia. The answer is **C**.

2. Deficiency of folic acid during early pregnancy is associated with increased risk of a neural tube defect in the newborn. In the United States, cereals and grains are supplemented with folic acid in an effort to decrease the incidence of neural tube defects. The answer is **E**.

3. The anemia most commonly associated with pregnancy is iron deficiency microcytic anemia. In this condition, oral iron supplementation is indicated. The answer is **C**.

4. Acute iron poisoning often causes severe gastrointestinal damage resulting from direct corrosive effects, shock from fluid loss in the gastrointestinal

tract, and metabolic acidosis from cellular dysfunction. The answer is **D.**

5. The iron stored in intestinal mucosal cells, macrophages and hepatocytes is in ferritin, a complex of iron and the protein apoferritin. The answer is **A.**

6. The kidney produces erythropoietin; patients with chronic renal insufficiency often require exogenous erythropoietin to avoid chronic anemia. The answer is **C.**

7. Filgrastim (G-CSF) stimulates the production and function of neutrophils, which are important cellular mediators of the innate immune system, the first line of defense against infection. The answer is **E.**

8. Deficiency of vitamin B_{12} (cobalamin) leads to a deficiency in tetrahydrofolate and subsequently a deficiency of the dTMP required for DNA synthesis. Homocysteine and N^5-methyltetrahydrofolate accumulate. The answer is **B.**

9. Oprelvekin (IL-11) stimulates platelet production and decreases the number of platelet transfusions required by patients undergoing bone marrow suppression therapy for cancer. The answer is **D.**

10. The success of transplantation with peripheral blood stem cells depends on infusion of adequate numbers of hematopoietic stem cells. Administration of G-CSF to the donor (in the case of autologous transplantation, the patient who also will be the recipient of the transplantation) greatly increases the number of hematopoietic stem cells harvested from the donor's blood. The answer is **B.**

SKILL KEEPER ANSWERS: ROUTES OF ADMINISTRATION (SEE CHAPTER 1)

All of the hematopoietic growth factors are proteins with molecular weights greater than 15,000. Like other proteinaceous drugs, the growth factors cannot be administered orally because they have such poor bioavailability. Their peptide bonds are destroyed by stomach acid and digestive enzymes.

Injections are required for the intravenous, intramuscular, and subcutaneous routes of administration. The intravenous route offers the fastest onset of drug action and shortest duration of drug action. Because the intravenous route can produce high blood levels, this route of administration has the greatest risk of producing concentration-dependent drug toxicity. Intramuscular injection has a quicker onset of action than subcutaneous injection, and larger volumes of injected fluid can be given. Because protective barriers can be breached by the needle or injection tubing used for drug injection, all 3 of these routes of administration carry a greater risk of infection than does oral drug administration.

CHECKLIST

When you complete this chapter, you should be able to:

☐ Name the 2 most common types of nutritional anemia and, for each, describe the most likely biochemical causes.

☐ Diagram the normal pathways of absorption, transport, and storage of iron in the human body.

☐ Name the anemias for which iron supplementation is indicated and those for which it is contraindicated.

☐ List the acute and chronic toxicities of iron.

☐ Sketch the dTMP cycle and show how deficiency of folic acid or deficiency of vitamin B_{12} affects the normal cycle.

☐ Explain the major hazard involved in the use of folic acid as sole therapy for megaloblastic anemia and indicate on a sketch of the dTMP cycle the biochemical basis of the hazard.

☐ Name 3–5 major hematopoietic growth factors that are used clinically and describe the clinical uses and toxicity of each.

☐ Explain the advantage of covalently attaching polyethylene glycol to filgrastim.

Drugs Used in Coagulation Disorders

34

The drugs used in clotting and bleeding disorders fall into 2 major groups: (1) drugs used to decrease clotting or dissolve clots already present in patients at risk for vascular occlusion and (2) drugs used to increase clotting in patients with clotting deficiencies. The first group, the anticlotting drugs, includes some of the most commonly used drugs in the United States. Anticlotting drugs are used in the treatment and prevention of myocardial infarction and other acute coronary syndromes, atrial fibrillation, ischemic stroke, and deep vein thrombosis (DVT). Within the anticlotting group, the anticoagulant and thrombolytic drugs are effective in treatment of both venous and arterial thrombosis, whereas antiplatelet drugs are used primarily for treatment of arterial disease.

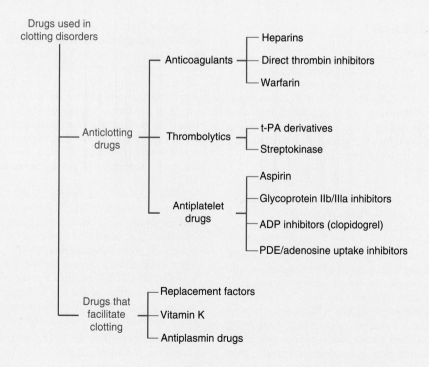

<table>
<tr><td colspan="2" align="center">HIGH-YIELD TERMS TO LEARN</td></tr>
<tr><td>Activated partial thromboplastin time (aPTT) test</td><td>Laboratory test used to monitor the anticoagulant effect of unfractionated heparin and direct thrombin inhibitors; prolonged when drug effect is adequate</td></tr>
<tr><td>Antithrombin III</td><td>An endogenous anticlotting protein that irreversibly inactivates thrombin and factor Xa. Its enzymatic action is markedly accelerated by the heparins</td></tr>
<tr><td>Clotting cascade</td><td>System of serine proteases and substrates in the blood that provides rapid generation of clotting factors in response to blood vessel damage</td></tr>
<tr><td>Glycoprotein IIb/IIIa (GPIIb/IIIa)</td><td>A protein complex on the surface of platelets. When activated, it aggregates platelets primarily by binding to fibrin. Endogenous factors including thromboxane A_2, ADP, and serotonin initiate a signaling cascade that activates GPIIb/IIIa</td></tr>
<tr><td>Heparin-induced thrombocytopenia (HIT)</td><td>A hypercoagulable state plus thrombocytopenia that occurs in a small number of individuals treated with unfractionated heparin for a week or more</td></tr>
<tr><td>LMW heparins</td><td>Fractionated preparations of heparin of molecular weight 2000–6000. Unfractionated heparin has a molecular weight range of 5000–30,000</td></tr>
<tr><td>Prothrombin time (PT) test</td><td>Laboratory test used to monitor the anticoagulant effect of warfarin; prolonged test when drug effect is adequate</td></tr>
</table>

ANTICOAGULANTS

A. CLASSIFICATION

Anticoagulants inhibit the formation of fibrin clots. Three major types of anticoagulants are available: heparin and related products, which must be used parenterally; direct thrombin inhibitors, which also must be used parenterally; and the orally active coumarin derivatives (eg, warfarin). Comparative properties of the heparins and warfarin are shown in Table 34–1.

B. HEPARIN

1. Chemistry—Heparin is a large sulfated polysaccharide polymer obtained from animal sources. Each batch contains molecules of varying size, with an average molecular weight of 15,000–20,000. Heparin is highly acidic and can be neutralized by basic molecules (eg, **protamine**). Heparin is given intravenously or subcutaneously to avoid the risk of hematoma associated with intramuscular injection.

Low-molecular-weight (LMW) fractions of heparin (eg, **enoxaparin**) have molecular weights of 2000–6000. LMW heparins have greater bioavailability and longer durations of action than unfractionated heparin; thus, doses can be given less frequently (eg, once or twice a day). They are given subcutaneously. **Fondaparinux** is a small synthetic drug that contains the biologically active pentasaccharide present in unfractionated and LMW heparins. It is administered subcutaneously once daily.

2. Mechanism and effects—Unfractionated heparin binds to endogenous **antithrombin III** (ATIII) via a key saccharide sequence. The heparin–ATIII complex combines with and irreversibly inactivates thrombin and several other factors, particularly factor Xa (Figure 34–1). In the presence of heparin, antithrombin III proteolyzes thrombin and factor Xa approximately 1000-fold faster than in its absence. Because it acts on preformed blood components, heparin provides anticoagulation immediately after administration. The action of heparin is monitored with the **activated partial thromboplastin time (aPTT)** laboratory test.

LMW heparins and fondaparinux, like unfractionated heparin, bind ATIII. These complexes have the same inhibitory effect on factor Xa as the unfractionated heparin–ATIII complex. However, the short-chain heparin–ATIII and fondaparinux–ATIII complexes provide a more selective action because they fail to affect thrombin. The aPTT test does not reliably measure the anticoagulant effect of the LMW heparins and fondaparinux; this is a potential problem, especially in renal failure, in which their clearance may be decreased.

3. Clinical use—Because of its rapid effect, heparin is used when anticoagulation is needed immediately (eg, when starting therapy). Common uses include treatment of DVT, pulmonary embolism, and acute myocardial infarction. Heparin is used in combination with thrombolytics for revascularization and in combination with glycoprotein IIb/IIIa inhibitors during angioplasty

Table 34–1. Properties of heparins and warfarin.

Property	Heparins	Warfarin
Structure	Large acidic polymers	Small lipid-soluble molecule
Route of administration	Parenteral	Oral
Site of action	Blood	Liver
Onset of action	Rapid (minutes)	Slow (days); limited by half-lives of preexisting normal factors
Mechanism of action	Activates antithrombin III, which proteolyzes factors including thrombin and factor Xa	Impairs posttranslational modification of factors II, VII, IX and X
Monitoring	aPTT for unfractionated heparin but not LMW heparins	PT
Antidote	Protamine for unfractionated heparin but much less effective for LMW heparins	Vitamin K_1, plasma
Use	Mostly acute, over days	Chronic, over weeks to months
Use in pregnancy	Yes	No

and placement of coronary stents. Because it does not cross the placental barrier, it is the drug of choice when an anticoagulant must be used in pregnancy. LMW heparins and fondaparinux have similar clinical applications.

4. Toxicity—Increased bleeding is the most common adverse effect of heparin and related molecules; the bleeding may result in hemorrhagic stroke. **Protamine** can lessen the risk of serious bleeding that can result

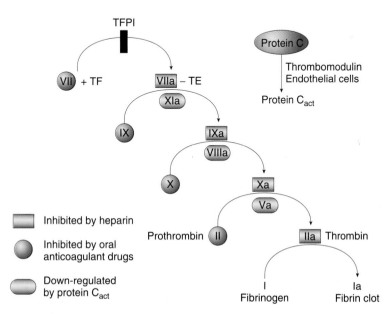

Figure 34–1. A model of the coagulation cascade, including its inhibition by the activated form of the protein C. Tissue factor (TF) is important in initiating the cascade. Tissue factor pathway inhibitor (TFPI) inhibits the action of the VIIa–TF complex. (Reproduced, with permission, from Katzung BG, editor: *Basic & Clinical Pharmacology,* 10th ed. McGraw-Hill, 2007.)

from excessive unfractionated heparin. Protamine only partially reverses the effects of LMW heparins and does not affect the action of fondaparinux. Unfractionated heparin causes moderate transient thrombocytopenia in many patients and severe thrombocytopenia and thrombosis (heparin-induced thrombocytopenia or HIT) in a small percentage of patients who produce an antibody that binds to a complex of heparin and platelet factor 4. LMW heparins and fondaparinux are less likely to cause this immune-mediated thrombocytopenia. Prolonged use of unfractionated heparin is associated with osteoporosis.

C. DIRECT THROMBIN INHIBITORS

1. Chemistry and pharmacokinetics—Direct thrombin inhibitors are based on proteins made by *Hirudo medicinalis,* the medicinal leech. **Lepirudin** is the recombinant form of the leech protein hirudin, while **desirudin** and **bivalirudin** are modified forms of hirudin. **Argatroban** is a small molecule with a short half-life. All 4 drugs are administered parenterally.

2. Mechanism and effects—The protein analogs of lepirudin bind simultaneously to the active site of thrombin and to thrombin substrates. Argatroban binds solely to the thrombin active site. Unlike the heparins, these drugs inhibit both soluble thrombin and the thrombin enmeshed within developing clots. Bivalirudin also inhibits platelet activation.

3. Clinical use—Direct thrombin inhibitors are used as alternatives to heparin primarily in patients with heparin-induced thrombocytopenia. Bivalirudin also is used in combination with aspirin during percutaneous coronary angioplasty. Like unfractionated heparin, the action of these drugs is monitored with the aPTT laboratory test.

4. Toxicity—Like other anticoagulants, the direct thrombin inhibitors can cause bleeding. No reversal agents exist. Prolonged infusion of lepirudin can induce antibodies that form a complex with lepirudin and prolong its action, and can induce anaphylactic reactions.

D. WARFARIN AND OTHER COUMARIN ANTICOAGULANTS

1. Chemistry and pharmacokinetics—**Warfarin** and other coumarin anticoagulants are small, lipid-soluble molecules that are readily absorbed after oral administration. Warfarin is highly bound to plasma proteins (>99%), and its elimination depends on metabolism by cytochrome P450 enzymes.

2. Mechanism and effects—Warfarin and other coumarins interfere with the normal posttranslational modification of clotting factors in the liver, a process that depends on vitamin K. The vitamin K-dependent factors include thrombin and factors VII, IX, and X (Figure 34–1). Because the clotting factors have half-lives

of 8–60 h in the plasma, an anticoagulant effect is observed only after sufficient time has passed for elimination of the normal preformed factors. The action of warfarin can be reversed with vitamin K, but recovery requires the synthesis of new normal clotting factors and is, therefore, slow (6–24 h). More rapid reversal can be achieved by transfusion with fresh or frozen plasma that contains normal clotting factors. The effect of warfarin is monitored by the **prothrombin time** (**PT**) test.

3. Clinical use—Warfarin is used for chronic anticoagulation in all of the clinical situations described previously for heparin except in pregnant women.

4. Toxicity—Bleeding is the most important adverse effect of warfarin. Early in therapy, a period of hypercoagulability with subsequent dermal vascular necrosis can occur. This is due to deficiency of protein C, an endogenous vitamin K-dependent anticoagulant with a short half-life. Warfarin can cause bone defects and hemorrhage in the developing fetus and, therefore, is contraindicated in pregnancy.

Because warfarin has a narrow therapeutic window, its involvement in drug interactions is of major concern. Cytochrome P450-inducing drugs (eg, carbamazepine, phenytoin, rifampin, barbiturates) increase warfarin's clearance and reduce the anticoagulant effect of a given dose. Cytochrome P450 inhibitors (eg, amiodarone, selective serotonin reuptake inhibitors, cimetidine) reduce warfarin's clearance and increase the anticoagulant effect of a given dose.

THROMBOLYTIC AGENTS

A. CLASSIFICATION AND PROTOTYPES

The thrombolytic drugs used most commonly are either forms of the endogenous **tissue plasminogen activator** (**t-PA**; eg, **alteplase**, tenecteplase, and reteplase) or a protein synthesized by streptococci (**streptokinase**). All are given intravenously.

B. MECHANISM OF ACTION

Plasmin is an endogenous fibrinolytic enzyme that degrades clots by splitting fibrin into fragments (Figure 34–2). The thrombolytic enzymes catalyze the conversion of the inactive precursor, **plasminogen**, to plasmin.

1. Tissue plasminogen activator—t-PA is an enzyme that directly converts plasminogen to plasmin (Figure 34–2). It has little activity unless it is bound to fibrin, which, in theory, should make it selective for the plasminogen that has already bound to fibrin (ie, in a clot) and should result in less danger of widespread production of plasmin and spontaneous bleeding. In fact, t-PA's selectivity appears to be quite limited. **Alteplase** is normal human plasminogen activator. **Reteplase** is a mutated form of human t-PA with similar effects but a slightly faster onset of action and longer duration of action. **Tenecteplase** is another mutated form of t-PA with a longer half-life.

2. Streptokinase—Streptokinase is obtained from bacterial cultures. Although not itself an enzyme, streptokinase forms a complex with endogenous plasminogen; the plasminogen in this complex undergoes a conformational change that allows it to rapidly convert free plasminogen into plasmin. Unlike the forms of t-PA, streptokinase does not show selectivity for fibrin-bound plasminogen.

C. CLINICAL USE

The major application of the thrombolytic agents is as an alternative to percutaneous coronary angioplasty in the emergency treatment of coronary artery thrombosis. Under ideal conditions (ie, treatment within 6 h), these agents can promptly recanalize the occluded coronary vessel. Very prompt use (ie, within 3 h of the first symptoms) of t-PA in patients with ischemic stroke is associated with a significantly better clinical outcome. Cerebral hemorrhage must be positively ruled out before such use. The thrombolytic agents are also used in cases of severe pulmonary embolism.

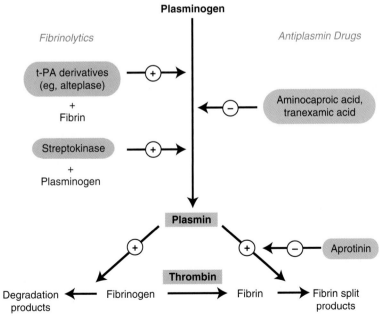

Figure 34–2. Diagram of the fibrinolytic system. The useful thrombolytic drugs are shown on the left. These drugs increase the formation of plasmin, the major fibrinolytic enzyme. Antiplasmin drugs are shown on the right. Aminocaproic acid and tranexamic acid inhibit plasmin formation, while aprotinin inhibits plasmin's enzymatic activity. (Redrawn and reproduced, with permission, from Katzung BG, editor: *Basic & Clinical Pharmacology,* 10th ed. McGraw-Hill, 2007.)

D. Toxicity

Bleeding is the most important hazard and has about the same frequency with all of these drugs. Cerebral hemorrhage is the most serious manifestation. Streptokinase, a bacterial protein, can evoke the production of antibodies that cause it to lose its effectiveness or induce severe allergic reactions on subsequent therapy. Patients who have had streptococcal infections may have preformed antibodies to the drug. Because they are human proteins, the recombinant forms of t-PA are not subject to this problem. However, they are much more expensive than streptokinase and not much more effective.

ANTIPLATELET DRUGS

Platelet aggregation contributes to the clotting process and is especially important in clots that form in the arterial circulation. Platelets appear to play a central role in pathologic coronary and cerebral artery occlusion. Platelet aggregation is triggered by a variety of endogenous mediators that include the prostaglandin thromboxane, adenosine diphosphate (ADP), thrombin, and fibrin. Substances that increase intracellular cyclic adenosine monophosphate (cAMP; eg, the prostaglandin prostacyclin, adenosine) inhibit platelet aggregation.

A. Classification and Prototypes

Antiplatelet drugs include **aspirin** and other NSAIDs, glycoprotein IIb/IIIa receptor inhibitors (**abciximab, tirofiban,** and **eptifibatide**), antagonists of ADP receptors (**clopidogrel** and **ticlopidine**), and inhibitors of phosphodiesterase 3 (**dipyridamole** and **cilostazol**) (Figure 34–3).

B. Mechanism of Action

Aspirin and other NSAIDs inhibit thromboxane synthesis by blocking the enzyme cyclooxygenase (COX; Chapter 18). Thromboxane A_2 is a potent stimulator of platelet aggregation. Aspirin, an irreversible COX inhibitor, is particularly effective. Because platelets lack the machinery for synthesis of new protein, inhibition by aspirin persists for several days, until new platelets are formed. Other NSAIDs, which cause a less persistent antiplatelet effect (hours), are not employed as antiplatelet drugs and, in fact, can interfere with the antiplatelet effect of aspirin when used in combination with aspirin.

Abciximab is a monoclonal antibody that reversibly inhibits the binding of fibrin and other ligands to the platelet **glycoprotein IIb/IIIa receptor,** a cell surface protein involved in platelet cross-linking. Eptifibatide and tirofiban also reversibly block the glycoprotein IIb/IIIa receptor.

Clopidogrel and the older drug ticlopidine irreversibly inhibit the platelet ADP receptor and thereby prevent ADP-mediated platelet aggregation.

Dipyridamole and the newer cilostazol appear to have a dual mechanism of action. They prolong the platelet-inhibiting action of intracellular cAMP by inhibiting phosphodiesterase 3, an enzyme that degrades cAMP. They also inhibit the uptake of adenosine by endothelial cells and erythrocytes and thereby increase the plasma concentration of adenosine. Adenosine acts through platelet adenosine A_2 receptors to increase platelet cAMP and inhibit aggregation.

C. Clinical Use

Aspirin is used to prevent further infarcts in individuals who have had 1 or more myocardial infarcts and may also reduce the incidence of first infarcts. The drug is used extensively to prevent transient ischemic attacks (TIAs), ischemic stroke, and other thrombotic events.

The glycoprotein IIb/IIIa inhibitors prevent restenosis after coronary angioplasty and are used in acute coronary syndromes (eg, unstable angina and non-Q-wave acute myocardial infarction).

Clopidogrel and ticlopidine are effective in preventing TIAs and ischemic strokes, especially in patients who cannot tolerate aspirin. Clopidogrel is routinely used to prevent thrombosis in patients who have recently received a coronary artery stent.

Dipyridamole and cilostazol are used to treat intermittent claudication, a manifestation of peripheral arterial disease.

D. Toxicity

Aspirin and other NSAIDs cause gastrointestinal and CNS effects (Chapter 36). All antiplatelet drugs significantly enhance the effects of other anticlotting agents. The major toxicities of the glycoprotein IIb/IIIa receptor blocking drugs are bleeding and, with chronic use, thrombocytopenia. Ticlopidine is used rarely because it causes bleeding in up to 5% of patients, severe neutropenia in about 1%, and very rarely **thrombotic thrombocytopenic purpura** (TTP), a syndrome characterized by the disseminated formation of small thrombi, platelet consumption, and thrombocytopenia. Clopidogrel is less hematotoxic. The most common adverse effects of dipyridamole and cilostazol are headaches and palpitations.

DRUGS USED IN BLEEDING DISORDERS

Inadequate blood clotting can result from vitamin K deficiency, genetically determined errors of clotting factor synthesis (eg, hemophilia), a variety of drug-induced conditions, and thrombocytopenia. Treatment involves administration of vitamin K, preformed clotting factors, or antiplasmin drugs. Thrombocytopenia can be treated by administration of platelets or by administration of oprelvekin, the recombinant form of the megakaryocyte growth factor interleukin-11 (Chapter 33).

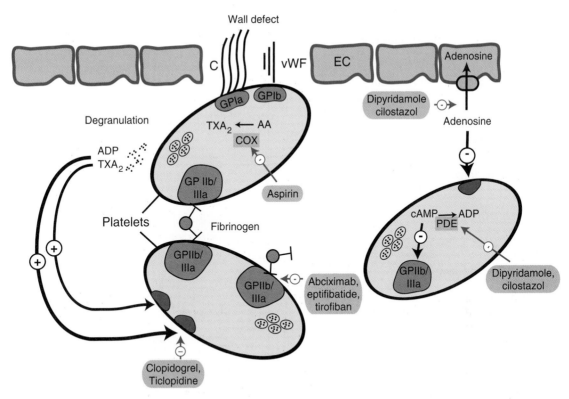

Figure 34–3. Antiplatelet drug mechanisms. At the site of blood vessel wall defects and damage endothelial cells (EC), the exposure of collagen (C) and von Willebrand factor (vWF) activates platelets by binding to platelet membrane glycoproteins (GP) 1a and 1b. Platelet activation triggers degranulation and the release of adenosine diphosphate (ADP) and thromboxane A_2 (TXA_2), which act through platelet receptors to modify GPIIb/IIIa so it is able to bind fibrinogen and cross-link platelets. Aspirin inhibits the production of TXA_2 by irreversibly inhibiting cyclooxygenase (COX). Abciximab, eptifibatide, and tirofiban inhibit the binding of GPIIb/IIIa to fibrinogen, while clopidogrel and ticlopidine irreversibly inhibit the ADP receptor. Dipyridamole and cilostazol inhibit GPIIb/IIIa activation by inhibiting the phosphodiesterase enzyme (PDE) that degrades cAMP and by inhibiting the uptake by EC of adenosine, an endogenous inhibitor of platelet function. (Redrawn and reproduced, with permission, from Katzung BG, editor: *Basic & Clinical Pharmacology,* 10th ed. McGraw-Hill, 2007.)

A. VITAMIN K

Deficiency of vitamin K, a fat-soluble vitamin, is most common in older individuals with abnormalities of fat absorption and in newborns, who are at risk of vitamin K deficiency bleeding. The deficiency is readily treated with oral or parenteral **phytonadione (vitamin K_1).** In the United States, all newborns receive an injection of phytonadione. Large doses of vitamin K_1 are used to reverse the anticoagulant effect of excess warfarin.

B. CLOTTING FACTORS AND DESMOPRESSIN

The most important agents used to treat hemophilia are fresh plasma and purified human blood clotting factors, especially **factor VIII** (for hemophilia A) and **factor IX** (for hemophilia B), which are either purified from blood products or produced by recombinant DNA technology. These products are extremely expensive and carry a risk of immunologic reactions and, in the case of factors purified from blood products, infection (although most known bloodborne pathogens are removed by chemical treatment of the plasma extracts.)

The vasopressin V_2 receptor agonist **desmopressin acetate** (Chapter 37) increases the plasma concentration of von Willebrand factor and factor VIII. It is used to prepare patients with mild hemophilia A or von Willebrand disease for elective surgery.

C. ANTIPLASMIN AGENTS

Antiplasmin agents are valuable for the prevention or management of acute bleeding episodes in patients with

KEY DRUGS		
Subclass	**Prototypes**	**Other Significant Agents**
Anticoagulants		
Heparins	Unfractionated heparin	LMW heparins (enoxaparin, dalteparin, tinzaparin)
Direct thrombin inhibitors	Lepirudin	Bivalirudin, argatroban
	Fondaparinux	
Coumadin derivatives	Warfarin	
Thrombolytic drugs	Alteplase	Reteplase, tenecteplase
	Streptokinase	
Antiplatelet drugs	Aspirin	
	Abciximab	Eptifibatide, tirofiban
	Clopidogrel	Ticlopidine
	Dipyridamole	Cilostazol
Drugs used in bleeding disorders		
Vitamin K	Phytonadione (vitamin K_1)	
Drugs that increase clotting factor concentrations	Factor VIII	Factor IX
	Desmopressin	
Antiplasmin drugs	Aminocaproic acid	Tranexamic acid
	Aprotinin	

hemophilia and others with a high risk of bleeding disorders. **Aminocaproic acid** and **tranexamic acid** are orally active agents that inhibit fibrinolysis by inhibiting plasminogen activation (Figure 34–2). **Aprotinin** is a serine protease inhibitor that inhibits fibrinolysis by plasmin and by the plasmin-streptokinase complex. It is approved for use in patients undergoing coronary artery bypass grafting who are at high risk of excessive blood loss. Its use is associated with increased risk of myocardial infarction, stroke, and renal damage.

QUESTIONS

1–3. A 58-year-old business executive is brought to the emergency department 2 h after the onset of severe chest pain during a vigorous tennis game. She has a history of poorly controlled mild hypertension and elevated blood cholesterol but does not smoke. ECG changes confirm the diagnosis of myocardial infarction. The decision is made to attempt to open her occluded artery.

1. Conversion of plasminogen to plasmin is accelerated by
   (A) Aminocaproic acid
   (B) Heparin
   (C) Lepirudin
   (D) Reteplase
   (E) Warfarin

2. If a fibrinolytic drug is used for treatment of this woman's acute myocardial infarction, the adverse drug effect that is most likely to occur is
   (A) Acute renal failure
   (B) Development of antiplatelet antibodies
   (C) Encephalitis secondary to liver dysfunction
   (D) Hemorrhagic stroke
   (E) Neutropenia

3. If this patient undergoes a percutaneous coronary angiography procedure and placement of a stent in a coronary blood vessel, she may be given eptifibatide. The mechanism of eptifibatide anticlotting action is
   (A) Activation of antithrombin III
   (B) Blockade of posttranslational modification of clotting factors
   (C) Inhibition of thromboxane production
   (D) Irreversible inhibition of platelet ADP receptors
   (E) Reversible inhibition of glycoprotein IIb/IIIa receptors

4. The following graph shows the plasma concentration of free warfarin as a function of time in weeks for a

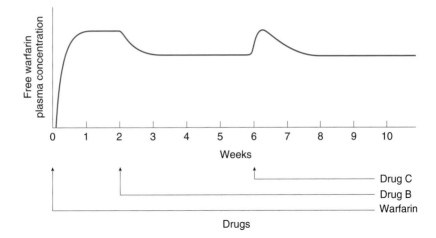

patient who was treated with 2 other agents, drugs B and C, on a daily basis at constant dosage starting at the times shown. The most accurate explanation for the observed changes in warfarin concentration is that

(A) Drug B displaces warfarin from plasma proteins; drug C displaces warfarin from tissue binding sites

(B) Drug B inhibits hepatic metabolism of warfarin; drug C displaces drug B from tissue binding sites

(C) Drug B stimulates hepatic metabolism of warfarin; drug C displaces warfarin from plasma protein

(D) Drug B increases renal clearance of warfarin; drug C inhibits hepatic metabolism of drug B

5–7. A 65-year-old man is brought to the emergency department 30 min after the onset of right-sided weakness and aphasia (difficulty speaking). Imaging studies ruled out cerebral hemorrhage as the cause of his acute symptoms of stroke.

5. Prompt administration of which of the following drugs is most likely to improve this patient's clinical outcome?

(A) Abciximab
(B) Alteplase
(C) Factor VIII
(D) Streptokinase
(E) Vitamin K

6. Over the next 2 days, the patient's symptoms resolved completely. To prevent a recurrence of this disease, the patient is most likely to be treated indefinitely with

(A) Aminocaproic acid
(B) Aspirin
(C) Enoxaparin
(D) Lepirudin
(E) Warfarin

7. If the patient is unable to tolerate the drug identified in Question 6, he may be treated with clopidogrel. Relative to ticlopidine, clopidogrel

(A) Has a shorter duration of action
(B) Is less likely to cause neutropenia
(C) Is more likely to induce antiplatelet antibodies
(D) Is more likely to precipitate serious bleeding
(E) Will have a greater antiplatelet effect

8–9. A 67-year-old woman presents with pain in her left thigh muscle. Duplex ultrasonography indicates the presence of deep vein thrombosis (DVT) in the affected limb.

8. The decision was made to treat this woman with enoxaparin. Relative to unfractionated heparin, enoxaparin

(A) Can be used without monitoring the patient's aPTT
(B) Has a shorter duration of action
(C) Is less likely to have a teratogenic effect
(D) Is more likely to be given intravenously
(E) Is more likely to cause thrombosis and thrombocytopenia

9. During the next week, the patient was started on warfarin and her heparin was discontinued. Two months later, she returned after a severe nosebleed. Laboratory analysis revealed an INR (international normalized ratio) of 7.0 (INR value in such a warfarin-treated patient should be 2.5–3.5). To prevent severe hemorrhage, the warfarin should be discontinued and this patient should be treated immediately with

(A) Aminocaproic acid
(B) Desmopressin
(C) Factor VIII
(D) Protamine
(E) Vitamin K_1

10. A patient develops severe thrombocytopenia in response to treatment with unfractionated heparin and still requires parenteral anticoagulation. The patient is most likely to be treated with

(A) Abciximab
(B) Aprotinin
(C) Lepirudin
(D) Plasminogen
(E) Vitamin K_2

ANSWERS

1. Reteplase is the only thrombolytic drug listed. Heparin and warfarin are anticoagulants that affect activation or formation of clotting factors. Lepirudin is a direct inhibitor of thrombin, and aminocaproic acid is an inhibitor, not an activator, of the conversion of plasminogen to plasmin. The answer is **D**.

2. The most common serious adverse effect of the fibrolytics is bleeding, especially in the cerebral circulation. The fibrinolytics do not usually have serious effects on the renal, hepatic, or hematologic systems. Unlike heparin, they do not induce antiplatelet antibodies. The answer is **D**.

3. Eptifibatide is a reversible inhibitor of glycoprotein IIb/IIIa, a protein on the surface of platelets that serves as a key regulator of platelet aggregation. Glycoprotein IIb/IIIa receptor antagonists help prevent platelet-induced occlusion of coronary stents. The answer is **E**.

4. A drug that increases metabolism (clearance) of the anticoagulant will lower the steady-state plasma concentration (both free and bound forms), whereas one that displaces the anticoagulant will increase the plasma level of the free form only until elimination of the drug has again lowered it to the steady-state level. The answer is **C**.

5. Alteplase improves the clinical outcome in patients with ischemic stroke if given within 3 h after the onset of symptoms, after ruling out hemorrhagic stroke. Use of streptokinase results in unacceptably high rates of bleeding. Glycoprotein IIb/IIIa receptor inhibitors like abciximab have not been tested in ischemic stroke. The answer is **B**.

6. Aspirin, an irreversible inhibitor of platelet cyclooxygenase, prevents recurrence of TIAs and ischemic stroke. The answer is **B**.

7. Ticlopidine and clopidogrel have similar mechanisms of action and therapeutic efficacy. The key difference between these 2 drugs is that clopidogrel is less likely to cause hematologic adverse effects (neutropenia, TTP) and, therefore, does not require routine monitoring of blood cell counts during therapy. The answer is **B**.

8. Enoxaparin is an LMW heparin. LMW heparins have a longer half-life than standard heparin and a more consistent relationship between dose and therapeutic effect. Enoxaparin is given subcutaneously, not intravenously. It is less, not more, likely to cause thrombosis and thrombocytopenia. Neither LMW heparins nor standard heparin are teratogenic. The aPTT is not useful for monitoring the effects of LMW heparins. The answer is **A**.

9. The elevated INR indicates excessive anticoagulation with a high risk of hemorrhage. Warfarin should be discontinued and vitamin K_1 administered to accelerate formation of vitamin K-dependent factors. The answer is **E**.

10. Direct thrombin inhibitors such as lepirudin and argatroban provide parenteral anticoagulation similar to that achieved with heparin, but the direct thrombin inhibitors do not induce formation of antiplatelet antibodies. The answer is **C**.

SKILL KEEPER ANSWERS: TREATMENT OF ATRIAL FIBRILLATION (SEE CHAPTERS 13 AND 14)

1. *The β adrenoceptor-blocking drugs (class II; eg, propranolol, acebutolol) and calcium channel-blocking drugs (class IV; eg, verapamil, diltiazem) are useful for treating atrial fibrillation because they slow atrioventricular (AV) nodal conduction and thereby help control ventricular rate. Digoxin is also sometimes used because it increases the effective refractory period in AV nodal tissue and decreases AV nodal conduction velocity.*

2. *With warfarin, one is always concerned about pharmacodynamic and pharmacokinetic drug interactions. None of these antiarrhythmic drugs are likely to cause a pharmacodynamic interaction with warfarin. However, many other drugs inhibit cytochrome P450 enzymes and increase warfarin's antithrombotic effect. Patients taking such drugs usually need to decrease their dose of warfarin.*

CHECKLIST

When you complete this chapter, you should be able to:

☐ List the 3 major classes of anticlotting drugs and compare their utility in venous and arterial thromboses.

☐ Name 3 types of anticoagulants and describe their mechanisms of action.

☐ Explain why the onset of warfarin's action is relatively slow.

☐ Compare the oral anticoagulants, standard heparin, and LMW heparins in terms of their pharmacokinetics, mechanisms, and toxicities.

☐ Give several examples of warfarin's role in pharmacokinetic and pharmacodynamic drug interactions.

☐ Diagram the role of activated platelets at the site of a damaged blood vessel wall and show where the 4 major classes of antiplatelet drugs act.

☐ Compare the pharmacokinetics, clinical uses, and toxicities of the major antiplatelet drugs.

☐ List 3 different drugs used to treat disorders of excessive bleeding.

Drugs Used in the Treatment of Hyperlipidemias

35

Atherosclerosis is the leading cause of death in the Western world. Drugs discussed in this chapter prevent the sequelae of atherosclerosis (heart attacks, angina, peripheral arterial disease, and stroke) and decrease mortality in patients with a history of cardiovascular disease and hyperlipidemia. Although the drugs are generally safe and effective, they can cause problems, including drug–drug interactions and toxic reactions in skeletal muscle and the liver.

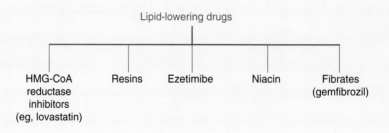

HYPERLIPOPROTEINEMIA

A. PATHOGENESIS

Premature or accelerated development of atherosclerosis is strongly associated with elevated levels of certain plasma lipoproteins, especially the low-density lipoproteins (LDL) that participate in cholesterol transport. A *depressed* level of high-density lipoproteins (HDL) is also associated with increased risk of atherosclerosis. In some families, hypertriglyceridemia is similarly correlated with atherosclerosis. Chylomicronemia, the occurrence of chylomicrons in the serum while fasting, is a recessive trait that is correlated with a high incidence of acute pancreatitis and managed by restriction of total fat intake (Table 35–1).

Regulation of plasma lipoprotein levels involves a complex interplay of dietary fat intake, hepatic processing, and utilization in peripheral tissues (Figure 35–1). Primary disturbances in regulation occur in a number of

genetic conditions involving mutations in apolipoproteins, their receptors, transport mechanisms, and lipid-metabolizing enzymes. Secondary disturbances are associated with a Western diet, many endocrine conditions, and diseases of the liver or kidneys.

B. TREATMENT STRATEGIES

1. Diet—Cholesterol and saturated fats are the primary dietary factors that contribute to elevated levels of plasma lipoproteins. Dietary measures designed to reduce the total intake of these substances are the first method of management and may be sufficient to reduce lipoprotein levels to a safe range. Because alcohol raises triglyceride and very-low-density lipoprotein (VLDL) levels, it should be avoided by patients with hypertriglyceridemia.

2. Drugs—For an individual patient, the choice of drug treatment is based upon the lipid abnormality. The drugs that are most effective at lowering LDL cholesterol include

HIGH-YIELD TERMS TO LEARN

Lipoproteins	Macromolecular complexes in the blood that serve to transport lipids
Apolipoproteins	Proteins located on the surface of lipoproteins; they play critical roles in the regulation of lipoprotein metabolism and uptake into cells
Low-density lipoprotein (LDL)	Cholesterol-rich lipoprotein whose regulated uptake by hepatocytes and other cells requires functional LDL receptors; elevated LDL concentrations are associated with atherosclerosis
High-density lipoprotein (HDL)	Cholesterol-rich lipoprotein that transports cholesterol from the tissues to the liver; low concentrations are associated with atherosclerosis
Very-low-density lipoprotein (VLDL)	Triglyceride- and cholesterol-rich lipoprotein secreted by the liver that transports triglycerides to the periphery; precursor of LDL
HMG-CoA reductase	3-Hydroxy-3-methylglutaryl-coenzyme A reductase; the enzyme that catalyzes the rate-limiting step in cholesterol biosynthesis
Lipoprotein lipase (LPL)	An enzyme found primarily on the surface of endothelial cells. It clips off free fatty acids from triglycerides in lipoproteins; the free fatty acids are taken up into cells
Proliferator-activated receptor-alpha (PPAR-α)	One of a family of nuclear transcription regulators that participates in the regulation of metabolic processes

the HMG-CoA reductase inhibitors, resins, ezetimibe, and niacin. The fibric acid derivatives (eg, gemfibrozil) and niacin are most effective at lowering triglyceride and VLDL concentrations and raising HDL cholesterol concentrations (Table 35–2).

HMG-CoA REDUCTASE INHIBITORS

A. MECHANISM AND EFFECTS

The rate-limiting step in hepatic cholesterol synthesis is conversion of hydroxymethylglutaryl coenzyme A (**HMG-CoA**) to mevalonate by HMG-CoA reductase. The "**statins**" are structural analogs of HMG-CoA that competitively inhibit the enzyme (Figure 35–2). Lovastatin and simvastatin are prodrugs, whereas the other HMG-CoA reductase inhibitors (atorvastatin, fluvastatin, pravastatin, rosuvastatin) are active as given.

Although the inhibition of hepatic cholesterol synthesis contributes a small amount to the total serum cholesterol-lowering effect of these drugs, a much greater effect derives from the response to a reduction in a tightly regulated hepatic pool of cholesterol. The liver compensates by increasing the number of high-affinity LDL receptors, which clear LDL and VLDL remnants from the blood (Figure 35–1). HMG-CoA reductase inhibitors also have direct anti-atherosclerotic effects, and it has been shown that they prevent bone loss.

B. CLINICAL USE

Statins can reduce LDL cholesterol levels dramatically (Table 35–2), especially when used in combination with other cholesterol-lowering drugs (Table 35–1). These drugs are used commonly because they are effective and well tolerated. Large clinical trials have shown that they reduce the risk of coronary events and mortality in patients with ischemic heart disease.

Rosuvastatin, atorvastatin, and simvastatin have greater maximal efficacy than the other HMG-CoA reductase inhibitors. These drugs also reduce triglycerides and increase HDL cholesterol in patients with triglycerides levels that are >250 mg/dL and with reduced HDL cholesterol levels. Fluvastatin has less maximal efficacy than the other drugs in this group.

C. TOXICITY

Mild elevations of serum aminotransferases are common but are not often associated with hepatic damage. Patients with preexisting liver disease may have more severe reactions. An increase in creatine kinase (released from skeletal muscle) is noted in about 10% of patients; in a few, severe muscle pain and even rhabdomyolysis may occur. HGM-CoA reductase inhibitors are metabolized by the cytochrome P450 system; drugs or foods (eg, grapefruit juice) that inhibit cytochrome P450 activity increase the risk of hepatotoxicity and myopathy. Because of evidence that the HMG-CoA reductase inhibitors are teratogenic, these drugs should be avoided in pregnancy.

Table 35–1. Primary hyperlipoproteinemias and their drug treatment.

Condition/Cause	Manifestations, Cause	Single Drug	Drug Combination
Primary chylomicronemia	Chylomicrons, VLDL increased; deficiency in LPL or apoC-II	Niacin, fibrate	Niacin plus fibrate
Familial hypertriglyceridemia			
Severe	VLDL, chylomicrons increased; decreased clearance of VLDL	Niacin, fibrate	Niacin plus fibrate
Moderate	VLDL increased, chylomicrons may be increased; increased production of VLDL	Niacin, fibrate	
Familial combined hyperlipoproteinemia	Increased hepatic apoB and VLDL production		
	VLDL increased	Niacin, fibrate	
	LDL increased	Niacin, statin, ezetimibe	Two or 3 of the individual drugs
	VLDL, LDL increased	Niacin, reductase inhibitor	Niacin or fibrate plus statin or ezetimibe
Familial dysbetalipoproteinemia	VLDL remnants, chylomicron remnants increased; deficiency in apoE	Fibrate, niacin	Fibrate plus niacin, or niacin plus statin
Familial hypercholesterolemia	LDL increased; defect in LDL receptors		
Heterozygous		Statin, resin, niacin, ezetimibe	Two or 3 of the individual drugs
Homozygous		Niacin, statin, ezetimibe	Niacin plus statin plus ezetimibe

Modified and reproduced, with permission, from Katzung BG, editor: *Basic & Clinical Pharmacology,* 10th ed. McGraw-Hill, 2007.

SKILL KEEPER: ANGINA (SEE CHAPTER 12)

The antihyperlipidemic drugs, especially the HMG-CoA reductase inhibitors, are commonly used to treat patients with ischemic heart disease. One of the most common manifestations of ischemic heart disease and coronary atherosclerosis is angina.

1. *What are the 3 major forms of angina?*
2. *Name the 3 major drug groups used to treat angina and specify which form of angina each is useful for.*

The Skill Keeper Answers appear at the end of the chapter.

RESINS

A. MECHANISM AND EFFECTS

Normally, over 90% of bile acids, metabolites of cholesterol, are reabsorbed in the gastrointestinal tract and returned to the liver for reuse. Bile acid-binding resins (**cholestyramine, colestipol,** and **colesevelam**) are large nonabsorbable polymers that bind bile acids and similar steroids in the intestine and prevent their absorption (Figure 35–2).

By preventing the recycling of bile acids, resins divert hepatic cholesterol to synthesis of new bile acids, thereby reducing the amount of cholesterol in a tightly regulated pool. A compensatory increase in the synthesis of high-affinity LDL receptors increases the removal of LDL lipoproteins from the blood.

The resins cause a modest reduction in LDL cholesterol (Table 35–2) but have little effect on HDL cholesterol or triglycerides. In some patients with a genetic condition that predisposes them to hypertriglyceridemia

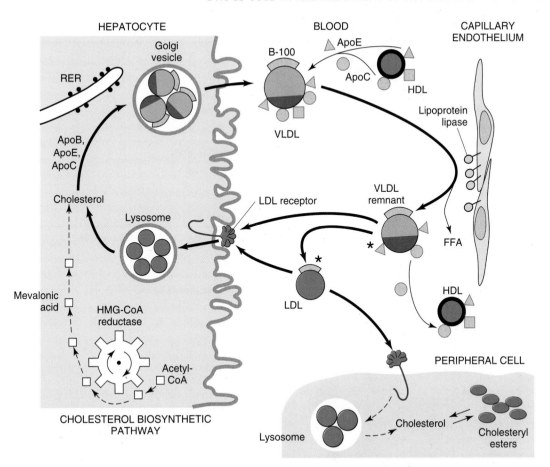

Figure 35–1. Metabolism of lipoproteins of hepatic origin. The heavy arrows show the primary pathways. Nascent VLDLs are secreted via the Golgi apparatus. They acquire additional C apolipoproteins and apo E from HDL. VLDLs are converted to VLDL remnants by lipolysis via lipoprotein lipase associated with capillaries in peripheral tissues. In the process, C apolipoproteins and a portion of the apo E are given back to HDL. Some of the VLDL remnants are converted to LDL by further loss of triglycerides and loss of apo E. A major pathway for LDL degradation involves the endocytosis of LDL by LDL receptors in the liver and the peripheral tissues, for which apo B-100 is the ligand. Dark color denotes cholesteryl esters; light color, triglycerides; the asterisk denotes a functional ligand for LDL receptors; triangles indicate apo E; circles and squares represent C apolipoproteins; RER denotes rough endoplasmic reticulum. (Reproduced, with permission, from Katzung BG, editor: *Basic & Clinical Pharmacology,* 10th ed. McGraw-Hill, 2007.)

and hypercholesterolemia (familial combined hyperlipidemia), resins increase triglycerides and VLDL.

B. CLINICAL USE

The resins are used in patients with hypercholesterolemia (Table 35–1). They have also been used to reduce pruritus in patients with cholestasis and bile salt accumulation.

C. TOXICITY

Adverse effects include bloating, constipation, and an unpleasant gritty taste. Absorption of vitamins (eg,

vitamin K, dietary folates) and drugs (eg, digitalis, thiazides, warfarin, pravastatin, fluvastatin) is impaired by the resins.

EZETIMIBE

A. MECHANISM AND EFFECTS

Ezetimibe is a prodrug that is converted in the liver to the active glucuronide form. This active metabolite inhibits a transporter that mediates gastrointestinal uptake of cholesterol and phytosterols (plant sterols that normally enter gastrointestinal epithelial cell but then are immediately transported back into the intestinal lumen.)

Table 35–2. Lipid-modifying effects of antihyperlipidemic drugs.

Drug or Drug Group	LDL Cholesterol	HDL Cholesterol	Triglycerides
Statins			
Atorvastatin, rosuvastatin, simvastatin	−25 to 50%	+5 to +15%	↓↓
Lovastatin, pravastatin	−25 to −40%	+5 to +10%	↓
Fluvastatin	−20 to −30%	+5 to +10%	↓
Resins	−15 to −25%	+5 to +10%	±[a]
Ezetimibe	−20%	+5%	±
Niacin	−15 to −25%	+25 to +35%	↓↓
Gemfibrozil	10 to −15%[b]	+15 to +20%	↓↓

Modified and reproduced, with permission, from McPhee SJ, Papadakis MA, Tierney LM, editors: *Current Medical Diagnosis & Treatment,* 46th ed. McGraw-Hill, 2006.
LDL, low-density lipoprotein; HDL, high-density lipoprotein; ±, variable, if any.
[a]Resins can increase triglycerides in some patients with combined hyperlipidemia.
[b]Gemfibrozil and other fibrates can increase LDL cholesterol in patients with combined hyperlipidemia.

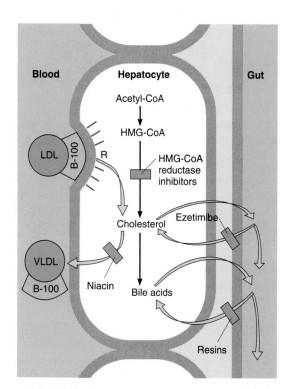

Figure 35–2. Sites of action of cholesterol-lowering drugs. R, LDL receptors. (Reproduced, with permission, from Katzung BG, editor: *Basic & Clinical Pharmacology,* 10th ed. McGraw-Hill, 2007.)

By preventing absorption of dietary cholesterol and cholesterol that is excreted in bile, ezetimibe reduces the cholesterol in the tightly regulated hepatic pool. A compensatory increase in the synthesis of high-affinity LDL receptors increases the removal of LDL lipoproteins from the blood.

As monotherapy, ezetimibe reduces LDL cholesterol by about 18% (Table 35–2). When combined with an HMG-CoA reductase inhibitor, it is even more effective.

B. CLINICAL USE

Ezetimibe is used for treatment of hypercholesterolemia (Table 35–1) and phytosterolemia, a rare genetic disorder that results from impaired export of phytosterols.

C. TOXICITY

Ezetimibe is well tolerated. When combined with HMG-CoA reductase inhibitors, it may increase the risk of hepatic toxicity. Serum concentrations of the glucuronide form are increased by fibrates and reduced by cholestyramine.

NIACIN (NICOTINIC ACID)

A. MECHANISM AND EFFECTS

Through multiple actions, niacin (but not nicotinamide) reduces LDL cholesterol, triglycerides and VLDL, and also increases HDL cholesterol. In the liver, niacin reduces VLDL synthesis, which in turn reduces LDL levels (Figures 35–1 and 35–2). In adipose tissue, niacin appears to activate a signaling pathway that reduces hormone-sensitive lipase activity and thus decreases plasma fatty acid and triglyceride levels. Consequently, LDL formation is reduced, and there is a decrease in LDL cholesterol (see Table 35–2). Increased clearance of VLDL by the lipoprotein lipase associated with capillary endothelial cells has also been demonstrated and probably accounts for the reduction in plasma triglyceride concentrations. Niacin appears to increase HDL levels by increasing plasma concentrations of apoA-I, the major lipoprotein in HDL. Finally, niacin decreases circulating fibrinogen and increases tissue plasminogen activator.

B. CLINICAL USE

Because it lowers serum LDL cholesterol and triglyceride concentrations and increases HDL cholesterol concentrations, niacin has wide clinical utility in the treatment of hypercholesterolemia, hypertriglyceridemia, and low levels of HDL cholesterol (Table 35–1).

C. TOXICITY

Cutaneous flushing is a common adverse effect. Pretreatment with aspirin or other NSAIDs reduces the intensity of this flushing, suggesting that it is mediated by prostaglandin release. Tolerance to the flushing reaction usually develops within a few days. Dose-dependent nausea and abdominal discomfort often occur. Pruritus and other skin conditions are reported. Moderate elevations of liver enzymes and even severe hepatotoxicity may occur. Hyperuricemia occurs in about 20% of patients, and carbohydrate tolerance may be moderately impaired.

FIBRIC ACID DERIVATIVES

A. MECHANISM AND EFFECTS

Fibric acid derivatives (eg, **gemfibrozil**, fenofibrate) are ligands for the peroxisome proliferator-activated receptor-alpha (**PPAR-α**) protein, a receptor that regulates transcription of genes involved in lipid metabolism.

This interaction with PPAR-α results in increased synthesis by adipose tissue of lipoprotein lipase, which associates with capillary endothelial cells and enhances clearance of triglyceride-rich lipoproteins (Figure 35–1). In the liver, fibrates stimulate fatty acid oxidation, which limits the supply of triglycerides and decreases VLDL synthesis. They also decrease expression of apoC-III, which impedes the clearance of VLDL and increases the expression of apoA-I, which in turn increases HDL levels. In most patients, fibrates have little or no effect on LDL concentrations. However, LDL often increases LDL cholesterol in patients with a genetic condition called familial combined hyperlipoproteinemia, which is associated with a combined increase in VLDL and LDL.

B. CLINICAL USE

Gemfibrozil and other fibrates are used to treat hypertriglyceridemia (Table 35–1). Because these drugs have only a modest ability to reduce LDL cholesterol and can increase LDL cholesterol in some patients, they often are combined with other cholesterol-lowering drugs for treatment of patients with elevated concentrations of both LDL and VLDL.

C. TOXICITY

Nausea is the most common adverse effect with all members of this subgroup. Skin rashes are common with gemfibrozil. A few patients show decreases in white blood count or hematocrit, and these drugs can potentiate the action of anticoagulants. There is an increased risk of cholesterol gallstones; these drugs should be used with caution in patients with a history of cholelithiasis. When used in combination with reductase inhibitors, the fibrates significantly increase the risk of myopathy.

COMBINATION THERAPY

All patients with hyperlipidemia are treated first with dietary modification, but this is often insufficient and drugs must be added. Drug combinations are often

---

KEY DRUGS		
Subclass	**Prototypes**	**Other Significant Agents**
HMG-CoA reductase inhibitors	Lovastatin	Atorvastatin, pravastatin, simvastatin, rosuvastatin, fluvastatin
Bile acid-binding resins	Cholestyramine	Colestipol, colesevelam
Cholesterol uptake inhibitor	Ezetimibe	
Nicotinic acid	Niacin	
Fibrates	Gemfibrozil	Fenofibrate

required to achieve the maximum lowering possible with minimum toxicity and to achieve the desired effect on the various lipoproteins (LDL, VLDL, and HDL).

Certain drug combinations provide advantages (Table 35–1), whereas others present specific challenges. Because resins interfere with the absorption of certain HMG-CoA reductase inhibitors (pravastatin, cerivastatin, atorvastatin, and fluvastatin), these must be given at least 1 h before or 4 h after the resins. The combination of reductase inhibitors with either fibrates or niacin increases the risk of myopathy.

QUESTIONS

1. Increased serum levels of which of the following is associated with a *decreased* risk of atherosclerosis?
   (A) Cholesterol
   (B) LDL
   (C) HDL
   (D) Triglyceride
   (E) VLDL

2. A 58-year-old man with a history of hyperlipidemia was treated with a drug. The chart below shows the results of the patient's fasting lipid panel before treatment and 6 mo after initiating drug therapy. Normal values are also shown. Which of the following drugs is most likely to be the one that this man received?
   (A) Colestipol
   (B) Ezetimibe
   (C) Gemfibrozil
   (D) Lovastatin
   (E) Niacin

3–6. A 35-year-old woman appears to have familial combined hyperlipidemia. Her serum concentrations of total cholesterol, LDL cholesterol, and triglyceride are elevated. Her serum concentration of HDL cholesterol is somewhat reduced.

3. Which of the following drugs is most likely to increase this patient's triglyceride and VLDL cholesterol concentrations when used as monotherapy?
   (A) Atorvastatin
   (B) Cholestyramine

   (C) Ezetimibe
   (D) Gemfibrozil
   (E) Niacin

4. If this patient is pregnant, which of the following drugs should be avoided because of a risk of harming the fetus?
   (A) Cholestyramine
   (B) Ezetimibe
   (C) Fenofibrate
   (D) Niacin
   (E) Pravastatin

5. The patient is started on gemfibrozil. A major mechanism of action of gemfibrozil is
   (A) Increased excretion of bile acid salts
   (B) Increased expression of high-affinity LDL receptors
   (C) Increased secretion of VLDL by the liver
   (D) Increased triglyceride hydrolysis by lipoprotein lipase
   (E) Reduced uptake of dietary cholesterol

6. When used as monotherapy, a major toxicity of gemfibrozil is increased risk of
   (A) Bloating and constipation
   (B) Cholelithiasis
   (C) Hyperuricemia
   (D) Liver damage
   (E) Severe cardiac arrhythmia

7–10. A 43-year-old man has heterozygous familial hypercholesterolemia. His serum concentrations of total cholesterol and LDL are markedly elevated. His serum concentration of HDL cholesterol, VLDL cholesterol, and triglycerides are normal or slightly elevated. The patient's mother and older brother died of myocardial infarctions before the age of 50. This patient recently experienced mild chest pain when walking up stairs and has been diagnosed as having angina of effort. The patient is somewhat overweight. He drinks alcohol most evenings and smokes about 1 pack of cigarettes per week.

7. Consumption of alcohol is associated with which of the following changes in serum lipid concentrations?

Time of Lipid Measurement	Triglyceride	Total Cholesterol	LDL Cholesterol	VLDL Cholesterol	HDL Cholesterol
Before treatment	1000	640	120	500	20
Six months after starting treatment	300	275	90	150	40
Normal values	< 150	< 200	< 130	< 30	> 35

(A) Decreased chylomicrons
(B) Decreased HDL cholesterol
(C) Decreased VLDL cholesterol
(D) Increased LDL cholesterol
(E) Increased triglyceride

8. If the patient has a history of gout, which of the following drugs is most likely to exacerbate this condition?
(A) Colestipol
(B) Ezetimibe
(C) Gemfibrozil
(D) Niacin
(E) Simvastatin

9. After being counseled about lifestyle and dietary changes, the patient was started on atorvastatin. During his treatment with atorvastatin, it is important to routinely monitor serum concentrations of
(A) Blood urea nitrogen
(B) Alanine and aspartate aminotransferase
(C) Platelets
(D) Red blood cells
(E) Uric acid

10. Six months after beginning atorvastatin, the patient's total and LDL cholesterol concentrations remained above normal, and he continued to have anginal attacks despite good adherence to his antianginal medications. His physician decided to add ezetimibe. The major recognized mechanism of action of ezetimibe is
(A) Decreased lipid synthesis in adipose tissue
(B) Decreased secretion of VLDL by the liver
(C) Decreased gastrointestinal absorption of cholesterol
(D) Increased endocytosis of HDL by the liver
(E) Increased lipid hydrolysis by lipoprotein lipase

ANSWERS

1. Increased serum concentrations of LDL and total cholesterol are associated with *increased* risk of atherosclerosis. High serum concentration of HDL cholesterol is associated with a decrease in the risk of atherosclerotic disease. The answer is **C.**

2. This patient presents with striking hypertriglyceridemia, elevated VLDL cholesterol, and depressed HDL cholesterol. Six months after drug treatment was started, his triglyceride and VLDL cholesterol have dropped dramatically and his HDL cholesterol level has doubled. The drug that is most likely to have achieved all of these desirable changes, particularly the large increase in HDL cholesterol, is niacin. Although gemfibrozil lowers triglyceride and VLDL concentrations, it does not cause such large increases in HDL cholesterol and decreases in LDL cholesterol. The answer is **E.**

3. In some patients with familial combined hyperlipidemia and elevated VLDL, the resins increase VLDL and triglyceride concentrations even though they also lower LDL cholesterol. The answer is **B.**

4. The HMG-CoA reductase inhibitors are contraindicated in pregnancy because of the risk of teratogenic effects. The answer is **E.**

5. A major mechanism recognized for gemfibrozil is increased activity of the lipoprotein lipase associated with capillary endothelial cells. Gemfibrozil and other fibrates decrease VLDL secretion, presumably by stimulating hepatic fatty acid oxidation. The answer is **D.**

6. A major toxicity of the fibrates is increased risk of gallstone formation, which may be due to enhanced biliary excretion of cholesterol. The answer is **B.**

7. Chronic ethanol ingestion can increase serum concentrations of VLDL and triglyceride. This is one of the factors that places patients with alcoholism at risk of pancreatitis. Chronic ethanol ingestion also has the possibly beneficial effect of raising, not

SKILL KEEPER ANSWERS: ANGINA (SEE CHAPTER 12)

1. *The 3 major forms of angina are (1) angina of effort, which is associated with a fixed plaque that partially occludes 1 or more coronary arteries; (2) vasospastic angina, which involves unpredictably timed, reversible coronary spasm; and (3) unstable angina, which often immediately precedes a myocardial infarction and requires emergency treatment.*

2. *The 3 major drug groups used in angina are nitrates, calcium channel blockers, and β-blockers. Nitrates are used in all 3 types of angina. Calcium channel blockers are useful for treatment of angina of effort and vasospastic angina. They can be added to β-blockers and nitroglycerin in patients with refractory unstable angina. Beta-blockers are not useful in vasospastic angina or for an acute attack of angina of effort. They are primarily used for prophylaxis of angina of effort and also in emergency treatment of acute coronary syndromes.*

decreasing, serum HDL concentrations. The answer is **E**.

8. Niacin can exacerbate both hyperuricemia and glucose intolerance. The answer is **D**.

9. The 2 primary adverse effects of the HMG-CoA reductase inhibitors are hepatotoxicity and myopathy. Patients taking these drugs should have liver function tests performed before starting therapy and at regular intervals during therapy. Serum concentrations of alanine and aspartate aminotransferase are used as markers of hepatocellular toxicity. The answer is **B**.

10. The major recognized effect of ezetimibe is inhibition of absorption of cholesterol in the intestine. The answer is **C**.

CHECKLIST

When you complete this chapter, you should be able to:

☐ Describe the proposed role of lipoproteins in the formation of atherosclerotic plaques.

☐ Describe the dietary management of hyperlipidemia.

☐ List the 5 main classes of drugs used to treat hyperlipidemia. For each, describe the mechanism of action, effects on serum lipid concentrations, and adverse effects.

☐ On the basis of a set of baseline serum lipid values, propose a rational drug treatment regimen.

☐ Argue the merits of combined drug therapy for some diseases and list 3 rational drug combinations.

NSAIDs, Acetaminophen, & Drugs Used in Rheumatoid Arthritis and Gout

36

Inflammation is a complex response to cell injury that primarily occurs in vascularized connective tissue and often involves the immune response. The mediators of inflammation function to eliminate the cause of cell injury and clear away debris, in preparation for tissue repair. Unfortunately, inflammation also causes pain and, in instances in which the cause of cell injury is not eliminated, can result in a chronic condition of pain and tissue damage such as that seen in rheumatoid arthritis. The nonsteroidal anti-inflammatory drugs (NSAIDs) and the nonopioid analgesic acetaminophen are often effective in controlling inflammatory pain. Other treatment strategies applied to the reduction of inflammation are targeted at immune processes. These include disease-modifying antirheumatic drugs (DMARDs), glucocorticoids, and colchicine. Gout is an inflammatory joint disease caused by precipitation of uric acid crystals. Treatment of acute episodes targets inflammation, whereas treatment of chronic gout targets both inflammatory processes and the production and elimination of uric acid.

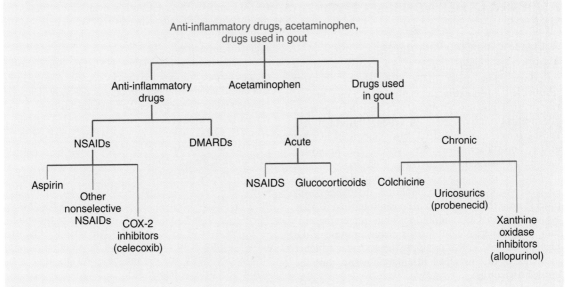

HIGH-YIELD TERMS TO LEARN

Antipyretic	A drug that reduces fever (eg, aspirin, NSAIDs, acetaminophen)
Cyclooxygenase (COX)	The enzyme at the head of the enzymatic pathway for prostaglandin synthesis (see drug classification figure, Chapter 18)
Cytotoxic drug	Drugs that interfere with essential cell processes, especially DNA maintenance and replication and cell division. Such drugs generally kill rapidly dividing cells; primarily used for cancer chemotherapy and immunosuppression (Chapters 55 and 56)
Disease-modifying antirheumatic drugs (DMARDs)	Diverse group of drugs that modify the inflammatory processes underlying rheumatoid arthritis; they have a slow (weeks to months) onset of clinical effects and also are known as slow-acting antirheumatic drugs, or SAARDs
Nonsteroidal anti-inflammatory drugs (NSAIDs)	Inhibitors of cyclooxygenase; the term nonsteroidal was introduced to differentiate them from steroid drugs that mediate anti-inflammatory effects through activation of glucocorticoid receptors (eg, cortisol; Chapter 39)
Reye's syndrome	A rare syndrome of rapid liver degeneration and encephalitis in children treated with aspirin during a viral infection
Tumor necrosis factor-α (TNF-α)	A cytokine that plays a central role in inflammation
Uricosuric agent	A drug that increases the renal excretion of uric acid
Xanthine oxidase	A key enzyme in the purine metabolism pathway that ends with the production of uric acid

ASPIRIN & OTHER NONSELECTIVE NSAIDS

A. CLASSIFICATION AND PROTOTYPES

Aspirin (acetylsalicylic acid) is the prototype of the salicylates. The other older nonselective NSAIDs (**ibuprofen, indomethacin,** many others) vary primarily in their potency, analgesic and anti-inflammatory effectiveness, and duration of action. Ibuprofen and naproxen have moderate effectiveness; indomethacin has greater anti-inflammatory effectiveness; and **ketorolac** has greater analgesic effectiveness. **Celecoxib** was the first member of a newer NSAID subgroup, the cyclooxygenase-2 (COX-2)-selective inhibitors that were developed in an attempt to lessen the gastrointestinal toxicity associated with COX inhibition while preserving efficacy. Unfortunately, clinical trials involving some of the highly selective COX-2 inhibitors have shown a higher incidence of cardiovascular thrombotic events than the nonselective drugs.

B. MECHANISM OF ACTION

As noted in Chapter 18, cyclooxygenase is the enzyme that converts arachidonic acid into the endoperoxide precursors of prostaglandins, important mediators of inflammation. Cyclooxygenase has at least 2 isoforms:

COX-1 and COX-2. COX-1 is primarily expressed in noninflammatory cells, whereas COX-2 is expressed in activated lymphocytes, polymorphonuclear cells, and other inflammatory cells.

Aspirin and nonselective NSAIDs inhibit both cyclooxygenase isoforms and thereby decrease prostaglandin and thromboxane synthesis throughout the body. Release of prostaglandins necessary for homeostatic function is disrupted, as is release of prostaglandins involved in inflammation. The COX-2-selective inhibitors have less effect on the prostaglandins involved in homeostatic function, particularly those in the gastrointestinal tract.

The major difference between the mechanisms of action of aspirin and other NSAIDs is that aspirin (but not its active metabolite, salicylate) acetylates and thereby irreversibly inhibits cyclooxygenase, whereas the inhibition produced by other NSAIDs is reversible. The irreversible action of aspirin results in a longer duration of its antiplatelet effect and is the basis for its use as an antiplatelet drug (Chapter 34).

C. EFFECTS

Arachidonic acid derivatives are important mediators of inflammation; cyclooxygenase inhibitors reduce the manifestations of inflammation, although they have no effect on underlying tissue damage or immunologic reactions.

These inhibitors also suppress the prostaglandin synthesis in the CNS that is stimulated by pyrogens and thereby reduces fever (antipyretic action). The analgesic mechanism of these agents is less well understood. Activation of peripheral pain sensors may be diminished as a result of reduced production of prostaglandins in injured tissue; in addition, a central mechanism is operative. Cyclooxygenase inhibitors also interfere with the homeostatic function of prostaglandins. Most importantly, they reduce prostaglandin-mediated cytoprotection in the gastrointestinal tract and autoregulation of renal function.

D. PHARMACOKINETICS AND CLINICAL USE

1. Aspirin—Aspirin has 3 therapeutic dose ranges: The low range (< 300 mg/day) is effective in reducing platelet aggregation; intermediate doses (300–2400 mg/day) have antipyretic and analgesic effects; and high doses (2400–4000 mg/day) are used for an anti-inflammatory effect. Aspirin is readily absorbed and is hydrolyzed in blood and tissues to acetate and salicylic acid. Salicylate is a reversible nonselective inhibitor of cyclooxygenase. Elimination of salicylate is first order at low doses, with a half-life of 3–5 h. At high (anti-inflammatory) doses, half-life increases to 15 h or more and elimination becomes zero order. Excretion is via the kidney.

2. Other NSAIDs—The other NSAIDs are well absorbed after oral administration. Ibuprofen has a half-life of about 2 h, is relatively safe, and is the least expensive of the older, nonselective NSAIDs. Indomethacin is a potent NSAID with increased toxicity. Naproxen and piroxicam are noteworthy because of their longer half-lives (12–24 h), which permit less frequent dosing. These other NSAIDs are used for the treatment of mild to moderate pain, especially the pain of musculoskeletal inflammation such as that seen in arthritis and gout. Selected NSAIDs are also used to treat other conditions, including dysmenorrhea, headache, and patent ductus arteriosus in premature infants. Ketorolac is notable as a drug used mainly as a systemic analgesic, not as an anti-inflammatory (although it has typical nonselective NSAID properties). It is the only NSAID available in a parenteral formulation. Nonselective NSAIDs reduce polyp formation in patients with primary familial adenomatous polyposis. Long-term use of NSAIDs reduces the risk of colon cancer.

E. TOXICITY

1. Aspirin—The most common adverse effect from therapeutic anti-inflammatory doses of aspirin is gastric upset. Chronic use can result in gastric ulceration, upper gastrointestinal bleeding, and renal effects, including acute failure and interstitial nephritis. Aspirin increases the bleeding time. When prostaglandin synthesis is inhibited by even small doses of aspirin, persons with aspirin hypersensitivity (especially associated with nasal polyps) can experience asthma from the increased synthesis of leukotrienes. This type of hypersensitivity to aspirin precludes treatment with any NSAID. At higher doses of aspirin, tinnitus, vertigo, hyperventilation, and respiratory alkalosis are observed. At very high doses, the drug causes metabolic acidosis, dehydration, hyperthermia, collapse, coma, and death. Children with viral infections who are treated with aspirin are at increased risk for Reye's syndrome, a rare but serious syndrome of rapid liver degeneration and encephalopathy.

2. Nonselective NSAIDs—Like aspirin, these agents are associated with significant gastrointestinal disturbance, but the incidence is lower than with aspirin. There is a risk of renal damage with any of the NSAIDs, especially in patients with preexisting renal disease. Because these drugs are cleared by the kidney, renal damage results in higher, more toxic serum concentrations. Use of parenteral ketorolac is generally restricted to 72 h because of the risk of gastrointestinal and renal damage with longer administration. Serious hematologic reactions have been noted with indomethacin.

3. COX-2-selective inhibitors—The COX-2-selective inhibitors (celecoxib, rofecoxib, valdecoxib) have a *reduced* risk of gastrointestinal effects, including gastric ulcers and serious gastrointestinal bleeding. The COX-2 inhibitors carry the same risk of renal damage as nonselective COX inhibitors, presumably because COX-2 contributes to homeostatic renal effects. Clinical trial data suggest that highly selective COX-2 inhibitors such as rofecoxib and valdecoxib carry an increased risk of myocardial infarction and stroke. The increased risk of arterial thrombosis is believed to be due to the COX-2 inhibitors having a greater inhibitory effect on endothelial prostacyclin (PGI_2) formation than on platelet thromboxane A_2 formation. Prostacyclin promotes vasodilation and inhibits platelet aggregation, whereas TXA_2 has the opposite effects. Several COX-2 inhibitors have been removed from the market, and the others are now labeled with warnings about the increased risk of thrombosis.

ACETAMINOPHEN

A. CLASSIFICATION AND PROTOTYPE

Acetaminophen is the only over-the-counter non-anti-inflammatory analgesic commonly available in the United States. Phenacetin, a toxic prodrug that is metabolized to acetaminophen, is still available in some other countries.

B. MECHANISM OF ACTION

The mechanism of analgesic action of acetaminophen is unclear. The drug is only a weak COX-1 and COX-2 inhibitor in peripheral tissues, which accounts for its lack of anti-inflammatory effect. Evidence suggests that acetaminophen may inhibit a third enzyme, COX-3, in the CNS.

C. EFFECTS

Acetaminophen is an analgesic and antipyretic agent; it lacks anti-inflammatory or antiplatelet effects.

D. PHARMACOKINETICS AND CLINICAL USE

Acetaminophen is effective for the same indications as intermediate-dose aspirin. Acetaminophen is, therefore, useful as an aspirin substitute, especially in children with viral infections and in individuals with any type of aspirin intolerance. Acetaminophen is well absorbed orally and metabolized in the liver. Its half-life, which is 2–3 h in persons with normal hepatic function, is unaffected by renal disease.

E. TOXICITY

In therapeutic dosages, acetaminophen has negligible toxicity in most individuals. However, when taken in overdose or by patients with severe liver impairment, the drug is a dangerous hepatotoxin. The mechanism of toxicity involves oxidation to cytotoxic intermediates by phase I cytochrome P450 enzymes. This occurs if substrates for phase II conjugation reactions (acetate and glucuronide) are lacking (Chapter 4). Prompt administration of **acetylcysteine**, a sulfhydryl donor, may be lifesaving after an overdose. People who regularly consume 3 or more alcoholic drinks per day are at increased risk of acetaminophen-induced hepatotoxicity (Chapters 4 and 23).

SKILL KEEPER: OPIOID ANALGESICS AND ANTAGONISTS (SEE CHAPTER 31)

Although the NSAIDs and acetaminophen are extremely useful for the treatment of mild to moderate pain, adequate control of more intense pain often requires treatment with an opioid.

1. *Name 1 strong, 1 moderate, and 1 weak opioid drug.*
2. *Briefly describe the most common adverse effects of strong and moderate opioids.*
3. *What drug should be administered in the event of an opioid overdose?*

The Skill Keeper Answers appear at the end of the chapter.

DISEASE-MODIFYING ANTIRHEUMATIC DRUGS (DMARDS)

A. CLASSIFICATION

This heterogeneous group of agents (Table 36–1) has anti-inflammatory actions in several connective tissue diseases. They are called disease-modifying drugs because some evidence shows slowing or even reversal of joint damage, an effect never seen with NSAIDs. They are also called slow-acting antirheumatic drugs (SAARDs) because it may take 6 weeks to 6 months for their benefits to become apparent. **Corticosteroids** can be considered anti-inflammatory drugs with an intermediate rate of action (ie, slower than NSAIDs but faster than the other DMARDs). However, the corticosteroids are too toxic for routine chronic use (Chapter 39) and are reserved for temporary control of severe exacerbations and long-term use in patients with severe disease not controlled by other agents.

B. MECHANISMS OF ACTION AND EFFECTS

The mechanisms of action of most of these drugs in treating rheumatoid arthritis are poorly understood. Cytotoxic drugs (eg, **methotrexate**) probably act by reducing the numbers of immune cells available to maintain the inflammatory response; many of these drugs are also used in the treatment of cancer (Chapter 55). Other drugs appear to interfere with the activity of T lymphocytes (eg, **sulfasalazine, hydroxychloroquine, cyclosporine,** leflunomide, mycophenolate mofetil, abatacept), B lymphocytes (**rituximab**) or macrophages (gold compounds). In recent years, drugs that inhibit the action of tumor necrosis factor-α (TNF-α including **infliximab**, adalimumab, and **etanercept**, have also shown efficacy in rheumatoid arthritis. The immunosuppressant effects of these drugs are discussed in more detail in Chapter 56.

C. PHARMACOKINETICS AND CLINICAL USE

Sulfasalazine, hydroxychloroquine, methotrexate, cyclosporine, penicillamine, and leflunomide are given orally. Anti-TNF-α drugs are given by injection. Gold compounds are available for parenteral use (gold sodium thiomalate and aurothioglucose) and for oral administration (auranofin).

Increasingly, DMARDs, particularly low doses of methotrexate, are initiated fairly early in patients with moderate to severe rheumatoid arthritis in an attempt to ameliorate disease progression. Some of these drugs are also used in other rheumatic diseases such as lupus erythematosus, arthritis associated with Sjögren's syndrome, and juvenile rheumatoid arthritis and in other immunologic disorders (Chapter 56).

D. TOXICITY

All disease-modifying agents can cause severe or fatal toxicities. Careful monitoring of patients who take these

Table 36–1. Some slow-acting antirheumatic drugs.

Drug	Other Clinical Uses	Toxicity When Used for Rheumatoid Arthritis
Methotrexate	Anticancer	Nausea, mucosal ulcers, hematotoxicity, teratogenicity
Cyclosporine	Tissue transplantation	Nephrotoxicity, hypertension, liver toxicity
Hydroxychloroquine, chloroquine	Antimalarial	Rash, gastrointestinal disturbance, ocular toxicity
Sulfasalazine	Inflammatory bowel disease	Rash, gastrointestinal disturbance, dizziness, headache, leukopenia
Anti-TNF-α drugs (Infliximab, etanercept, adalimumab)	Inflammatory bowel disease	Macrophage-dependent infection (eg, activation of latent tuberculosis), formation of antibodies to double-stranded DNA and antinuclear antibodies, vasculitis
Leflunomide		Teratogen, hepatotoxicity, gastrointestinal disturbance, skin reactions
Gold compounds		Many adverse effects, including diarrhea, dermatitis, hematologic abnormalities (including aplastic anemia)
Penicillamine	Chelating agent	Many adverse effects, including proteinuria, dermatitis, gastrointestinal disturbance, hematologic abnormalities (including aplastic anemia)

drugs is mandatory. Their major adverse effects are listed in Table 36–1.

DRUGS USED IN GOUT

A. CLASSIFICATION AND PROTOTYPES

Gout is associated with increased serum concentrations of uric acid. Acute attacks involve joint inflammation initiated by precipitation of uric acid crystals. Treatment strategies include (1) reducing inflammation during acute attacks (with colchicine, NSAIDs, or glucocorticoids; Figure 36–1); (2) accelerating renal excretion of uric acid with uricosuric drugs (probenecid or sulfinpyrazone); and (3) reducing (with allopurinol or febuxostat) the conversion of purines to uric acid by xanthine oxidase (Figure 36–2).

B. ANTI-INFLAMMATORY DRUGS USED FOR GOUT

1. Mechanisms—Potent NSAIDs such as **indomethacin** are effective in inhibiting the inflammation of acute gouty arthritis. These agents act through the reduction of prostaglandin formation and the inhibition of crystal phagocytosis by macrophages (Figure 36–1). **Colchicine,** a selective inhibitor of microtubule assembly, reduces leukocyte migration and phagocytosis; the drug may also reduce production of leukotriene B$_4$ and decrease free radical formation.

2. Effects—NSAIDs and glucocorticoids reduce the synthesis of mediators of inflammation by inflammatory

cells in the gouty joint. Because it reacts with tubulin and interferes with microtubule assembly, colchicine is a general mitotic poison. Tubulin is necessary for normal cell division, motility, and many other processes.

3. Pharmacokinetics and clinical use—Indomethacin or a glucocorticoid is preferred for the treatment of acute gouty arthritis. Although colchicine can be used for acute attacks, the doses required cause significant gastrointestinal disturbance, particularly diarrhea. Lower doses of colchicine are used to prevent attacks of gout in patients with a history of multiple acute attacks. Colchicine is also of value in the management of Mediterranean fever, a disease of unknown cause characterized by fever, hepatitis, peritonitis, pleuritis, arthritis, and, occasionally, amyloidosis. Indomethacin, some glucocorticoids, and colchicine are used orally; parenteral preparations of glucocorticoids and colchicine are also available.

4. Toxicity—Indomethacin can cause renal damage or bone marrow depression. Short courses of glucocorticoids can cause behavioral changes and impaired glucose control. Because colchicine can severely damage the liver and kidney, dosage must be carefully limited and monitored. Overdose is often fatal.

C. URICOSURIC AGENTS

1. Mechanism—Normally, over 90% of the uric acid filtered by the kidney is reabsorbed in the proximal tubules. Uricosuric agents (**probenecid, sulfinpyrazone**)

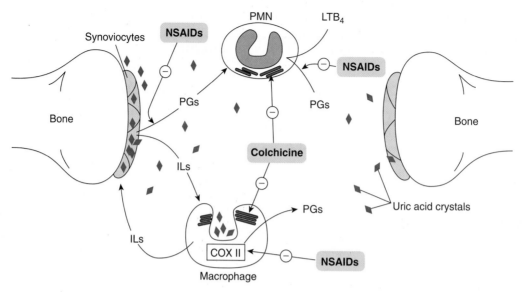

Figure 36–1. Sites of action of some anti-inflammatory drugs in a gouty joint. Synoviocytes damaged by uric acid crystals release prostaglandins (PGs), interleukins (ILs), and other mediators of inflammation. Polymorphonuclear leukocytes (PMNs), macrophages, and other inflammatory cells enter the joint and also release inflammatory substances, including leukotrienes (eg, LTB_4), that attract additional inflammatory cells. Colchicine acts on microtubules in the inflammatory cells. NSAIDs act on cyclooxygenase-2 in all of the cells of the joint.

are weak acids that compete with uric acid for reabsorption by the weak acid transport mechanism in the proximal tubules and thereby increase uric acid excretion. At low doses, these agents may also compete with uric acid for **secretion** by the tubule and, occasionally, can elevate, rather than reduce, serum uric acid concentration.

Elevation of uric acid levels by this mechanism occurs with aspirin (another weak acid) over much of its dose range.

2. Effects—Uricosuric drugs inhibit the **secretion** of a large number of other weak acids (eg, penicillin,

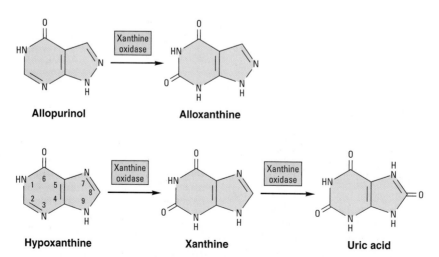

Figure 36–2. The action of xanthine oxidase in uric acid synthesis and metabolism of allopurinol. (Reproduced, with permission, from Katzung BG, editor: *Basic & Clinical Pharmacology,* 10th ed. McGraw-Hill, 2007.)

methotrexate) in addition to inhibiting the reabsorption of uric acid.

3. Pharmacokinetics and clinical use—Uricosuric drugs are used orally to treat chronic gout. These drugs are of no value in acute episodes.

4. Toxicity—Uricosuric drugs can precipitate an attack of acute gout during the early phase of their action. This can be avoided by simultaneously administering colchicine or indomethacin. Because they are sulfonamides, the uricosuric drugs may share allergenicity with other classes of sulfonamide drugs (diuretics, antimicrobials, oral hypoglycemic drugs).

D. XANTHINE OXIDASE INHIBITORS

1. Mechanism—The production of uric acid can be reduced by inhibition of **xanthine oxidase**, the enzyme that converts hypoxanthine to xanthine and xanthine to uric acid (Figure 36–2). Allopurinol is converted to oxypurinol (alloxanthine) by xanthine oxidase; alloxanthine is an irreversible suicide inhibitor of the enzyme. The newer drug **febuxostat** is a nonpurine inhibitor of xanthine oxidase that is more selective than allopurinol and alloxanthine, which inhibit other enzymes involved in purine and pyrimidine metabolism.

2. Effects—Inhibition of xanthine oxidase increases the concentrations of the more soluble hypoxanthine and xanthine and decreases the concentration of the less soluble uric acid. As a result, there is less likelihood of precipitation of uric acid crystals in joints and tissues. Clinical trials suggest that febuxostat is more effective than allopurinol in lowering serum uric acid.

3. Pharmacokinetics and clinical use—The xanthine oxidase inhibitors are given orally in the management of chronic gout. Like uricosuric agents, these drugs are usually withheld for 1–2 weeks after an acute episode of gouty arthritis and are administered in combination with colchicine or an NSAID to avoid an acute attack. Allopurinol is also used as an adjunct to cancer chemotherapy to slow the formation of uric acid from purines released by the death of large numbers of neoplastic cells.

4. Toxicity and drug interactions—Allopurinol causes gastrointestinal upset, rash, and, rarely, peripheral neuritis, vasculitis, or bone marrow dysfunction, including aplastic anemia. It inhibits the metabolism of mercaptopurine and azathioprine, drugs that depend on xanthine oxidase for elimination. Febuxostat can cause liver function abnormalities, headache, and gastrointestinal upset.

QUESTIONS

1. Among NSAIDs, aspirin is unique because it
   (A) Irreversibly inhibits its target enzyme
   (B) Prevents episodes of gouty arthritis with long-term use
   (C) Reduces fever
   (D) Reduces the risk of colon cancer
   (E) Selectively inhibits the COX-2 enzyme

2. An analgesic and antipyretic drug that lacks an anti-inflammatory action is

KEY DRUGS		
Subclass	**Prototypes**	**Other Significant Agents**
Anti-inflammatory drugs		
Salicylates	Aspirin	
Nonselective NSAIDS	Ibuprofen	Indomethacin, ketorolac, naproxen, many others
COX-2 inhibitors	Celecoxib	
Disease-modifying antirheumatic drugs	Methotrexate	See Table 36–1
Acetaminophen class	Acetaminophen	
Drugs used in gout		
Anti-inflammatory drugs	Colchicine	
	NSAIDs	
	Glucocorticoids	
Uricosurics	Probenecid	Sulfinpyrazone
Xanthine oxidase inhibitors	Allopurinol	Febuxostat

(A) Acetaminophen
(B) Celecoxib
(C) Colchicine
(D) Indomethacin
(E) Probenecid

3. Aspirin overdose is characterized by a syndrome of
(A) Bone marrow suppression and possibly aplastic anemia
(B) Fever, hepatic dysfunction, and encephalopathy
(C) Hyperthermia, metabolic acidosis, and coma
(D) Rapid, fulminant hepatic failure
(E) Rash, interstitial nephritis, and acute renal failure

4. Which of the following drugs is MOST likely to increase serum concentrations of conventional doses of methotrexate, a weak acid that is primarily cleared in the urine?
(A) Acetaminophen
(B) Allopurinol
(C) Colchicine
(D) Hydroxychloroquine
(E) Probenecid

5. The main advantage of ketorolac over aspirin is that ketorolac
(A) Can be combined more safely with an opioid such as codeine
(B) Can be obtained as an over-the-counter agent
(C) Does not prolong the bleeding time
(D) Is available in a parenteral formulation that can be injected intramuscularly or intravenously
(E) Is less likely to cause acute renal failure in patients with some preexisting degree of renal impairment

6. The most likely cause of death associated with an overdose of acetaminophen is
(A) Arrhythmia
(B) Hemorrhagic stroke
(C) Liver failure
(D) Noncardiogenic pulmonary edema
(E) Ventilatory failure

7–8. A 52-year-old woman presented with intense pain, warmth, and redness in the first toe on her left foot. Examination of fluid withdrawn from the inflamed joint revealed crystals of uric acid.

7. In the treatment of this woman's acute attack of gout, a high dose of colchicine will reduce the pain and inflammation. However, many physicians prefer to treat acute gout with a corticosteroid or indomethacin because high doses of colchicine are likely to cause
(A) Behavioral changes that include psychosis
(B) High blood pressure

(C) Rash
(D) Severe diarrhea
(E) Sudden gastrointestinal bleeding

8. Over the next 7 mo, the patient had 2 more attacks of acute gout. Her serum concentration of uric acid was elevated. The decision was made to put her on chronic drug therapy to try to prevent subsequent attacks. Which of the following drugs could be used to decrease this woman's rate of production of uric acid?
(A) Allopurinol
(B) Aspirin
(C) Colchicine
(D) Hydroxychloroquine
(E) Probenecid

9–10. A 54-year-old woman presented with signs and symptoms consistent with an early stage of rheumatoid arthritis. The decision was made to initiate NSAID therapy.

9. Which of the following patient characteristics is the most compelling reason for avoiding the use of celecoxib in the treatment of her arthritis?
(A) History of alcohol abuse
(B) History of gout
(C) History of myocardial infarction
(D) History of osteoporosis
(E) History of peptic ulcer disease

10. Although the patient's disease was adequately controlled with an NSAID and methotrexate for some time, her symptoms began to worsen and radiologic studies of her hands indicated progressive destruction in the joints of several fingers. Treatment with another second-line agent for rheumatoid arthritis was considered. This drug is available only in a parenteral formulation; its mechanism of anti-inflammatory action is antagonism of tumor necrosis factor. The drug being considered is
(A) Cyclosporine
(B) Etanercept
(C) Penicillamine
(D) Phenylbutazone
(E) Sulfasalazine

ANSWERS

1. Aspirin differs from other NSAIDs by **irreversibly** inhibiting cyclooxygenase. The answer is **A.**

2. Acetaminophen is the only drug that fits this description. Indomethacin is a nonselective COX inhibitor and celecoxib is a COX-2 inhibitor; both have analgesic, antipyretic, and anti-inflammatory effects. Colchicine is a drug used for gout that also has an

anti-inflammatory action. Probenecid is a uricosuric drug that promotes the excretion of uric acid.
The answer is **A.**

3. Salicylate intoxication is associated with metabolic
acidosis, dehydration, and hyperthermia. If these
problems are not corrected, coma and death ensue.
The answer is **C.**

4. Like other weak acids, Methotrexate depends on
active tubular excretion in the proximal tubule for
efficient elimination. Probenecid competes with
methotrexate for binding to the proximal tubule
transporter and thereby decreases the rate of clearance of methotrexate. The answer is **E.**

5. Ketorolac exerts typical NSAID effects. It prolongs
the bleeding time and can impair renal function,
especially in a patient with preexisting renal disease.
Its primary use is as a **parenteral** agent for pain
management, especially for treatment of postoperative patients. The answer is **D.**

6. In overdose, acetaminophen causes fulminant liver
failure due to its conversion by hepatic cytochrome
P450 enzymes to a highly reactive metabolite. The
answer is **C.**

7. At doses needed to treat acute gout, colchicine
frequently causes significant diarrhea. Such gastrointestinal effects are less likely with the lower
doses used in chronic gout. The answer is **D.**

8. Allopurinol is the only drug listed that decreases
production of uric acid. Probenecid increases uric
acid excretion. Colchicine and hydroxychloroquine
do not affect uric acid metabolism. Aspirin actually
slows renal secretion of uric acid and raises uric acid
blood levels. It should not be used in gout. The
answer is **A.**

SKILL KEEPER ANSWERS: OPIOIDS (SEE CHAPTER 31)

1. *Morphine is the prototype of the strong opioids. Fentanyl is a strong agent with a rapid onset that is commonly used in the hospital. Methadone is a strong agonist used in mainte-nance programs for patients addicted to opi-oids. Codeine, oxycodone, and hydrocodone are moderate agonists, whereas propoxyphene is a weak agonist.*

2. *Constipation and sedation occur with thera-peutic doses; constipation should be managed with stool softeners. In overdose, opioids cause a triad of pinpoint pupils, coma, and respiratory depression.*

3. *Naloxone, a nonselective opioid receptor antagonist, is an antidote for opioid overdose.*

9. Celecoxib is a COX-2-selective inhibitor. Although
the COX-2 inhibitors have the advantage over
nonselective NSAIDs of reduced gastrointestinal
toxicity, there are clinical data suggesting that they
are more likely to cause arterial thrombotic events.
A history of myocardial infarction would be a compelling reason to avoid a COX-2 inhibitory. The
answer is **C.**

10. Etanercept is a recombinant protein that binds to
tumor necrosis factor and prevents its inflammatory
effects. The answer is **B.**

CHECKLIST

When you complete this chapter, you should be able to:

☐ Describe the effects of aspirin on prostaglandin synthesis.

☐ Contrast the functions of COX-1 and COX-2.

☐ Compare the actions and toxicity of aspirin, the older nonselective NSAIDs, and the COX-2-selective drugs.

☐ Explain why several of the highly selective COX-2 inhibitors have been withdrawn from the market.

☐ Describe the toxic effects of aspirin.

☐ Describe the effects and the major toxicity of acetaminophen.

☐ Name 5 slow-acting antirheumatic drugs and describe their toxicity.

☐ Contrast the pharmacologic treatment of acute and chronic gout.

☐ Describe the mechanisms of action and toxicity of 3 different drug groups used in gout.

PART VII
Endocrine Drugs

Hypothalamic & Pituitary Hormones | 37

The hormones produced by the hypothalamus and pituitary gland are key regulators of metabolism, growth, and reproduction. Preparations of these hormones, including products made by recombinant DNA technology and drugs that mimic or block their effects, are used in the treatment of a variety of endocrine disorders.

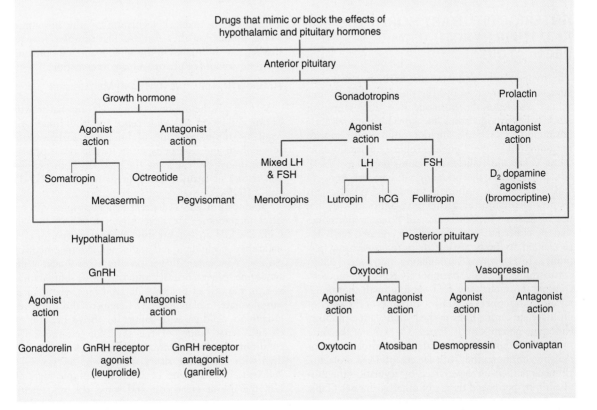

HIGH-YIELD TERMS TO LEARN

Acromegaly	A syndrome of GH excess in adults that is characterized by abnormal growth of tissues—particularly connective tissue—metabolic abnormalities, and cardiac dysfunction
Central diabetes insipidus	A syndrome of polyuria, polydipsia, and hypernatremia caused by inadequate production of vasopressin
Gigantism	A syndrome of GH excess in children and adolescents with open long bone epiphyses that results in excessive height
Gonadotropins	The 2 anterior pituitary hormones (luteinizing hormone [LH] and follicle-stimulating hormone [FSH]) that regulate reproduction in males and females
Insulin-like growth factor-1 (IGF-1)	A growth factor that is the primary mediator of GH effects
Prolactinoma	Pituitary tumor that secretes excessive amounts of prolactin and is associated with a syndrome of infertility and galactorrhea
Tocolytics	Drug used to inhibit preterm labor (eg, the oxytocin receptor antagonist atosiban; magnesium sulfate; nifedipine; β_2 agonists)

ANTERIOR PITUITARY HORMONES AND THEIR HYPOTHALAMIC REGULATORS

The hypothalamic and pituitary hormones and their antagonists are often grouped according to the anatomic site of release of the hormone that they mimic or block—the hypothalamus for gonadotropin-releasing hormone (GnRH); the anterior pituitary for growth hormone (GH), the 2 gonadotropins, luteinizing hormone (LH) and follicle-stimulating hormone (FSH), and prolactin; or the posterior pituitary for oxytocin and vasopressin (antidiuretic hormone [ADH]). This chapter focuses on the agents used commonly. It does not discuss the hypothalamic and pituitary hormones that are either not used clinically or are used rarely for specialized diagnostic testing (thyrotropin-releasing hormone [TRH], thyroid-stimulating hormone [TSH], corticotropin-releasing hormone [CRH], adrenocorticotropic hormone [ACTH], and growth hormone-releasing hormone [GHRH]). Hormones of the anterior pituitary are central links in the hypothalamic-pituitary endocrine system (or axis; Figure 37–1). All of the anterior pituitary hormones are under the control of a hypothalamic hormone and, with the exception of prolactin, all mediate their ultimate effects by regulating the production by peripheral tissues of other hormones (Table 37–1). Four anterior pituitary hormones (TSH, LH, FSH, and ACTH) and their hypothalamic regulators are subject to feedback regulation by the hormones whose production they control. The complex systems that regulate hormones of the anterior pituitary provide multiple avenues of pharmacologic intervention.

A. GROWTH HORMONE (GH) AND MECASERMIN

1. GH—Growth hormone is required for normal growth during childhood and adolescence and is an important regulator throughout life of lipid and carbohydrate metabolism and lean body mass. Its effects are primarily mediated by regulating the production in peripheral tissues of **insulin-like growth factor 1 (IGF-1)** and **2 (IGF-2)**.

Somatropin and somatrem (somatotropin with an extra methionine) are recombinant forms of human GH. The GH analogs are used in the treatment of GH deficiency in children and adults and the treatment of children with either Turner's syndrome or Prader-Willi syndrome, genetic diseases associated with short stature and, in the case of Prader-Willi syndrome, obesity and carbohydrate intolerance. GH treatment also improves growth in children with failure to thrive because of chronic renal failure or the small-for-gestational-age condition. The most controversial use of GH is for children with **idiopathic short stature** who are not GH deficient. In this group of children, multiple years of GH therapy at great cost and some risk of toxicity results in a small (1–3 inches) average increase in final adult height.

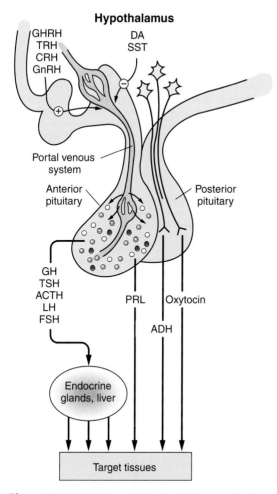

Hypothalamus

GHRH
TRH
CRH
GnRH

DA
SST

Portal venous system

Anterior pituitary

Posterior pituitary

GH
TSH
ACTH
LH
FSH

PRL   Oxytocin

ADH

Endocrine glands, liver

Target tissues

Figure 37–1. The hypothalamic-pituitary endocrine system. Hypothalamic factors regulate the release of anterior pituitary hormones. Pituitary hormones either stimulate the release of other hormones or act directly on target tissues. (ACTH, adrenocorticotropic hormone; ADH, antidiuretic hormone [vasopressin]; CRH, corticotropin-releasing hormone; DA, dopamine; FSH, follicle-stimulating hormone; GH, growth hormone; GHRH, growth-hormone releasing hormone; GnRH, gonadotropin-releasing hormone; LH, luteinizing hormone; PRL, prolactin; SST, somatostatin; TRH, thyrotropin-releasing hormone; TSH, thyroid-stimulating hormone.) (Reproduced, with permission, from Katzung BG, editor: *Basic & Clinical Pharmacology*, 10th ed. McGraw-Hill, 2007.)

In adults, GH has efficacy in treatment of AIDS-associated wasting and GH deficiency, and it may improve gastrointestinal function in patients who have undergone intestinal resection and have subsequently developed a malabsorption syndrome. GH is a popular component of antiaging programs even though studies in model animal systems have consistently found that analogs of GH and IGF-1 shorten lifespan. GH is also used by athletes for a purported increase in muscle mass and athletic performance and is one of the drugs banned by the Olympic Committee and professional sports associations. Recombinant bovine GH is used in dairy cattle to increase milk production.

Adults generally tolerate GH less well than children. Adverse effects include peripheral edema, myalgia, and arthralgia.

2. Mecasermin—A small group of children with growth failure unresponsive to GH therapy are deficient in IGF-1 and a binding protein (insulin-like growth factor-binding protein-3) that maintains an adequate half-life of the IGF-1. Mecasermin, a complex of recombinant human IGF-1 and the binding protein, is administered parenterally to children with IGF-1 deficiency. Its most important toxicity is hypoglycemia, which can be prevented by consumption of a snack or meal shortly before mecasermin administration.

B. GROWTH HORMONE ANTAGONISTS

Growth hormone-secreting pituitary adenomas cause **acromegaly** in adults and, rarely, **gigantism** in children and adolescents who have not completed their growth phase. Pharmacologic treatment of GH excess seeks to inhibit GH secretion or interfere with GH effects.

1. Octreotide—Somatostatin, a 14-amino-acid peptide, inhibits the release of GH, glucagon, insulin, and gastrin. Octreotide, a long-acting synthetic analog of somatostatin, is used to treat acromegaly, carcinoid, gastrinoma, glucagonoma, and other endocrine tumors. Regular octreotide must be administered subcutaneously 2 to 4 times daily. Once a brief course of regular octreotide has been demonstrated to be effective and tolerated, a slow-release intramuscular formulation is administered every 4 weeks for long-term therapy. Octreotide causes significant gastrointestinal disturbances, gallstones, and cardiac conduction abnormalities.

2. Dopamine D_2 receptor antagonists—Dopamine D_2 receptor antagonists such as **bromocriptine** are more effective at inhibiting prolactin release than inhibiting GH release (see below). However, high doses of D_2 receptor antagonists have some efficacy in the treatment of small GH-secreting tumors.

3. Pegvisomant—Pegvisomant is a GH receptor antagonist that is approved for treatment of acromegaly. Normally, GH, which has 2 distinct receptor binding sites, initiates cellular signaling cascades by dimerizing 2 GH receptors. Pegvisomant is a long-acting derivative of a mutant GH that is able to cross-link GH receptors but

Table 37–1. Links between hypothalamic, anterior pituitary, and target organ hormone or mediator.[a]

Anterior Pituitary Hormone	Hypothalamic Hormone	Target Organ	Primary Target Organ Hormone or Mediator
Growth hormone (GH, somatotropin)	Growth hormone-releasing hormone (GHRH) (+) Somatostatin (–)	Liver, muscle, bone, kidney, and others	Insulin-like growth factor-1 (IGF-1)
Thyroid-stimulating hormone (TSH)	Thyrotropin-releasing hormone (TRH) (+)	Thyroid	Thyroxine, triiodothyronine
Adrenocorticotropin (ACTH)	Corticotropin-releasing hormone (CRH) (+)	Adrenal cortex	Glucocorticoids, mineralo-corticoids, androgens
Follicle-stimulating hormone (FSH) Luteinizing hormone (LH)	Gonadotropin-releasing hormone (GnRH) (+)[b]	Gonads	Estrogen, progesterone, testosterone
Prolactin (PRL)	Dopamine (–)	Breast	—

(+), stimulant; (–), inhibitor.
[a]All of these hormones act through G protein-coupled receptors except growth hormone and prolactin, which act through JAK/STAT receptors.
[b]Endogenous GnRH, which is released in pulses, stimulates LH and FSH release. When administered continuously as a drug, GnRH and its analogs inhibit LH and FSH release.
Reproduced, with permission, from Katzung BG, editor: *Basic & Clinical Pharmacology,* 10th ed. McGraw–Hill, 2007.

is incapable of inducing the conformational changes required for receptor activation.

C. FOLLICLE-STIMULATING HORMONE (FSH), LUTEINIZING HORMONE, AND THEIR ANALOGS

In women, FSH directs follicle development, while FSH and LH collaborate in the regulation of ovarian steroidogenesis. In men, FSH is the primary regulator of spermatogenesis, whereas LH is the main stimulus for testicular androgen production. The gonadotropins and their analogs are used in combination to stimulate spermatogenesis in infertile men and to induce ovulation in women with anovulation that is not responsive to less complicated treatments (Chapter 40).

Ovulation induction protocols are increasingly complex. They require significant close monitoring to ensure successful insemination or retrieval of mature oocytes and to avoid the 2 most serious complications of ovulation induction—multiple pregnancies and the ovarian hyperstimulation syndrome, a syndrome of ovarian enlargement, ascites, hypovolemia, and possibly shock. All ovulation induction protocols that employ gonadotropins have 3 basic steps. First, endogenous gonadotropin production is inhibited by administration of a GnRH agonist or antagonist (see below). Second, follicle development is driven by daily injections of a preparation with FHS activity (menotropins, FSH, or an FSH analog). Last, the final stage of oocyte maturation is induced with an injection of LH or the LH analog human chorionic gonadotropin (hCG). The treatment of male infertility

that is due to hypogonadism requires months of administration of a mixture of drugs with LH and FSH activity.

A variety of gonadotropin preparations are available. All are administered parenterally.

1. Menotropins—Menotropins are human gonadotropins that consist of a mixture of FSH and LH purified from the urine of postmenopausal women (who produce high levels of FSH and LH due to the disinhibition of pituitary gonadotropin production that results from cessation of ovarian steroidogenesis).

2. FSH and its analogs—Three forms of FSH are available. **Urofollitropin** is a purified preparation extracted from the urine of postmenopausal women. The 2 recombinant forms of human FSH—**follitropin alpha** and follitropin beta—differ from each in the composition of their carbohydrate side chains.

3. LH and its analogs—**Human chorionic gonadotropin (hCG),** the placental protein that supports the corpus luteum during the early stages of pregnancy, has a structure that is nearly identical to LH and mediates its effects through activation of LH receptors. hCG purified from human urine or recombinant hCG is used commonly for an LH activity. **Lutropin,** a recombinant form of human LH, is also available.

D. GONADOTROPIN-RELEASING HORMONE (GNRH) AND ITS ANALOGS

GnRH is a decapeptide that stimulates gonadotropin release when it is secreted in a pulsatile pattern by the hypothalamus. **Leuprolide** was the first of a set of synthetic peptides with long-acting GnRH agonist activity. Other long-acting GnRH agonists include goserelin, histrelin, and nafarelin.

In men and women, steady dosing with these GnRH agonists inhibits gonadotropin release by causing downregulation of GnRH receptors in the pituitary cells that normally release gonadotropins. Continuous GnRH agonist treatment is used to suppress endogenous gonadotropin secretion in women undergoing ovulation induction with gonadotropins, in women with gynecologic disorders that benefit from ovarian suppression (eg, endometriosis, uterine leiomyomata), in children with precocious puberty, and in men with advanced prostate cancer.

In women, continuous treatment with a GnRH agonist causes the typical symptoms of menopause (hot flushes, sweats, headache). Long-term treatment is avoided because of the risk of bone loss and osteoporosis. In men treated continuously with a GnRH agonist, adverse effects include hot flushes, sweats, gynecomastia, reduced libido, decreased hematocrit, and reduced bone density. In men with prostate cancer and children with precocious puberty, the first few weeks of therapy can temporarily exacerbate the condition.

E. Gonadotropin-Releasing Hormone (GnRH) Antagonists

Ganirelix and **cetrorelix** are GnRH *antagonists* that can be used during ovulation induction in place of GnRH agonists to suppress endogenous gonadotropin production. Their immediate onset of antagonist activity permits a shortened course of therapy, and there is some evidence that they are less likely to cause the ovarian hyperstimulation syndrome. These GnRH antagonists may also be effective in disorders that are currently treated with GnRH agonists, including endometriosis and uterine leiomyomata in women and prostate cancer in men.

F. Prolactin Antagonists (Dopamine D_2 Receptor Agonists)

The anterior pituitary hormone prolactin regulates lactation. In women and men, hyperprolactinemia and an associated syndrome of infertility and galactorrhea can result from prolactin-secreting adenomas. Dopamine is the physiologic inhibitor of prolactin release (Figure 37–1). Prolactin-secreting adenomas usually retain their sensitivity to dopamine. In hyperprolactinemia, **bromocriptine** and other orally active D_2 dopamine receptor agonists (eg, cabergoline, pergolide; Chapter 16) are effective in reducing serum prolactin concentrations and restoring fertility. As mentioned above, high doses of a dopamine agonist can also be used in the treatment of acromegaly.

POSTERIOR PITUITARY HORMONES

A. Oxytocin

Oxytocin is a nonapeptide synthesized in cell bodies in the paraventricular nuclei of the hypothalamus and transported through the axons of these cells to the posterior pituitary (Figure 37–1). Oxytocin is an effective stimulant of uterine contraction and is used intravenously to induce or reinforce labor. **Atosiban** is an antagonist of the oxytocin receptor that is used in some countries as a **tocolytic**, a drug used to treat preterm labor.

B. Vasopressin (Antidiuretic Hormone [ADH])

Vasopressin is synthesized in neuronal cell bodies in the hypothalamus and released from nerve terminals in the posterior pituitary (Figure 37–1). As discussed in Chapter 15, vasopressin acts through V_2 receptors to increase the insertion of water channels in the apical membranes of collecting duct cells in the kidney and to thereby provide an antidiuretic effect. Extrarenal V_2-like receptors regulate the release of coagulation factor VIII and von Willebrand factor (Chapter 34). **Desmopressin,** a selective agonist of V_2 receptors, is administered orally, nasally, or parenterally in patients with pituitary diabetes insipidus and in patients with mild hemophilia A or von Willebrand disease.

Vasopressin also contracts vascular smooth muscle by activating V_1 receptors. Because of this vasoconstrictor effect, vasopressin is sometimes used to treat patients with bleeding from esophageal varices or colon diverticula.

KEY DRUGS

Subclass	Prototypes	Other Significant Agents
GH analogs	Somatropin	Somatrem
IGF-1 analog	Mecasermin	
GH antagonists		
Somatostatin analog	Octreotide	
Dopamine D$_2$ receptor agonists	Bromocriptine	
GH receptor antagonist	Pegvisomant	
Gonadotropin analogs		
Mixed LH and FSH	Menotropins	
FSH	Follitropin	Urofollitropin
LH	hCG	Lutropin
GnRH analogs	Gonadorelin	
	Leuprolide	Goserelin, histrelin, nafarelin
GnRH receptor antagonists	Ganirelix	Cetrorelix
Prolactin antagonists (dopamine D$_2$ receptor agonists)	Bromocriptine	Cabergoline, pergolide, quinagolide
Oxytocin agonist	Oxytocin	
Oxytocin antagonist	Atosiban	
Vasopressin agonist	Desmopressin	
Vasopressin antagonist	Conivaptan	Tolvaptan

Several antagonists of vasopressin receptors (eg, **conivaptan,** tolvaptan) have been developed to offset the fluid retention that results from the excessive production of vasopressin associated with hyponatremia or acute heart failure (Chapter 15).

QUESTIONS

1. A drug that is purified from the urine of postmenopausal women and used to promote spermatogenesis in infertile men is
   (A) Desmopressin
   (B) Gonadorelin
   (C) Goserelin
   (D) Somatropin
   (E) Urofollitropin

2. A 29-year-old woman in her 41st week of gestation had been in labor for 12 h. Although her uterine contractions had been strong and regular initially, they had diminished in force during the past hour. To facilitate this woman's labor and delivery, she would be treated with

   (A) Dopamine
   (B) Leuprolide
   (C) Oxytocin
   (D) Prolactin
   (E) Vasopressin

3. A 3-year-old boy with failure to thrive and metabolic disturbances was found to have an inactivating mutation in the gene that encodes the growth hormone receptor. The drug that is most likely to promote improve his metabolic function and promote his growth is
   (A) Atosiban
   (B) Bromocriptine
   (C) Mecasermin
   (D) Octreotide
   (E) Somatropin

4. An important difference between leuprolide and ganirelix is that ganirelix
   (A) Can be administered as an oral formulation
   (B) Can be used alone to restore fertility to hypogonadal men and women

(C) Immediately reduces gonadotropin secretion

(D) Initially stimulates pituitary production of LH and FSH

(E) Must be administered in a pulsatile fashion

5. A 27-year-old woman with amenorrhea, infertility, and galactorrhea was treated with a drug that successfully restored ovulation and menstruation. Before being given the drug, the woman was carefully questioned about previous mental health problems, which she did not have. She was advised to take the drug orally. The drug used to treat this patient was probably

(A) Bromocriptine

(B) Desmopressin

(C) Human gonadotropin hormone

(D) Leuprolide

(E) Octreotide

6. Who is LEAST likely to be treated with somatropin?

(A) A 3-year-old cow on a dairy farm

(B) A 4-year-old girl with an XO genetic genotype

(C) A 4-year-old boy with chronic renal failure and growth deficiency

(D) A 10-year-old boy with polydipsia and polyuria

(E) A 37-year-old patient with AIDS-related wasting syndrome

7. A 3-year-old girl presented with hirsutism, breast enlargement, and a height and bone age that was more consistent with an age of 9. Diagnostic testing revealed precocious puberty. The most appropriate drug treatment is

(A) Atosiban

(B) Follitropin

(C) Leuprolide

(D) Octreotide

(E) Pegvisomant

8. A 47-year-old man exhibited signs and symptoms of acromegaly. Radiologic studies showed the presence of a large pituitary tumor. Surgical treatment of the tumor was only partially effective in controlling his disease. At this point, which of the following drugs is most likely to be used as pharmacologic therapy?

(A) Cosyntropin

(B) Desmopressin

(C) Leuprolide

(D) Octreotide

(E) Somatropin

9. A 37-year-old woman with infertility due to obstructed fallopian tubes was undergoing ovulation induction in preparation for in vitro fertilization. After 10 days of treatment with leuprolide, the next step in the procedure is most likely to involve 10–14 days of treatment with

(A) Bromocriptine

(B) Follitropin

(C) Gonadorelin

(D) hCG

(E) Pergolide

10. A 7-year-old boy underwent successful chemotherapy and cranial radiation for treatment of acute lymphocytic leukemia. One month after the completion of therapy, the patient presented with excessive thirst and urination plus hypernatremia. Laboratory testing revealed pituitary diabetes insipidus. To correct these problems, this patient is likely to be treated with

(A) Corticotropin

(B) Desmopressin

(C) hCG

(D) Menotropins

(E) Thyrotropin

ANSWERS

1. Spermatogenesis in males requires the action of FSH and LH. Urofollitropin, which is purified from the urine of postmenopausal women, is used clinically to provide FSH activity. The answer is **E.**

2. Oxytocin is an effective stimulant of uterine contraction that is routinely used to augment labor. The answer is **C.**

3. This child's condition is due to the inability of GH to stimulate the production of insulin-like growth factors, the ultimate mediators of GH effects. Mecasermin, a combination of recombinant IGF-1 and the binding protein that protects IGF-1 from immediate destruction, will help correct the IGF deficiency. Because of the inactive GH receptors, somatropin will not be effective. The answer is **C.**

4. Leuprolide is an agonist of GnRH receptors, whereas ganirelix is an antagonist. Although both drugs can be used to inhibit gonadotropin release, ganirelix does so immediately, whereas leuprolide does so only after about 1 week of sustained activity. The answer is **C.**

5. Bromocriptine, a dopamine receptor agonist, is used to treat the amenorrhea-galactorrhea syndrome, which is a consequence of hyperprolactinemia. Because of its central dopaminergic effects, the drug should not be used in patients with a history of schizophrenia or other forms of psychotic illness. The answer is **A.**

6. Somatropin, recombinant human GH, promotes growth in children with Turner's syndrome (an XO genetic genotype) or chronic renal failure. It also helps combat the AIDS-associated wasting syndrome. Bovine GH promotes milk production in cows. GH would not be appropriate for the boy with

polydipsia and polyuria, which is probably symptomatic of a form of diabetes. The answer is **D.**

7. In precocious puberty, the hypothalamic-pituitary-
gonadal axis becomes prematurely active for reasons that are not understood. Treatment involves
suppressing gonadotropin secretion with continuous administration of a long-acting GnRH agonist
such as leuprolide. The answer is **C.**

8. Octreotide, a somatostatin analog, has some efficacy
in reducing the excess GH production that causes
acromegaly. The answer is **D.**

9. Once the patient's endogenous gonadotropin production has been inhibited through continuous
administration of the GnRH agonist leuprolide, the
next step in ovulation induction is the administration
of a drug with FSH activity to stimulate follicle maturation. Follitropin is recombinant FSH. The only
other drug listed that is used in ovulation induction is
hCG, but this is a LH analog. The answer is **B.**

10. Pituitary diabetes insipidus results from deficiency in
vasopressin. It is treated with desmopressin, a peptide
agonist of vasopressin V_2 receptors. The answer is **B.**

SKILL KEEPER ANSWERS: DRUGS THAT CAUSE HYPERPROLACTINEMIA (SEE CHAPTER 29)

1. *Drugs that block dopamine D_2 receptors cause
hyperprolactinemia by blocking the inhibitory
effects of endogenous dopamine on the pituitary cells that release prolactin.*

2. *The older antipsychotic drugs (eg, phenothiazines, haloperidol), with their strong
dopamine D_2 receptor-blocking activity, are
most likely to be the pharmacologic cause of
hyperprolactinemia (see Chapter 29). This
adverse effect is less likely with the newer
antipsychotic drugs (eg, olanzapine). Drugs or
drug groups that cause hyperprolactinemia
through mechanisms that are not well characterized include methyldopa (an antihypertensive), amphetamines, tricyclic and other types of
antidepressants, and opioids.*

CHECKLIST

When you complete this chapter, you should be able to:

☐ Diagram the hypothalamic-pituitary endocrine system and indicate the sites of release of and links between the
hormones in the system.

☐ Describe the drugs used as substitutes for the natural pituitary hormones and list their clinical uses.

☐ List the gonadotropin analogs and GnRH agonists and antagonists and describe their clinical use in treating male
and female infertility, endometriosis, and prostate cancer.

☐ Describe the drugs used for treatment of acromegaly and hyperprolactinemia.

Thyroid & Antithyroid Drugs

The thyroid secretes 2 types of hormones: iodine-containing amino acids (thyroxine and triiodothyronine) and a peptide (calcitonin). Thyroxine and triiodothyronine have broad effects on growth, development, and metabolism. Calcitonin is important in calcium metabolism and is discussed in Chapter 42. This chapter describes the drugs used in the treatment of hypothyroidism and hyperthyroidism.

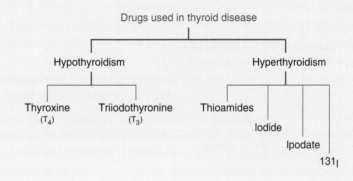

THYROID HORMONES

A. SYNTHESIS & TRANSPORT OF THYROID HORMONES

The thyroid secretes 2 iodine-containing hormones: thyroxine (T_4) and triiodothyronine (T_3). The iodine necessary for the synthesis of these molecules comes from food or iodide supplements. Iodide ion is actively taken up by and highly concentrated in the thyroid gland, where it is converted to elemental iodine by thyroidal peroxidase (Figure 38–1). The protein **thyroglobulin** serves as a scaffold for thyroid hormone synthesis. Tyrosine residues in thyroglobulin are iodinated to form monoiodotyrosine (MIT) or diiodotyrosine (DIT). Within thyroglobulin, 2 molecules of DIT combine to form T_4, while 1 molecule each of MIT and DIT combine to form T_3. Proteolysis of thyroglobulin liberates the T_4 and T_3 that is then released from the thyroid. After release from the gland, T_4 and T_3 are transported in the blood by **thyroxine-binding globulin,** a protein synthesized in the liver.

Thyroid function is controlled by the pituitary through the release of thyrotropin (thyroid-stimulating hormone [TSH]) and by the availability of iodide. Thyrotropin stimulates the uptake of iodide as well as synthesis and release of thyroid hormone. It also has a growth-promoting effect that causes thyroid cell hyperplasia and an enlarged gland (**goiter**). High levels of thyroid hormones inhibit the release of TSH, providing an effective negative feedback control mechanism. In **Graves' disease**, an autoimmune disorder, B lymphocytes produce an antibody that activates the TSH receptor and causes a syndrome of hyperthyroidism called **thyrotoxicosis**. Because these lymphocytes are not susceptible to negative feedback, patients with Graves' disease can have very high blood concentrations of thyroid hormone at the same time that their blood concentrations of TSH are very low.

HIGH-YIELD TERMS TO LEARN

Goiter	Enlargement of the thyroid gland
Graves' disease	Autoimmune disorder that results in hyperthyroidism during the early phase and can progress to hypothyroidism if there is destruction of the gland in later phases
Thyroglobulin	A protein synthesized in the thyroid gland; its tyrosine residues are used to synthesize thyroid hormones
Thyroid-stimulating hormone (TSH)	The anterior pituitary hormone that regulates thyroid gland growth, uptake of iodine and synthesis of thyroid hormone
Thyroid storm	Severe thyrotoxicosis
Thyrotoxicosis	Medical syndrome caused by an excess of thyroid hormone (Table 38–1)
Thyroxine-binding globulin (TBG)	Protein synthesized in the liver that transports thyroid hormone in the blood

---

B. MECHANISMS OF ACTION OF T_4 AND T_3

T_3 is about 10 times more potent than T_4; because T_4 is converted to T_3 in target cells, the liver, and the kidneys, most of the effect of circulating T_4 is probably due to T_3. Thyroid hormone binds to intracellular receptors that control the expression of genes responsible for many metabolic processes. The proteins synthesized under T_3 control differ depending on the tissue involved; these proteins include, for example, Na^+/K^+ ATPase, specific contractile proteins in smooth muscle and the heart, enzymes involved in lipid metabolism, and important developmental components in the brain. T_3 may also have a separate membrane receptor-mediated effect in some tissues.

1. Effects of thyroid hormone—The organ-level actions of the thyroid hormones include normal growth and development of the nervous, skeletal, and reproductive systems and control of metabolism of fats, carbohydrates, proteins, and vitamins. The key features of excess thyroid activity (thyrotoxicosis) and hypothyroidism are listed in Table 38–1.

2. Clinical use—Thyroid hormone therapy can be accomplished with either T_4 or T_3. Synthetic

---

Table 38–1. Key features of thyrotoxicosis and hypothyroidism.

Thyrotoxicosis	Hypothyroidism
Warm, moist skin	Pale, cool, puffy skin
Sweating, heat intolerance	Sensation of being cold
Tachycardia, increased stroke volume, cardiac output, and pulse pressure	Bradycardia, decreased stroke volume, cardiac output, and pulse pressure
Dyspnea	Pleural effusions, hypoventilation, and CO_2 retention
Increased appetite	Reduced appetite
Nervousness, hyperkinesia, tremor	Lethargy, general slowing of mental processes
Weakness, increased deep tendon reflexes	Stiffness, decreased deep tendon reflexes
Menstrual irregularity, decreased fertility	Infertility, decreased libido, impotence, oligospermia
Weight loss	Weight gain
Exophthalmos (Graves' disease)	

levothyroxine (T_4) is usually the form of choice. T_3 (liothyronine) is faster acting but has a shorter half-life and is more expensive.

3. Toxicity—Toxicity is that of thyrotoxicosis (Table 38–1). Older patients, those with cardiovascular disease, and those with long-standing hypothyroidism are highly sensitive to the stimulatory effects of T_4 on the heart. Such patients should receive lower initial doses of T_4.

 SKILL KEEPER: THE CYCLIC AMP SECOND MESSENGER SYSTEM (CHAPTER 2)

Like many neurotransmitters and hormones, TSH mediates its effects in thyroid cells by activating the cAMP second messenger system. Draw a diagram that shows the key events in this pathway, beginning with the binding of an agonist to its receptor and ending with cellular responses. The Skill Keeper Answers appear at the end of the chapter.

ANTITHYROID DRUGS

A. THIOAMIDES

Methimazole and propylthiouracil (PTU) are small sulfur-containing thioamides that inhibit thyroid hormone synthesis by blocking iodination of the tyrosine residues of thyroglobulin and coupling of DIT and MIT (Figure 38–1). Because the thioamides do not inhibit the release of preformed thyroid hormone, their onset of activity is usually slow, often requiring 3–4 weeks for full effect. The thioamides can be used by the oral route and are effective in young patients with small glands and mild disease. Methimazole is preferred because it can be administered once per day. PTU is less likely than methimazole to cross the placenta and enter breast milk, but it should be used cautiously in pregnant and nursing women. Toxic effects include skin rash (common) and severe reactions (rare) such as vasculitis, agranulocytosis, hypoprothrombinemia, and liver dysfunction. These effects are usually reversible.

B. IODIDE SALTS AND IODINE

Iodide salts inhibit iodination of tyrosine and thyroid hormone release (Figure 38–1); these salts also decrease

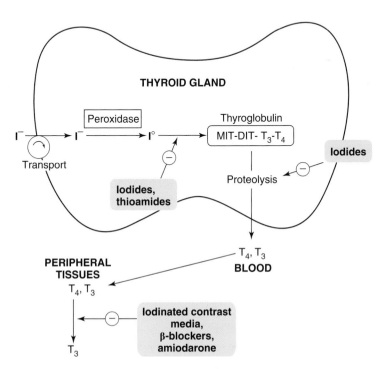

Figure 38–1. Sites of action of some antithyroid drugs. I⁻, iodide ion; I°, elemental iodine. Not shown: radioactive iodine (^{131}I), which destroys the gland through radiation.

the size and vascularity of the hyperplastic thyroid gland. Because iodide salts inhibit release as well as synthesis of the hormones, their onset of action occurs rapidly, within 2–7 days. However, the effects are transient; the thyroid gland "escapes" from the iodide block after several weeks of treatment. Iodide salts are used in the management of thyroid storm and to prepare patients for surgical resection of a hyperactive thyroid. The usual forms of this drug are Lugol's solution (iodine and potassium iodide) and saturated solution of potassium iodide. Adverse effects include rash, drug fever, metallic taste, bleeding disorders and, rarely, anaphylactic reactions.

C. RADIOACTIVE IODINE

Radioactive iodine (^{131}I) is taken up and concentrated in the thyroid gland so avidly that a dose large enough to severely damage the gland can be given without endangering other tissues. Unlike the thioamides and iodide salts, an effective dose of ^{131}I can produce a permanent cure of thyrotoxicosis without surgery. ^{131}I should not be used in pregnant or nursing women.

D. IODINATED RADIOCONTRAST MEDIA

Iodinated radiocontrast media (eg, oral diatrizoate or oral or intravenous iohexol) rapidly suppress the conversion of T_4 to T_3 in the liver, kidney, and other peripheral tissues (Figure 38–1). Inhibition of hormone release from the thyroid may also play a part. Iodinated radiocontrast media are useful for rapidly reducing T_3 concentrations in thyrotoxicosis.

E. OTHER DRUGS

Another class of drugs used in the treatment of thyrotoxicosis is the β-blockers. These agents are particularly useful in controlling the tachycardia and other cardiac abnormalities of severe thyrotoxicosis. **Propranolol** also inhibits the peripheral conversion of T_4 to T_3.

The iodine-containing antiarrhythmic drug **amiodarone** (Chapter 14) can cause hypothyroidism through its ability to block the peripheral conversion of T_4 to T_3. It also can cause hyperthyroidism either through an iodine-induced mechanism in persons with an underlying thyroid disease such as multinodular goiter or through an inflammatory mechanism that causes leakage of thyroid hormone into the circulation. Amiodarone-associated hypothyroidism is treated with thyroid hormone. Iodine-associated hyperthyroidism caused by amiodarone is treated with thioamides, whereas the inflammatory version is best treated with corticosteroids.

QUESTIONS

1–3. A 24-year-old woman was found to have mild hyperthyroidism due to Graves' disease. She appears to be in good health otherwise.

1. In Graves' disease, the cause of the hyperthyroidism is the production of an antibody that
   - **(A)** Activates the pituitary thyrotropin-releasing hormone (TRH) receptor and stimulates TSH release
   - **(B)** Activates the thyroid gland TSH receptor and stimulates thyroid hormone synthesis and release
   - **(C)** Activates thyroid hormone receptors in peripheral tissues
   - **(D)** Binds to thyroid gland thyroglobulin and accelerates its proteolysis and the release of its supply of T_4 to T_3
   - **(E)** Binds to thyroid binding globulin (TBG) and displaces bound T_4 to T_3

2. The decision is made to begin treatment with methimazole. Methimazole reduces serum concentration of T_3 primarily by
   - **(A)** Accelerating the peripheral metabolism of T_3
   - **(B)** Inhibiting the proteolysis of thyroid-binding globulin
   - **(C)** Inhibiting the secretion of TSH

KEY DRUGS

Subclass	Prototypes	Other Significant Agents
Thyroid hormones	Thyroxine (T_4)	Triiodothyronine (T_3)
Antithyroid drugs	Methimazole	Propylthiouracil
	Iodide salts ^{131}I	
	Diatrizoate	Iohexol
Miscellaneous	Propranolol	

(D) Inhibiting the uptake of iodide by cells in the thyroid

(E) Preventing the addition of iodine to tyrosine residues on thyroglobulin

3. Though rare, a serious toxicity associated with the thioamides is
(A) Agranulocytosis
(B) Lupus erythematosus-like syndrome
(C) Myopathy
(D) Torsades de pointes arrhythmia
(E) Thrombotic thrombocytic purpura (TTP)

4–5. A 56-year-old woman presented to the emergency department with tachycardia, shortness of breath, and chest pain. She had had shortness of breath and diarrhea for the past 2 days and was sweating and anxious. A relative reported that the patient had run out of methimazole 2 weeks earlier. A TSH measurement revealed a value of < 0.01 mIU/L (normal 0.4–4.0 mIU/L). The diagnosis of thyroid storm was made.

4. In the treatment of thyroid storm, it is important to use antithyroid drugs with a rapid onset of activity. A rapidly acting antithyroid drug that blocks the conversion of T_4 to T_3 is
(A) Diatrizoate
(B) Levothyroxine
(C) Propylthiouracil
(D) Triiodothyronine
(E) Radioactive iodine

5. A drug that is a useful adjuvant in the treatment of thyroid storm is
(A) Amiodarone
(B) Betamethasone
(C) Epinephrine
(D) Propranolol
(E) Radioactive iodine

6. A symptom that would be expected to occur in the event of chronic overdose with exogenous T_4 is
(A) Bradycardia
(B) Dry, puffy skin
(C) Large tongue and drooping of the eyelids
(D) Lethargy, sleepiness
(E) Weight loss

7. When initiating T_4 therapy for an elderly patient with long-standing hypothyroidism, it is important to begin with small doses to avoid
(A) A flare of exophthalmos
(B) Acute renal failure
(C) Hemolysis
(D) Overstimulation of the heart
(E) Seizures

DIRECTIONS: 8–10. The matching questions in this section consist of a list of 5 lettered options followed by several numbered items. For each numbered item, select the ONE lettered option that is most closely associated with it. Each lettered option may be selected once, more than once, or not at all.

(A) ^{131}I
(B) Diatrizoate
(C) Propranolol
(D) Propylthiouracil
(E) T_3

8. Produced in the peripheral tissues when T_4 is administered

9. Radiocontrast medium that is also useful in thyrotoxicosis

10. Produces a permanent reduction in thyroid activity

ANSWERS

1. The antibodies produced in Graves' disease activate thyroid gland TSH receptors. Their effects mimic those of TSH. The answer is **B**.

2. The thioamides (methimazole and propylthiouracil) primarily act in thyroid cells to prevent conversion of tyrosine residues in thyroglobulin to MIT or DIT. The answer is **E**.

3. Rarely, the thioamides cause severe adverse reactions that include agranulocytosis, vasculitis, hepatic damage, and hypoprothrombinemia. The answer is **A**.

4. Diatrizoate, an iodinated radiocontrast medium, has a rapid onset of antithyroid activity resulting from inhibition of the peripheral conversion of T_4 to T_3. The answer is **A**.

5. In thyroid storm, β-blockers such as propranolol are useful in controlling the tachycardia and other cardiac abnormalities, and propranolol also inhibits peripheral conversion of T_4 to T_3. The answer is **D**.

6. In hyperthyroidism, the metabolic rate increases and even though there is increased appetite, weight loss often occurs. The other choices are symptoms seen in hypothyroidism. The answer is **E**.

7. Patients with long-standing hypothyroidism, especially those who are elderly, are highly sensitive to the stimulatory effects of T_4 on cardiac function. Administration of regular doses can cause overstimulation of the heart and cardiac collapse. The answer is **D**.

8. T_4 is converted into T_3 in the periphery. The answer is **E**.

9. Diatrizoate is a radiocontrast agent. The answer is **B**.

10. Radioactive iodine is the only medical therapy that produces a permanent reduction of thyroid activity. The answer is **A**.

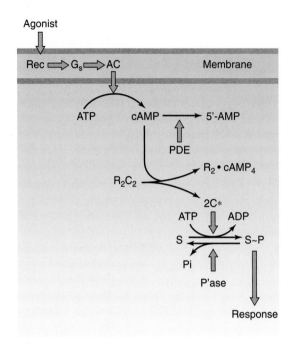

Your drawing should show that receptor (Rec) stimulation acts through the G protein G_s to activate the enzyme adenylyl cyclase (AC). Adenylyl cyclase converts ATP to cAMP, which binds to the regulatory subunit (R) of cAMP-dependent protein kinases and thereby frees the catalytic subunit (C) of the kinase so it can transfer phosphate from ATP to substrate proteins that mediate the ultimate cellular responses. These responses are varied and include immediately apparent effects that stem from phosphorylation of substrates such as enzymes and ion channels as well as delayed effects that follow changes in gene transcription. "Brakes" are applied to the pathway by phosphodiesterases (PDE) that hydrolyze cAMP and phosphatases (P'ase) that dephosphorylate substrates. The figure is reproduced, with permission, from Katzung BG, editor: Basic & Clinical Pharmacology, 10th ed. McGraw-Hill, 2007.

CHECKLIST

When you complete this chapter, you should be able to:

☐ Sketch the biochemical pathway for thyroid hormone synthesis and release and indicate the sites of action of antithyroid drugs.

☐ List the principal drugs used in the treatment of hypothyroidism.

☐ List the principal drugs used in the treatment of hyperthyroidism and compare the onset and duration of their action.

☐ Describe the major toxicities of thyroxine and the antithyroid drugs.

Corticosteroids & Antagonists

39

The corticosteroids are steroid hormones produced by the adrenal cortex. They consist of 2 major physiologic and pharmacologic groups: (1) glucocorticoids, which have important effects on intermediary metabolism, catabolism, immune responses, and inflammation; and (2) mineralocorticoids, which regulate sodium and potassium reabsorption in the collecting tubules of the kidney. This chapter reviews the glucocorticoids, the mineralocorticoids, and the adrenocorticosteroid antagonists.

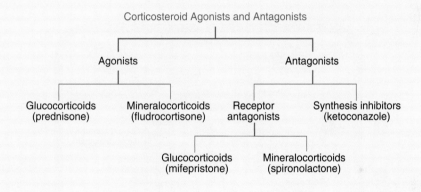

GLUCOCORTICOIDS

A. MECHANISM OF ACTION

Corticosteroids enter the cell and bind to cytosolic receptors that transport the steroid into the nucleus. The steroid-receptor complex alters gene expression by binding to glucocorticoid response elements (GREs) or mineralocorticoid-specific elements (Figure 39–1). Tissue-specific responses to steroids are made possible by the presence in each tissue of different protein regulators that control the interaction between the hormone-receptor complex and particular response elements.

B. ORGAN AND TISSUE EFFECTS

1. Metabolic effects—Glucocorticoids stimulate gluconeogenesis. As a result, blood glucose rises, muscle protein is catabolized, and insulin secretion is stimulated. Both lipolysis and lipogenesis are stimulated, with a net increase of fat deposition in certain areas (eg, the face [moon facies] and the shoulders and back [buffalo hump]).

2. Catabolic effects—Glucocorticoids cause muscle protein catabolism. In addition, lymphoid and connective tissue, fat, and skin undergo wasting under the influence of high concentrations of these steroids. Catabolic effects on bone can lead to osteoporosis. In children, growth is inhibited.

3. Immunosuppressive effects—Glucocorticoids inhibit cell-mediated immunologic functions, especially those dependent on lymphocytes. These agents are actively lymphotoxic and, as such, are important in the treatment of hematologic cancers. The drugs do not interfere with the development of normal acquired immunity but delay rejection reactions in patients with organ transplants.

HIGH-YIELD TERMS TO LEARN	
Addison's disease	Partial or complete loss of adrenocortical function, including loss of glucocorticoid and mineralocorticoid function
Adrenal suppression	A suppression of the ability of the adrenal cortex to produce corticosteroids. Most commonly is an iatrogenic effect of prolonged exogenous glucocorticoid treatment that results from inhibition by the glucocorticoid of the secretion of ACTH by the pituitary
Cushing's syndrome	A metabolic disorder caused by excess secretion of adrenocorticoid steroids, which is most commonly due to increased amounts of ACTH
Glucocorticoid	A substance, usually a steroid, that activates glucocorticoid receptors (eg, cortisol)
Mineralocorticoid	A substance, usually a steroid, that activates mineralocorticoid receptors (eg, aldosterone)

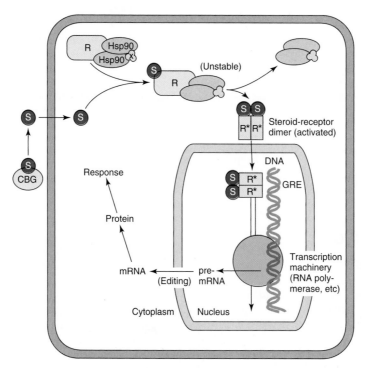

Figure 39–1. Mechanism of glucocorticoid action. This figure models the interaction of a steroid (S; eg, cortisol), with its receptor (R) and the subsequent events in a target cell. The steroid is present in the blood bound to the corticosteroid-binding globulin (CBG) but enters the cell as the free molecule. The intracellular receptor is bound to stabilizing proteins, including heat shock protein 90 (Hsp90) and several others (X). When the complex binds a molecule of steroid, the Hsp90 and associated molecules are released. The steroid-receptor complex enters the nucleus as a dimer, binds to the glucocorticoid response element (GRE) on the gene, and regulates gene transcription by RNA polymerase II and associated transcription factors. The resulting mRNA is edited and exported to the cytoplasm for the production of protein that brings about the final hormone response. (Reproduced, with permission, from Katzung BG, editor: *Basic & Clinical Pharmacology,* 10th ed. McGraw-Hill, 2007.)

4. Anti-inflammatory effects—Glucocorticoids have a dramatic effect on the distribution and function of leukocytes. These drugs increase neutrophils and decrease lymphocytes, eosinophils, basophils, and monocytes. The migration of leukocytes is also inhibited. The biochemical mechanisms underlying these cellular effects include the induced synthesis of an inhibitor of phospholipase A_2 (Chapter 18), decreased mRNA for COX-2, decreases in IL-2 and IL-3, and decreases in platelet activating factor (PAF), an inflammatory cytokine.

5. Other effects—Glucocorticoids such as cortisol are required for normal renal excretion of water loads. The glucocorticoids also have effects on the CNS. When given in large doses, these drugs may cause profound behavioral changes. Large doses also stimulate gastric acid secretion and decrease resistance to ulcer formation.

C. Important Glucocorticoids

1. Cortisol—The major natural glucocorticoid is cortisol (hydrocortisone). The physiologic secretion of cortisol is regulated by adrenocorticotropin (ACTH) and varies during the day (circadian rhythm); the peak occurs in the morning and the trough occurs about midnight. In the plasma, cortisol is 95% bound to corticosteroid-binding globulin (CBG). Given orally, cortisol is well absorbed from the gastrointestinal tract, is cleared by the liver, and has a short duration of action compared with its synthetic congeners (Table 39–1). Although it diffuses poorly across normal skin, cortisol is readily absorbed across inflamed skin and mucous membranes.

The cortisol molecule also has a small but significant salt-retaining (mineralocorticoid) effect. This is an important cause of hypertension in patients with a cortisol-secreting adrenal tumor or a pituitary ACTH-secreting tumor (Cushing's syndrome).

2. Synthetic glucocorticoids—The mechanism of action of these agents is identical to that of cortisol. A large number are available for use; prednisone and its active metabolite, prednisolone, dexamethasone, and triamcinolone are representative. Their properties (compared with cortisol) include longer half-life and duration of action, reduced salt-retaining effect, and better penetration of lipid barriers for topical activity (Table 39–1).

Special glucocorticoids have been developed for use in asthma (Chapter 20) and other conditions in which good surface activity on mucous membranes or skin is needed and systemic effects are to be avoided. **Beclomethasone** and **budesonide** readily penetrate the airway mucosa but have very short half-lives after they enter the blood, so that systemic effects and toxicity are greatly reduced.

D. Clinical Uses

1. Adrenal disorders—Glucocorticoids are essential to preserve life in patients with chronic adrenal cortical insufficiency (Addison's disease) and are necessary in acute adrenal insufficiency associated with life-threatening shock, infection, or trauma. Glucocorticoids are also used in certain types of congenital adrenal hyperplasia, in which synthesis of abnormal forms of corticosteroids are stimulated by ACTH. In these conditions, administration of a potent synthetic glucocorticoid suppresses ACTH secretion sufficiently to reduce the synthesis of the abnormal steroids.

2. Nonadrenal disorders—Many disorders respond to corticosteroid therapy. Some of these are inflammatory or immunologic in nature (eg, asthma, organ transplant rejection, collagen diseases, exophthalmos). Other applications include the treatment of hematopoietic cancers, neurologic disorders, chemotherapy-induced vomiting, hypercalcemia, and mountain sickness. Betamethasone, a glucocorticoid with a low degree of protein binding, is given to pregnant women in premature labor to hasten maturation of the fetal lungs. The degree of benefit differs considerably in different disorders, and the toxicity of corticosteroids given chronically limits their use.

Table 39–1. Properties of representative corticosteroids.

Agent	Duration of Action (hours)	Anti-inflammatory Potency[a]	Salt-retaining Potency[a]	Topical Activity
Primarily glucocorticoid Cortisol	8–12	1	1	0
Prednisone	12–24	4	0.3	(+)
Triamcinolone	15-24	5	0	+++
Dexamethasone	24–36	30	0	+++++
Primarily mineralocorticoid Aldosterone	1–2	0.3	3000	0
Fludrocortisone	8–12	10	125–250	0

[a]Relative to cortisol.

KEY DRUGS		
Subclass	**Prototypes**	**Other Significant Agents**
Agonists		
Glucocorticoids	Cortisol (hydrocortisone), prednisone	Dexamethasone, triamcinolone, beclomethasone
Mineralocorticoids	Aldosterone	Fludrocortisone
Antagonists		
Receptor agonists		
Glucocorticoid receptor	Mifepristone	
Mineralocorticoid receptor	Spironolactone	Eplerenone
Synthesis inhibitors	Ketoconazole	Aminoglutethimide, metyrapone

E. TOXICITY

Most of the toxic effects of the glucocorticoids are predictable from the effects already described. Some are life threatening and include metabolic effects (growth inhibition, diabetes, muscle wasting, osteoporosis), salt retention, and psychosis. Methods for minimizing these toxicities include local application (eg, aerosols for asthma), alternate-day therapy (to reduce pituitary suppression), and tapering the dose soon after achieving a therapeutic response. To avoid adrenal insufficiency in patients who have had long-term therapy, additional "stress doses" may need to be given during serious illness or before major surgery. Patients who are being withdrawn from glucocorticoids after protracted use should have their doses tapered slowly, over the course of several months, to allow recovery of normal adrenal function.

MINERALOCORTICOIDS

A. ALDOSTERONE

The major natural mineralocorticoid in humans is aldosterone, which has already been mentioned in connection with hypertension (Chapter 11) and control of its secretion by angiotensin II (Chapter 17). The secretion of aldosterone is regulated by ACTH and by the renin-angiotensin system and is very important in the regulation of blood volume and blood pressure (Figure 6–4). Aldosterone has a short half-life and little glucocorticoid activity (Table 39–1). Its mechanism of action is the same as that of the glucocorticoids.

B. OTHER MINERALOCORTICOIDS

Other mineralocorticoids include deoxycorticosterone, the naturally occurring precursor of aldosterone, and **fludrocortisone.** The latter has significant glucocorticoid activity. Because of its long duration of action (Table 39–1), fludrocortisone is favored for replacement therapy after adrenalectomy and in other conditions in which mineralocorticoid therapy is needed.

CORTICOSTEROID ANTAGONISTS

A. RECEPTOR ANTAGONISTS

Spironolactone and **eplerenone,** antagonists of aldosterone at its receptor, have been discussed in connection with the diuretics (Chapter 15). **Mifepristone (RU-486)** is a competitive inhibitor of glucocorticoid receptors as well as progesterone receptors (Chapter 40) and has been used in the treatment of Cushing's syndrome.

SKILL KEEPER: ALDOSTERONE ANTAGONISTS AND CONGESTIVE HEART FAILURE (CHAPTERS 13 AND 15)

Recent clinical trials have shown that the aldosterone receptor antagonists spironolactone and eplerenone decrease morbidity and mortality in patients who are taking other standard therapies.

1. *Why is aldosterone elevated in patients with congestive heart failure?*

2. *How does the increase in aldosterone contribute to the signs and symptoms of heart failure?*

3. *What happens to serum potassium concentrations in patients who are treated with aldosterone antagonists?*

The Skill Keeper Answers appear at the end of the chapter.

B. Synthesis Inhibitors

Several drugs are used in the treatment of adrenal cancer when surgical therapy is impractical or unsuccessful because of metastases. The most important of these drugs are **aminoglutethimide, metyrapone,** and **ketoconazole.**

Ketoconazole (an antifungal drug) inhibits the cytochrome P450 enzymes necessary for the synthesis of all steroids and is used in a number of conditions in which reduced steroid levels are desirable (eg, adrenal carcinoma, hirsutism, breast and prostate cancer). Aminoglutethimide blocks the conversion of cholesterol to pregnenolone and also inhibits synthesis of all hormonally active steroids. It can be used in conjunction with other drugs for treatment of steroid-producing adrenocortical cancer. Metyrapone inhibits the normal synthesis of cortisol but not that of cortisol precursors; the drug can be used in diagnostic tests of adrenal function.

QUESTIONS

1. Pharmacologic effects of exogenous glucocorticoids include
   (A) Increased muscle mass
   (B) Hypoglycemia
   (C) Inhibition of leukotriene synthesis
   (D) Improved wound healing
   (E) Increased excretion of salt and water

2. Toxic effects of long-term administration of a glucocorticoid include
   (A) A "lupus-like" syndrome
   (B) Adrenal gland neoplasm
   (C) Hepatotoxicity
   (D) Osteoporosis
   (E) Precocious puberty in children

3. A 46-year-old male patient has Cushing's syndrome that is due to the presence of an adrenal tumor. Which of the following drugs would be expected to reduce the signs and symptoms of this man's disease?
   (A) Betamethasone
   (B) Cortisol
   (C) Fludrocortisone
   (D) Ketoconazole
   (E) Triamcinolone

4. In the treatment of congenital adrenal hyperplasia in which there is excess production of cortisol precursors because of a lack of 21β-hydroxylase activity, the purpose of the administration of a synthetic glucocorticoid is

   (A) Inhibition of aldosterone synthesis
   (B) Normalization of renal function
   (C) Prevention of hypoglycemia
   (D) Recovery of normal immune function
   (E) Suppression of ACTH secretion

5. A glucocorticoid response element is
   (A) A protein regulator that controls the interaction between an activated steroid receptor and DNA
   (B) A short DNA sequence that binds tightly to RNA polymerase
   (C) A small protein that binds to an unoccupied steroid receptor protein and prevents it from becoming denatured
   (D) A specific nucleotide sequence that is recognized by a steroid hormone receptor-hormone complex
   (E) The portion of the steroid receptor that binds to DNA

6. Glucocorticoids have proved useful in the treatment of
   (A) Chemotherapy-induced vomiting
   (B) Chronic obstructive pulmonary disease
   (C) Hyperprolactinemia
   (D) Parkinson's disease
   (E) Type II diabetes

7. For patients who have been on long-term therapy with a glucocorticoid and who now wish to discontinue the drug, gradual tapering of the glucocorticoid is needed to allow recovery of
   (A) Depressed release of insulin from pancreatic B cells
   (B) Hematopoiesis in the bone marrow
   (C) Normal osteoblast function
   (D) The control by vasopressin of water excretion
   (E) The hypothalamic-pituitary-adrenal system

8–9. A 54-year-old man with advanced tuberculosis has developed signs of severe acute adrenal insufficiency.

8. This patient is likely to exhibit
   (A) A moon face
   (B) Dehydration
   (C) Hyperglycemia
   (D) Hypertension
   (E) Hyperthermia

9. The patient should be treated immediately. Which of the following combinations is most rational?
   (A) Aldosterone and fludrocortisone
   (B) Cortisol and fludrocortisone
   (C) Dexamethasone and metyrapone
   (D) Fludrocortisone and metyrapone
   (E) Triamcinolone and dexamethasone

10. A drug that blocks the glucocorticoid receptor is
    (A) Aminoglutethimide
    (B) Beclomethasone
    (C) Ketoconazole
    (D) Mifepristone
    (E) Spironolactone

ANSWERS

1. Glucocorticoids inhibit the production of both leukotrienes and prostaglandins. This is a key component of their anti-inflammatory action. The answer is **C**.

2. One of the metabolic effects of long-term glucocorticoid therapy is a net loss of bone, which can result in osteoporosis. The answer is **D**.

3. Ketoconazole inhibits many types of cytochrome P450 enzymes. It can be used to reduce the unregulated overproduction of corticosteroids by adrenal tumors. The answer is **D**.

4. A 21β-hydroxylase deficiency prevents normal synthesis of cortisol and causes accumulation of cortisol precursors. The hypothalamic-pituitary system responds to the abnormally low levels of cortisol by increasing ACTH release. High levels of ACTH induce adrenal hyperplasia and excess production of steroids, which are diverted to the androgen pathway to cause virilization of females and prepubertal males. A high dose of glucocorticoid is administered to suppress release of ACTH. The answer is **E**.

5. Activated steroid hormone receptors mediate their effects on gene expression by binding to hormone response elements, which are short sequences of DNA located near steroid-regulated genes. The answer is **D**.

6. Glucocorticoids are used in combination with other antiemetics to prevent chemotherapy-induced nausea and vomiting, which are commonly associated with anticancer drugs. The answer is **A**.

7. Exogenous glucocorticoids act at the hypothalamus and pituitary to suppress the production of CRF and ACTH. As a result, adrenal production of endogenous corticosteroids is suppressed. On discontinuance, the recovery of normal hypothalamic-pituitary-adrenal function occurs slowly. Glucocorticoid doses must be tapered slowly, over several months, to prevent adrenal insufficiency. The answer is **E**.

8. In acute adrenal insufficiency, there is loss of salt and water that is primarily due to reduced production of aldosterone. The loss of salt and water can lead to dehydration. The answer is **B**.

9. A rational combination of drugs should include agents with complementary effects (ie, a glucocorticoid and a mineralocorticoid). The combination with these characteristics is cortisol and fludrocortisone. (Note that although fludrocortisone may have sufficient glucocorticoid activity for a patient with mild disease, a patient in severe acute adrenal insufficiency needs a full glucocorticoid such as cortisol.) The answer is **B**.

10. Mifepristone is a competitive antagonist of glucocorticoid and progestin receptors. Ketoconazole and aminoglutethimide also antagonize corticosteroids; however, they act by inhibiting steroid hormone synthesis. The answer is **D**.

SKILL KEEPER ANSWERS: ALDOSTERONE ANTAGONISTS AND CONGESTIVE HEART FAILURE (CHAPTERS 13 AND 15)

1. *The reduction in cardiac output associated with heart failure decreases the effective arterial blood volume and renal blood flow. Decreased pressure in renal arterioles and increased sympathetic neural activity both stimulate renin release, which increases production of angiotensin II. Angiotensin II is a powerful stimulus of aldosterone secretion.*

2. *Acting through nuclear receptors in the epithelial cells that line renal collecting tubules, aldosterone promotes renal uptake of salt and water. This retention of salt and water exacerbates the peripheral and pulmonary edema that is associated with congestive heart failure, and it further overloads the weakened heart. In addition to these renal effects, aldosterone is also implicated in myocardial and vascular fibrosis and baroreceptor dysfunction.*

3. *The aldosterone antagonists are also known as "potassium-sparing diuretics" because, unlike other diuretics, they do not promote renal excretion of potassium. Because the excretion of potassium in the renal tubule is linked to the reuptake of sodium, the reduction in sodium uptake caused by spironolactone and eplerenone results in potassium retention and an increase in serum potassium.*

CHECKLIST

When you complete this chapter, you should be able to:

☐ Describe the major naturally occurring glucocorticosteroid and its actions.

☐ List several synthetic glucocorticoids and the differences between these agents and the naturally occurring hormone.

☐ Describe the actions of the naturally occurring mineralocorticoid and 1 synthetic agent in this subgroup.

☐ List the indications for the use of corticosteroids in adrenal and nonadrenal disorders.

☐ Name 3 drugs that interfere with the action or synthesis of corticosteroids and, for each, describe its mechanism of action.

Gonadal Hormones & Inhibitors

40

The gonadal hormones include the steroids of the ovary (estrogens and progestins) and testis (chiefly testosterone). Because of their importance as contraceptives, many synthetic estrogens and progestins have been produced. These include synthesis inhibitors, receptor antagonists, and some drugs with mixed effects (ie, agonist effects in some tissues and antagonist effects in other tissues). Mixed agonists with estrogenic effects are called selective estrogen receptor modulators (SERMs). Synthetic androgens, including those with anabolic activity, are also available for clinical use. A diverse group of drugs with antiandrogenic effects is used in the treatment of prostate cancer and benign prostatic hyperplasia in men and hyperandrogenism in women.

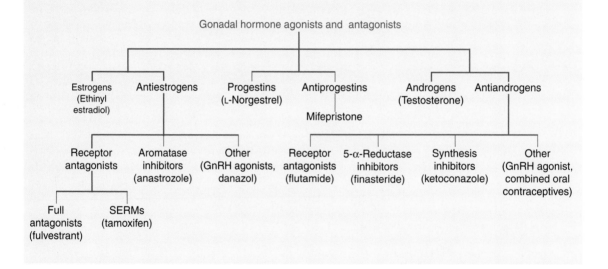

OVARIAN HORMONES

The ovary is the primary source of gonadal hormones in women during the childbearing years (ie, between puberty and menopause). When properly regulated by follicle-stimulating hormone (FSH) and luteinizing hormone (LH) from the pituitary, each menstrual cycle consists of the following events: A follicle in the ovary matures, secretes increasing amounts of estrogen, releases an ovum, and is transformed into a progesterone-secreting corpus luteum. If the ovum is not fertilized and implanted, the corpus luteum degenerates; the uterine endometrium, which has proliferated under the stimulation of estrogen and progesterone, is shed as part of the menstrual flow, and the cycle repeats. The mechanism of action of both estrogen and progesterone involves entry into cells, binding to cytosolic receptors, and translocation of the receptor–hormone complex into the nucleus, where it modulates gene expression (Figure 39–1).

A. ESTROGENS

The major ovarian estrogen in women is estradiol. Estradiol has low oral bioavailability but is available in a micronized form for oral use. It can also be administered

---

HIGH-YIELD TERMS TO LEARN

5α-Reductase	The enzyme that converts testosterone to dihydrotestosterone (DHT); it is inhibited by finasteride, a drug used to treat benign prostatic hyperplasia and prevent male-pattern hair loss in men
Anabolic steroid	Androgen receptor agonists used for anabolic effects (eg, weight gain, increased muscle mass)
Breakthrough bleeding	Vaginal bleeding that occurs outside of the period of regular menstrual bleeding
Combined oral contraceptive (COC or just OC)	Hormonal contraceptive administered orally that contains an estrogen and a progestin
Hirsutism	A male pattern of body hair growth (face, chest, abdomen) in females that results from hyperandrogenism
HRT	Hormone replacement therapy; refers to estrogen replacement for women who have lost ovarian function and nearly always involves combination therapy with estrogen and a progestin
SERM	Selective estrogen receptor modulator such as tamoxifen

---

via transdermal patch, vaginal cream, or intramuscular injection. Long-acting esters of estradiol that are converted in the body to estradiol (eg, estradiol cypionate) can be administered by intramuscular (IM) injection. Mixtures of conjugated estrogens from biologic sources (eg, Premarin) are used orally for hormone replacement therapy (HRT). Synthetic estrogens with high bioavailability (eg, **ethinyl estradiol**, mestranol) are used in hormonal contraceptives.

1. Effects—Estrogen is essential for normal female reproductive development. It is responsible for the growth of the genital structures (vagina, uterus, and uterine tubes) during childhood and for the appearance of secondary sexual characteristics and the growth spurt associated with puberty. Estrogen has many metabolic effects: It modifies serum protein levels and reduces bone resorption. It enhances the coagulability of blood and increases plasma triglyceride levels while reducing low-density lipoprotein (LDL) cholesterol. Continuous administration of estrogen, especially in combination with a progestin, inhibits the secretion of gonadotropins from the anterior pituitary (Figure 40–1).

2. Clinical use—Estrogens are used in the treatment of hypogonadism in young females (Table 40–1). Another use is as HRT in women with estrogen deficiency resulting from premature ovarian failure, menopause, or surgical removal of the ovaries. HRT ameliorates hot flushes and atrophic changes in the urogenital tract. It is effective also in preventing bone loss and osteoporosis. The estrogens are components of hormonal contraceptives (see later discussion).

3. Toxicity—In hypogonadal girls, the dose of estrogen must be adjusted carefully to prevent premature closure of the epiphyses of the long bones and short stature. When used as HRT, estrogen increases the risk of endometrial cancer; this effect is prevented by combining the estrogen with a progestin. Estrogen use by postmenopausal women is associated with a small increase in the risk of breast cancer and cardiovascular events (myocardial infarction, stroke). Dose-dependent toxicity includes nausea, breast tenderness, increased risk of migraine headache, thromboembolic events (eg, deep vein thrombosis), gallbladder disease, hypertriglyceridemia, and hypertension.

Diethylstilbestrol (DES), a nonsteroidal estrogenic compound, is associated with infertility, ectopic pregnancy, and vaginal adenocarcinoma in the daughters of women who were treated with the drug during pregnancy in a misguided attempt to prevent recurrent spontaneous abortion. These effects appear to be restricted to DES because there is no evidence that the estrogens and progestins in hormonal contraceptives have similar effects or other teratogenic effects.

B. PROGESTINS

Progesterone is the major progestin in humans. A micronized form is used orally for HRT, and progesterone-containing vaginal creams are also available. Synthetic progestins (eg, medroxyprogesterone) have improved oral bioavailability. The 19-nortestosterone compounds differ primarily in their degree of androgenic effects. Older drugs (eg, L-norgestrel and norethindrone) are

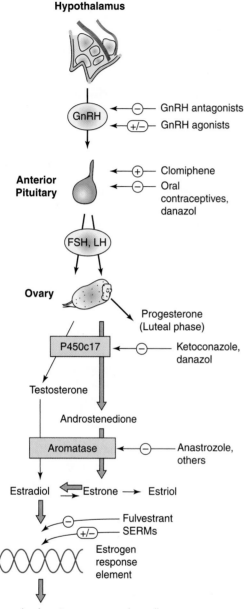

Figure 40–1. Control of estrogen and progesterone secretion and some sites of action of antiestrogens. In the follicular phase the ovary produces mainly estrogens; in the luteal phase it produces estrogens and progesterone. SERMS, selective estrogen receptor modulators. (Reproduced, with permission, from Katzung BG, editor: *Basic & Clinical Pharmacology*, 10th ed. McGraw-Hill, 2007.)

more androgenic than the newer progestins (eg, norgestimate, desogestrel).

1. Effects—Progesterone induces secretory changes in the endometrium and is required for the maintenance of pregnancy. The other progestins also stabilize the endometrium but do not support pregnancy. Progestins do not significantly affect plasma proteins, but they do affect carbohydrate metabolism and stimulate the deposition of fat. High doses suppress gonadotropin secretion and often cause anovulation in women.

2. Clinical use—Progestins are used as contraceptives, either alone or in combination with an estrogen. They are used in combination with an estrogen in HRT to prevent estrogen-induced endometrial cancer. Progesterone is used in assisted reproductive technology programs to promote and maintain pregnancy.

3. Toxicity—The toxicity of progestins is low. However, they may increase blood pressure and decrease high-density plasma lipoproteins (HDLs). Long-term use of high doses in premenopausal women is associated with a reversible decrease in bone density (a secondary effect of ovarian suppression and decreased ovarian production of estrogen) and delayed resumption of ovulation after termination of therapy.

C. Hormonal Contraceptives

Hormonal contraceptives contain either a combination of an estrogen and a progestin or a progestin alone. Hormonal contraceptives are available in a variety of preparations, including oral pills, long-acting injections, transdermal patches, vaginal rings, and intrauterine devices (IUDs) (Table 40–1). Three different types of **oral contraceptives** for women are available in the United States: combination estrogen-progestin tablets that are taken in constant dosage throughout the menstrual cycle (monophasic preparations); combination preparations (biphasic and triphasic) in which the progestin or estrogen dosage, or both, changes during the month (to more closely mimic hormonal changes in a menstrual cycle); and progestin-only preparations.

The **postcoital contraceptives** (also known as "emergency contraception") will prevent pregnancy if administered within 72 h after unprotected intercourse. Oral preparations containing a progestin (L-norgestrel) alone, estrogen alone, or the combination of an estrogen and a progestin are effective. The progestin-only preparation causes fewer side effects than the estrogen-containing preparations.

1. Mechanism of action—The combination hormonal contraceptives have several actions, including inhibition of ovulation (the primary action) and effects on the cervical mucus glands, uterine tubes, and endometrium that decrease the likelihood of fertilization and implantation. Progestin-only agents do not always inhibit ovulation and instead act through the

Table 40–1. Representative applications for the gonadal hormones and hormone antagonists.

Clinical Application	Drugs
Hypogonadism in girls, women	Conjugated estrogens, ethinyl estradiol, estradiol esters
Hormone replacement therapy	Estrogen component: conjugated estrogens, estradiol, estrone, estriol
	Progestin component: progesterone, medroxyprogesterone acetate
Oral hormonal contraceptive	Combined: ethinyl estradiol or mestranol plus a progestin
	Progestin only: norethindrone or norgestrel
Parenteral contraceptive	Medroxyprogesterone as a depot IM injection
	Ethinyl estradiol and noregestromin as a weekly patch
	Ethinyl estradiol and etonogestrel as a monthly vaginal ring
	L-Norgestrel as an intrauterine device (IUD)
	Etonogestrel as a subcutaneous implant
Postcoital contraceptive	L-Norgestrel, combined oral contraceptive
Intractable dysmenorrhea or uterine bleeding	Conjugated estrogens, ethinyl estradiol, oral contraceptive, GnRH agonist, depot injection of medroxyprogesterone acetate
Infertility	Clomiphene; hMG and hCG; GnRH analogs; progesterone; bromocriptine
Abortifacient	Mifepristone (RU 486) and misoprostol
Endometriosis	Oral contraceptive, depot injection of medroxyprogesterone acetate, GnRH agonist, danazol
Breast cancer	Tamoxifen, aromatase inhibitors (eg, anastrozole)
Osteoporosis in postmenopausal women	Conjugated estrogens, estradiol, raloxifene
Hypogonadism in boys, men; replacement therapy	Testosterone enanthate or cypionate; methyltestosterone; fluoxymesterone, testosterone (patch)
Anabolic protein synthesis	Oxandrolone, stanozolol
Prostate hyperplasia (benign)	Finasteride
Prostate carcinoma	GnRH agonist, androgen receptor antagonist (eg, flutamide)
Hirsutism	Combined oral contraceptive, spironolactone, flutamide, GnRH agonist

other mechanisms listed. The mechanisms of action of postcoital contraceptives are not well understood. When administered before the LH surge, they inhibit ovulation. They also affect cervical mucus, tubal function, and the endometrial lining.

2. Other clinical uses and beneficial effects— Combination hormonal contraceptives are used in young women with primary hypogonadism to prevent estrogen deficiency. Combinations of hormonal contraceptives and progestins are used to treat acne, hirsutism, dysmenorrhea, and endometriosis. Users of combination hormonal contraceptives have reduced risks of ovarian cysts, ovarian and endometrial cancer, benign breast disease, and pelvic inflammatory disease as well as a lower incidence of ectopic pregnancy, iron deficiency anemia, and rheumatoid arthritis.

3. Toxicity—The incidence of dose-dependent toxicity has fallen since the introduction of the low-dose combined oral contraceptives.

a. Thromboembolism—The major toxic effects of the combined hormonal contraceptives relate to the action of the estrogenic component on blood coagulation. There is a well-documented increase in the risk of thromboembolic events (myocardial infarction, stroke, deep vein thrombosis, pulmonary embolism) in older women, smokers, women with a personal or family history of such problems, and women with genetic defects that affect the production or function of clotting factors. However, the risk of thromboembolism incurred by the use of these drugs is usually less than that imposed by pregnancy.

b. Breast cancer—Evidence suggests that the lifetime risk of breast cancer in women who are current or past users of hormonal contraceptives is not changed, but there may be an earlier onset of breast cancer.

SKILL KEEPER: CYTOCHROME P450 AND HORMONAL CONTRACEPTIVES (SEE CHAPTERS 4 AND 61)

Hormonal contraceptives usually contain the lowest doses of the estrogen and progestin components that prevent pregnancy. The margin between effective and ineffective serum concentrations of the steroids is narrow, which presents a risk of unintended pregnancy resulting from drug–drug interactions. Most steroidal contraceptives are metabolized by cytochrome P450 isozymes.

1. *How many drugs can you identify that decrease the efficacy of hormonal contraceptives by increasing their metabolism?*

2. *When one of these drugs is prescribed for a woman who already is using a combined hormonal contraceptive, what should be done to prevent pregnancy?*

The Skill Keeper Answers appear at the end of the chapter.

---

c. Other toxicities—The low-dose combined oral and progestin-only contraceptives cause significant breakthrough bleeding, especially during the first few months of therapy. Other toxicities of the hormonal contraceptives include nausea, breast tenderness, headache, skin pigmentation, and depression. Preparations containing older, more androgenic progestins can cause weight gain, acne, and hirsutism. The high dose of estrogen in estrogen-containing postcoital contraceptives is associated with significant nausea.

ANTIESTROGENS AND ANTIPROGESTINS

A. SERMS

SERMs are mixed estrogen agonists that have estrogen agonist effects in some tissues and act as partial agonists or antagonists of estrogen in other tissues.

1. Tamoxifen—Tamoxifen is a SERM effective in the treatment of hormone-responsive breast cancer, where it acts as an *antagonist* to prevent receptor activation by endogenous estrogens (Figure 40–2). Prophylactic use of tamoxifen reduces the incidence of breast cancer in women who are at very high risk. As an *agonist* of endometrial receptors, tamoxifen promotes endometrial hyperplasia and increases the risk of endometrial cancer. The drug also causes hot flushes (an antagonist effect) and increases the risk of venous thrombosis (an agonist effect). Tamoxifen has more agonist than antagonist action on bone and thus prevents osteoporosis in postmenopausal women. **Toremifene** is structurally related to tamoxifen and has similar properties, indications, and toxicity.

2. Raloxifene—Raloxifene, approved for prevention and treatment of osteoporosis in postmenopausal women, has a partial agonist effect on bone. Like tamoxifen, raloxifene has antagonist effects in breast tissue and reduces the incidence of breast cancer in women who are at very high risk. Unlike tamoxifen, the drug has no estrogenic effects on endometrial tissue. Adverse effects include hot flushes (an antagonist effect) and an increased risk of venous thrombosis (an agonist effect).

3. Clomiphene—Clomiphene is a nonsteroidal compound with tissue-selective actions. It is used to induce ovulation in anovulatory women who wish to become pregnant. By selectively blocking estrogen receptors in the pituitary, clomiphene reduces negative feedback and increases FSH and LH output. The increase in gonadotropins stimulates ovulation.

B. PURE ESTROGEN RECEPTOR ANTAGONISTS

Fulvestrant is a pure estrogen receptor antagonist (in all tissues). It is used in the treatment of women with breast cancer that has developed resistance to tamoxifen.

C. SYNTHESIS INHIBITORS

1. Aromatase inhibitors—**Anastrozole** and related compounds (eg, letrozole) are nonsteroidal competitive inhibitors of aromatase, the enzyme required for the last step in estrogen synthesis. **Exemestane** is an irreversible aromatase inhibitor. These drugs are used in the treatment of breast cancer.

2. Danazol—Danazol inhibits several P450 enzymes involved in gonadal steroid synthesis and is a weak partial agonist of progestin, androgen, and glucocorticoid receptors. The drug is sometimes used in the treatment of endometriosis and fibrocystic disease of the breast.

D. GONADOTROPIN-RELEASING HORMONE ANALOGS

As discussed in Chapter 37, the continuous administration of gonadotropin-releasing hormone (GnRH) agonists (eg, **leuprolide**) suppresses gonadotropin secretion and thereby inhibits ovarian production of estrogens and progesterone. The GnRH agonists are used in combination with other agents in controlled ovarian hyperstimulation (Chapter 37) and are also used for treatment of precocious puberty in children and short-term (< 6 month) treatment of endometriosis and uterine fibroids in women. Treatment beyond 6 months in premenopausal women can result in decreased bone density.

E. ANTIPROGESTINS

Mifepristone (RU 486) is an orally active steroid antagonist of progesterone and glucocorticoids (Chapter 39). Its major use is as an abortifacient in early pregnancy (up to 49 days after the last menstrual period). The combination of mifepristone and the prostaglandin E analog misoprostol (Chapters 18 and 60) achieves a complete abortion in over 95% of early pregnancies. The most common complication is failure to induce a complete abortion. Side effects, which are primarily due to the misoprostol, include nausea, vomiting, and diarrhea plus the vaginal cramping and bleeding associated with passing the pregnancy.

ANDROGENS

Testosterone and related androgens are produced in the testis, the adrenal, and, to a small extent, the ovary. Testosterone is synthesized from progesterone and dehydroepiandrosterone (DHEA). In the plasma, testosterone is partly bound to sex hormone-binding globulin (SHBG), a transport protein. The hormone is converted in several organs (eg, prostate) to **dihydrotestosterone** (DHT), which is the active hormone in those tissues. Because of rapid hepatic metabolism, testosterone given orally has little effect. It may be given by injection in the form of long-acting esters or transdermal patch. Orally active variants are also available (Table 40–1).

Many androgens have been synthesized in an effort to increase the anabolic effect (see Effects, discussed later) without increasing androgenic action. **Oxandrolone** and **stanozolol** are examples of drugs that, in laboratory testing, have an increased ratio of anabolic–androgenic action. However, all of the so-called **anabolic steroids** have full androgenic agonist effects when used in humans.

A. MECHANISM OF ACTION

Like other steroid hormones, androgens enter cells and bind to cytosolic receptors. The hormone–receptor complex enters the nucleus and modulates the expression of target genes.

B. EFFECTS

Testosterone is necessary for normal development of the male fetus and infant and is responsible for the major changes in the male at puberty (growth of penis, larynx, and skeleton; development of facial, pubic, and axillary hair; darkening of skin; enlargement of muscle mass). After puberty, testosterone acts to maintain secondary sex characteristics, fertility, and libido. It also acts on hair cells to cause male-pattern baldness.

The major effect of androgenic hormones, in addition to development and maintenance of normal male characteristics, is an anabolic action that involves increased muscle size and strength and increased red blood cell production. Excretion of urea nitrogen is reduced, and nitrogen balance becomes more positive. Testosterone also helps maintain normal bone density.

C. CLINICAL USE

The primary clinical use of the androgens is for replacement therapy in hypogonadism (Table 40–1). Androgens have also been used to stimulate red blood cell production in certain anemias and to promote weight gain in patients with wasting syndromes (eg, AIDS patients). The anabolic effects have been exploited illicitly by athletes to increase muscle bulk and strength and perhaps enhance athletic performance.

D. TOXICITY

Use of androgens by females results in virilization (hirsutism, enlarged clitoris, deepened voice) and menstrual irregularity. In women who are pregnant with a female fetus, exogenous androgens can cause virilization of the fetus's external genitalia. Paradoxically, excessive doses in men can result in feminization (gynecomastia, testicular shrinkage, infertility) as a result of feedback inhibition of the pituitary and conversion of the exogenous androgens to estrogens. In both sexes, high doses of anabolic steroids can cause cholestatic jaundice, elevation of liver enzyme levels, and possibly hepatocellular carcinoma.

ANTIANDROGENS

Reduction of androgen effects is an important mode of therapy for both benign and malignant prostate disease, precocious puberty, hair loss, and hirsutism. Drugs are available that act at different sites in the androgen pathway (Figure 40–2).

A. RECEPTOR INHIBITORS

Flutamide and related drugs are nonsteroidal competitive antagonists of androgen receptors. These drugs are used to decrease the action of endogenous androgens in patients with prostate carcinoma. **Spironolactone,** a drug used principally as a potassium-sparing diuretic (Chapter 15), also inhibits androgen receptors and is used in the treatment of hirsutism in women.

B. 5α-REDUCTASE INHIBITORS

Testosterone is converted to DHT by the enzyme 5α-reductase. Some tissues, most notably prostate cells and hair follicles, depend on DHT rather than testosterone for androgenic stimulation. This enzyme is inhibited by **finasteride,** a drug used to treat benign prostatic hyperplasia and, at a lower dose, to prevent hair loss in men. Because the drug does not interfere with the action of testosterone, it is less likely than other antiandrogens to cause impotence, infertility, and loss of libido.

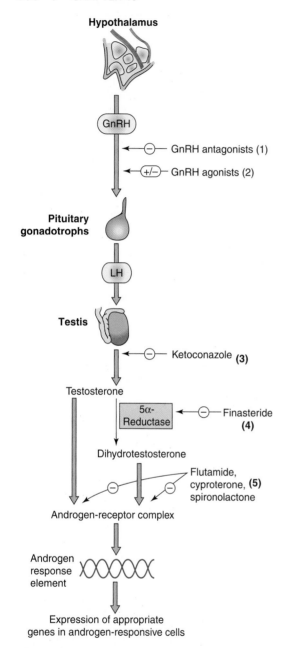

Figure 40–2. Control of androgen secretion and activity and some sites of action of antiandrogens: (1) competitive inhibition of GnRH receptors (see Chapter 37); (2) stimulation (+) or inhibition (–) by GnRH agonists; (3) inhibition of testosterone synthesis by ketoconazole; (4) inhibition of dihydrotestosterone production by finasteride; (5) inhibition of androgen binding at its receptor by flutamide and other drugs. (Modified and reproduced, with permission, from Katzung BG, editor: *Basic & Clinical Pharmacology,* 10th ed. McGraw-Hill, 2007.)

C. Gonadotropin-Releasing Hormone Analogs

Suppression of gonadotropin secretion, especially LH, reduces the production of testosterone. This can be effectively accomplished with long-acting depot preparations of **leuprolide** or similar gonadotropin-releasing hormone (GnRH) agonists (Chapter 37). These analogs are used in prostatic carcinoma. During the first week of therapy, an androgen receptor antagonist (eg, flutamide) is added to prevent the tumor flare that can result from the surge in testosterone synthesis caused by the initial agonistic action of the GnRH agonist. Within several weeks, testosterone production falls to low levels.

D. Combined Hormonal Contraceptives

Combined hormonal contraceptives are used in women with hirsutism. The estrogen in the contraceptive acts in the liver to increase the production of SHBG, which in turn reduces the concentration of the free androgen in the blood that is causing the male-pattern hair growth characteristic of hirsutism.

E. Inhibitors of Steroid Synthesis

Ketoconazole, an antifungal drug (Chapter 48), inhibits gonadal and adrenal steroid synthesis. The drug has been used to suppress adrenal steroid synthesis in patients with steroid-responsive metastatic prostate cancer.

QUESTIONS

1. The estrogen that is used in most combined hormonal contraceptives is
   (A) Clomiphene
   (B) Ethinyl estradiol
   (C) Estrone
   (D) DES
   (E) Norgestrel

2. A 23-year-old woman desires a combined oral contraceptive for pregnancy protection. A factor that would lead a health professional to recommend an alternative form of contraception is that the woman
   (A) Has evidence of hirsutism
   (B) Has a history of gastroesophageal reflux disease and is currently taking omeprazole
   (C) Has a history of pelvic inflammatory disease
   (D) Has a history of migraine headache that is well controlled by sumatriptan
   (E) Plans to use this contraceptive for about 1 year and will then attempt to become pregnant

3. Men who use large doses of anabolic steroids are at increased risk of
   (A) Anemia
   (B) Cholestatic jaundice and elevation of aspartate transaminase levels in the blood
   (C) Hirsutism

KEY DRUGS

Subclass	Prototype	Other Significant Agents
Estrogens	Ethinyl estradiol	Conjugated estrogens, estrone, estriol, mestranol
Progestins	Norgestrel, medroxyprogesterone	Progesterone, norgestimate, norethindrone
Antiestrogens and antiprogestins		
SERMs	Tamoxifen, raloxifene	Clomiphene
Aromatase inhibitors	Anastrozole	Letrozole
Synthesis inhibitor	Danazol	
Antiprogestin	Mifepristone (RU 486)	
GnRH agonist	Leuprolide	
Androgens	Testosterone	Methyltestosterone, fluoxymesterone
Anabolic steroids	Oxandrolone	Stanozolol
Antiandrogens		
Receptor antagonist	Flutamide	Bicalutamide
5α-Reductase inhibitor	Finasteride	
Synthesis inhibitor	Ketoconazole	
Other	GnRH analogs, combined oral contraceptives	

(D) Hyperprolactinemia
(E) Testicular enlargement

4. A 50-year-old woman with a positive mammogram undergoes lumpectomy and a small carcinoma is removed. Biochemical analysis of the cancer reveals the presence of estrogen and progesterone receptors. After this procedure, she will probably receive
(A) Danazol
(B) Flutamide
(C) Leuprolide
(D) Mifepristone
(E) Tamoxifen

5. A 60-year-old man is found to have a prostate lump and an elevated prostate-specific antigen (PSA) blood test. Magnetic resonance imaging suggests several enlarged lymph nodes in the lower abdomen, and x-ray film reveals 2 radiolucent lesions in the bony pelvis. This patient is likely to be treated with
(A) Anastrozole
(B) Desogestrel
(C) Flutamide
(D) Methyltestosterone
(E) Oxandrolone

6. A young woman complains of abdominal pain at the time of menstruation. Careful evaluation indicates the presence of significant endometrial deposits on the pelvic peritoneum. The most appropriate therapy for this patient is
(A) Flutamide, orally
(B) Medroxyprogesterone acetate by intramuscular injection
(C) Norgestrel as an IUD
(D) Oxandrolone by intramuscular injection
(E) Raloxifene orally

7. Diethylstilbestrol (DES) should never be used in pregnant women because it is associated with
(A) Deep vein thrombosis
(B) Feminization of the external genitalia of male offspring
(C) Infertility and development of vaginal cancer in female offspring
(D) Miscarriages
(E) Virilization of the external genitalia of female offspring

8. The unique property of SERMs is that they
(A) Act as agonists in some tissues and antagonists in other tissues
(B) Activate a unique plasma membrane-bound receptor
(C) Have both estrogenic and progestational agonist activity

(D) Inhibit the aromatase enzyme required for estrogen synthesis

(E) Produce estrogenic effects without binding to estrogen receptors

9. Finasteride has efficacy in the prevention of male-pattern baldness by virtue of its ability to
(A) Competitively antagonize androgen receptors
(B) Decrease the release of gonadotropins
(C) Increase the serum concentration of SHBG
(D) Inhibit the synthesis of testosterone
(E) Reduce the production of DHT

10. A 52-year-old postmenopausal patient has evidence of low bone mineral density. She and her physician are considering therapy with raloxifene or a combination of conjugated estrogens and medroxyprogesterone acetate. Which of the following patient characteristics is MOST likely to lead them to select raloxifene?
(A) Previous hysterectomy
(B) Recurrent vaginitis
(C) Rheumatoid arthritis
(D) Strong family history of breast cancer
(E) Troublesome hot flushes

ANSWERS

1. Ethinyl estradiol, a synthetic estrogen with good bioavailability, is the estrogenic component of most combined oral contraceptives, the transdermal contraceptive, and the vaginal ring contraceptive. The answer is **B**.

2. Estrogen-containing hormonal contraceptives increase the risk of episodes of migraine headache. The answer is **D**.

3. In men, large doses of anabolic steroids are associated with liver impairment, including cholestasis and elevation of serum concentrations of transaminases. The answer is **B**.

4. Tamoxifen has proved useful in adjunctive therapy of breast cancer; the drug decreases the rate of recurrence of cancer. The answer is **E**.

5. Antiandrogen drugs are used to treat metastatic prostate cancer because they have efficacy, whereas conventional cytotoxic drugs do not. Flutamide is a competitive antagonist of the androgen receptor that is used in combination with a GnRH agonist in the treatment of men with prostate cancer. The answer is **C**.

6. In endometriosis, suppression of ovarian function and production of gonadal steroids are useful. Intramuscular injection of relatively large doses of medroxyprogesterone provides 3 mo of an ovarian

suppressive effect because of inhibition of pituitary production of gonadotropins. The answer is **B**.

7. DES is a nonsteroidal estrogen agonist. Several decades ago, misguided use of the drug in pregnant women appears to have resulted in fetal damage that predisposed female offspring to infertility and a rare form of vaginal cancer. For this reason, the drug should be avoided in pregnant women. Other estrogenic drugs do not appear to have these same effects. Although estrogens do increase the risk of deep vein thrombosis, this is not the reason why DES should be avoided. The answer is **C**.

8. SERMs such as tamoxifen and raloxifene exhibit tissue-specific estrogenic and antiestrogenic effects. The answer is **A**.

9. Finasteride inhibits 5α-reductase, the enzyme that converts testosterone to DHT, the principal androgen in androgen-sensitive hair follicles. The answer is **E**.

10. Conjugated estrogens and raloxifene both improve bone mineral density and protect against osteoporosis. The 2 advantages of raloxifene over full estrogen

SKILL KEEPER ANSWERS: CYTOCHROME P450 AND HORMONAL CONTRACEPTIVES (SEE CHAPTERS 4 AND 61)

1. *Gonadal steroids and their derivatives are metabolized primarily by the cytochrome P450 3A4 (CYP3A4) family of enzymes. Inducers of CYP3A4 include barbiturates, carbamazepine, corticosteroids, griseofulvin, nelfinavir, phenytoin, pioglitazone, rifampin, and rifabutin. The potential reduction in contraceptive efficacy of hormonal contraceptives by carbamazepine and phenytoin are of particular importance because these drugs are known teratogens. St. John's wort, an unregulated herbal product, contains an ingredient that induces CYP3A4 enzymes and can reduce the efficacy of hormonal contraceptives.*

2. *To prevent an unwanted pregnancy, it would be advisable to use a combined hormonal contraceptive pill with a higher dose of estrogen (eg, a formulation containing 50 mcg of ethinyl estradiol). Alternatively, or additionally, women may use a barrier form of contraception or switch to an IUD.*

receptor agonists are that raloxifene has antagonist effects in breast tissue and lacks an agonistic effect in endometrium. If a patient's uterus was removed by surgery, the difference in the endometrial effect is moot. In patients with a strong family history of breast cancer, raloxifene may be a better choice than a full estrogen agonist because it will not further increase the woman's risk of breast cancer and may even lower her risk. The answer is D.

CHECKLIST

When you complete this chapter, you should be able to:

☐ Describe the hormonal changes that occur during the menstrual cycle.

☐ Name 3 estrogens and 4 progestins. Describe their pharmacologic effects, clinical uses, and toxicity.

☐ List the benefits and hazards of hormonal contraceptives.

☐ List the benefits and hazards of postmenopausal estrogen therapy.

☐ Describe the use of gonadal hormones and their antagonists in the treatment of cancer in women and men.

☐ List or describe the toxic effects of anabolic steroids used to build muscle mass.

☐ Name 2 SERMs and describe their unique properties.

Pancreatic Hormones, Antidiabetic Agents, & Glucagon

41

In the endocrine pancreas, the islets of Langerhans contain at least 4 different types of endocrine cells, including A (alpha, glucagon producing), B (beta, insulin and amylin producing), D (delta, somatostatin producing), and F (pancreatic polypeptide producing). Of these, the B (insulin producing) cells are the most numerous.

The most common pancreatic disease requiring pharmacologic therapy is diabetes mellitus, a deficiency of insulin production or effect. Diabetes is treated with several parenteral formulations of insulin and oral or parenteral noninsulin antidiabetic agents. Glucagon, a hormone that affects the liver, cardiovascular system, and gastrointestinal tract, can be used to treat severe hypoglycemia.

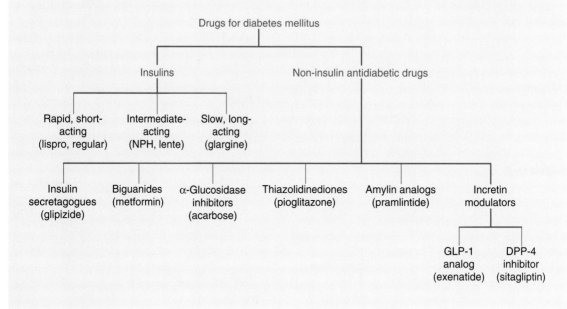

DIABETES MELLITUS

Two major forms of diabetes mellitus have been identified. Type 1 diabetes usually has its onset during childhood and results from autoimmune destruction of pancreatic B cells.

Type 2 diabetes is a progressive disorder characterized by increasing insulin resistance and diminishing insulin secretory capacity. Type 2 diabetes is frequently associated with obesity and is much more common than type 1 diabetes. Although type 2 diabetes usually has its onset in

HIGH-YIELD TERMS TO LEARN

Alpha-glucosidase	An enzyme in the gastrointestinal tract that converts complex starches and oligosaccharides to monosaccharides; inhibited by acarbose and miglitol
B cells in the islets of Langerhans	Insulin-producing cells in the endocrine pancreas; also commonly called beta cells
Hypoglycemia	Dangerously lowered serum glucose concentration; a toxic effect of high insulin concentrations and the secretagogue class of oral antidiabetic drugs
Lactic acidosis	Acidemia due to excess serum lactic acid; can result from excess production or decreased metabolism of lactic acid
Type 1 diabetes mellitus	A form of chronic hyperglycemia caused by immunologic destruction of pancreatic beta cells
Type 2 diabetes mellitus	A form of chronic hyperglycemia initially caused by resistance to insulin; often progresses to insulin deficiency

adulthood, the incidence in children and adolescents in the United States is rising dramatically, in parallel with the increase in obesity in children and adolescents.

The clinical history and course of these 2 forms differ considerably, but treatment in both cases requires careful attention to diet, fasting and postprandial blood glucose concentrations, and serum concentrations of hemoglobin A_{1c}, a glycosylated hemoglobin that serves as a marker of glycemia. Type 1 diabetes requires treatment with insulin. The early stages of type 2 diabetes usually can be controlled with noninsulin antidiabetic drugs. However, patients in the later stages of type 2 diabetes often require the addition of insulin to their drug regimen.

INSULIN

A. PHYSIOLOGY

Insulin is synthesized as the prohormone **proinsulin,** an 86-amino-acid single-chain polypeptide. Cleavage of proinsulin and cross-linking result in the 2-chain 51-peptide insulin molecule and a 31-amino-acid residual C-peptide. Neither proinsulin nor C-peptide appears to have any physiologic actions.

B. EFFECTS

Insulin has important effects in almost every tissue of the body. When activated by the hormone, the insulin receptor, a transmembrane tyrosine kinase, phosphorylates itself and a variety of intracellular proteins when activated by the hormone. The major target organs for insulin action include:

1. Liver—Insulin increases the storage of glucose as glycogen in the liver. This involves the insertion of additional GLUT2 glucose transport molecules in cell plasma membranes; increased synthesis of the enzymes pyruvate kinase, phosphofructokinase, and glucokinase; and suppression of several other enzymes. Insulin also decreases protein catabolism.

2. Skeletal muscle—Insulin stimulates glycogen synthesis and protein synthesis. Glucose transport into muscle cells is facilitated by insertion of GLUT4 transporters into cell plasma membranes.

3. Adipose tissue—Insulin facilitates triglyceride storage by activating plasma lipoprotein lipase, increasing glucose transport into cells via GLUT4 transporters, and reducing intracellular lipolysis.

C. INSULIN PREPARATIONS

Human insulin is manufactured by bacterial recombinant DNA technology. The available forms provide 4 rates of onset and durations of effect that range from rapid-acting to long-acting (Figure 41–1). The goals of insulin therapy are to control both basal and postprandial (after a meal) glucose levels while minimizing the risk of hypoglycemia. Insulin formulations with different rates of onset and effect are often combined to achieve these goals.

1. Rapid-acting—Three injected insulin analogs (**insulin lispro**, insulin aspart, and insulin glulisine) and the inhaled form of insulin have rapid onsets and early peaks of activity (Figure 41–1) that permit control of postprandial glucose levels. The 3 injectable rapid-acting insulins have small alterations in their primary amino acid sequences that speed their entry into the circulation without affecting their interaction with the insulin receptor. The rapid-acting insulins are injected immediately before a meal and are the preferred insulin

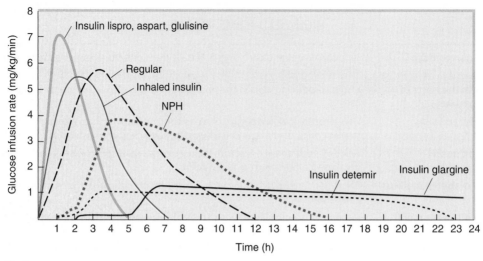

Figure 41–1. Extent and duration of action of various types of insulin as indicated by the glucose infusion rates (mg/kg/min) required to maintain a constant glucose concentration. The durations of action shown are typical of an average dose of 0.2–0.3 U/kg; with the exception of insulin lispro, aspart, and glulisine, duration increases considerably when dosage is increased. (Reproduced, with permission, from Katzung BG, editor: *Basic & Clinical Pharmacology,* 10th ed. McGraw–Hill, 2007.)

for continuous subcutaneous infusion devices. They also can be used for emergency treatment of uncomplicated diabetic ketoacidosis.

2. Short-acting—**Regular insulin** is used intravenously in emergencies or administered subcutaneously in ordinary maintenance regimens, alone or mixed with intermediate- or long-acting preparations. Before the development of rapid-acting insulins, it was the primary form of insulin used for controlling postprandial glucose concentrations, but it required administration 1 h or more before a meal.

3. Intermediate-acting—Neutral protamine Hagedorn insulin (**NPH insulin**) is a combination of regular insulin and protamine (a highly basic protein also used to reverse the action of unfractionated heparin, Chapter 34) that exhibits a delayed onset and peak of action (Figure 41–1). NPH insulin is often combined with regular and rapid-acting insulins.

4. Long-acting—**Insulin glargine** and insulin detemir are modified forms of human insulin that provide a peakless basal insulin level lasting more than 20 h, which helps control basal glucose levels without producing hypoglycemia.

5. Insulin delivery systems—The standard mode of insulin therapy is subcutaneous injection with conventional disposable needles and syringes. More convenient means of administration are also available.

Portable pen-sized injectors are used to facilitate subcutaneous injection. Some contain replaceable cartridges, whereas others are disposable.

Continuous subcutaneous insulin infusion devices avoid the need for multiple daily injections and provide flexibility in the scheduling of patients' daily activities. Programmable pumps deliver a constant 24-h basal rate, and manual adjustments in the rate of delivery can be made to accommodate changes in insulin requirements (eg, before meals or exercise).

An inhaled formulation of insulin can be used to cover mealtime insulin requirements.

D. HAZARDS OF INSULIN USE

The most common complication is **hypoglycemia**, resulting from excessive insulin effect. To avoid the brain damage that may result from hypoglycemia, prompt administration of glucose (sugar or candy by mouth, glucose by vein) or of glucagon (by intramuscular injection) is essential. Patients with advanced renal disease, the elderly, and children younger than 7 years are most susceptible to the detrimental effects of hypoglycemia.

The most common form of insulin-induced immunologic complication is the formation of antibodies to insulin or noninsulin protein contaminants, which results in resistance to the action of the drug or allergic reactions. With the current use of highly purified human insulins, immunologic complications are uncommon.

NONINSULIN ANTIDIABETIC DRUGS

Four well-established groups of oral antidiabetic drugs are used most commonly to treat type 2 diabetes. These include **insulin secretagogues**, the **biguanide metformin**,

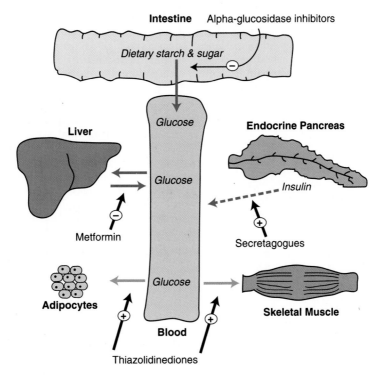

Figure 41–2. Major actions of the principal oral antidiabetic drugs used to treat type 2 diabetes.

thiazolidinediones, and α-glucosidase inhibitors (Figure 41–2). Three novel agents—pramlintide, exenatide, and sitagliptin—target endogenous regulators of glucose homeostasis. The durations of action of important members of these groups are listed in Table 41–1.

A. Insulin Secretagogues

1. **Mechanism and effects**—Insulin secretagogues stimulate the release of endogenous insulin by promoting closure of potassium channels in the pancreatic B cell membrane. Channel closure depolarizes the cell and triggers insulin release. Insulin secretagogues are not effective in patients who lack functional pancreatic B cells.

The older insulin secretagogues are in the chemical class known as **sulfonylureas.** The second-generation sulfonylureas (**glyburide, glipizide, glimepiride**) are considerably more potent and used more commonly than the older agents (**tolbutamide, chlorpropamide,** others). **Repaglinide**, a meglitinide, and **nateglinide,** a D-phenylalanine derivative, are the newest insulin secretagogues. Both have a rapid onset and short duration of action that make them useful for administration just before a meal to control postprandial glucose levels.

2. **Toxicities**—The insulin secretagogues, especially those with a high potency (eg, glyburide and glipizide), can precipitate hypoglycemia, although the risk is less than that associated with the insulins. The older

Table 41–1. Duration of action of representative oral antidiabetic drugs.

Drug	Duration of Action (hours)
Secretagogues	
Chlorpropamide	Up to 60
Tolbutamide	6–12
Glimepiride	12–24
Glipizide	10–24
Glyburide	10–24
Repaglinide	4–5
Biguanides	
Metformin	10–12
Thiazolidinediones	
Pioglitazone	15–24
Rosiglitazone	>24
α-Glucosidase inhibitors	
Acarbose	3–4
Miglitol	3–4
Incretin modifiers	
Sitagliptin	8–14

sulfonylureas (tolbutamide and chlorpropamide) are extensively bound to serum proteins, and drugs that compete for protein binding may enhance their hypoglycemic effects. Occasionally these drugs cause rash or other allergic reactions. Weight gain is common and is especially undesirable in the large fraction of patients with type 2 diabetes who already are overweight.

B. BIGUANIDES

1. Mechanism and effects—**Metformin**, the primary member of the biguanide group, reduces postprandial and fasting glucose levels. Biguanides inhibit hepatic and renal gluconeogenesis (Figure 41–2). Other effects include stimulation of glucose uptake and glycolysis in peripheral tissues, slowing of glucose absorption from the gastrointestinal tract, and reduction of plasma glucagon levels. The molecular mechanism of biguanide action is poorly understood but may involve activation of an AMP-stimulated protein kinase.

In patients with insulin resistance, metformin reduces endogenous insulin production presumably through enhanced insulin sensitivity. Because of this insulin-sparing effect and because it does not increase weight—unlike insulin, secretagogues, or the thiazolidinediones—metformin is increasingly the drug of first choice in overweight patients with type 2 diabetes. Recent clinical trials suggest that metformin reduces the risk of diabetes in high-risk patients. Metformin is also used to restore fertility in anovulatory women with polycystic ovary disease (PCOD) and evidence of insulin resistance.

2. Toxicities—Unlike the sulfonylureas, the biguanides do not cause hypoglycemia. Their most common toxicity is gastrointestinal distress (nausea, diarrhea), and they can cause lactic acidosis, especially in patients with renal or liver disease, alcoholism, or conditions that predispose to tissue anoxia and lactic acid production (eg, chronic cardiopulmonary dysfunction).

C. THIAZOLIDINEDIONES

1. Mechanism and effects—The thiazolidinediones, **rosiglitazone** and **pioglitazone**, increase target tissue sensitivity to insulin by activating the peroxisome proliferator-activated receptor-gamma nuclear receptor (**PPAR-γ receptor**). This nuclear receptor regulates the transcription of genes encoding proteins involved in carbohydrate and lipid metabolism. A primary effect of the thiazolidinediones is increasing glucose uptake in muscle and adipose tissue (Figure 41–2). They also inhibit hepatic gluconeogenesis, and have effects on lipid metabolism and the distribution of body fat. Thiazolidinediones reduce both fasting and postprandial hyperglycemia. They are used as monotherapy or in combination with insulin or other oral antidiabetic drugs. Like metformin, the thiazolidinediones have been shown to reduce the risk of diabetes in high-risk patients, and are used to restore fertility in anovulatory women with PCOD and evidence of insulin resistance.

2. Toxicities—When these drugs are used alone, hypoglycemia is extremely rare. Thiazolidinediones can cause fluid retention, which presents as mild anemia and edema and may increase the risk of heart failure. Recent data has linked rosiglitazone to increased risk of myocardial infarction. The original thiazolidinedione (troglitazone) was removed from the market in several countries because of hepatotoxicity. Rosiglitazone and pioglitazone have not been linked to serious liver dysfunction but still require routine monitoring of liver function. Female patients taking thiazolidinediones appear to have an increased risk of bone fractures. Pioglitazone and troglitazone induce cytochrome P450 activity (especially the 3A4 isozyme) and can reduce the serum concentrations of drugs that are metabolized by these enzymes (eg, oral contraceptives, cyclosporine).

D. α-GLUCOSIDASE INHIBITORS

1. Mechanism and effects—**Acarbose** and miglitol are carbohydrate analogs that act within the intestine to inhibit α-**glucosidase,** an enzyme necessary for the conversion of complex starches, oligosaccharides, and disaccharides to the monosaccharides that can be transported out of the intestinal lumen and into the bloodstream. As a result of slowed absorption, postprandial hyperglycemia is reduced. These drugs lack an effect on fasting blood sugar. Both drugs can be used as monotherapy or in combination with other antidiabetic drugs. They are taken just before a meal. Like metformin and the thiazolidinediones, the α-glucosidase inhibitors have been shown to prevent type 2 diabetes in prediabetic individuals.

2. Toxicities—The primary adverse effects of the α-glucosidase inhibitors include flatulence, diarrhea, and abdominal pain resulting from increased fermentation of unabsorbed carbohydrate by bacteria in the colon. Patients taking an α-glucosidase inhibitor who experience hypoglycemia should be treated with oral glucose (dextrose) and not sucrose, because the absorption of sucrose will be delayed.

E. PRAMLINTIDE

Pramlintide is an injectable synthetic analog of **amylin**, a 37-amino acid hormone produced by pancreatic B cells. Amylin contributes to glycemic control by activating high-affinity receptors that are a complex of the calcitonin receptor and a receptor-activity modifying receptor (RANK). Pramlintide suppresses glucagon release, slows gastric emptying, and works in the CNS to reduce appetite. After subcutaneous injection, it is rapidly absorbed and has a short duration of action. It is used in combination with insulin to control postprandial glucose levels. The major adverse effects associated with pramlintide are hypoglycemia and gastrointestinal disturbances.

F. EXENATIDE

Glucagon-like peptide-1 (**GLP-1**) is a member of the **incretin** family of peptide hormones, which are released from endocrine cells in the epithelium of the bowel in response to food. The incretins augment glucose-stimulated insulin release from pancreatic B cells, retard gastric emptying, inhibit glucagon secretion, and produce a feeling of satiety. The GLP-1 receptor is a G protein-coupled receptor (GPCR) that increases cAMP and also increases the free intracellular concentration of calcium.

Exenatide, a long-acting injectable peptide analog of GLP-1, is used in combination with metformin or a sulfonylurea for treatment of type 2 diabetes. The major adverse effects are gastrointestinal disturbances, particularly nausea during initial therapy, and hypoglycemia when exenatide is combined with a sulfonylurea.

G. SITAGLIPTIN

Sitagliptin is an oral inhibitor of dipeptidyl peptidase-4 (DPP-4), the enzyme that degrades GLP-1 and other incretins. It is approved for use in type 2 diabetes as monotherapy or in combination with metformin or a thiazolidinedione. Like exenatide, sitagliptin promotes insulin release, inhibits glucagon secretion, delays gastric emptying, and has an anorexic effect. The most common adverse effects associated with sitagliptin are headache, nasopharyngitis, and upper respiratory tract infection.

TREATMENT OF DIABETES MELLITUS

A. TYPE 1 DIABETES

Therapy of type 1 diabetes involves dietary instruction, parenteral insulin (a mixture of shorter- and longer-acting forms to maintain control of basal and postprandial glucose levels) and possibly pramlintide for improved control of postprandial glucose levels, plus careful attention by the patient to factors that change insulin requirements: exercise, infections, other forms of stress, and deviations from the regular diet. Large clinical studies indicate that **tight control** of blood sugar, by frequent blood sugar testing and insulin injections, reduces the incidence of vascular complications, including renal and retinal damage. The risk of hypoglycemic reactions is increased in tight control regimens but not enough to obviate the benefits of better control.

B. TYPE 2 DIABETES

Because type 2 diabetes is usually a progressive disease, therapy for an individual patient generally escalates over time. It begins with weight reduction and dietary control. Initial drug therapy usually is oral monotherapy with metformin, a second-generation sulfonylurea (glyburide, glipizide, or glimepiride) or, less commonly, a thiazolidinedione. Although initial responses to monotherapy usually are good, secondary failure within 5 years is common. Increasingly, noninsulin antidiabetics are being used in combination with each other or with insulin to achieve better glycemic control and minimize toxicity. Because type 2 diabetes involves both insulin resistance and inadequate insulin production, it makes sense to combine an agent that augments insulin's action (metformin, a thiazolidinedione, or an α-glucosidase inhibitor) with one that augments the insulin supplies (insulin secretagogue or insulin). Long-acting drugs (sulfonylureas, metformin, thiazolidinediones, exenatide, sitagliptin, some insulin formulations) help control both fasting and postprandial blood glucose levels, whereas short-acting drugs (α-glucosidase inhibitors, repaglinide, pramlintide, rapid-acting insulins) primarily target postprandial levels. As is the case for type 1 diabetes, clinical trials have shown that tight control of blood glucose trials in patients with type 2 diabetes reduces the risk of vascular complications.

SKILL KEEPER: DIABETES AND HYPERTENSION (SEE CHAPTER 11)

Diabetes is linked to hypertension in several important ways. Obesity predisposes patients to hypertension as well as to type 2 diabetes, so many patients suffer from both diseases. Both diseases damage the kidney and predispose patients to coronary artery disease. A large clinical trial of patients with type 2 diabetes suggests that poorly controlled hypertension exacerbates the microvascular disease caused by long-standing diabetes. Because of these links, it is important to consider the treatment of hypertension in diabetic patients.

1. *Identify the major drug groups used for chronic treatment of essential hypertension.*

2. *Which of these drug groups have special implications for the treatment of diabetic patients?*

The Skill Keeper Answers appear at the end of the chapter.

<table>
<tr><th colspan="3" align="center">KEY DRUGS</th></tr>
</table>

Subclass	Prototypes	Other Significant Agents
Insulins		
Rapid-acting	Insulin lispro	Insulin aspart, insulin glulisine
Short-acting	Regular insulin	
Intermediate-acting	NPH insulin	
Long-acting	Insulin glargine	Insulin detemir
Insulin secretagogues		
Sulfonylureas	Glipizide, glimepiride, glyburide	Chlorpropamide, tolbutamide
Meglitinide	Repaglinide	
D-Phenylalanine derivative	Nateglinide	
Biguanides	Metformin	
Thiazolidinediones	Pioglitazone, rosiglitazone	
α-Glucosidase inhibitors	Acarbose	Miglitol
Amylin analog	Pramlintide	
Incretin modifiers		
GLP-1 analog	Exenatide	
DPP-4 inhibitor	Sitagliptin	

HYPERGLYCEMIC DRUGS: GLUCAGON

A. GLUCAGON

1. Chemistry, mechanism, and effects—Glucagon is a protein hormone secreted by the A cells of the endocrine pancreas. Acting through G protein-coupled receptors in heart, smooth muscle, and liver, glucagon increases heart rate and force of contraction, increases hepatic glycogenolysis and gluconeogenesis, and relaxes smooth muscle. The smooth muscle effect is particularly marked in the gut.

2. Clinical uses—Glucagon is used to treat severe hypoglycemia in diabetics, but its hyperglycemic action requires intact hepatic glycogen stores. The drug is given intramuscularly or intravenously. In the management of severe β-blocker overdose, glucagon may be the most effective method for stimulating the depressed heart because it increases cardiac cAMP without requiring access to β receptors (Chapter 59).

QUESTIONS

1–2. A 13-year-old boy with type 1 diabetes is brought to the hospital complaining of dizziness. Laboratory findings include severe hyperglycemia, ketoacidosis, and a blood pH of 7.15.

1. To achieve rapid control of the severe ketoacidosis in this diabetic boy, the appropriate antidiabetic agent to use is
   (A) Crystalline zinc insulin
   (B) Glyburide
   (C) Insulin glargine
   (D) NPH insulin
   (E) Tobutamide

2. The most likely complication of insulin therapy in this patient is
   (A) Dilutional hyponatremia
   (B) Hypoglycemia
   (C) Increased bleeding tendency
   (D) Pancreatitis
   (E) Severe hypertension

3. A 24-year-old woman with type 1 diabetes wishes to try tight control of her diabetes to improve her long-term prognosis. Which of the following regimens is MOST appropriate?
   (A) Morning injections of mixed insulin lispro and insulin aspart
   (B) Evening injections of mixed regular insulin and insulin glargine
   (C) Morning and evening injections of regular insulin, supplemented by small amounts of NPH insulin at mealtimes

(D) Morning injections of insulin glargine, supplemented by small amounts of insulin lispro at mealtimes

(E) Morning injection of NPH insulin and evening injection of regular insulin

4. Which one of the following drugs promotes the release of endogenous insulin?
   (A) Acarbose
   (B) Glipizide
   (C) Metformin
   (D) Miglitol
   (E) Pioglitazone

5. An important effect of insulin is
   (A) Increased conversion of amino acids into glucose
   (B) Increased gluconeogenesis
   (C) Increased glucose transport into cells
   (D) Inhibition of lipoprotein lipase
   (E) Stimulation of glycogenolysis

6. A 54-year-old obese patient with type 2 diabetes and a history of alcoholism probably should not receive metformin because it can increase the risk of
   (A) A disulfiram-like reaction
   (B) Excessive weight gain
   (C) Hypoglycemia
   (D) Lactic acidosis
   (E) Serious hepatotoxicity

7. Which of the following drugs is taken during the first part of a meal for the purpose of delaying the absorption of dietary carbohydrates?
   (A) Acarbose
   (B) Exenatide
   (C) Glipizide
   (D) Pioglitazone
   (E) Repaglinide

8. The PPAR-γ receptor that is activated by thiazolidinediones increases tissue sensitivity to insulin by
   (A) Activating adenylyl cyclase and increasing the intracellular concentration of cAMP
   (B) Inactivating a cellular inhibitor of the GLUT2 glucose transporter
   (C) Inhibiting acid glucosidase, a key enzyme in glycogen breakdown pathways
   (D) Regulating transcription of genes involved in glucose utilization
   (E) Stimulating the activity of a tyrosine kinase that phosphorylates the insulin receptor

9. Which of the following drugs is MOST likely to cause hypoglycemia when used as monotherapy in the treatment of type 2 diabetes?
   (A) Acarbose
   (B) Glyburide

(C) Metformin
(D) Miglitol
(E) Rosiglitazone

10. Which of the following patients is MOST likely to be treated with intravenous glucagon?
    (A) An 18-year-old woman who took an overdose of cocaine and now has a blood pressure of 190/110
    (B) A 27-year-old woman with severe diarrhea caused by a flare in her inflammatory bowel disease
    (C) A 57-year-old woman with type 2 diabetes who has not taken her glyburide for the past 3 days
    (D) A 62-year-old man with severe bradycardia and hypotension resulting from ingestion of an overdose of atenolol
    (E) A 74-year-old man with lactic acidosis as a complication of severe infection and shock

ANSWERS

1. Oral antidiabetic agents are inappropriate in this patient because he has insulin-dependent diabetes. He needs a rapid-acting insulin preparation that can be given intravenously (see Table 41–1). The answer is **A.**

2. Because of the risk of brain damage, the most important complication of insulin therapy is hypoglycemia. The other choices are not common effects of insulin. The answer is **B.**

3. Insulin regimens for close control usually take the form of establishing a basal level of insulin with a small amount of a long-acting preparation (eg, insulin glargine) and supplementing the insulin levels, when called for by food intake, with short-acting insulin lispro. Less tight control may be achieved with 2 injections of intermediate-acting insulin per day. Because intake of glucose is mainly during the day, long-acting insulins are usually given in the morning, not at night. The answer is **D.**

4. Glipizide is a second-generation sulfonylurea that promotes insulin release by closing potassium channels in pancreatic B cells. The answer is **B.**

5. Insulin lowers serum glucose concentration in part by driving glucose into cells, particularly into muscle cells. The answer is **C.**

6. Biguanides, especially the older drug phenformin, have been associated with lactic acidosis. Thus, metformin should be avoided in patients with conditions that increase the risk of lactic acidosis, including alcoholism. The answer is **D.**

7. To be absorbed, carbohydrates must be converted into monosaccharides by the action of α-glucosidase

enzymes in the gastrointestinal tract. Acarbose inhibits α-glucosidase and, when present during digestion, delays the uptake of carbohydrates. The answer is **A.**

8. The PPAR-γ receptor belongs to a family of nuclear receptors. When activated, these receptors translocate to the nucleus, where they regulate the transcription of genes encoding proteins involved in the metabolism of carbohydrate and lipids. The answer is **D.**

9. The insulin secretagogues, including the sulfonylurea glyburide, can cause hypoglycemia as a result of their ability to increase serum insulin levels. The biguanides, thiazolidinediones, and α-glucosidase inhibitors are euglycemics that are unlikely to cause hypoglycemia when used alone. The answer is **B.**

10. Glucagon acts through cardiac glucagon receptors to stimulate the rate and force of contraction of the heart. Because this bypasses cardiac β adrenoceptors, glucagon is useful in the treatment of β-blocker-induced cardiac depression. The answer is **D.**

SKILL KEEPER ANSWERS:
DIABETES AND HYPERTENSION
(CHAPTER 11)

1. *The major antihypertensive drug groups are (a) β adrenoceptor blockers; (b) α_1 selective adrenoceptor blockers (eg, prazosin); (c) centrally acting sympathoplegics (eg, clonidine or methyldopa); (d) calcium channel blockers (eg, diltiazem, nifedipine, verapamil); (e) angiotensin-converting enzyme (ACE) inhibitors (eg, captopril); (f) angiotensin receptor antagonists (eg, losartan); and (g) thiazide diuretics.*

2. *ACE inhibitors slow the progression of diabetic nephropathy and help stabilize renal function. Angiotensin receptor antagonists may have similar protective effects in diabetic patients. Beta adrenoceptor blockers can mask the symptoms of hypoglycemia in diabetic patients. However, many patients with diabetes and cardiovascular disease are successfully treated with these drugs. A large clinical trial showed that control of hypertension decreases diabetes-associated microvascular disease. This trial included many patients being maintained on β adrenoceptor blockers. Thiazide diuretics impair the release of insulin and tissue utilization of glucose, so they are not drugs of first choice for patients with diabetes.*

CHECKLIST

When you complete this chapter, you should be able to:

☐ Describe the effects of insulin on hepatocytes, muscle, and adipose tissue.

☐ List the types of insulin preparations and their durations of action.

☐ Describe the major hazards of insulin therapy.

☐ List the prototypes and describe the mechanisms of action, key pharmacokinetic features, and toxicities of the major classes of agents used to treat type 2 diabetes.

☐ Give 3 examples of rational drug combinations for treatment of type 2 diabetes mellitus.

☐ Describe the clinical uses of glucagon.

Drugs That Affect Bone Mineral Homeostasis

Calcium and phosphorus, the 2 major elements of bone, are crucial not only for the mechanical strength of the skeleton but also for the normal function of many other cells in the body. Accordingly, a complex regulatory mechanism has evolved to tightly regulate calcium and phosphate homeostasis. Parathyroid hormone (PTH) and vitamin D are primary regulators, whereas calcitonin, glucocorticoids, and estrogens play secondary roles. These hormones or drugs that mimic or suppress their actions are used in the treatment of bone mineral disorders (eg, osteoporosis, rickets, osteomalacia, Paget's disease), as are several nonhormonal agents.

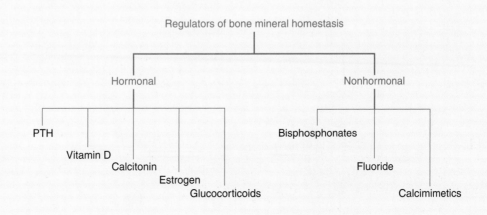

HORMONAL REGULATORS OF BONE MINERAL HOMEOSTASIS

A. PTH

PTH, an 84-amino-acid peptide, acts on membrane G protein-coupled receptors to increase cAMP in bone and renal tubular cells. In the kidney, PTH inhibits calcium excretion, promotes phosphate excretion, and stimulates the production of active vitamin D metabolites (Figure 42–1, Table 42–1). In bone, PTH promotes bone turnover by increasing the activity of both osteoclasts and osteoblasts. At the continuous high concentrations seen in hyperparathyroidism, the net effect of elevated PTH is increased bone resorption, hypercalcemia, and hyperphosphatemia. However, low intermittent doses of PTH produce a net increase in bone formation; this is

HIGH-YIELD TERMS TO LEARN	
Hyperparathyroidism	A condition of PTH excess characterized by hypercalcemia, bone pain, cognitive abnormalities, and renal stones. Primary disease results from parathyroid gland dysfunction. Secondary disease most commonly results from chronic kidney disease
Osteoblast	Bone cell that promotes bone *formation*
Osteoclast	Bone cell that promotes bone *resorption*
Osteomalacia	A condition of abnormal mineralization of adult bone secondary to nutritional deficiency of vitamin D or inherited defects in the formation or action of active vitamin D metabolites
Osteoporosis	Abnormal loss of bone with increased risk of fractures, spinal deformities, and loss of stature; remaining bone histologically normal
Paget's disease	A bone disorder, of unknown origin, characterized by excessive bone destruction and disorganized repair. Complications include skeletal deformity, musculoskeletal pain, kidney stones, and organ dysfunction secondary to pressure from bony overgrowth
Rickets	The same as osteomalacia, but when it occurs in the growing skeleton

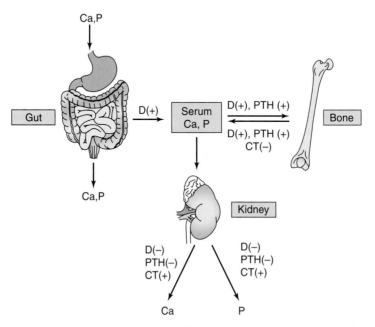

Figure 42–1. Effects of active metabolites of vitamin D *(D)*, parathyroid hormone *(PTH)*, and calcitonin *(CT)* on calcium and phosphorus homeostasis. Active metabolites of vitamin D increase absorption of calcium from both gut and bone, whereas PTH increases reabsorption from bone. Vitamin D metabolites and PTH both reduce urinary excretion of calcium. (Reproduced and modified, with permission, from Katzung BG, editor: *Basic & Clinical Pharmacology*, 10th ed. McGraw-Hill, 2007.)

Table 42–1. Actions of PTH and active vitamin D metabolites on intestine, kidney, and bone.

Organ	PTH	Active Vitamin D Metabolites
Intestine	Indirectly increases calcium and phosphate absorption by increasing vitamin D metabolites	Increased calcium and phosphate absorption
Kidney	Decreased calcium excretion, increased phosphate excretion	Increased resorption of calcium and phosphate but usually net increase in urinary calcium due to effects in GI tract and bone
Bone	Calcium and phosphate resorption increased by continuous high concentrations. Low intermittent doses increase bone formation	Direct effect is increased calcium and phosphate resorption; indirect effect is promoting mineralization by increasing the availability of calcium and phosphate
Net effect on serum levels	Serum calcium increased, serum phosphate decreased	Serum calcium and phosphate both increased

Reproduced and modified, with permission, from Katzung BG, editor: *Basic & Clinical Pharmacology,* 10th ed. McGraw-Hill, 2007.

the basis of the use of **teriparatide**, a recombinant truncated form of PTH, for parenteral treatment of osteoporosis.

The synthesis and secretion of PTH is primarily regulated by the serum concentration of free ionized calcium; a drop in free ionized calcium stimulates PTH release. Active metabolites of vitamin D play a secondary role in regulating PTH secretion by inhibiting PTH synthesis.

B. VITAMIN D

Vitamin D, a fat-soluble vitamin, can be synthesized in the skin from 7-dehydrocholesterol under the influence of ultraviolet light or absorbed from the diet in the natural form (vitamin D_3, **cholecalciferol**) or the plant form (vitamin D_2, **ergocalciferol**). Active metabolites are formed in the liver (25-hydroxyvitamin D or calcifediol) and kidney (1,25-dihydroxyvitamin D or **calcitriol** plus other metabolites). Renal synthesis of active vitamin D metabolites is stimulated by PTH and inhibited by phosphate and vitamin D metabolites. The action of vitamin D metabolites is mediated by activation of 1 or possibly a family of nuclear receptors that regulate gene expression.

Active vitamin D metabolites cause a net increase in serum concentrations of calcium and phosphate by increasing intestinal absorption and bone resorption and decreasing renal excretion (see Figure 42–1, Table 42–1). Because their effect in the GI tract and bone is greater than their effect in the kidney, they also increase urinary calcium. Active vitamin D metabolites are required for normal mineralization of bone; deficiencies cause rickets in growing children adolescents and osteomalacia in adults. Vitamin D metabolites inhibit PTH secretion directly and indirectly, by increasing serum calcium.

Vitamin D, vitamin D metabolites, and synthetic derivatives (Table 42–2) are used to treat deficiency states, including nutritional deficiency, intestinal osteodystrophy, chronic kidney or liver disease, hypoparathyroidism, and nephrotic syndrome. They are also used, in combination with calcium supplementation, to prevent and treat osteoporosis in older women and men. Topical formulations are used in psoriasis, a hyperproliferative skin disorder. The 2 forms of vitamin D—cholecalciferol and ergocalciferol—are available as oral supplements and are commonly added to dairy products and other foods. In patients with conditions that impair vitamin D activation (chronic kidney disease, liver disease, hypoparathyroidism), an active form of vitamin D such as calcitriol is required. In the

Table 42–2. Vitamin D and its clinically available metabolites and analogs.

Chemical Name	Generic Name
Vitamin D_3	Cholecalciferol
Vitamin D_2	Ergocalciferol
1,25-Dihydroxyvitamin D_3	Calcitriol
1α-Hydroxyvitamin D_2	Doxercalciferol
19-nor-1,25-Dihydroxyvitamin D_2	Paricalcitol
Calcipotriene	Calcipotriol

Reproduced and modified, with permission, from Katzung BG, editor: *Basic & Clinical Pharmacology,* 10th ed. McGraw-Hill, 2007.

treatment of secondary hyperparathyroidism associated with chronic kidney disease, calcitriol reduces PTH levels, corrects hypocalcemia, and improves bone disease, but it can also result in hypercalcemia and hypercalciuria through direct effects on intestinal, bone and renal handling of calcium and phosphate. Several forms of active vitamin D that selectively inhibit PTH formation while posing less risk of hypercalcemia have been developed. 1α-Hydroxyvitamin D_2 (**doxercalciferol**) is a prodrug that is converted in the liver to 1,25-dihyroxyvitamin D while 19-nor-1,25-dihydroxyvitamin D_2 (**paricalcitol**) and **calcipotriene** (calcipotriol) are analogs of calcitriol. All cause less hypercalcemia and, in patients with normal renal function, less hypercalciuria than calcitriol. Oral and parenteral doxercalciferol and oral paricalcitol are approved for treatment of secondary hyperparathyroidism in patients with chronic kidney disease. Calcipotriene (calcipotriol) is approved for topical treatment of psoriasis. These and other analogs are being investigated for use in various malignancies and inflammatory disorders.

The primary toxicity caused by chronic overdose with vitamin D or its active metabolites is hypercalcemia, hyperphosphatemia and hypercalciuria.

C. CALCITONIN

Calcitonin, a peptide hormone secreted by the thyroid gland, decreases serum calcium and phosphate by inhibiting bone resorption and inhibiting renal excretion of these minerals (see Figure 42–1). Bone formation is not impaired initially, but ultimately it is reduced. The hormone has been used in conditions in which an acute reduction of serum calcium is needed (eg, Paget's disease and hypercalcemia). Calcitonin is approved for treatment of osteoporosis and has been shown to increase bone mass and to reduce spine fractures. However, it is not as effective as teriparatide or bisphosphonates (below). Although human calcitonin is available, salmon calcitonin is most often selected for clinical use because of its longer half-life and greater potency. Calcitonin is administered by injection or as a nasal spray.

D. ESTROGENS

Estrogens and selective estrogen receptor modulators (SERMs; eg, **raloxifene**) can prevent or delay bone loss in postmenopausal women (Chapter 40). Their action may involve the inhibition of PTH-stimulated bone resorption.

E. GLUCOCORTICOIDS

The glucocorticoids (Chapter 39) inhibit bone mineral maintenance. As a result, chronic systemic use of these drugs is a common cause of osteoporosis in adults. However, these hormones are useful in the intermediate-term treatment of hypercalcemia.

SKILL KEEPER: DIURETICS AND CALCIUM (SEE CHAPTER 15)

The kidney is a key regulator of serum calcium concentrations. Several diuretics affect the kidney's handling of filtered calcium.

1. *Which 2 classes of diuretics have opposite effects on calcium elimination?*
2. *What mechanisms are responsible for their opposing effects?*
3. *What is the clinical importance of these effects?*

The Skill Keeper Answers appear at the end of the chapter.

NONHORMONAL AGENTS

A. BISPHOSPHONATES

The bisphosphonates (**alendronate, etidronate, ibandronate, pamidronate, risedronate, tiludronate,** and **zoledronic acid**) are short-chain organic polyphosphate compounds that reduce both the resorption and the formation of bone by an action on the basic hydroxyapatite crystal structure. The bisphosphonates have other complex cellular effects, including effects on vitamin D production and calcium absorption from the gastrointestinal tract, and direct effects on osteoclasts, including inhibition of farnesyl pyrophosphate synthase, an enzyme that appears to play a critical role in osteoclast survival. Bisphosphonates are used to manage the hypercalcemia associated with some malignancies and to treat Paget's disease. Chronic bisphosphonate therapy is used commonly to prevent and treat all forms of osteoporosis. It has been shown to increase bone density and reduce fractures.

Pamidronate, zoledronic acid, or etidronate are available for parenteral treatment of hypercalcemia associated with Paget's disease and malignancies. Etidronate and the other bisphosphonates listed above are available as oral medications. Oral bioavailability of bisphosphonates is low (< 10%), and food impairs their absorption. In the prevention or treatment of osteoporosis with alendronate, risedronate, or ibandronate, once-weekly or once-monthly administration of a relatively large dose of a bisphosphonate is as efficacious as daily administration of a smaller dose and does not result in more toxicity. The primary toxicity of the low bisphosphonate doses used for osteoporosis is gastric and esophageal irritation. To reduce esophageal irritation, patients are advised to take the drugs with large quantities of water and avoid situations that permit esophageal reflux. The higher doses of bisphosphonates used to treat hypercalcemia have been associated with renal impairment and osteonecrosis of the jaw.

B. Calcimimetics

Cinacalcet lowers PTH by activating the calcium-sensing receptor in the parathyroid gland. It is used for oral treatment of secondary hyperparathyroidism in chronic kidney disease and for the treatment of hypercalcemia in patients with parathyroid carcinoma. Its toxicities include hypocalcemia and adynamic bone disease, a condition of profoundly decreased bone cell activity.

C. Fluoride

Appropriate concentrations of fluoride ion in drinking water or as an additive in toothpaste have a well-documented ability to reduce dental caries. Chronic exposure to the ion, especially in high concentrations, may increase new bone synthesis. It is not clear, however, whether this new bone is normal in strength. Clinical trials of fluoride in patients with osteoporosis have not demonstrated a reduction in fractures. Acute toxicity of fluoride (usually caused by ingestion of rat poison) is manifested by gastrointestinal and neurologic symptoms.

D. Other Drugs With Effects on Serum Calcium and Phosphate

Gallium nitrate is effective in managing the hypercalcemia associated with some malignancies and possibly Paget's disease. It acts by inhibiting bone resorption. To prevent nephrotoxicity, patients need to be well hydrated and to have good renal output. The antibiotic **plicamycin (mithramycin)** has been used to reduce serum calcium and bone resorption in Paget's disease and hypercalcemia. Because of the risk of serious toxicity (eg, thrombocytopenia, hemorrhage, hepatic and renal damage), plicamycin is mainly restricted to short-term treatment of serious hypercalcemia. Several diuretics, most notably **thiazide diuretics** and **furosemide,** can affect serum and urinary calcium levels (see this chapter's Skill Keeper). The phosphate-binding gel **sevelamer** is used in combination with calcium supplements and dietary phosphate restriction to treat hyperphosphatemia, a common complication of renal failure, hypoparathyroidism, and vitamin D intoxication.

QUESTIONS

1. A drug that is routinely added to calcium supplements and milk for the purpose of preventing rickets in children and osteomalacia in adults is
   (A) Cholecalciferol
   (B) Calcitriol
   (C) Gallium nitrate
   (D) Sevelamer
   (E) Plicamycin

2. A drug that is useful for the treatment of hypercalcemia in Paget's disease is
   (A) Fluoride
   (B) Hydrochlorothiazide

KEY DRUGS

Subclass	Prototypes	Other Significant Agents
PTH analog	Teriparatide	
Vitamin D, metabolites and analogs		
Vitamin D	Cholecalciferol	Ergocalciferol
Vitamin D metabolites	Calcitriol	Doxercalciferol
Vitamin D analogs	Paricalcitol	Calcipotriene
Calcitonin	Calcitonin	
Estrogens	Raloxifene	
Bisphosphonates	Alendronate	Pamidronate, risedronate, and others
Calcimimetics	Cinacalcet	
Miscellaneous agents for treating hypercalcemia, hypercalciuria, or hyperphosphatemia	Glucocorticoids Gallium nitrate Plicamycin Furosemide Thiazide diuretics Sevelamer	

(C) Pamidronate
(D) Raloxifene
(E) Teriparatide

3. The active metabolites of vitamin D act through a nuclear receptor to
(A) Decrease the absorption of calcium from bone
(B) Increase PTH formation
(C) Increase renal production of erythropoietin
(D) Increase the absorption of calcium from the gastrointestinal tract
(E) Lower the serum phosphate concentration

4. Which of the following conditions is an indication for the use of raloxifene?
(A) Chronic kidney failure
(B) Hypoparathyroidism
(C) Intestinal osteodystrophy
(D) Postmenopausal osteoporosis
(E) Rickets

5–7. A 58-year-old postmenopausal woman was sent for dual-energy x-ray absorptiometry to evaluate the bone mineral density of her lumbar spine, femoral neck, and total hip. The test results revealed significantly low bone mineral density in all sites.

5. Chronic use of which of the following medications is MOST likely to have contributed to this woman's osteoporosis?
(A) Lovastatin
(B) Metformin
(C) Prednisone
(D) Propranolol
(E) Thiazide diuretic

6. If this patient began oral therapy with alendronate, she would be advised to drink large quantities of water with the tablets and remain in an upright position for at least 30 min and until eating the first meal of the day. These instructions would be given to decrease the risk of
(A) Cholelithiasis
(B) Diarrhea
(C) Constipation
(D) Erosive esophagitis
(E) Pernicious anemia

7. The patient's condition was not sufficiently controlled with alendronate, so she began therapy with a nasal spray containing a protein that inhibits bone resorption. The drug contained in the nasal spray was
(A) Calcitonin
(B) Calcitriol
(C) Cinacalcet
(D) Cortisol
(E) Teriparatide

8-10. A 67-year-old man with chronic kidney disease was found to have an elevated serum PTH concentration and a low serum concentration of 25-hydroxyvitamin D, the metabolite of vitamin D formed in the liver. He was successfully treated with ergocalciferol. Unfortunately, his kidney disease progressed so that he required dialysis and his serum PTH concentration became markedly elevated.

8. The drug that is MOST likely to lower this patient's serum PTH concentration is
(A) Calcitriol
(B) Cholecalciferol
(C) Furosemide
(D) Gallium nitrate
(E) Risedronate

9. Although the drug therapy was effective at lowering serum PTH concentrations, the patient experienced several episodes of hypercalcemia. He was switched to a vitamin D analog that suppresses PTH with less risk of hypercalcemia. The drug MOST likely used was
(A) Calcitriol
(B) Cholecalciferol
(C) Furosemide
(D) Paricalcitol
(E) Risedronate

10. In the treatment of patients like this with secondary hyperparathyroidism due to chronic kidney disease, cinacalcet is an alternative to vitamin D-based drugs. Cinacalcet lowers PTH by
(A) Activating a steroid receptor that inhibits expression of the PTH gene
(B) Activating the calcium-sensing receptor in parathyroid cells
(C) Activating transporters in the GI tract that are involved in calcium absorption
(D) Inducing the liver enzyme that converts vitamin D_3 to 25-hydroxyvitamin D_3
(E) Inhibiting the farnesyl pyrophosphate synthase found in osteoclasts

ANSWERS

1. The 2 forms of vitamin D—cholecalciferol and ergocalciferol—are commonly added to calcium supplements and dairy products. Calcitriol, the active 1,25-dihydroxyvitamin D_3 metabolite, would prevent vitamin D deficiency and is available as an oral formulation. However, because it is not subject to the complex mechanisms that regulate endogenous production of active vitamin D metabolites, it is not suitable for widespread use. The answer is **A.**

2. Paget's disease is characterized by excessive bone resorption, poorly organized bone formation, and

hypercalcemia. Bisphosphonates and calcitonin are first-line treatments. Pamidronate is a powerful bisphosphonate used parenterally to treat hypercalcemia. The answer is **C.**

3. The active metabolites of vitamin D increase serum calcium and phosphate by promoting calcium and phosphate uptake from the gastrointestinal tract, increasing bone resorption, and decreasing renal excretion of both electrolytes. They inhibit, rather than stimulate, PTH formation. The answer is **D.**

4. Raloxifene, a SERM, is approved for use in postmenopausal women with osteoporosis. The answer is **D.**

5. Long-term therapy with glucocorticoids such as prednisone is associated with a reduction in bone mineral density and an increased risk of fractures. The other drugs are not known to have significant effects on bone or serum calcium. The answer is **C.**

6. Oral bisphosphonates such as alendronate can irritate the esophagus and stomach. The risk of this toxicity is reduced by drinking water and by remaining in an upright position for 30 min after taking the medication. The answer is **D.**

7. Calcitonin is a peptide hormone that prevents bone resorption. Salmon calcitonin is available as a nasal spray or a parenteral form for injection. The answer is **A.**

8. In patients with chronic kidney disease that requires dialysis, the impaired production of active vitamin D metabolites compounded with elevated serum phosphate due to renal impairment leads to secondary hyperparathyroidism. Administration of the active vitamin D metabolite calcitriol acts directly on the parathyroid to inhibit PTH production. Cholecalciferol, a form of vitamin D, is not effective in patients with advanced renal disease who cannot form adequate amounts of active vitamin D metabolites. The answer is **A.**

9. Paricalcitol is an analog of 1,25-dihyroxyvitamin D_3 (calcitriol) that lowers serum PTH at doses that only rarely precipitate hypercalcemia. The molecular basis of this selective action is poorly understood but is of value in the management of hyperparathyroidism and psoriasis. The answer is **D.**

10. Cinacalcet is a member of a novel class of drugs that activate the calcium-sensing receptor in parathyroid cells. When this receptor is activated by cinacalcet or free ionized calcium, it activates a signaling pathway that suppresses PTH synthesis and release. The answer is **B.**

SKILL KEEPER ANSWERS: DIURETICS AND CALCIUM (SEE CHAPTER 15)

1. *Loop diuretics (eg, furosemide) and thiazide diuretics have opposite effects on urine calcium concentrations; loop diuretics increase urine concentrations of calcium, whereas the thiazides decrease urine calcium.*

2. *Loop diuretics inhibit the $Na^+/K^+/2Cl^-$ cotransporter in apical membranes of the thick ascending limb of the loop of Henle (see Figure 15–3). By disrupting the positive lumen-positive potential that normally serves as the driving force for resorption of Mg^{2+} and Ca^{2+}, loop diuretics inhibit Mg^{2+} and Ca^{2+} resorption, leaving more Mg^{2+} and Ca^{2+} in the urine and less in the blood. In the distal convoluted tubule where thiazides act, Ca^{2+} is actively resorbed through the concerted action of an apical Ca^{2+} channel and a basolateral Na^+/Ca^{2+} exchanger (see Figure 15–4). The system is under control of the PTH. When thiazides inhibit the Na^+/Cl^- transporter in cells that line the distal convoluted tubule, they lower the intracellular concentration of sodium and thereby enhance the Na^+/Ca^{2+} exchange that occurs on the basolateral surface. This, in turn, creates a greater driving force for passage of Ca^{2+} through the apical membrane calcium channels. The net effect is enhanced resorption of calcium.*

3. *In patients with hypercalcemia, treatment with a loop diuretic plus saline promotes calcium excretion and lowers serum calcium. In patients with intact regulatory function, increases in calcium resorption promoted by thiazides have minor impact on serum calcium because of buffering in bone and gut. However, thiazides can unmask hypercalcemia in patients with diseases that disrupt normal calcium regulation (eg, hyperparathyroidism, sarcoidosis, carcinoma). Thiazide diuretics are also used for treatment of individuals who are prone to kidney stone formation as a result of idiopathic hypercalciuria. In such individuals, it is crucial that primary hyperparathyroidism is ruled out before thiazide treatment is initiated.*

CHECKLIST

When you complete this chapter, you should be able to:

☐ Identify the major and minor endogenous regulators of bone mineral homeostasis.

☐ Sketch the pathway and sites of formation of 1,25-dihydroxyvitamin D.

☐ Compare and contrast the clinical uses and effects of the major forms of vitamin D and its active metabolites.

☐ Describe the major effects of PTH and vitamin D derivatives on the intestine, the kidney, and bone.

☐ Describe the agents used in the treatment of hypercalcemia and the agents used in the treatment of osteoporosis.

☐ Recall the effects of adrenal and gonadal steroids on bone structure and the actions of diuretics on serum calcium levels.

PART VIII
Chemotherapeutic Drugs

The emergence of **microbial resistance** poses a constant challenge to the use of antimicrobial drugs. Mechanisms underlying microbial resistance to cell wall synthesis inhibitors include the production of antibiotic-inactivating enzymes, changes in the structure of target receptors, increased efflux via drug transporters, and decreases in the permeability of microbes' cellular membranes to antibiotics. Strategies designed to combat microbial resistance include the use of adjunctive agents that can protect against antibiotic inactivation, the use of antibiotic combinations, the introduction of new (and often expensive) chemical derivatives of established antibiotics, and efforts to avoid the indiscriminate use or misuse of antibiotics.

Beta-Lactam Antibiotics & Other Cell Wall Synthesis Inhibitors

43

Penicillins and cephalosporins are the major antibiotics that inhibit bacterial cell wall synthesis. They are called beta-lactams because of the unusual 4-member ring that is common to all their members. The beta-lactams include some of the most effective, widely used, and well-tolerated agents available for the treatment of microbial infections. Vancomycin, fosfomycin, and bacitracin also inhibit cell wall synthesis but are not nearly as important as the beta-lactam drugs. The selective toxicity of the drugs discussed in this chapter is mainly due to specific actions on the synthesis of a cellular structure that is unique to the microorganism. More than 50 antibiotics that act as cell wall synthesis inhibitors are currently available, with individual spectra of activity that afford a wide range of clinical applications.

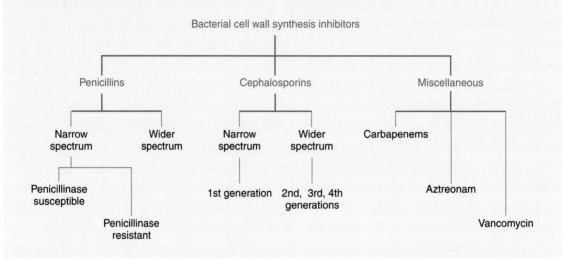

PENICILLINS

A. CLASSIFICATION

All penicillins are derivatives of 6-aminopenicillanic acid and contain a beta-lactam ring structure that is essential for antibacterial activity. Penicillin subclasses have additional chemical substituents that confer differences in antimicrobial activity, susceptibility to acid and enzymatic hydrolysis, and biodisposition.

B. PHARMACOKINETICS

Penicillins vary in their resistance to gastric acid and, therefore, vary in their oral bioavailability. Parenteral formulations of ampicillin, piperacillin, and ticarcillin

---

HIGH-YIELD TERMS TO LEARN

Bactericidal	An antimicrobial drug that can eradicate an infection in the absence of host defense mechanisms; kills bacteria
Bacteriostatic	An antimicrobial drug that inhibits antimicrobial growth but requires host defense mechanisms to eradicate the infection; does not kill bacteria
Beta-lactam antibiotics	Drugs with structures containing a beta-lactam ring: includes the penicillins, cephalosporins, and carbapenems. This ring must be intact for antimicrobial action
Beta-lactamases	Bacterial enzymes (penicillinases, cephalosporinases) that hydrolyze the beta-lactam ring of certain penicillins and cephalosporins
Beta-lactamase inhibitors	Potent inhibitors of some bacterial beta-lactamases used in combinations to protect hydrolyzable penicillins from inactivation
Minimal inhibitory concentration (MIC)	Lowest concentration of antimicrobial drug capable of inhibiting growth of an organism in a defined growth medium
Penicillin-binding proteins (PBPs)	Bacterial cytoplasmic membrane proteins that act as the initial receptors for penicillins and other beta-lactam antibiotics
Peptidoglycan	Chains of polysaccharides and polypeptides that are cross-linked to form the bacterial cell wall
Selective toxicity	More toxic to the invader than to the host; a property of useful antimicrobial drugs
Transpeptidases	Bacterial enzymes involved in the cross-linking of linear peptidoglycan chains, the final step in cell wall synthesis

---

are available for injection. Penicillins are polar compounds and are not metabolized extensively. They are usually excreted unchanged in the urine via glomerular filtration and tubular secretion; the latter process is inhibited by probenecid. Nafcillin is excreted mainly in the bile and ampicillin undergoes enterohepatic cycling. The plasma half-lives of most penicillins vary from 30 min to 1 h. Procaine and benzathine forms of penicillin G are administered intramuscularly and have long plasma half-lives because the active drug is released very slowly into the bloodstream. Most penicillins cross the blood-brain barrier only when the meninges are inflamed.

C. MECHANISMS OF ACTION AND RESISTANCE

Beta-lactam antibiotics are **bactericidal** drugs. They act to inhibit cell wall synthesis by the following steps (Figure 43–1): (1) binding of the drug to specific enzymes (**penicillin-binding proteins [PBPs]**) located in the bacterial cytoplasmic membrane; (2) inhibition of the **transpeptidation reaction** that cross-links the linear peptidoglycan chain constituents of the cell wall; and (3) activation of **autolytic** enzymes that cause lesions in the bacterial cell wall.

Enzymatic hydrolysis of the beta-lactam ring results in loss of antibacterial activity. The formation of **beta-lactamases (penicillinases)** by most staphylococci and many gram-negative organisms is a major mechanism of bacterial resistance. Inhibitors of these bacterial enzymes (eg, clavulanic acid, sulbactam, tazobactam) are often used in combination with penicillins to prevent their inactivation. Structural change in target PBPs is another mechanism of resistance and is responsible for methicillin resistance in staphylococci and for resistance to penicillin G in pneumococci (eg, penicillin-resistant *Streptococcus pneumoniae* [PRSP]) and enterococci. In some gram-negative rods (eg, *Pseudomonas aeruginosa*), changes in the porin structures in the outer cell wall membrane may contribute to resistance by impeding access of penicillins to PBPs.

D. CLINICAL USES

1. Narrow-spectrum penicillinase-susceptible agents—**Penicillin G** is the prototype of a subclass of penicillins that have a limited spectrum of antibacterial activity and are susceptible to beta-lactamases. Clinical uses include therapy of infections caused by common streptococci, meningococci, gram-positive bacilli, and spirochetes. Many strains of pneumococci are now resistant to penicillins (PRSP strains). Most strains of *Staphylococcus aureus* and a significant number of strains of *Neisseria gonorrhoeae* are resistant via production of beta-lactamases. Although no longer suitable for treatment of gonorrhea, penicillin G remains

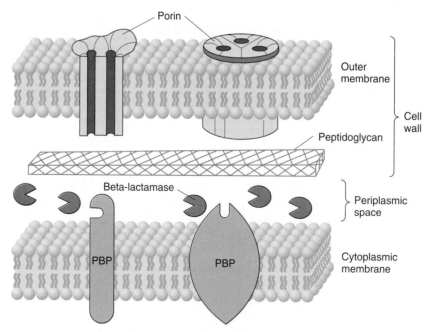

Figure 43–1. Beta-lactams and bacterial cell wall synthesis. The outer membrane shown in this simplified diagram is present only in gram-negative organisms. It is penetrated by proteins (porins) that are permeable to hydrophilic substances such as beta-lactam antibiotics. The peptidoglycan chains (mureins) are cross-linked by transpeptidases located in the cytoplasmic membrane, closely associated with penicillin-binding proteins (PBPs). Beta-lactam antibiotics bind to PBPs and inhibit transpeptidation, the final step in cell wall synthesis. They also activate autolytic enzymes that cause lesions in the cell wall. Beta-lactamases, which inactivate beta-lactam antibiotics, may be present in the periplasmic space or on the outer surface of the cytoplasmic membrane. (Reproduced, with permission, from Katzung BG, editor: *Basic & Clinical Pharmacology,* 10th ed. McGraw-Hill, 2007.)

the drug of choice for syphilis. Activity against enterococci is enhanced by aminoglycoside antibiotics. **Penicillin V** is an oral drug used mainly in oropharyngeal infections.

2. Very-narrow-spectrum penicillinase-resistant drugs—This subclass of penicillins includes **methicillin** (the prototype, but rarely used due to its nephrotoxic potential), **nafcillin,** and **oxacillin.** Their primary use is in the treatment of known or suspected staphylococcal infections. Methicillin-resistant (MR) staphylococci (*S aureus* [MRSA] and *S epidermidis* [MRSE]) are resistant to all penicillins and are often resistant to multiple antimicrobial drugs.

3. Wider spectrum penicillinase-susceptible drugs

    a. Ampicillin and amoxicillin—These drugs comprise a penicillin subgroup that has a wider spectrum of antibacterial activity than penicillin G but remains susceptible to penicillinases. Their clinical uses include indications similar to penicillin G as well as infections resulting from enterococci, *Listeria monocytogenes, Escherichia coli, Proteus mirabilis, Haemophilus*

influenzae, and *Moraxella catarrhalis,* although resistant strains occur. When used in combination with inhibitors of penicillinases (eg, clavulanic acid), their antibacterial activity is often enhanced. In enterococcal and listerial infections, ampicillin is synergistic with aminoglycosides.

    b. Piperacillin and ticarcillin—These drugs have activity against several gram-negative rods, including *Pseudomonas, Enterobacter,* and in some cases *Klebsiella* species. Most drugs in this subgroup have synergistic actions when used with aminoglycosides against such organisms. Piperacillin and ticarcillin are susceptible to penicillinases and are often used in combination with penicillinase inhibitors to enhance their activity.

E. TOXICITY

1. Allergy—Allergic reactions include urticaria, severe pruritus, fever, joint swelling, hemolytic anemia, nephritis, and anaphylaxis. About 5–10% of persons with a history of penicillin reaction have an allergic response when given a penicillin again. Methicillin causes interstitial nephritis, and nafcillin is associated with neutropenia. Antigenic determinants include degradation products of penicillins such as penicilloic acid. Complete **cross-allergenicity** between different penicillins should be assumed. Ampicillin frequently causes maculopapular skin rash that does not appear to be an allergic reaction.

2. Gastrointestinal disturbances—Nausea and diarrhea may occur with oral penicillins, especially with ampicillin. Gastrointestinal upsets may be caused by direct irritation or by overgrowth of gram-positive organisms or yeasts. Ampicillin has been implicated in pseudomembranous colitis.

CEPHALOSPORINS

A. CLASSIFICATION

The cephalosporins are derivatives of 7-aminocephalosporanic acid and contain the beta-lactam ring structure. Many members of this group are in clinical use. They vary in their antibacterial activity and are designated first-, second-, third-, or fourth-generation drugs according to the order of their introduction into clinical use.

B. PHARMACOKINETICS

Several cephalosporins are available for oral use, but most are administered parenterally. Cephalosporins with side chains may undergo hepatic metabolism, but the major elimination mechanism for drugs in this class is renal excretion via active tubular secretion. Cefoperazone and ceftriaxone are excreted mainly in the bile. Most first- and second-generation cephalosporins do not enter the cerebrospinal fluid even when the meninges are inflamed.

C. MECHANISMS OF ACTION AND RESISTANCE

Cephalosporins bind to PBPs on bacterial cell membranes to inhibit bacterial cell wall synthesis by mechanisms similar to those of the penicillins. Cephalosporins are bactericidal against susceptible organisms.

Structural differences from penicillins render cephalosporins less susceptible to penicillinases produced by staphylococci, but many bacteria are resistant through the production of other beta-lactamases that can inactivate cephalosporins. Resistance can also result from decreases in membrane permeability to cephalosporins and from changes in PBPs. Methicillin-resistant staphylococci are also resistant to cephalosporins.

D. CLINICAL USES

1. First-generation drugs—**Cefazolin** (parenteral) and **cephalexin** (oral) are examples of this subgroup. They are active against gram-positive cocci, including staphylococci and common streptococci. Many strains of *E coli* and *K pneumoniae* are also sensitive. Clinical uses include treatment of infections caused by these organisms and surgical prophylaxis in selected conditions. These drugs have minimal activity against gram-negative cocci, enterococci, methicillin-resistant staphylococci, and most gram-negative rods.

2. Second-generation drugs—Drugs in this subgroup usually have slightly less activity against gram-positive organisms than the first-generation drugs but have an extended gram-negative coverage. Marked differences in activity occur among the drugs in this subgroup. Examples of clinical uses include infections caused by the anaerobe *Bacteroides fragilis* (**cefotetan, cefoxitin**) and sinus, ear, and respiratory infections caused by *H influenzae* or *M catarrhalis* (**cefamandole, cefuroxime, cefaclor**).

3. Third-generation drugs—Characteristic features of third-generation drugs (eg, **ceftazidime, cefoperazone, cefotaxime**) include increased activity against gram-negative organisms resistant to other beta-lactam drugs and ability to penetrate the blood-brain barrier (except cefoperazone and cefixime). Most are active against *Providencia, Serratia marcescens,* and beta-lactamase-producing strains of *H influenzae* and *Neisseria*; they are less active against *Enterobacter* strains that produce extended-spectrum beta-lactamases. Ceftriaxone and cefotaxime are currently the most active cephalosporins against penicillin-resistant pneumococci (PRSP strains), but resistance has been reported. Individual drugs also have activity against *Pseudomonas* (**cefoperazone, ceftazidime**) and *B fragilis* (**ceftizoxime**). Drugs in this subclass should usually be reserved for treatment of serious infections. **Ceftriaxone** (parenteral) and **cefixime** (oral), currently drugs of choice in gonorrhea, are exceptions. Likewise, in acute otitis media, a single injection of ceftriaxone is usually as effective as a 10-day course of treatment with amoxicillin.

4. Fourth-generation drugs—**Cefepime** is more resistant to beta-lactamases produced by gram-negative organisms, including *Enterobacter, Haemophilus, Neisseria,* and some penicillin-resistant pneumococci. Cefepime combines the gram-positive activity of first-generation agents with the wider gram-negative spectrum of third-generation cephalosporins.

E. TOXICITY

1. Allergy—Cephalosporins cause a range of allergic reactions from skin rashes to anaphylactic shock. These reactions occur less frequently with cephalosporins than with penicillins. Complete cross-hypersensitivity between different cephalosporins should be assumed. Cross-reactivity between penicillins and cephalosporins is incomplete (5–10%), so penicillin-allergic patients are sometimes treated successfully with a cephalosporin. However, patients with a history of *anaphylaxis* to penicillins should not be treated with a cephalosporin.

2. Other adverse effects—Cephalosporins may cause pain at intramuscular injection sites and phlebitis after intravenous administration. They may increase the nephrotoxicity of aminoglycosides when the two are administered together. Drugs containing a methylthiotetrazole group (eg, cefamandole, cefoperazone, cefotetan) may cause hypoprothrombinemia and disulfiram-like reactions with ethanol.

OTHER BETA-LACTAM DRUGS

A. AZTREONAM

Aztreonam is a **monobactam** that is resistant to beta-lactamases produced by certain gram-negative rods, including *Klebsiella, Pseudomonas,* and *Serratia.* The drug has no activity against gram-positive bacteria or anaerobes. It is an inhibitor of cell wall synthesis, preferentially binding to a specific penicillin-binding protein (PBP3), and is synergistic with aminoglycosides.

Aztreonam is administered intravenously and is eliminated via renal tubular secretion. Its half-life is prolonged in renal failure. Adverse effects include gastrointestinal upset with possible superinfection, vertigo and headache, and rare hepatotoxicity. Although skin rash may occur, there is no cross-allergenicity with penicillins.

B. IMIPENEM, MEROPENEM, AND ERTAPENEM

These drugs are **carbapenems** (chemically different from penicillins but retaining the beta-lactam ring structure) with low susceptibility to beta-lactamases. They have wide activity against gram-positive cocci (including some penicillin-resistant pneumococci), gram-negative rods, and anaerobes. For pseudomonal infections, they are often used in combination with an aminoglycoside. The carbapenems are administered parenterally and are especially useful for infections caused by organisms resistant to other antibiotics. However, MRSA strains of staphylococci are resistant. They are currently drugs of choice for infections caused by *Enterobacter.*

Imipenem is rapidly inactivated by renal dehydropeptidase I and is administered in fixed combination with cilastatin, an inhibitor of this enzyme. Cilastatin increases the plasma half-life of imipenem and inhibits the formation of a potentially nephrotoxic metabolite.

Adverse effects of imipenem-cilastatin include gastrointestinal distress, skin rash, and, at very high plasma levels, CNS toxicity (confusion, encephalopathy, seizures). There is partial cross-allergenicity with the penicillins. **Meropenem** is similar to imipenem except that it is not metabolized by renal dehydropeptidases and is less likely to cause seizures. **Ertapenem** has a long half-life but is less active against *Pseudomonas,* and its intramuscular injection causes pain and irritation.

C. BETA-LACTAMASE INHIBITORS

Clavulanic acid, sulbactam, and **tazobactam** are used in fixed combinations with certain hydrolyzable penicillins. They are most active against plasmid-encoded beta-lactamases such as those produced by gonococci, streptococci, *E coli,* and *H influenzae.* They are not good inhibitors of inducible chromosomal beta-lactamases formed by *Enterobacter, Pseudomonas,* and *Serratia.*

OTHER CELL WALL OR MEMBRANE-ACTIVE AGENTS

A. VANCOMYCIN

Vancomycin is a bactericidal glycoprotein that binds to the D-Ala-D-Ala terminal of the nascent peptidoglycan pentapeptide side chain and inhibits transglycosylation. This action prevents elongation of the peptidoglycan chain and interferes with cross-linking. Resistance in strains of enterococci (vancomycin-resistant enterococci [VRE]) and staphylococci (vancomycin-resistant *S aureus* [VRSA]) involves a decreased affinity of vancomycin for the binding site because of the replacement of the terminal D-Ala by D-lactate. Vancomycin has a narrow spectrum of activity and is used for serious infections caused by drug-resistant gram-positive organisms, including methicillin-resistant staphylococci (MRSA) and in combination with a third-generation cephalosporin such as ceftriaxone for penicillin-resistant pneumococci (PRSP). Vancomycin is also a backup drug to metronidazole for treatment of infections caused by *Clostridium difficile.* **Teicoplanin,** another glycopeptide, has similar characteristics.

Vancomycin-resistant enterococci are increasing and pose a potentially serious clinical problem because such organisms usually exhibit multiple-drug resistance. Vancomycin-inermediate (VISA) strains of *S aureus* resulting in treatment failures have also been reported. Vancomycin is not absorbed from the gastrointestinal tract and may be given orally for bacterial enterocolitis. When given parenterally, vancomycin penetrates most tissues and is eliminated unchanged in the urine. Dosage modification is mandatory in patients with renal impairment. Toxic effects of vancomycin include chills, fever, phlebitis, ototoxicity, and nephrotoxicity. Rapid intravenous infusion may cause diffuse flushing ("red man syndrome") from histamine release.

B. FOSFOMYCIN

Fosfomycin is an antimetabolite inhibitor of cytosolic enolpyruvate transferase. This action prevents the formation of *N*-acetylmuramic acid, an essential precursor molecule for peptidoglycan chain formation. Resistance to fosfomycin occurs via decreased intracellular accumulation of the drug.

Fosfomycin is excreted by the kidney, with urinary levels exceeding the **minimal inhibitory concentrations (MICs)** for many urinary tract pathogens. In a single dose, the drug is less effective than a 7-day course of treatment with fluoroquinolones. With multiple dosing, resistance emerges rapidly and diarrhea is common. Fosfomycin may be synergistic with beta-lactam and quinolone antibiotics in specific infections.

KEY DRUGS

Subclass	Prototypes	Other Significant Agents
Penicillins		
Limited spectrum	Penicillin G	Penicillin V
Beta-lactamase resistant	Methicillin	Nafcillin, oxacillin
Wider spectrum	Ampicillin	Amoxicillin, piperacillin, ticarcillin
Cephalosporins		
First generation	Cefazolin	Cephradine
Second generation	Cefamandole	Cefaclor, cefotetan, cefoxitin
Third generation	Cefoperazone	Cefotaxime, ceftazidime, ceftriaxone
Fourth generation	Cefipime	
Carbapenems	Imipenem	Ertapenem, meropenem
Monobactam	Aztreonam	
Beta-lactamase inhibitors	Clavulanic acid	Sulbactam, tazobactam
Other agents	Vancomycin	Bacitracin, cycloserine, daptomycin, fosfomycin

C. BACITRACIN

Bacitracin is a peptide antibiotic that interferes with a late stage in cell wall synthesis in gram-positive organisms. Because of its marked nephrotoxicity, the drug is limited to topical use.

D. CYCLOSERINE

Cycloserine is an antimetabolite that blocks the incorporation of D-Ala into the pentapeptide side chain of the peptidoglycan. Because of its potential neurotoxicity (tremors, seizures, psychosis), cycloserine is only used to treat tuberculosis caused by organisms resistant to first-line antituberculous drugs.

E. DAPTOMYCIN

Daptomycin is a novel cyclic lipopeptide with spectrum similar to vancomycin but active against vancomycin-resistant strains of enterococci and staphylococci. The drug is eliminated via the kidney. Creatine phosphokinase activity should be monitored since daptomycin may cause myopathy.

QUESTIONS

1. Which statement about the biodisposition of penicillins and cephalosporins is *not* accurate?
    (A) Oral bioavailability is affected by lability in gastric acid
    (B) Most third-generation cephalosporins cross the blood-brain barrier
    (C) Nafcillin and ceftriaxone are eliminated mainly via biliary secretion
    (D) Procaine penicillin G is used via intramuscular injection
    (E) Renal tubular reabsorption of beta-lactams is inhibited by probenecid

2. The primary mechanism of antibacterial action of cephalosporins involves inhibition of
    (A) Beta-lactamases
    (B) Cell membrane synthesis
    (C) Reactions involving transpeptidation
    (D) Synthesis of *N*-acetylmuramic acid
    (E) Transglycosylation

3–4. A 21-year-old man was seen in a clinic with a complaint of dysuria and urethral discharge of yellow pus. He had a painless clean-based ulcer on the penis and nontender enlargement of the regional lymph nodes. Gram stain of the urethral exudate showed gram-negative diplococci within polymorphonucleocytes. The patient informed the clinic staff that he was unemployed and had not eaten a meal for 2 days.

3. The most appropriate treatment of gonorrhea in this patient is
    (A) Amoxicillin orally for 7 days
    (B) Ceftriaxone intramuscularly as a single dose
    (C) Procaine penicillin G intramuscularly as a single dose plus 1 g of probenecid
    (D) Tetracycline orally for 7 days
    (E) Vancomycin intramuscularly as a single dose

4. Immunofluorescent microscopic examination of fluid expressed from the penile chancre of this

patient revealed treponemes. Because he appears to be infected with *Treponema pallidum,* the best course of action would be to
(A) Treat with vancomycin
(B) Treat with oral tetracycline for 7 days
(C) Inject intramuscular benzathine penicillin G
(D) Give a single oral dose of fosfomycin
(E) Give no other antibiotics because drug treatment of gonorrhea provides coverage for incubating syphilis

5. Which statement about imipenem is accurate?
   (A) Has a narrow spectrum of antibacterial action
   (B) Is used in fixed combination with sulbactam
   (C) Is highly susceptible to beta-lactamases produced by *Enterobacter* species
   (D) In renal dysfunction, dosage reductions are necessary to avoid seizures
   (E) Is active against methicillin-resistant staphylococci

6. An elderly debilitated patient has a fever believed to be due to an infection. He has extensive skin lesions, scrapings of which reveal the presence of large numbers of gram-positive cocci. The drug to use for treatment of this patient is
   (A) Amoxicillin
   (B) Aztreonam
   (C) Cefoxitin
   (D) Nafcillin
   (E) Penicillin G

7. A 36-year-old woman recently treated for leukemia is admitted to the hospital with malaise, chills, and high fever. Gram stain of blood reveals the presence of gram-negative bacilli. The initial diagnosis is bacteremia, and parenteral antibiotics are indicated. The records of the patient reveal that she had a severe urticarial rash, hypotension, and respiratory difficulty after oral penicillin V about 6 mo ago. The drug regimen for empiric treatment is
   (A) Ampicillin plus sulbactam
   (B) Aztreonam
   (C) Cefazolin
   (D) Imipenem plus cilastatin
   (E) Ticarcillin plus clavulanic acid

8–10. A 52-year-old man (weight, 70 kg) is brought to the hospital emergency department in a confused and delirious state. He has had an elevated temperature for more than 24 h, during which time he had complained of a severe headache and had suffered from nausea and vomiting. Lumbar puncture reveals an elevated opening pressure, and cerebrospinal fluid findings include elevated protein, decreased glucose, and increased neutrophils. Gram stain of a smear of cerebrospinal fluid reveals gram-positive diplococci, and a preliminary diagnosis is made

of purulent meningitis. The microbiology report informs you that, for approximately 15% of *S pneumoniae* isolates in the community, the minimal inhibitory concentration for penicillin G is greater than 2 mcg/mL.

8. Treatment of this patient should be initiated immediately with intravenous administration of
   (A) Ampicillin-sulbactam
   (B) Cefoperazone
   (C) Cefotaxime plus vancomycin
   (D) Cefoxitin
   (E) Nafcillin

9. The molecular basis for the resistance of pneumococci to penicillin G is
   (A) Beta-lactamase production
   (B) Changes in penicillin binding proteins
   (C) Decreased intracellular accumulation of penicillin G
   (D) Changes in the D-Ala-D-Ala building block of peptidoglycan precursor
   (E) Changes in porin structure

10. If this patient had been 82 years old and the Gram stain of the smear of cerebrospinal fluid had revealed gram-positive rods resembling diphtheroids, the antibiotic regimen for empiric treatment would include
    (A) Ampicillin
    (B) Cefazolin
    (C) Fosfomycin
    (D) Ticarcillin
    (E) Vancomycin

11. Which statement about cefotetan is accurate?
    (A) It is active against MRSA strains
    (B) It is the drug of choice in community-acquired pneumonia
    (C) It decreases prothrombin time
    (D) It is a third-generation cephalosporin
    (E) It has an antibacterial spectrum that includes *Bacteroides fragilis*

12. A patient needs antibiotic treatment for native valve, culture-positive infective enterococcal endocarditis. His medical history includes a severe anaphylactic reaction to penicillin G during the past year. The best approach would be treatment with
    (A) Amoxicillin-clavulanate
    (B) Aztreonam
    (C) Cefazolin plus gentamicin
    (D) Meropenem
    (E) Vancomycin

13. This drug has activity against many strains of *P aeruginosa.* However, when it is used alone, resistance has emerged during the course of treatment. The drug should not be used in penicillin-allergic

patients. Its activity against gram-negative rods is enhanced if it is given in combination with tazobactam.
 (A) Amoxicillin
 (B) Aztreonam
 (C) Imipenem
 (D) Piperacillin
 (E) Vancomycin

14. Which statement about vancomycin is accurate?
 (A) It is bacteriostatic
 (B) It binds to PBPs
 (C) It is not susceptible to penicillinase
 (D) It has the advantage of oral bioavailability
 (E) Staphylococcal enterocolitis occurs commonly with its use

15. Which statement about ampicillin is NOT accurate?
 (A) Antibacterial activity is enhanced by sulbactam
 (B) Causes maculopapular rashes
 (C) Drug of choice for *L monocytogenes* infection
 (D) Eradicates most strains of MRSA
 (E) May cause pseudomembranous colitis

ANSWERS

1. Procaine penicillin G is given by intramuscular injection but is rarely used now owing to resistance on the part of gonococci and pneumococci. The elimination half-lives of many beta-lactam antibiotics are prolonged by probenecid, which inhibits their proximal tubular *secretion*. The answer is **E**.

2. The cephalosporins bind to PBPs acting at the transpeptidation stage of cell wall synthesis (the final step) to inhibit peptidoglycan cross-linking. Like penicillins, they also activate autolysins, which break down the bacterial cell wall. Synthesis of *N*-acetylmuramic acid is inhibited by fosfomycin. Vancomycin inhibits transglycosylase, preventing elongation of peptidoglycan chains. The answer is **C**.

3. Currently, the treatments of choice for gonorrhea include a single dose of ceftriaxone (intramuscularly). Because of the high incidence of beta-lactamase-producing gonococci, the use of penicillin G or amoxicillin is no longer appropriate for gonorrhea. Similarly, many strains of gonococci are resistant to tetracyclines. Alternative drugs (not listed) for gonorrhea include spectinomycin (see Chapter 45) and in some cases a fluoroquinolone (see Chapter 46). The answer is **B**.

4. This patient with gonorrhea also has primary syphilis. The penile chancre, the enlarged nontender lymph nodes, and the microscopic identification of treponemes in fluid expressed from the lesion are essentials of diagnosis. Although a single dose of ceftriaxone may cure incubating syphilis, it cannot be relied on for treating primary syphilis. The most appropriate course of action in this patient is to administer a single intramuscular injection of 2.4 million units of benzathine penicillin G. For penicillin-allergic patients, oral doxycycline or tetracycline for 15 days is effective in most cases (see Chapter 44). However, lack of compliance may be a problem with oral therapy. Fosfomycin and vancomycin have no significant activity against spirochetes. The answer is **C**.

5. Imipenem has a wide spectrum of activity that includes anaerobes and many beta-lactamase-producing gram-negative rods, including *Enterobacter*. It is not active against MRSA strains. The drug is hydrolyzed by renal dehydropeptidases and is given in combination with cilastatin, an inhibitor of this enzyme. Severe CNS toxicity, including seizures, will occur if the dose of imipenem is not reduced in patients with renal impairment. The answer is **D**.

6. Bacterial lesions of the skin are often caused by staphylococci or streptococci and may lead to systemic infections; they should be treated promptly. Virtually all strains of *S aureus* produce penicillinase, so amoxicillin and penicillin G would not be effective. Aztreonam is only active against gram-negative bacilli, and the second-generation cephalosporin (cefoxitin) has limited activity against gram-positive organisms. Nafcillin is resistant to penicillinases and has activity against many strains of *S aureus* (but not MRSA strains) and common streptococci. The answer is **D**.

7. Each of the drugs listed has activity against some gram-negative bacilli. All penicillins should be avoided in patients with a history of allergic reactions to any individual penicillin drug. Cephalosporins should also be avoided in patients who have had anaphylaxis or other severe hypersensitivity reactions after use of a penicillin. There is no cross-reactivity between the penicillins and aztreonam. The answer is **B**.

8. Pneumococcal isolates with a minimal inhibitory concentration for penicillin G of greater than 2 μg/mL are highly resistant. Such strains are not killed by the concentrations of penicillin G or ampicillin that can be achieved in the cerebrospinal fluid. Nafcillin has minimal activity against penicillin-resistant pneumococci. Cefotaxime and ceftriaxone (not listed) are the most active cephalosporins against penicillin-resistant pneumococci, and the addition of vancomycin or rifampin is recommended in the case of highly resistant strains. Cefoperazone does not readily cross the blood-brain barrier. The answer is **C**.

9. Pneumococcal resistance to penicillin is due to changes in the chemical structures of penicillin-binding proteins located in the bacterial cytoplasmic membrane. A similar mechanism underlies the resistance of staphylococci to methicillin (MRSA strains). A structural alteration in the D-Ala-D-Ala component of the pentapeptide side chains of peptidoglycans is the basis for a mechanism of resistance to vancomycin. The answer is **B.**

10. Diphtheroid-like gram-positive rods in the cerebrospinal fluid smear of an elderly patient are indicative of *L monocytogenes*. *Listeria* infections are more common in neonates, elderly patients, and those who have been treated with immunosuppressive agents. Treatment consists of ampicillin with or without gentamicin. The answer is **A.**

11. No currently available cephalosporin agents have activity against MRSA strains, and they are not drugs of choice in community-acquired pneumonia. The second-generation drugs cefotetan and cefoxitin have activity against anaerobes. Cephalosporins containing the methylthiotetrazole ring (cefamandole, cefotetan, cefoperazone) may cause hypoprothrombinemia and disulfiram-like interactions with ethanol. The answer is **E.**

12. In patients who have had a severe reaction to a penicillin, it is inadvisable to administer a cephalosporin or a carbapenem such as meropenem. Aztreonam has no significant activity against gram-positive cocci, so the logical treatment in this case is vancomycin, often with an aminoglycoside for synergistic activity against enterococci. The answer is **E.**

13. The drugs listed with activity against *P aeruginosa* are aztreonam, imipenem, and piperacillin. When any of these drugs are used as sole agents in pseudomonal infections, resistance can emerge rapidly. Aztreonam is safe in patients with established allergy to the penicillins. Piperacillin has greater activity against beta-lactamase-producing gram-negative rods when used with tazobactam. The answer is **D.**

14. Vancomycin is a bactericidal glycoprotein. It inhibits cell wall synthesis but does not bind to PBPs and is not susceptible to beta-lactamases. Vancomycin is not absorbed after oral administration and is used by this route in the treatment of colitis caused by *C difficile* and staphylococci. Vancomycin has useful activity against strains of methicillin-resistant staphylococci. The answer is **C.**

15. Ampicillin disturbs normal microflora and may cause yeast infections or colitis resulting from staphylococcal or clostridial overgrowths. Maculopapular rashes occur frequently, especially if ampicillin is administered to patients with viral infections. Sulbactam (a penicillinase inhibitor) enhances activity, but no penicillin has activity against MRSA strains. The answer is **D.**

CHECKLIST

When you complete this chapter, you should be able to:

☐ Describe the mechanism of antibacterial action of beta-lactam antibiotics.

☐ Describe 3 mechanisms underlying the resistance of bacteria to beta-lactam antibiotics.

☐ Identify the prototype drugs in each subclass of penicillins and describe their antibacterial activity and clinical uses.

☐ Identify the 4 subclasses of cephalosporins and describe their antibacterial activities and clinical uses.

☐ List the major adverse effects of the penicillins and the cephalosporins.

☐ Identify the important features of aztreonam, imipenem, and meropenem.

☐ Describe the clinical uses and toxicities of vancomycin.

Chloramphenicol, Tetracyclines, Macrolides, Clindamycin, Streptogramins, & Linezolid

44

The antimicrobial drugs reviewed in this chapter selectively inhibit bacterial protein synthesis. The mechanisms of protein synthesis in microorganisms are not identical to those of mammalian cells. Bacteria have 70S ribosomes, whereas mammalian cells have 80S ribosomes. Differences exist in ribosomal subunits and in the chemical composition and functional specificities of component nucleic acids and proteins. Such differences form the basis for the selective toxicity of these drugs against microorganisms without causing major effects on protein synthesis in mammalian cells.

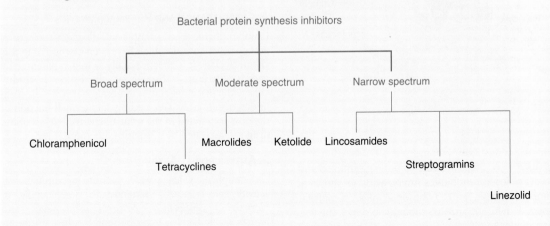

INHIBITORS OF MICROBIAL PROTEIN SYNTHESIS

Drugs that inhibit protein synthesis vary considerably in terms of chemical structures and their spectrum of antimicrobial activity. Chloramphenicol, tetracyclines, and the aminoglycosides (see Chapter 45) were the first inhibitors of bacterial protein synthesis to be discovered. Because they had a broad spectrum of antibacterial activity and were thought to have low toxicities, they were overused. Many once highly susceptible bacterial

species have become resistant, and most of these drugs are now used for more selected targets. Erythromycin, an older macrolide antibiotic, has a narrower spectrum of action but continues to be active against several important pathogens. Azithromycin and clarithromycin, semisynthetic macrolides, have some distinctive properties compared with erythromycin, as does clindamycin. Newer drugs, which include streptogramins, linezolid, telithromycin, and tigecycline (a tetracycline analog), have activity against certain bacteria that have developed resistance to older antibiotics.

MECHANISMS OF ACTION

Most of the antibiotics reviewed in this chapter are bacteriostatic inhibitors of protein synthesis acting at the ribosomal level (Figure 44–1). With the exception of tetracyclines, the binding sites for these antibiotics are on the 50S ribosomal subunit. Chloramphenicol inhibits transpeptidation (catalyzed by peptidyl transferase) by blocking the binding of the aminoacyl moiety of the charged transfer RNA (tRNA) molecule to the acceptor site on the ribosome-messenger (mRNA) complex. Thus, the peptide at the donor site cannot be transferred to its amino acid acceptor. Macrolides, telithromycin, and clindamycin, which share a common

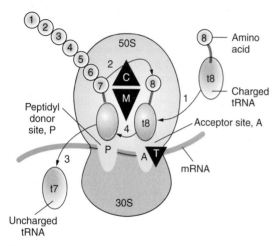

Figure 44–1. Steps in bacterial protein synthesis and targets of several antibiotics. Amino acids are shown as numbered circles. The 70S ribosomal mRNA complex is shown with its 50S and 30S subunits. In step 1, the charged tRNA unit carrying amino acid 8 binds to the acceptor site A on the 70S ribosome. The peptidyl tRNA at the donor site, with amino acids 1 through 7, then binds the growing amino acid chain to amino acid 8 (transpeptidation, step 2). The uncharged tRNA left at the donor site is released (step 3), and the new 8-amino acid chain with its tRNA shifts to the peptidyl site (translocation, step 4). The antibiotic binding sites are shown schematically as triangles. Chloramphenicol (C) and macrolides (M) bind to the 50S subunit and block transpeptidation (step 2). The tetracyclines (T) bind to the 30S subunit and prevent binding of the incoming charged tRNA unit (step 1). (Reproduced, with permission, from Katzung BG, editor: *Basic & Clinical Pharmacology*, 10th ed. McGraw-Hill, 2007.)

binding site on the 50S ribosome, also block transpeptidation. Tetracyclines bind to the 30S ribosomal subunit, preventing binding of amino acid-charged tRNA to the acceptor site of the ribosome-mRNA complex.

Streptogramins are bactericidal for most susceptible organisms. They bind to the 50S ribosomal subunit, constricting the exit channel on the ribosome through which nascent polypeptides are extruded. In addition, tRNA synthetase activity is inhibited, leading to a decrease in free tRNA within the cell. Linezolid is mainly bacteriostatic. The drug binds to a unique site on the 50S ribosome, inhibiting initiation by blocking formation of the tRNA-ribosome-mRNA ternary complex.

Selective toxicity of these protein synthesis inhibitors against microorganisms may be explained by target differences. Chloramphenicol does not bind to the 80S ribosomal RNA of mammalian cells, although it can inhibit the functions of *mitochondrial* ribosomes, which contain 70S ribosomal RNA. Tetracyclines have little effect on mammalian protein synthesis because an active efflux mechanism prevents their intracellular accumulation.

CHLORAMPHENICOL

A. CLASSIFICATION AND PHARMACOKINETICS

Chloramphenicol has a simple and distinctive structure, and no other antimicrobials have been discovered in this chemical class. It is effective orally as well as parenterally and is distributed throughout all tissues; it readily crosses the placental and blood-brain barriers. The drug undergoes enterohepatic cycling, and a small fraction of the dose is excreted in the urine unchanged. Most of the drug is inactivated by a hepatic glucuronosyltransferase.

B. ANTIMICROBIAL ACTIVITY

Chloramphenicol has a wide spectrum of antimicrobial activity and is usually bacteriostatic. Some strains of *Haemophilus influenzae, Neisseria meningitidis,* and *Bacteroides* are highly susceptible, and for these organisms chloramphenicol may be bactericidal. It is not active against *Chlamydiae* species. Resistance to chloramphenicol, which is plasmid mediated, occurs through the formation of acetyltransferases that inactivate the drug.

C. CLINICAL USES

Because of its toxicity, chloramphenicol has very few uses as a systemic drug. It is a backup drug for severe infections caused by *Salmonella* species and for the treatment of pneumococcal and meningococcal meningitis in beta-lactam-sensitive persons. Chloramphenicol is sometimes used for rickettsial diseases and for infections caused by anaerobes such as *Bacteroides fragilis.* The drug is commonly used as a topical antimicrobial agent.

D. TOXICITY

1. Gastrointestinal disturbances—These may occur from direct irritation and from superinfections, especially candidiasis.

2. Bone marrow—Inhibition of red cell maturation leads to a decrease in circulating erythrocytes. This action is dose dependent and reversible. Aplastic anemia is a rare idiosyncratic reaction (approximately 1 case in 25,000–40,000 patients treated). It is usually irreversible and may be fatal.

3. Gray baby syndrome—This syndrome occurs in infants and is characterized by decreased red blood cells, cyanosis, and cardiovascular collapse. Neonates, especially those who are premature, are deficient in hepatic glucuronosyltransferase and are, therefore, very sensitive to doses of this drug that would be tolerated in older infants.

4. Drug interactions—Chloramphenicol inhibits hepatic drug-metabolizing enzymes, increasing the elimination half-lives of drugs including phenytoin, tolbutamide, and warfarin.

TETRACYCLINES

A. CLASSIFICATION

Drugs in this class are broad-spectrum bacteriostatic antibiotics that have, with the exception of tigecycline, only minor differences in their activities against specific organisms.

B. PHARMACOKINETICS

Oral absorption is variable, especially for the older drugs, and may be impaired by foods and multivalent cations (calcium, iron, aluminum). Several tetracyclines are formulated for intravenous use. Tetracyclines have a wide tissue distribution and cross the placental barrier. All of the tetracyclines undergo enterohepatic cycling. Doxycycline is excreted mainly in feces; the other drugs are eliminated primarily in the urine. The half-lives of doxycycline and minocycline are longer than those of other tetracyclines. Tigecycline, formulated only for IV use, is eliminated in the bile and has a half-life of 30–36 h.

C. ANTIBACTERIAL ACTIVITY

Tetracyclines are broad-spectrum antibiotics with activity against gram-positive and gram-negative bacteria; species of *Rickettsia*, *Chlamydia*, and *Mycoplasma*; and some protozoa.

However, resistance to most tetracyclines is widespread. Resistance mechanisms include the development of mechanisms (efflux pumps) for active extrusion of tetracyclines and the formation of ribosomal protection proteins that interfere with tetracycline binding. These mechanisms do not confer resistance to tigecycline in most organisms, with the exception of the multidrug efflux pumps of *Proteus* and *Pseudomonas* species.

D. CLINICAL USES

1. Primary uses—Tetracyclines are recommended in the treatment of infections caused by *Mycoplasma pneumoniae* (in adults), *Chlamydia*, *Rickettsia*, and *Vibrio* species. Doxycycline is currently an alternative to macrolides in the initial treatment of community-acquired pneumonia.

2. Secondary uses—Tetracyclines are alternative drugs in the treatment of syphilis. They are also used in the treatment of respiratory infections caused by susceptible organisms, for prophylaxis against infection in chronic bronchitis, in the treatment of leptospirosis, and in the treatment of acne.

3. Selective uses—Specific tetracyclines are used in the treatment of gastrointestinal ulcers caused by *Helicobacter pylori* (tetracycline), in Lyme disease (doxycycline), and in the meningococcal carrier state (minocycline). Doxycycline is also used for the prevention of malaria and in the treatment of amebiasis (Chapter 53). Demeclocycline inhibits the renal actions of antidiuretic hormone (ADH) and is used in the management of patients with ADH-secreting tumors (Chapter 15).

4. Tigecycline—Unique features of this derivative of minocycline include a broad spectrum of action, which includes organisms resistant to standard tetracyclines. The antimicrobial activity of tigecycline includes gram-positive cocci resistant to methicillin (MRSA strains) and vancomycin (VRE strains), beta-lactamase producing gram-negative bacteria, anaerobes, chlamydiae, and mycobacteria.

E. TOXICITY

1. Gastrointestinal disturbances—Effects on the gastrointestinal system range from mild nausea and diarrhea to severe, possibly life-threatening colitis. Disturbances in the normal flora lead to candidiasis (oral and vaginal) and, more rarely, to bacterial superinfections with *S aureus* or *Clostridium difficile*.

2. Bony structures and teeth—Fetal exposure to tetracyclines may lead to tooth enamel dysplasia and irregularities in bone growth. Although usually contraindicated in pregnancy, there may be situations in which the benefit of tetracyclines outweigh the risk. Treatment of younger children may cause enamel dysplasia and crown deformation when permanent teeth appear.

3. Hepatic toxicity—High doses of tetracyclines, especially in pregnant patients and those with preexisting hepatic disease, may impair liver function and lead to hepatic necrosis.

4. Renal toxicity—One form of renal tubular acidosis, Fanconi's syndrome, has been attributed to the use of out-dated tetracyclines. Although not directly nephrotoxic, tetracyclines may exacerbate preexisting renal dysfunction.

5. Photosensitivity—Tetracyclines, especially deme-clocycline, may cause enhanced skin sensitivity to ultraviolet light.

6. Vestibular toxicity—Dose-dependent reversible dizziness and vertigo have been reported with doxycy-cline and minocycline.

MACROLIDES

A. CLASSIFICATION AND PHARMACOKINETICS

The macrolide antibiotics (**erythromycin, azithromycin, and clarithromycin**) are large cyclic lactone ring structures with attached sugars. The drugs have good oral bioavailability, but azithromycin absorption is impeded by food. Macrolides distribute to most body tissues, but azithromycin is unique in that the levels achieved in tissues and in phagocytes are considerably higher than those in the plasma. The elimination of erythromycin via biliary excretion) and clarithromycin (via hepatic metabolism and urinary excretion of intact drug) is fairly rapid (half-lives of 2 and 6 h, respectively). Azithromycin is eliminated slowly (half-life 2–4 days), mainly in the urine as unchanged drug.

B. ANTIBACTERIAL ACTIVITY

Erythromycin has activity against many species of *Campylobacter, Chlamydia, Mycoplasma, Legionella,* gram-positive cocci, and some gram-negative organisms. The spectra of activity of azithromycin and clarithromycin are similar but include greater activity against species of *Chlamydia, Mycobacterium avium* complex, and *Toxoplasma.*

Resistance to the macrolides in gram-positive organisms involves efflux pump mechanisms and the production of a methylase that adds a methyl group to the ribosomal binding site. Cross-resistance between individual macrolides is complete. In the case of methylase-producing microbial strains, there is partial cross-resistance with other drugs that bind to the same ribosomal site as macrolides, including clindamycin and streptogramins. Resistance in *Enterobacteriaceae* is the result of formation of drug-metabolizing esterases.

C. CLINICAL USES

Erythromycin is effective in the treatment of infections caused by *M pneumoniae, Corynebacterium, Campylobacter jejuni, Chlamydia trachomatis, Chlamydophila pneumoniae, Legionella pneumophila, Ureaplasma urealyticum,* and *Bordetella pertussis.* The drug is also active against gram-positive cocci (but not penicillin-resistant *Streptococcus pneumoniae* [PRSP] strains) and beta-lactamase-producing

staphylococci (but not methicillin-resistant *S aureus* [MRSA] strains).

Azithromycin has a similar spectrum of activity but is more active against *H influenzae, Moraxella catarrhalis,* and *Neisseria.* Because of its long half-life, a single dose of azithromycin is effective in the treatment of urogenital infections caused by *C trachomatis,* and a 4-day course of treatment has been effective in community-acquired pneumonia.

Clarithromycin has almost the same spectrum of antimicrobial activity and potential clinical uses as erythromycin. The drug is also used for prophylaxis against and treatment of *M avium* complex and as a component of drug regimens for ulcers caused by *H pylori.*

D. TOXICITY

Adverse effects include gastrointestinal irritation (common) via stimulation of motolin receptors, skin rashes, and eosinophilia. A hypersensitivity-based acute cholestatic hepatitis may occur with erythromycin estolate. Hepatitis is rare in children, but there is an increased risk with erythromycin estolate in the pregnant patient. Erythromycin inhibits several forms of hepatic cytochrome P450 and can increase the plasma levels of anticoagulants, carbamazepine, cisapride, digoxin, and theophylline. Similar drug interactions have also occurred with clarithromycin. The lactone ring structure of azithromycin is slightly different from that of other macrolides, and drug interactions are uncommon because azithromycin does not inhibit hepatic cytochrome P450.

TELITHROMYCIN

Telithromycin is a ketolide structurally related to macrolides. The drug has the same mechanism of action as erythromycin and a similar spectrum of antimicrobial activity. However, some macrolide-resistant strains are susceptible to telithromycin because it binds more tightly to ribosomes and is a poor substrate for bacterial efflux pumps that mediate resistance. The drug can be used for community-acquired pneumonia, including infections caused by multidrug-resistant organisms. Telithromycin is given orally once daily and is eliminated in the bile and the urine. Unfortunately, the use of telithromycin is limited by its adverse effects, which include severe hepatotoxicity, visual disturbances, and fainting episodes.

CLINDAMYCIN

A. CLASSIFICATION AND PHARMACOKINETICS

Clindamycin inhibits bacterial protein synthesis via a mechanism similar to that of the macrolides, although it is not chemically related. Mechanisms of resistance include methylation of the binding site on the 50S ribosomal subunit and enzymatic inactivation. Gram-negative aerobes are intrinsically resistant because of poor penetration of clindamycin through the outer membrane. Cross-resistance between clindamycin and macrolides is common. Good tissue penetration occurs after oral absorption. Clindamycin undergoes hepatic metabolism and both intact drug and metabolites are eliminated by biliary and renal excretion.

B. CLINICAL USE AND TOXICITY

The main use of clindamycin is in the treatment of severe infections caused by certain anaerobes such as *Bacteroides*. Clindamycin has been used as a backup drug against gram-positive cocci and is currently recommended for prophylaxis of endocarditis in valvular disease patients who are allergic to penicillin. The drug is also active against *Pneumocystis jiroveci* and is used in combination with pyrimethamine for AIDS-related toxoplasmosis. The toxicity of clindamycin includes gastrointestinal irritation, skin rashes, neutropenia, hepatic dysfunction, and possible superinfections such as *C difficile* pseudomembranous colitis.

STREPTOGRAMINS

Quinupristin-dalfopristin, a combination of 2 streptogramins, is bactericidal (see prior discussion of mechanism of action) and has a duration of antibacterial activity longer than the half-lives of the 2 compounds (postantibiotic effects). Antibacterial activity includes penicillin-resistant pneumococci, methicillin-resistant (MRSA) and vancomycin-resistant staphylococci (VRSA), and resistant *E faecium*; *E faecalis* is intrinsically resistant via an efflux transport mechanism. Administered intravenously, the combination product may cause pain and an arthralgia-myalgia syndrome. Streptogramins are potent inhibitors of CYP3A4 and increase plasma levels of many drugs, including astemizole, cisapride, cyclosporine, diazepam, nonnucleoside reverse transcriptase inhibitors, and warfarin.

LINEZOLID

The first of a new class of antibiotics (oxazolidinones), linezolid is active against drug-resistant gram-positive cocci, including strains resistant to penicillins (eg, MRSA, PRSP) and vancomycin (eg, VRE). The drug is also active against *L monocytogenes* and corynebacteria. Linezolid binds to a unique site located on the 23S ribosomal RNA of the 50S ribosomal subunit, and there is currently no cross-resistance with other protein synthesis inhibitors. Resistance (rare to date) involves a decreased affinity of linezolid for its binding site. Linezolid is available in both oral and parenteral formulations and should be reserved for treatment of infections caused by multidrug-resistant gram-positive bacteria. The drug is metabolized by the liver and has an elimination half-life of 4–6 h. Thrombocytopenia and neutropenia occur, most commonly in immunosuppressed patients.

QUESTIONS

1. A 2-year-old child is brought to the hospital after ingesting pills that a parent had used for bacterial dysentery when traveling outside the United States. The child has been vomiting for more than 24 h and has had diarrhea with green stools. He is now lethargic with an ashen color. Other signs and symptoms include hypothermia, hypotension, and abdominal distention. The drug most likely to be the cause of this problem is
   (A) Ampicillin
   (B) Chloramphenicol
   (C) Clindamycin
   (D) Doxycycline
   (E) Erythromycin

KEY DRUGS

Subclass	Prototype	Other Significant Agents
Chloramphenicol	Chloramphenicol	
Tetracyclines	Tetracycline	Demeclocycline, doxycycline, minocycline tigecycline
Macrolides	Erythromycin	Azithromycin, clarithromycin
Ketolides	Telithromycin	
Lincomycins	Lincomycin	Clindamycin
Streptogramins	Quinupristin-dalfopristin	
Oxazoladinones	Linezolid	

2. The mechanism of antibacterial action of tetracyclines involves
   (A) Binding to a component of the 50S ribosomal subunit
   (B) Block of binding of aminoacyl-tRNA to bacterial ribosomes
   (C) Inhibition of DNA-dependent RNA polymerase
   (D) Inhibition of translocase activity
   (E) Selective inhibition of ribosomal peptidyl transferases

3. A 24-year-old woman has primary syphilis. She has a history of penicillin hypersensitivity, so tetracycline will be used to treat the infection. Which statement about the proposed drug treatment of this patient is accurate?
   (A) Antacids will not affect absorption of the drug
   (B) Azithromycin would not be effective in treatment of this patient
   (C) For full effectiveness, tetracycline must be taken for 15 days
   (D) She should eat plenty of yogurt to prevent vaginal candidiasis
   (E) Tetracycline is a potent inhibitor of hepatic drug metabolizing enzymes

4. Clarithromycin and erythromycin have very similar spectra of antimicrobial activity. The major advantage of clarithromycin is that it
   (A) Eradicates mycoplasmal infections in a single dose
   (B) Is active against strains of streptococci that are resistant to erythromycin
   (C) Is more active against *M avium* complex
   (D) Is not an inhibitor of liver drug-metabolizing enzymes
   (E) Is active against methicillin-resistant strains of staphylococci

5. A primary mechanism underlying the resistance of gram-positive organisms to macrolide antibiotics is
   (A) Decreased activity of uptake mechanisms
   (B) Decreased drug permeability of the cytoplasmic membrane
   (C) Formation of drug-inactivating acetyltransferases
   (D) Formation of esterases that hydrolyze the lactone ring
   (E) Methylation of binding sites on the 50S ribosomal subunit

6. A 26-year-old woman was treated for gonorrhea at a neighborhood clinic. Since she was allergic to beta-lactams, a single intramuscular injection of spectinomycin was administered, and she was given a prescription for oral doxycycline to be taken for 7 days. Two weeks later she returns to the clinic with mucopurulent cervicitis. On questioning, she admits that she did not have the prescription filled because she had no money. The best course of action at this point would be to
   (A) Delay drug treatment until the infecting organism is identified
   (B) Give her the money for the prescription
   (C) Treat her with a single oral dose of cefixime
   (D) Treat her with a single oral dose of azithromycin
   (E) Write a prescription for oral erythromycin for 7 days

7. A 55-year-old patient with a prosthetic heart valve is to undergo a periodontal procedure involving scaling and root planing. Several years ago, the patient had a severe allergic reaction to procaine penicillin G. Regarding prophylaxis against bacterial endocarditis, which one of the following is most appropriate?
   (A) Administer amoxicillin orally 10 min before the procedure
   (B) Administer clindamycin orally 1 h before the procedure
   (C) Administer erythromycin orally 1 h before the procedure and 4 h after the procedure
   (D) Administer vancomycin orally 15 min before the procedure
   (E) No prophylaxis is needed because this patient is in the negligible risk category

8–10. A 24-year-old woman comes to a clinic with complaints of dry cough, headache, fever, and malaise, which have lasted 3 or 4 days. She appears to have some respiratory difficulty, and chest examination reveals rales but no other obvious signs of pulmonary involvement. However, extensive patchy infiltrates are seen on chest x-ray film. Gram stain of expectorated sputum fails to reveal any bacterial pathogens. The patient informs the attending physician that her husband is not sick but that a colleague at work has symptoms similar to those she is experiencing. The patient has no history of serious medical problems. The patient is taking loratadine for allergies, multivitamins, and supplementary iron tablets. She is an avid consumer of coffee and caffeinated beverages. The physician makes an initial diagnosis of community-acquired pneumonia.

8. Regarding the management of this patient, which drug is most suitable ?
   (A) Amoxicillin
   (B) Clindamycin
   (C) Doxycycline
   (D) Linezolid
   (E) Vancomycin

9. If this patient were to be treated with erythromycin, she should
   (A) Avoid exposure to sunlight
   (B) Avoid taking supplementary iron tablets
   (C) Decrease her intake of caffeinated beverages
   (D) Have her plasma urea nitrogen or creatinine checked before treatment
   (E) Temporarily discontinue the antihistamine

10. This patient should not be treated with telithromycin because the drug causes
    (A) Auditory dysfunction
    (B) Hepatotoxicity
    (C) Hyperkalemia
    (D) Myasthenia gravis
    (E) Seizures

11. In a patient with culture-positive enterococcal bacteremia who has failed to respond to vancomycin because of resistance, the treatment most likely to be effective is
    (A) Clarithromycin
    (B) Erythromycin
    (C) Linezolid
    (D) Minocycline
    (E) Ticarcillin

12. Which statement about doxycycline is accurate?
    (A) It is bactericidal
    (B) It is excreted mainly in the urine
    (C) It has an elimination half-life of less than 2 h
    (D) It is more active than tetracycline against *H pylori*
    (E) It is used in Lyme disease

13. Concerning streptogramins, which statement is accurate?
    (A) They are active in treatment of infections caused by *E faecalis*
    (B) They are used in the management of infections caused by multidrug-resistant streptococci
    (C) They are bacteriostatic
    (D) They induce formation of hepatic drug-metabolizing enzymes
    (E) Severe hepatotoxicity with these agents has led to FDA drug alerts

14. Which drug inhibits bacterial protein synthesis, has a narrow spectrum of activity, has been used in the management of abdominal abscess caused by *Bacteroides fragilis*, and may cause antibiotic-associated colitis?
    (A) Chloramphenicol
    (B) Clarithromycin
    (C) Clindamycin
    (D) Minocycline
    (E) Ticarcillin

ANSWERS

1. Chloramphenicol causes a dose-dependent suppression of erythropoiesis. Although the gray baby syndrome was initially described in neonates, a similar syndrome has occurred with overdosage of chloramphenicol in older children and adults, especially those with hepatic dysfunction. The answer is **B.**

2. Tetracyclines inhibit bacterial protein synthesis by interfering with the binding of aminoacyl-tRNA molecules to bacterial ribosomes. Peptidyl transferase is inhibited by chloramphenicol. The answer is **B.**

3. Azithromycin is a backup drug to penicillin G for treatment of syphilis, as is tetracycline. The ingestion of antacids and of foods containing multivalent cations (yogurt contains calcium and magnesium) can interfere with gastrointestinal absorption of tetracyclines. Tetracyclines do not inhibit drug metabolism. The answer is **C.**

4. Clarithromycin can be administered less frequently than erythromycin, but it is not effective in single doses against susceptible organisms. Organisms resistant to erythromycin, including pneumococci and methicillin-resistant staphylococci, are also resistant to other macrolides. Drug interactions have occurred with clarithromycin through its ability to inhibit cytochrome P450. Clarithromycin is more active than erythromycin against *M avium* complex, *T gondii,* and *H pylori.* The answer is **C.**

5. Methylase production and methylation of the receptor site are established mechanisms of resistance of gram-positive organisms to macrolide antibiotics. Such enzymes may be inducible by macrolides or constitutive; in the latter case, cross-resistance occurs between macrolides and clindamycin. Increased expression of efflux pumps is also a mechanism of macrolide resistance. Esterase formation is a mechanism of macrolide resistance seen in coliforms. The answer is **E.**

6. Cervicitis or urethritis that appears 2–3 weeks after treatment of gonorrhea is often caused by *C trachomatis.* Such infections may have been acquired at the same time as gonorrhea but develop more slowly because of the long incubation period of chlamydial infection. Treatment with oral doxycycline for 7 days would have eradicated *C trachomatis* and most other organisms commonly associated with nongonococcal cervicitis or urethritis. Given the limited compliance of this patient, the best course of action would be the administration (in the clinic) of a single oral dose of azithromycin. The answer is **D.**

7. This patient is in the high-risk category for bacterial endocarditis and should receive prophylactic

antibiotics before many dental procedures. The American Heart Association recommends that clindamycin be used in patients allergic to penicillins. Oral erythromycin is not recommended because it is no more effective than clindamycin and causes more gastrointestinal side effects. Intravenous vancomycin (not oral), sometimes with gentamicin, is recommended for prophylaxis in high-risk penicillin-allergic patients undergoing genitourinary and lower gastrointestinal surgical procedures. Complete cross-allergenicity must be assumed between individual penicillins. The answer is **B.**

8. It is often difficult to establish a definite cause of community-acquired pneumonia (CAP). Approximately 85% of CAP cases are caused by typical pathogens, such as *S pneumoniae, H influenzae,* or *M catarrhalis,* and 15% are due to the nonzoonotic atypical pathogens, such as *Legionella* species, *Mycoplasma* species, or *C pneumoniae.* Currently, monotherapy coverage of both typical and atypical pathogens in CAP is preferred to double-drug therapy. Preferred initial monotherapy includes a macrolide, doxycycline, or a quinolone active against respiratory pathogens (Chapter 46). Amoxicillin, clindamycin, linezolid, and vancomycin have low activity against atypical pathogens in CAP. The answer is **C.**

9. The inhibition of liver cytochrome P450 by erythromycin has led to serious drug interactions. Although erythromycin does not inhibit loratadine metabolism, it does inhibit the CYP1A2 form of cytochrome P450, which metabolizes methylxanthines. Consequently, cardiac and CNS toxicity may occur with excessive ingestion of caffeine. Unlike the tetracyclines, the oral absorption of erythromycin is not affected by cations and the drug does not cause photosensitivity. Because erythromycin undergoes biliary excretion, there is little reason to assess renal function before treatment. The answer is **C.**

10. The use of telithromycin has been linked to a significant number of cases of liver injury or failure, including several deaths. Its use should be restricted to community-acquired pneumonia due to pneumococci resistant to other antibiotics. Telithromycin also causes blurred vision and fainting episodes. It exacerbates, but does not cause, myasthenia gravis. The answer is **B.**

11. There is no regimen that is reliably bactericidal for infections caused by vancomycin-resistant enterococcus. However, regimens reported to be effective include ampicillin + ciprofloxacin + gentamicin, daptomycin + vancomycin, and linezolid as a single agent. The answer is **C.**

12. Tetracyclines are bacteriostatic drugs. Elimination of doxycycline is via nonrenal mechanisms, and the drug has a half-life of > 12 h, which allows for once-daily dosing. Doxycycline is no more active than tetracycline against *H pylori.* However, doxycycline is more effective against pathogens associated with acute exacerbations of chronic bronchitis (pneumococci, *H influenzae, M catarrhalis*) and has better activity in Lyme disease than other tetracyclines. The answer is **E.**

13. The combination of quinupristin-dalfopristin is bactericidal against many drug-resistant gram-positive cocci, including multidrug-resistant streptococci, MRSA, and vancomycin-resistant enterococci. The streptogramins have activity against *E faecium* (not *E faecalis*). The drugs are potent *inhibitors* of CYP3A4 and interfere with the metabolism of many other drugs. The streptogramins are not hepatotoxic. The answer is **B.**

14. Carbapenems (not listed), chloramphenicol, clindamycin, and ticarcillin (with clavulanic acid) are alternative drugs for infections caused by *B fragilis.* Chloramphenicol is a broad-spectrum antibiotic, and ticarcillin inhibits bacterial cell wall synthesis. The drug of choice currently for infections due to *B fragilis* is metronidazole (Chapter 50). The answer is **C.**

CHECKLIST

When you complete this chapter, you should be able to:

☐ Explain (1 sentence per drug class) how these agents inhibit bacterial protein synthesis.

☐ Identify the primary mechanisms of resistance to each of these drug classes.

☐ Name the most important agents in each drug class and list 3 clinical uses of each.

☐ Recall distinctive pharmacokinetic features of the major drugs.

☐ List the characteristic toxic effects of the major drugs in each class.

Aminoglycosides

MODES OF ANTIBACTERIAL ACTION

In the treatment of microbial infections with antibiotics, multiple daily dosage regimens traditionally have been designed to maintain serum concentrations above the minimal inhibitory concentration (MIC) for as long as possible. However, the in vivo effectiveness of some antibiotics, including aminoglycosides, results from a **concentration-dependent** killing action. As the plasma level is increased above the MIC, aminoglycosides kill an increasing proportion of bacteria and do so at a more rapid rate. Many antibiotics, including penicillins and cephalosporins, cause **time-dependent** killing of microorganisms, wherein their in vivo efficacy is directly related to time above MIC and becomes independent of concentration once the MIC has been reached.

Aminoglycosides are also capable of exerting a **postantibiotic effect** such that their killing action continues when their plasma levels have declined below measurable levels. Consequently, aminoglycosides have greater efficacy when administered as a single large dose than when given as multiple smaller doses. The toxicity (in contrast to the antibacterial efficacy) of aminoglycosides depends both on a critical plasma concentration and on the time that such a level is exceeded. The time above such a threshold will be shorter with administration of a single large dose of an aminoglycoside than when multiple smaller doses are given. These concepts form the basis for once-daily aminoglycoside dosing protocols, which can be more effective and less toxic than traditional dosing regimens.

PHARMACOKINETICS

Aminoglycosides are structurally related amino sugars attached by glycosidic linkages. They are polar compounds, not absorbed after oral administration and must be given intramuscularly, or intravenously for systemic effect. They have limited tissue penetration and do not readily cross the blood-brain barrier. Glomerular filtration is the major mode of excretion, and plasma levels of these drugs are greatly affected by changes in renal function. Excretion of aminoglycosides is directly proportionate to creatinine clearance. With normal renal function the elimination half-life of aminoglycosides is 2–3 h.

Dosage adjustments must be made in renal insufficiency to avoid toxic accumulation. Monitoring of plasma levels of aminoglycosides can be valuable for safe and effective dosage selection and adjustment. For traditional dosing regimens (2 or 3 times daily), peak serum levels are measured 30–60 min after administration and trough levels just before the next dose.

MECHANISM OF ACTION

Aminoglycosides are bactericidal inhibitors of protein synthesis. Their penetration through the bacterial cell envelope is partly dependent on oxygen-dependent active transport, and they have minimal activity against strict anaerobes. Aminoglycoside transport can be enhanced by cell wall synthesis inhibitors, which may be the basis of antimicrobial synergism. Inside the cell, aminoglycosides bind to the 30S ribosomal subunit and interfere with protein synthesis in at least 3 ways: (1) They block formation of the initiation complex; (2) they cause misreading of the code on the mRNA template; and (3) they inhibit translocation (Figure 45–1). Aminoglycosides may also disrupt polysomal structure, resulting in nonfunctional monosomes.

MECHANISMS OF RESISTANCE

Streptococci, including *Streptococcus pneumoniae,* and enterococci are relatively resistant to gentamicin and most other aminoglycosides owing to failure of the drugs to penetrate into the cell. However, the primary mechanism of resistance to aminoglycosides, especially in gram-negative bacteria, involves the plasmid-mediated formation of inactivating enzymes. These enzymes are **group transferases** that catalyze the acetylation of amine functions and the transfer of phosphoryl or adenylyl groups to the oxygen atoms of hydroxyl groups on the aminoglycoside. Individual aminoglycosides have varying susceptibilities to such enzymes. For example, transferases produced by enterococci can inactivate amikacin, gentamicin, and tobramycin but not streptomycin. Currently, **netilmicin** is less susceptible to such enzymes, and the drug may be active against more strains of organisms than other aminoglycosides.

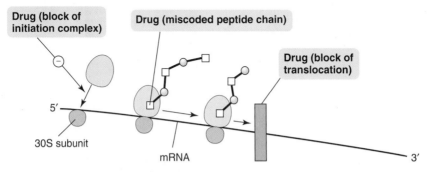

Normal bacterial cell

Figure 45–1. Putative mechanisms of action of the aminoglycosides. Normal protein synthesis is shown in the top panel. At least 3 different aminoglycoside effects have been described, as shown in the bottom panel: block of formation of the initiation complex; miscoding of amino acids in the emerging peptide chain due to misreading of the mRNA; and block of translocation on mRNA. Block of movement of the ribosome may occur after the formation of a single initiation complex, resulting in an mRNA chain with only a single ribosome on it, a so-called monosome.

CLINICAL USES

The main differences among the individual aminoglycosides lie in their activities against specific organisms, particularly gram-negative rods. **Gentamicin, tobramycin, and amikacin** are important drugs for the treatment of serious infections caused by aerobic gram-negative bacteria, including *Escherichia coli* and *Enterobacter, Klebsiella, Proteus, Providencia, Pseudomonas,* and *Serratia* species. These aminoglycosides also have activity against strains of *Haemophilus influenzae, Moraxella catarrhalis,* and *Shigella* species, although they are not drugs of choice for infections caused by these organisms. In most cases, aminoglycosides are used in combination with a beta-lactam antibiotic. When used alone, aminoglycosides are not reliably effective in the treatment of infections caused by gram-positive cocci. Antibacterial synergy may occur when aminoglycosides are used in combination with cell wall synthesis inhibitors. Examples include their combined use with penicillins in the treatment of pseudomonal, listerial, and enterococcal infections.

Streptomycin in combination with penicillin is often more effective in enterococcal carditis than regimens that

include other aminoglycosides. It is also used in the treatment of tuberculosis, plague, and tularemia. Other aminoglycosides are usually effective in these conditions. Multidrug-resistant (MDR) strains of *Mycobacterium tuberculosis* that are resistant to streptomycin may be susceptible to amikacin. Because of the risk of ototoxicity, streptomycin should not be used when other drugs will serve. Owing to their toxic potential, **neomycin and kanamycin** are restricted to topical or oral use (eg, to eliminate bowel flora).

Netilmicin is usually reserved for treatment of serious infections caused by organisms resistant to the other aminoglycosides.

Spectinomycin is an aminocyclitol related to the aminoglycosides. It is a backup drug, administered intramuscularly as a single dose for the treatment of gonorrhea, most commonly in patients allergic to beta-lactams.

TOXICITY

A. Ototoxicity

Auditory or vestibular damage (or both) may occur with any aminoglycoside and may be irreversible. Auditory

KEY DRUGS		
Subclass	**Prototype**	**Other Significant Agents**
Aminoglycosides		
Systemic	Gentamicin	Amikacin, netilmicin, tobramycin
Local	Neomycin	Gentamicin, kanamycin
Aminocyclitol	Spectinomycin	

impairment is more likely with amikacin and kanamycin; vestibular dysfunction is more likely with gentamicin and tobramycin. Ototoxicity risk is proportionate to the plasma levels and thus is especially high if dosage is not appropriately modified in a patient with renal dysfunction. Ototoxicity may be increased by the use of loop diuretics. Because ototoxicity has been reported after fetal exposure, the aminoglycosides are contraindicated in pregnancy unless their potential benefits are judged to outweigh risk.

B. NEPHROTOXICITY

Renal toxicity usually takes the form of acute tubular necrosis. This adverse effect, which is often reversible, is more common in elderly patients and in those concurrently receiving amphotericin B, cephalosporins, or vancomycin. Gentamicin and tobramycin are the most nephrotoxic.

C. NEUROMUSCULAR BLOCKADE

Although rare, a curare-like block may occur at high doses of aminoglycosides and may result in respiratory paralysis. It is usually reversible by treatment with calcium and neostigmine, but ventilatory support may be required.

D. SKIN REACTIONS

Allergic skin reactions may occur in patients, and contact dermatitis may occur in personnel handling the drug. Neomycin is the agent most likely to cause this adverse effect.

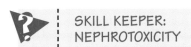

SKILL KEEPER: NEPHROTOXICITY

One of the characteristics of aminoglycoside antibiotics is their nephrotoxic potential. What other drugs can you identify that are known to have adverse effects on renal function? The Skill Keeper Answer appears at the end of the chapter.

QUESTIONS

1. Which statement about the mechanism of action of aminoglycosides is accurate?
   - **(A)** They are bacteriostatic
   - **(B)** They bind to the 50S ribosomal subunit
   - **(C)** They cause misreading of the code on the mRNA template
   - **(D)** They inhibit peptidyl transferase
   - **(E)** They stabilize polysomes

2. A 70-kg patient with creatinine clearance of greater than 90 mL/min has a gram-negative infection. Amikacin is administered intramuscularly at a dose of 5 mg/kg every 8 h, and the patient begins to respond. After 2 days, creatinine clearance declines to 30 mL/min. Assuming that no information is available about amikacin plasma levels, what would be the most reasonable approach to management of the patient at this point?
   - **(A)** Administer 5 mg/kg every 12 h
   - **(B)** Decrease the dosage to 120 mg every 8 h
   - **(C)** Decrease the dose to a daily total of 100 mg
   - **(D)** Discontinue amikacin and switch to gentamicin
   - **(E)** Maintain the patient on the present dosage and test auditory function

3. Which of the following statements about the clinical uses of the aminoglycosides is NOT accurate?
   - **(A)** Aminoglycosides are often used in combination with cephalosporins in the empiric treatment of life-threatening bacterial infections
   - **(B)** Gentamicin is used with ampicillin for synergistic effects in the treatment of enterococcal endocarditis
   - **(C)** Netilmicin is more likely to be effective than streptomycin in the treatment of a hospital-acquired infection caused by *Serratia marcescens*
   - **(D)** Owing to their polar nature, aminoglycosides are not absorbed following oral administration
   - **(E)** The spectrum of antimicrobial activity of aminoglycosides includes *Bacteroides fragilis*

4. Which statement about bacterial resistance to aminoglycosides is accurate?
   (A) Bacteria resistant to aminoglycosides have characteristic alterations in the pathway of folic acid synthesis
   (B) Clinical resistance mainly occurs through plasmid-mediated formation of group transferase enzymes
   (C) Emergence of resistance during the course of drug treatment is common
   (D) Resistance is due to the production of peptidyl transferases
   (E) Staphylococci resistant to methicillin (MRSA) are usually sensitive to aminoglycosides

5. Which antibiotic is the most effective agent in the treatment of an infection due to enterococci if used in combination with penicillin G?
   (A) Amikacin
   (B) Gentamicin
   (C) Neomycin
   (D) Spectinomycin
   (E) Streptomycin

6. Regarding the antibacterial action of gentamicin, which statement is accurate?
   (A) Antibacterial activity of the drug is often reduced by the presence of an inhibitor of cell wall synthesis
   (B) Antibacterial action of gentamicin is not concentration dependent
   (C) Gentamicin continues to exert antibacterial effects even after plasma levels decrease below detectable levels
   (D) Efficacy of the drug is directly proportionate to the time that the plasma level of the drug is greater than the minimal inhibitory concentration
   (E) The antibacterial action of gentamicin is time-dependent

7. An adult patient (weight, 70 kg) has bacteremia suspected to be due to a gram-negative rod. Tobramycin is to be administered using a once-daily dosing regimen, and the loading dose must be calculated to achieve a peak plasma level of 20 mg/L. Assume that the patient has normal renal function. Pharmacokinetic parameters of tobramycin in this patient are as follows: $V_d = 20$ L; $t_{1/2} = 3$ h; CL = 80 mL/min. What loading dose should be given?
   (A) 100 mg
   (B) 200 mg
   (C) 300 mg
   (D) 400 mg
   (E) 800 mg

8. Which drug is most likely to be effective against multidrug-resistant strains of *M tuberculosis*, including those resistant to streptomycin?

   (A) Amikacin
   (B) Clarithromycin
   (C) Gentamicin
   (D) Meropenem
   (E) Spectinomycin

9. A 67-year-old man is seen in a hospital emergency department complaining of pain in and behind the right ear. Physical examination shows edema of the external otic canal with purulent exudate and weakness of the muscles on the right side of the face. The patient informs the physician that he is a diabetic. Gram stain of the exudate from the ear shows many polymorphonucleocytes and gram-negative rods and samples are sent to the microbiology laboratory for culture and drug susceptibility testing. A preliminary diagnosis is made of external otitis. At this point, which of the following is most appropriate?
   (A) Analgesics should be prescribed for pain, but antibiotics should be withheld pending the results of cultures
   (B) The patient should be sent home with a prescription for oral cefaclor
   (C) The patient should be hospitalized and treatment started with gentamicin plus ticarcillin
   (D) The patient should be hospitalized and treatment started with intravenous imipenem-cilastatin
   (E) The patient should be hospitalized and treatment started with spectinomycin

10. Regarding the toxicity of gentamicin, which statement is accurate?
    (A) Gentamicin is more likely to cause ototoxic effects than renal damage
    (B) Ototoxicity due to gentamicin includes vestibular dysfunction, which is often irreversible
    (C) Ototoxicity is reduced if loop diuretics are used to facilitate gentamicin excretion
    (D) Systemic neomycin is usually safer than gentamicin
    (E) With traditional dosage regimens, the earliest sign of nephrotoxicity is a reduced blood creatinine

11. Which statement about neomycin is accurate?
    (A) Adjunctive use in treatment of tuberculosis
    (B) Drug of choice in Rocky Mountain spotted fever
    (C) Least nephrotoxic aminoglycoside
    (D) Metabolized by hepatic enzymes
    (E) Used in hepatic coma

12. Streptomycin has no useful activity in the treatment of
    (A) Bubonic plague
    (B) Brucellosis
    (C) Lyme disease

(D) Tuberculosis

(E) Tularemia

13. This drug has pharmacodynamic and pharmacokinetic properties almost identical to those of gentamicin, but has poor activity in combination with penicillin against enterococci.
(A) Amikacin
(B) Erythromycin
(C) Netilmycin
(D) Spectinomycin
(E) Tobramycin

14. Your 23-year-old female patient is pregnant and has gonorrhea. The medical history includes anaphylaxis following exposure to amoxicillin. Worried about compliance, you would like to treat this patient with a single dose, so you choose
(A) Cefixime
(B) Ceftriaxone
(C) Ciprofloxacin
(D) Spectinomycin
(E) Tetracycline

15. In the empiric treatment of severe bacterial infections of unidentified etiology, this drug, often used in combination with an aminoglycoside, provides coverage against many staphylococci
(A) Amoxicillin
(B) Clavulanic acid
(C) Erythromycin
(D) Nafcillin
(E) Tetracycline

16. Which statement about "once-daily" dosing with aminoglycosides is NOT accurate?
(A) Dosage adjustment is less important in renal insufficiency
(B) It is convenient for outpatient therapy
(C) It is often less toxic than conventional (multiple) dosing regimens
(D) Less nursing time is required for drug administration
(E) Underdosing is less of a problem

ANSWERS

1. Aminoglycosides are bactericidal inhibitors of protein synthesis binding to specific components of the 30S ribosomal subunit. Their actions include block of the formation of the initiation complex, miscoding, and polysomal breakup. Peptidyl transferase is inhibited by chloramphenicol, not aminoglycosides. The answer is **C**.

2. Monitoring plasma drug levels is important when aminoglycosides are used. In this case, the patient seems to be improving, so a decrease of the amikacin dose in proportion to decreased creatinine clearance is most appropriate. Because creatinine clearance is only one third of the starting value, a dose reduction should be made to one third of that given initially. The answer is **B**.

3. The intracellular accumulation of aminoglycoside by bacteria is oxygen dependent. Anaerobic bacteria are innately resistant. The answer is **E**.

4. Clinical resistance to aminoglycosides results from the formation of drug-metabolizing transferases. The emergence of resistance during drug treatment is rare. Aminoglycosides are not active against staphylococci resistant to methicillin. The answer is **B**.

5. When used in combination with penicillin G, streptomycin continues to be a useful agent for treating enterococcal infections. About 15% of enterococcal isolates that are resistant to gentamicin and the other systemic aminoglycosides remain susceptible to streptomycin. The answer is **E**.

6. The antibacterial action of aminoglycosides is concentration-dependent rather than time-dependent. The activity of the drug continues to increase as its plasma level rises above the minimal inhibitory concentration (MIC). When the plasma level of gentamicin falls below the MIC, the drug continues to exert antibacterial effects for several hours, exerting a postantibiotic effect. Inhibitors of bacterial cell wall synthesis often exert synergistic effects with aminoglycosides, possibly by increasing the intracellular accumulation of the aminoglycoside. The answer is **C**.

7. The loading dose of any drug is calculated by multiplying the desired plasma concentration (mg/L) by the volume of distribution (L). The answer is **D**.

8. Strains of multidrug-resistant *M tuberculosis* resistant to streptomycin are usually susceptible to amikacin. None of the other drugs listed (including gentamicin) have significant antitubercular activity. In the treatment of tuberculosis, amikacin or streptomycin are always used in combination regimens with other antitubercular agents. The answer is **A**.

9. The diabetic patient with external otitis is at special risk because of the danger of spread to the middle ear and possibly the meninges, so hospitalization is advisable, especially in the elderly. Likely pathogens include *E coli* and *Pseudomonas aeruginosa,* and coverage must be provided for these and possibly other gram-negative rods. The combination of an aminoglycoside plus a wider spectrum penicillin is most suitable in this case and is synergistic against many pseudomonas strains. Imipenem-cilastatin is also possible, but resistant strains of *Pseudomonas aeruginosa* have emerged during treatment. Cefaclor lacks antipseudomonal activity. The answer is **C**.

10. The incidence of nephrotoxic effects with gentamicin is 2 to 3 times greater than the incidence of ototoxicity. With traditional dosage regimens, the first indication of potential nephrotoxicity is an increase in trough serum levels of aminoglycosides, which is followed by an increase in blood creatinine. Although ototoxicity resulting from gentamicin usually involves irreversible effects on vestibular function, hearing loss can also occur. Ototoxicity is enhanced by loop diuretics. The answer is **B**.

11. When used parenterally, neomycin causes renal damage and ototoxicity. It is used topically and for local actions, including gastrointestinal tract infections and sterilization prior to bowel surgery. In hepatic coma, neomycin is used (with decreased protein intake) to suppress coliform bacteria, thus reducing ammonia intoxication. The answer is **E**.

12. Streptomycin is the drug of choice for treatment of plague and tularemia and has important adjunctive value in tuberculosis. Gentamicin (plus tetracycline) is usually preferred in brucellosis, but streptomycin is a backup drug. Aminoglycosides have minimal activity in Lyme disease, which is usually treated with either doxycycline or amoxicillin. The answer is **C**.

13. Tobramycin is almost identical to gentamicin in both its pharmacodynamic and pharmacokinetic properties. However, it is much less active than either gentamicin or streptomycin when used in combination with a penicillin in the treatment of enterococcal endocarditis. The answer is **E**.

14. Spectinomycin (2 g intramuscularly) is the appropriate choice in this case. Avoid cephalosporins in patients with a history of severe hypersensitivity to penicillins, and avoid fluoroquinolones (see Chapter 46) in pregnancy. Tetracyclines have been used in the past for gonorrhea, but not as single doses, and they too should be avoided in pregnancy. The answer is **D**.

15. In most cases involving the empiric use of aminoglycosides, coverage for possible staphylococcal infection would involve combined use with nafcillin or a cephalosporin (not listed). Amoxicillin is susceptible to penicillinases produced by most staphylococci, and although clavulanic acid is an inhibitor of these enzymes it would not be used independently of a penicillin. The answer is **D**.

16. In "once-daily dosing" with aminoglycosides, the selection of an appropriate dose is particularly critical in patients with renal insufficiency. The aminoglycosides are eliminated by the kidney in proportion to creatinine clearance. Knowledge of the degree of insufficiency, based on plasma creatinine (or BUN), is essential for estimation of the appropriate single daily dose of an aminoglycoside. The answer is **A**.

SKILL KEEPER ANSWER: NEPHROTOXICITY

Drugs with nephrotoxic potential include ACE inhibitors, acetazolamide, aminoglycosides, aspirin, amphotericin B, cyclosporine, furosemide, gold salts, lithium, methicillin, methoxyflurane, NSAIDs, pentamidine, sulfonamides, tetracyclines (degraded), thiazides, and triamterene.

CHECKLIST

When you complete this chapter, you should be able to:

☐ Describe 3 actions of aminoglycosides on protein synthesis and 2 mechanisms of resistance to this class of drugs.

☐ List the major clinical applications of aminoglycosides and identify their 2 main toxicities.

☐ Describe aminoglycoside pharmacokinetic characteristics with reference to their renal clearance and potential toxicity.

☐ Understand time-dependent and concentration-dependent killing actions of antibiotics and what is meant by "postantibiotic effect."

Sulfonamides, Trimethoprim, & Fluoroquinolones

46

Sulfonamides and trimethoprim are antimetabolites selectively toxic to microorganisms because they interfere with folic acid synthesis. Sulfonamides continue to be used selectively as individual antimicrobial agents, although resistance is common. The combination of a sulfonamide with trimethoprim causes a sequential blockade of folic acid synthesis. This results in a synergistic action against a wide spectrum of microorganisms; resistance occurs but has been relatively slow in development.

Fluoroquinolones, which selectively inhibit microbial nucleic acid metabolism, also have a broad spectrum of antimicrobial activity that includes many common pathogens. Resistance has emerged to the older antibiotics in this class, but has been offset to some extent by the introduction of newer fluoroquinolones with expanded activity against common pathogenic organisms.

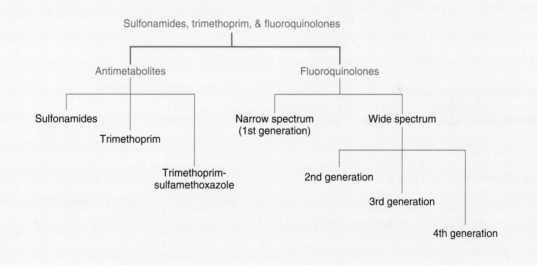

ANTIFOLATE DRUGS

A. CLASSIFICATION AND PHARMACOKINETICS

1. Sulfonamides—The sulfonamides are weakly acidic compounds that have a common chemical nucleus resembling *p*-aminobenzoic acid (PABA). Members of this group differ mainly in their pharmacokinetic properties and clinical uses. Pharmacokinetic features include modest tissue penetration, hepatic metabolism, and excretion of both intact drug and acetylated metabolites in the urine. Solubility may be decreased in acidic urine, resulting in precipitation of the drug or its metabolites. Because of the solubility limitation, a combination of 3 separate sulfonamides (**triple sulfa**) has

HIGH-YIELD TERMS TO LEARN	
Antimetabolite	A drug that, through chemical similarity, is able to interfere with the role of an endogenous compound in cellular metabolism.
Sequential blockade	The combined action of 2 drugs that inhibit sequential steps in a pathway of bacterial metabolism
DNA gyrase	Bacterial topisomerase responsible for negative supercoiling of double-stranded DNA that balances the positive supercoiling of DNA replication, acts as a "swivel," preventing damage to the DNA strand
Topoisomerase IV	Bacterial topisomerase initiating decatenation, the mechanism by which 2 daughter DNA molecules are separated at the conclusion of DNA replication

been used to reduce the likelihood that any one drug will precipitate. The sulfonamides may be classified as short acting (eg, sulfisoxazole), intermediate acting (eg, sulfamethoxazole), and long acting (eg, sulfadoxine). Sulfonamides bind to plasma proteins at sites shared by bilirubin and by other drugs.

2. Trimethoprim—This drug is structurally similar to folic acid. It is a weak base and is trapped in acidic environments, reaching high concentrations in prostatic and vaginal fluids. A large fraction of trimethoprim is excreted unchanged in the urine. The half-life of this drug is similar to that of sulfamethoxazole (10–12 h).

B. MECHANISMS OF ACTION

1. Sulfonamides—The sulfonamides are bacteriostatic inhibitors of folic acid synthesis. As antimetabolites of PABA, they are competitive inhibitors of dihydropteroate synthase (Figure 46–1). They can also act as substrates for this enzyme, resulting in the synthesis of nonfunctional forms of folic acid. The selective toxicity of sulfonamides results from the inability of mammalian cells to synthesize folic acid; they must use preformed folic acid that is present in the diet.

2. Trimethoprim—Trimethoprim is a selective inhibitor of bacterial dihydrofolate reductase that prevents formation of the active tetrahydro form of folic acid (Figure 46–1). Bacterial dihydrofolate reductase is 4 to 5 orders of magnitude more sensitive to inhibition by trimethoprim than the mammalian enzyme.

3. Trimethoprim plus sulfamethoxazole—When the 2 drugs are used in combination, antimicrobial synergy results from the **sequential blockade** of folate synthesis (Figure 46–1). The drug combination is bactericidal against susceptible organisms.

C. RESISTANCE

Bacterial resistance to sulfonamides is common and may be plasmid mediated. It can result from decreased intracellular accumulation of the drugs, increased production

of PABA by bacteria, or a decrease in the sensitivity of dihydropteroate synthase to the sulfonamides. Clinical resistance to trimethoprim most commonly results from the production of dihydrofolate reductase that has a reduced affinity for the drug.

D. CLINICAL USE

1. Sulfonamides—The sulfonamides are active against gram-positive and gram-negative organisms, *Chlamydiae*, and *Nocardia*. Specific members of the sulfonamide group are used by the following routes for the conditions indicated:

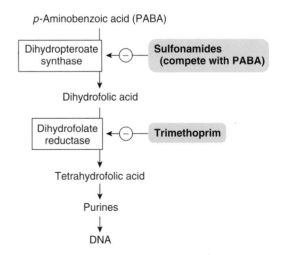

Figure 46–1. Inhibitory effects of sulfonamides and trimethoprim on folic acid synthesis. Inhibition of 2 successive steps in the formation of tetrahydrofolic acid constitutes sequential blockade and results in antibacterial synergy. (Modified and reproduced, with permission, from Katzung BG, editor: *Basic & Clinical Pharmacology*, 10th ed. McGraw-Hill, 2007.)

a. Simple urinary tract infections—Oral (eg, triple sulfa, sulfisoxazole).

b. Ocular infections—Topical (eg, sulfacetamide).

c. Burn infections—Topical (eg, mafenide, silver sulfadiazine).

d. Ulcerative colitis, rheumatoid arthritis—Oral (eg, sulfasalazine).

e. Toxoplasmosis—Oral sulfadiazine plus pyrimethamine (a dihydrofolate reductase inhibitor) plus folinic acid

2. Trimethoprim-sulfamethoxazole (TMP-SMX)—This drug combination is effective orally in the treatment of urinary tract infections and in respiratory, ear, and sinus infections caused by *Haemophilus influenzae* and *Moraxella catarrhalis*. In the immunocompromised patient, TMP-SMX is used for infections due to *Aeromonas hydrophila* and is the drug of choice for prevention and treatment of pneumocystis pneumonia. An intravenous formulation is available for patients unable to take the drug by mouth. TMP-SMX is also the drug of choice in nocardiosis, a possible backup drug for cholera, typhoid fever, and shigellosis, and has been used in the treatment of infections caused by methicillin-resistant staphylococci and *Listeria monocytogenes*.

E. TOXICITY OF SULFONAMIDES

1. Hypersensitivity—Allergic reactions, including skin rashes and fever, occur commonly. Cross-allergenicity between the individual sulfonamides should be assumed and may also occur with chemically related drugs (eg, oral hypoglycemics, thiazides). Exfoliative dermatitis, polyarteritis nodosa, and Stevens-Johnson syndrome have occurred rarely.

2. Gastrointestinal—Nausea, vomiting, and diarrhea occur commonly. Mild hepatic dysfunction can occur, but hepatitis is uncommon.

3. Hematotoxicity—Although such effects are rare, sulfonamides can cause granulocytopenia, thrombocytopenia, and aplastic anemia. Acute hemolysis may occur in persons with glucose-6-phosphate dehydrogenase deficiency.

4. Nephrotoxicity—Sulfonamides may precipitate in the urine at acidic pH, causing crystalluria and hematuria.

5. Drug interactions—Competition with warfarin and methotrexate for plasma protein binding transiently increases the plasma levels of these drugs. Sulfonamides can displace bilirubin from plasma proteins, with the risk of kernicterus in the neonate if used in the third trimester of pregnancy.

F. TOXICITY OF TRIMETHOPRIM

Trimethoprim may cause the predictable adverse effects of an antifolate drug, including megaloblastic anemia, leukopenia, and granulocytopenia. These effects are usually ameliorated by supplementary folinic acid. The combination of TMP-SMX may cause any of the adverse effects associated with the sulfonamides. AIDS patients given TMP-SMX have a high incidence of adverse effects, including fever, rashes, leukopenia, and diarrhea.

FLUOROQUINOLONES

A. CLASSIFICATION

Fluoroquinolines are classified by "generation" based on their antimicrobial spectrum of activity. **Norfloxacin,** a first-generation fluoroquinolone derived from nalidixic acid, has activity against the common pathogens that cause urinary tract infections. **Ciprofloxacin** and **ofloxacin** (second-generation fluoroquinolones) have greater activity against gram-negative bacteria and are also active against the gonococcus, many gram-positive cocci, mycobacteria, and agents of atypical pneumonia (eg, *Mycoplasma pneumoniae, Chlamydophila pneumoniae*). Third-generation fluoroquinolones (**levofloxacin, gatifloxacin**) are slightly less active than ciprofloxacin and ofloxacin against gram-negative bacteria but have greater activity against gram-positive cocci, including *S pneumoniae* and some strains of enterococci and MRSA. The most recently introduced drugs (eg, **gemifloxacin**, **moxifloxacin**) are the broadest spectrum fluoroquinolones to date, with enhanced activity against anaerobes.

B. PHARMACOKINETICS

All of the fluoroquinolones have good oral bioavailability (antacids containing multivalent cations may interfere) and penetrate most body tissues. However, norfloxacin does not achieve adequate plasma levels for use in most systemic infections. Elimination of most fluoroquinolones is through the kidneys via active tubular secretion, which can be blocked by probenecid. Dosage reductions are usually needed in renal dysfunction except for moxifloxacin, which is eliminated partly by hepatic metabolism and also by biliary excretion. Half-lives of fluoroquinolones are usually in the range of 3–8 h.

C. MECHANISM OF ACTION

The fluoroquinolones interfere with bacterial DNA synthesis by inhibiting topoisomerase II (DNA gyrase), especially in gram-negative organisms and topoisomerase IV, especially in gram-positive organisms. They block the relaxation of supercoiled DNA that is catalyzed by DNA gyrase, a step required for normal transcription and duplication. Inhibition of topoisomerase IV by fluoroquinolones interferes with the separation of replicated chromosomal DNA during cell division. Fluoroquinolones are usually bactericidal against susceptible organisms. Like aminoglycosides, the fluoroquinolines exhibit postantibiotic effects, whereby bacterial growth continues to be inhibited even after the plasma concentration of the drug has fallen below the minimum inhibitory concentration of the bacterium (see Chapter 45).

D. Resistance

Fluoroquinolone resistance has emerged rapidly in the case of second-generation fluoroquinolones especially in *Campylobacter jejuni* and gonococci, but also in gram-positive cocci (eg, MRSA), *Pseudomonas aeruginosa* and *Serratia* species. Mechanisms of resistance include decreased intracellular accumulation of the drug via the production of efflux pumps or changes in porin structure (in gram-negative bacteria). Efflux mechanisms appear to be responsible for resistance in strains of *M tuberculosis, S aureus,* and *S pneumoniae.* Changes in the sensitivity of the target enzymes via point mutations in the antibiotic binding regions are also established to confer resistance against specific fluoroquinolones. Mutations in the quinolone resistance-determining region of the *gyrA* gene that encodes DNA gyrase is responsible for resistance in gonococci.

E. Clinical Use

Fluoroquinolones are effective in the treatment of infections of the urogenital and gastrointestinal tracts caused by gram-negative organisms, including gonococci, *E coli, Klebsiella pneumoniae, Campylobacter jejuni, Enterobacter, Pseudomonas aeruginosa, Salmonella,* and *Shigella* species. They have been used widely for respiratory tract, skin, and soft tissue infections, but their effectiveness is now variable because of the emergence of resistance. Ciprofloxacin and ofloxacin are alternatives to third-generation cephalosporins in gonorrhea (though resistance is increasing), administered in single oral doses.

Ofloxacin will eradicate accompanying organisms such as *Chlamydia trachomatis,* but a 7-day course of treatment is required. Levofloxacin has activity against most organisms associated with community-acquired pneumonia, including chlamydiae, mycoplasma, and legionella species. Gemifloxacin and moxifloxacin have the widest spectrum of activity, which includes both gram-positive and gram-negative organisms, atypical pneumonia agents, and some anaerobic bacteria. Fluoroquinolones have also been used in the meningococcal carrier state, in the treatment of tuberculosis, and in prophylactic management of neutropenic patients.

F. Toxicity

Gastrointestinal distress is the most common side effect. The fluoroquinolones may cause skin rashes, headache,

SKILL KEEPER: PROLONGATION OF THE QT INTERVAL (SEE CHAPTER 14)

Grepafloxacin was withdrawn from clinical use in the United States because of serious cardiotoxicity. The currently available fluoroquinolones are contraindicated in patients taking drugs that prolong the QT interval. What other drugs can you recall that have this characteristic effect to increase the duration of the ventricular action potential? The Skill Keeper Answer appears at the end of the chapter.

KEY DRUGS

Subclass	Prototypes	Other Significant Agents
Sulfonamides		
Oral agents	Sulfisoxazole	Sulfadiazine
Local agents	Sulfacetamide	Silver sulfadiazine
Combination	Trimethoprim-sulfamethoxazole (TMP-SMX)	
Folate reductase inhibitors	Trimethoprim	Pyrimethamine
Fluoroquinolones		
First generation	Norfloxacin	
Second generation	Ciprofloxacin	Ofloxacin
Third generation	Levofloxacin	
Fourth generation	Moxifloxacin	Gemifloxacin

dizziness, insomnia, abnormal liver function tests, phototoxicity, and both tendinitis and tendon rupture. Opportunistic infections caused by *C albicans* and streptococci have occurred. The fluoroquinolones are not recommended for use in children or in pregnancy because they have caused cartilage problems in developing animals. Fluoroquinolones may increase the plasma levels of theophylline and other methylxanthines, enhancing their toxicity. Newer fluoroquinolones (gemifloxacin, levofloxacin, moxifloxacin)prolong the QT_c interval. They should be avoided in patients with known QT_c prolongation and patients on certain antiarrhymthic drugs (Chapter 14).

QUESTIONS

1. Which statement about sulfonamides is accurate?
   (A) Cross-allergenicity may occur between sulfonamides and penicillins
   (B) Crystalluria due to sulfonamides is most likely to occur at high urinary pH
   (C) Dysfunction of the basal ganglia may occur in the newborn if sulfonamides are administered late in pregnancy
   (D) Sulfonamides are bactericidal
   (E) Sulfonamides inhibit bacterial dihydrofolate reductase

2. The combination of trimethoprim and sulfamethoxazole is effective against which opportunistic infection in the AIDS patient?
   (A) Disseminated herpes simplex
   (B) Cryptococcal meningitis
   (C) Toxoplasmosis
   (D) Oral candidiasis
   (E) Tuberculosis

3. A 24-year-old woman has returned from a vacation abroad suffering from traveler's diarrhea, and her problem has not responded to antidiarrheal drugs. A pathogenic gram-negative bacillus is suspected. Which drug is most likely to be effective in the treatment of this patient?
   (A) Ampicillin
   (B) Levofloxacin
   (C) Sulfacetamide
   (D) Trimethoprim
   (E) Vancomycin

4. Which statement about the clinical use of sulfonamides is false?
   (A) Resistant bacterial strains may have decreased intracellular accumulation of sulfonamides
   (B) Sulfonamides have activity against *C trachomatis* and can be used topically for the treatment of chlamydial infections of the eye

   (C) Sulfonamides are effective in Rocky Mountain spotted fever in patients allergic to tetracyclines
   (D) Sulfonamides are minimally effective as sole agents in the treatment of chronic prostatitis
   (E) Sulfonamide resistance can occur in some strains of bacteria because of increased production of PABA

5. A 31-year-old man has gonorrhea. He has no drug allergies, but a few years ago acute hemolysis followed use of an antimalarial drug. The physician is concerned that the patient has an accompanying urethritis caused by *C trachomatis,* although no cultures or enzyme tests have been performed. Which of the following drugs is most likely to be effective against both gonococci and *C trachomatis* in this patient?
   (A) Cefixime
   (B) Norfloxacin
   (C) Ofloxacin
   (D) Spectinomycin
   (E) Sulfamethoxazole

6. Which statement about the fluoroquinolones is accurate?
   (A) Antacids increase the oral bioavailability of fluoroquinolones
   (B) Gonococcal resistance to fluoroquinolones may involve changes in DNA gyrase
   (C) Modification of moxifloxacin dosage is required in patients if creatinine clearance is less than 50 mL/min
   (D) A fluoroquinolone is the drug of choice for treatment of an uncomplicated urinary tract infection in a 7-year-old girl
   (E) The fluoroquinolones are contraindicated in hepatic dysfunction

7. A 55-year-old man complains of periodic bouts of diarrhea with lower abdominal cramping and intermittent rectal bleeding. Seen in the clinic, he appears well nourished, with blood pressure in the normal range. Examination reveals moderate abdominal pain and tenderness. His current medications are limited to loperamide for his diarrhea. Sigmoidoscopy reveals mucosal edema, friability, and some pus. Laboratory findings include mild anemia and decreased serum albumin. Microbiologic examination via stool cultures and mucosal biopsies do not reveal any evidence for bacterial, amebic, or cytomegalovirus involvement. A preliminary diagnosis is made of mild to moderate ulcerative colitis. The most appropriate drug to use in this patient is
   (A) Ciprofloxacin
   (B) Ganciclovir
   (C) Metronidazole

(D) Sulfasalazine

(E) Trimethoprim-sulfamethoxazole

8. Which statement about the combination of trimethoprim plus sulfamethoxazole (TMP-SMX) is false?

(A) It is an alternative to ampicillin in the treatment of listeriosis

(B) It is appropriate for the treatment of a community-acquired pneumonia

(C) It is effective in the treatment of pneumonia caused by *Pneumocystis jiroveci*

(D) Fever and pancytopenia occur frequently when these drugs are used in AIDS patients

(E) The drugs produce a sequential blockade of folic acid synthesis

9. Which adverse effect is most likely to occur with sulfonamides?

(A) Fanconi's aminoaciduria syndrome

(B) Hematuria

(C) Kernicterus in the newborn

(D) Neurologic dysfunction

(E) Skin reactions

10. Which drug is effective in the treatment of nocardiosis and, in combination with pyrimethamine, is prophylactic against *Pneumocystis jiroveci* infections in AIDS patients?

(A) Ampicillin

(B) Clindamycin

(C) Norfloxacin

(D) Sulfadiazine

(E) Trimethoprim

11. Which statement about ciprofloxacin is accurate?

(A) It is active against most MRSA strains of staphylococci

(B) Clinical antagonism occurs if it is used with inhibitors of dihydrofolate reductase

(C) It should not be used for "first-time" urinary tract infections

(D) Organisms associated with middle ear infections are highly resistant

(E) Tendinitis and tendon rupture may occur during treatment

12. Supplementary folinic acid may prevent anemia in folate-deficient persons who use this drug, a weak base that achieves tissue levels similar to those in plasma

(A) Ciprofloxacin

(B) Norfloxacin

(C) Ofloxacin

(D) Sulfacetamide

(E) Trimethoprim

ANSWERS

1. Make sure you know the specific enzymes in bacterial folic acid synthesis that are inhibited by sulfonamides and trimethoprim: Sulfonamides (bacteriostatic) inhibit dihydropteroate synthase, not dihydrofolate reductase, the enzyme inhibited by trimethoprim. There is no cross-hypersensitivity between sulfonamides and beta-lactam antibiotics. Sulfonamides are weak acids, and crystalluria is more likely at low urine pH. The answer is **C**.

2. Trimethoprim-sulfamethoxazole is not effective in the treatment of infections caused by viruses, fungi, or mycobacteria. However, the drug combination is active against certain protozoans, including *Toxoplasma,* and can be used for both prevention and treatment of toxoplasmosis in the AIDS patient. The answer is **C**.

3. The fluoroquinolones are very effective in diarrhea caused by bacterial pathogens, including *E coli, Shigella,* and *Salmonella.* None of the other drugs listed would be appropriate. Many coliforms are now resistant to ampicillin. Sulfacetamide is a topical agent used for bacterial conjunctivitis. Although trimethoprim is available as a single drug, resistance may emerge during treatment unless it is used for urinary tract infections, where high concentrations are achieved. Vancomycin has no activity against gram-negative bacilli. The answer is **B**.

4. Sulfonamides have minimal therapeutic actions in rickettsial infections. Chloramphenicol may be used for Rocky Mountain spotted fever in patients with established allergy or other contraindication to tetracyclines. The answer is **C**.

5. Although cefixime in a single oral dose is effective in gonorrhea (Chapter 43), it has no activity against organisms causing nongonococcal urethritis. Spectinomycin (Chapter 45) is active against most gonococci, but will not eradicate a urogenital chlamydial infection. Norfloxacin is the least active fluoroquinolone and is minimally effective in gonorrhea. However, other fluoroquinolones, including ofloxacin, are effective in both gonorrhea and chlamydial urethritis. This patient could also be treated by single oral doses of cefixime and azithromycin (not listed). Sulfamethoxazole would not be useful and may cause acute hemolysis in this patient. The answer is **C**.

6. Antacids can decrease oral bioavailability of fluoroquinolones. Neither hepatic nor renal dysfunction is a *contraindication* to the use of fluoroquinolones. Most fluoroquinolones undergo renal elimination, and dosage should be modified with creatinine

clearance < 50 mL/min. Moxifloxacin elimination occurs mainly via the liver. The fluoroquinolones should not be used to treat uncomplicated first-time urinary tract infections in children. Because of possible effects on cartilage, fluoroquinolones are not recommended for use in developing children. In this child, the infection is almost certainly due to a strain of *E coli* that is sensitive to many other drugs, including beta-lactam antibiotics. The answer is **B**.

7. In the absence of any evidence pointing toward a definite microbial cause for the colitis in this patient, a drug that decreases inflammation is indicated. Sulfasalazine has significant anti-inflammatory action, and its oral use results in symptomatic improvement in 50–75% of patients. The drug is also used for its anti-inflammatory effects in rheumatoid arthritis. The answer is **D**.

8. TMP-SMX is not reliably active against most of the microorganisms associated with a community-acquired pneumonia. Drugs currently recommended in otherwise healthy ambulatory patients include an oral macrolide (eg, azithromycin) or doxycycline. For older patients or those with comorbid illness, a fluoroquinolone with enhanced activity versus pneumococci is preferred. The answer is **B**.

9. The most common adverse effect of sulfonamides is a skin rash caused by hypersensitivity. CNS effects and hematuria occur less frequently. Sulfonamides are usually avoided in the third trimester of pregnancy or in neonates, so kernicterus is rare. Fanconi's syndrome is associated with the use of outdated tetracyclines. The answer is **E**.

10. Sulfadiazine and TMP-SMX are drugs of choice in nocardiosis. In combination with pyrimethamine (an effective dihydrofolate reductase inhibitor in protozoa), sulfadiazine is effective in toxoplasmosis and is prophylactic against pneumocystis pneumonia in the AIDS patient. However, TMP-SMX is more commonly used for the latter purpose. The answer is **D**.

11. Ciprofloxacin is commonly used for the treatment of urinary tract infections and is active against most strains of common causative agents of otitis media, including *H influenzae* and pneumococci. However, up to 50% of strains of MRSA are now resistant to ciprofloxacin. No clinical antagonism has been reported between fluoroquinolones and inhibitors of folic acid synthesis. The answer is **E**.

12. Trimethoprim is the only weak base listed (fluoroquinolones and sulfonamides are acidic compounds), and its high lipid solubility at blood pH allows penetration of the drug into prostatic and vaginal fluid to reach levels similar to those in plasma. Leukopenia and thrombocytopenia may occur in folate deficiency when the drug is used alone or in combination with sulfamethoxazole. Fluoroquinolones do not exacerbate symptoms of folic acid deficiency. The answer is **E**.

SKILL KEEPER ANSWER: PROLONGATION OF THE QT INTERVAL (SEE CHAPTER 14)

The most important drugs that prolong the QT interval are antiarrhythmics. These include drugs from class IA and class III, including amiodarone, bretylium, disopyramide, procainamide, quinidine, and sotalol. You may recall that although group IA drugs are classified as Na^+ channel blockers, they also block K^+ channels and prolong the duration of the ventricular action potential. Other drugs implicated in QT prolongation include mefloquine, pentamidine, thioridazine, and ziprasidone.

CHECKLIST

When you complete this chapter, you should be able to:

☐ Describe how sulfonamides and trimethoprim affect bacterial folic acid synthesis and how resistance to the antifolate drugs occurs.

☐ Identify major clinical uses of sulfonamides and trimethoprim, singly and in combination, and describe their characteristic pharmacokinetic properties and toxic effects.

☐ Describe how fluoroquinolones inhibit nucleic acid synthesis, and identify mechanisms involved in bacterial resistance to these agents.

☐ List the major clinical uses of fluoroquinolones and describe their characteristic pharmacokinetic properties and toxic effects.

Antimycobacterial Drugs

47

The chemotherapy of infections caused by *Mycobacterium tuberculosis, M leprae,* and *M avium-intracellulare* is complicated by numerous factors, including (1) limited information about the mechanisms of antimycobacterial drug actions; (2) the development of resistance; (3) the intracellular location of mycobacteria; (4) the chronic nature of mycobacterial disease, which requires protracted drug treatment and is associated with drug toxicities; and (5) patient compliance. Chemotherapy of mycobacterial infections almost always involves the use of drug combinations to delay the emergence of resistance and to enhance antimycobacterial efficacy.

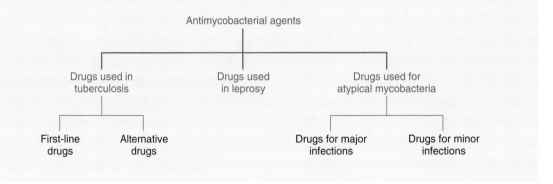

DRUGS FOR TUBERCULOSIS

The major drugs used in tuberculosis are **isoniazid (INH), rifampin, ethambutol, pyrazinamide,** and **streptomycin.** Actions of these agents on *M tuberculosis* are bactericidal or bacteriostatic depending on drug concentration and strain susceptibility. Appropriate drug treatment involves antibiotic susceptibility testing of mycobacterial isolates. Initiation of treatment of pulmonary tuberculosis usually involves a 3- or 4-drug combination regimen depending on the known or anticipated rate of resistance to isoniazid (INH). Directly observed therapy (DOT) regimens are recommended in noncompliant patients and in drug-resistant tuberculosis.

A. Isoniazid

1. Mechanisms—Isoniazid (INH) is a structural congener of pyridoxine. Its mechanism of action involves inhibition of mycolic acids, characteristic components of mycobacterial cell walls. Resistance can emerge rapidly if the drug is used alone. High-level resistance is associated with deletion in the *katG* gene that codes for a catalase-peroxidase involved in the bioactivation of INH. Low-level resistance occurs via deletions in the *inhA* gene that encodes the "target enzyme," an acyl carrier protein reductase. INH is bactericidal for actively growing tubercle bacilli, but is less effective against dormant organisms.

2. Pharmacokinetics—INH is well absorbed orally and penetrates cells to act on intracellular mycobacteria. The liver metabolism of INH is by acetylation and is under genetic control. Patients may be fast or slow inactivators of the drug. INH half-life in "fast acetylators" is 60–90 min; in "slow acetylators" it may be 3–4 h. The proportion of fast acetylators is higher among people of Asian origin (including Native Americans) than those of

European or African origin. Fast acetylators may require higher dosage than slow acetylators for equivalent therapeutic effects.

3. Clinical use—INH is the single most important drug used in tuberculosis and is a component of most drug combination regimens. In the treatment of latent infection (formerly known as "prophylaxis") including skin test converters, and for close contacts of patients with active disease, INH is given as the sole drug.

4. Toxicity and interactions—Neurotoxic effects are common and include peripheral neuritis, restlessness, muscle twitching, and insomnia. These effects can be alleviated by administration of pyridoxine (25–50 mg/day orally). INH is hepatotoxic and may cause abnormal liver function tests, jaundice, and hepatitis. Fortunately, hepatotoxicity is rare in children. INH may inhibit the hepatic metabolism of drugs (eg, carbamazepine, phenytoin, warfarin). Hemolysis has occurred in patients with glucose-6-phosphate dehydrogenase deficiency. A lupus-like syndrome has been reported.

SKILL KEEPER: GENOTYPIC VARIATIONS IN DRUG METABOLISM (SEE CHAPTER 4)

Genotypic variants occur with regard to the metabolism of isoniazid. What other drugs exhibit such variation, and what enzymes are involved in their metabolism? What are the clinical consequences of genetic polymorphisms in drug metabolism? The Skill Keeper Answers appear at the end of the chapter.

B. RIFAMPIN

1. Mechanisms—Rifampin, a derivative of rifamycin, is bactericidal against *M tuberculosis*. The drug inhibits DNA-dependent RNA polymerase (encoded by the *rpo* gene) in *M tuberculosis* and many other microorganisms. Resistance via changes in drug sensitivity of the polymerase often emerges rapidly if the drug is used alone.

2. Pharmacokinetics—When given orally, rifampin is well absorbed and is distributed to most body tissues, including the CNS. The drug undergoes enterohepatic cycling and is partially metabolized in the liver. Both free drug and metabolites, which are orange colored, are eliminated mainly in the feces.

3. Clinical uses—In the treatment of tuberculosis, rifampin is almost always used in combination with other

drugs. However, rifampin can be used as the sole drug in treatment of latent tuberculosis in INH-intolerant patients or in close contacts of patients with INH-resistant strains of the organism. In leprosy, rifampin given monthly delays the emergence of resistance to dapsone. Rifampin may be used with vancomycin for infections due to resistant staphylococci (MRSA strains) or pneumococci (PRSP strains). Other uses of rifampin include the meningococcal and staphylococcal carrier states.

4. Toxicity and interactions—Rifampin commonly causes light chain proteinuria and may impair antibody responses. Occasional side effects include skin rashes, thrombocytopenia, nephritis, and liver dysfunction. If given less often than twice weekly, rifampin may cause a flulike syndrome and anemia. Rifampin strongly induces liver drug-metabolizing enzymes and enhances the elimination rate of many drugs, including anticonvulsants, contraceptive steroids, cyclosporine, ketoconazole, methadone, terbinafine, and warfarin. **Rifabutin**, another rifamycin, is less likely to cause drug interactions than rifampin and is equally effective as an antimycobacterial agent. It is usually preferred over rifampin in the treatment of tuberculosis or other mycobacterial infections in AIDS patients.

C. ETHAMBUTOL

1. Mechanisms—Ethambutol inhibits arabinosyl transferases (encoded by the *embCAB* operon) involved in the synthesis of arabinogalactan, a component of mycobacterial cell walls. Resistance occurs rapidly via mutations in the *emb* gene if the drug is used alone.

2. Pharmacokinetics—The drug is well absorbed orally and distributed to most tissues, including the CNS. A large fraction is eliminated unchanged in the urine. Dose reduction is necessary in renal impairment.

3. Clinical use—The main use of ethambutol is in tuberculosis, and it is always given in combination with other drugs.

4. Toxicity—The most common adverse effects are dose-dependent visual disturbances, including decreased visual acuity, red-green color blindness, optic neuritis, and possible retinal damage (from prolonged use at high doses). Most of these effects regress when the drug is stopped. Other toxic effects include headache, confusion, hyperuricemia, and peripheral neuritis.

D. PYRAZINAMIDE

1. Mechanisms—The mechanism of action of pyrazinamide is not known; however, its bacteriostatic action appears to require metabolic conversion via pyrazinamidases (encoded by the *pncA* gene) present in *M tuberculosis*. Resistance occurs via mutations in the gene that encodes enzymes involved in bioactivation of pyrazinamide and by increased expression of drug efflux systems. Resistance develops rapidly if the drug is used alone, but there is minimal cross-resistance with other antimycobacterial drugs.

2. Pharmacokinetics—Pyrazinamide is well absorbed orally and penetrates most body tissues, including the CNS. The drug is partly metabolized to pyrazinoic acid, and both parent molecule and metabolite are excreted in the urine. The plasma half-life of pyrazinamide is increased in hepatic or renal failure.

3. Clinical use—The combined use of pyrazinamide with other antituberculous drugs is an important factor in the success of "short-course" treatment regimens.

4. Toxicity—Approximately 40% of patients develop nongouty polyarthralgia. Hyperuricemia occurs commonly but is usually asymptomatic. Other adverse effects include myalgia, gastrointestinal irritation, maculopapular rash, hepatic dysfunction, porphyria, and photosensitivity reactions. Pyrazinamide should be avoided in pregnancy.

E. STREPTOMYCIN

This aminoglycoside is now used more frequently than before because of the growing prevalence of drug-resistant strains of *M tuberculosis*. Streptomycin is used principally in drug combinations for the treatment of life-threatening tuberculous disease, including meningitis, miliary dissemination, and severe organ tuberculosis. The pharmacodynamic and pharmacokinetic properties of streptomycin are similar to those of other aminoglycosides (see Chapter 45).

F. ALTERNATIVE DRUGS

Several drugs with antimycobacterial activity are used in cases that are resistant to first-line agents; they are considered second-line drugs because they are no more effective, and their toxicities are often more serious than those of the major drugs.

Amikacin is indicated for treatment of tuberculosis suspected to be caused by streptomycin-resistant or multi-drug-resistant mycobacterial strains. To avoid emergence of resistance, amikacin should always be used in combination drug regimens.

Ciprofloxacin and **ofloxacin** are often active against strains of *M tuberculosis* resistant to first-line agents. The fluoroquinolones should always be used in combination regimens with two or more other active agents.

Ethionamide is a congener of INH, but cross-resistance does not occur. The major disadvantage of ethionamide is severe gastrointestinal irritation and adverse neurologic effects at doses needed to achieve effective plasma levels.

p-Aminosalicylic acid (PAS) is rarely used because primary resistance is common. In addition, its toxicity includes gastrointestinal irritation, peptic ulceration,

hypersensitivity reactions, and effects on kidney, liver, and thyroid function.

Other drugs of limited use because of their toxicity include **capreomycin** (ototoxicity, renal dysfunction) and **cycloserine** (peripheral neuropathy, CNS dysfunction).

G. ANTITUBERCULAR DRUG REGIMENS

1. Standard regimens—For empiric treatment of pulmonary tuberculosis (in most areas of < 4% INH resistance), an initial 3-drug regimen of INH, rifampin, and pyrazinamide is recommended. If the organisms are fully susceptible to drugs (and the patient is HIV negative), pyrazinamide can be discontinued after 2 months and treatment continued for a further 4 months with a 2-drug regimen.

2. Alternative regimens—Alternative regimens in cases of fully susceptible organisms include INH + rifampin for 9 months, or INH + ethambutol for 18 months. Intermittent (2 or 3 × weekly) high-dose 4-drug regimens are also effective.

3. Resistance—If resistance to INH is > 4%, the initial drug regimen should include ethambutol or streptomycin. Tuberculosis resistant only to INH (the most common form of resistance) can be treated for 6 months with a regimen of rifampin + pyrazinamide + ethambutol or streptomycin. Multiple-drug resistant organisms (resistant to both INH and rifampin) should be treated with 3 or more drugs to which the organism is susceptible for a period of 18+ mo, including 12 mo after sputum cultures become negative.

DRUGS FOR LEPROSY

A. SULFONES

Dapsone (diaminodiphenylsulfone) remains the most active drug against *M leprae*. The mechanism of action of sulfones may involve inhibition of folic acid synthesis. Because of increasing reports of resistance, it is recommended that the drug be used in combinations with rifampin or clofazimine or both (see below). Dapsone can be given orally, penetrates tissues well, undergoes enterohepatic cycling, and is eliminated in the urine, partly as acetylated metabolites. Common adverse effects include gastrointestinal irritation, fever, skin rashes, and methemoglobinemia. Hemolysis may occur, especially in patients with glucose-6-phosphate dehydrogenase deficiency.

Acedapsone is a repository form of dapsone that provides inhibitory plasma concentrations for several months. In addition to its use in leprosy, dapsone is an alternative drug for the treatment of *Pneumocystis jiroveci* pneumonia in AIDS patients.

B. OTHER AGENTS

Drug regimens usually include combinations of dapsone with rifampin (or rifabutin, see prior discussion)

KEY DRUGS

Subclass	Prototypes	Other Significant Agents
Drugs for tuberculosis		
Pyridines	Isoniazid	Ethionamide, pyrazinamide
Rifamycins	Rifampin	Rifabutin
Diamines	Ethambutol	
Aminoglycosides	Streptomycin	Amikacin
Others		Ciprofloxacin, ofloxacin, aminosalicylic acid, capreomycin, cycloserine
Drugs for leprosy		
Sulfones	Dapsone	Acedapsone
Phenazines	Clofazime	
Others		Rifampin
Drugs for *M avium* complex		A combination of azithromycin or clarithromycin with ethambutol, with or without rifabutin is favored

plus or minus **clofazimine.** Clofazimine, a phenazine dye that may interact with DNA, causes gastrointestinal irritation and skin discoloration ranging from red-brown to nearly black.

DRUGS FOR ATYPICAL MYCOBACTERIAL INFECTIONS

M avium complex (MAC) is an important cause of disseminated infections in AIDS patients. Currently, clarithromycin or azithromycin with or without rifabutin is recommended for primary prophylaxis in patients with CD4 counts less than $50/\mu L$. Treatment of MAC infections requires a combination of drugs, with one favored regimen consisting of azithromycin or clarithromycin with ethambutol and rifabutin. Infections resulting from other atypical mycobacteria (eg, *M marinum, M ulcerans*), although sometimes asymptomatic, may be treated with the described antimycobacterial drugs (eg, ethambutol, rifampin) or other antibiotics (eg, erythromycin, amikacin).

QUESTIONS

1. The primary reason for the use of drug combinations in the treatment of tuberculosis is to
   (A) Delay or prevent the emergence of resistance
   (B) Enhance activity against metabolically inactive mycobacteria
   (C) Ensure patient compliance with the drug regimen
   (D) Provide prophylaxis against other bacterial infections
   (E) Reduce the incidence of adverse effects

2–5. A 21-year-old woman from Southeast Asia has been staying with family members in California for the past 3 mo and is looking after her sister's preschool children during the day. Because she has difficulty with the English language, her sister escorts her to the emergency department of a local hospital. She tells the staff that the patient has been feeling very tired for the past month, has a poor appetite, and has lost weight. Two weeks ago she had symptoms of the "flu," with fever and night sweats. The patient has been feeling better lately except for a cough that produces a greenish sputum, sometimes specked with blood. With the exception of rales in the left upper lobe, the physical examination of the patient is unremarkable and she does not seem to be acutely ill. Laboratory values show a white count of $12,000/\mu L$ and a hematocrit of 33%. Chest x-ray film reveals an infiltrate in the left upper lobe with a possible cavity. A Gram-stained smear of the sputum shows mixed flora with no dominance. An acid-fast stain reveals many thin rods of pinkish hue. A preliminary diagnosis is made of pulmonary tuberculosis. Sputum is sent to the laboratory for culture.

2. At this point, the most appropriate course of action is to
   (A) Hospitalize the patient and start treatment with isoniazid plus rifampin
   (B) Hospitalize the patient and start treatment with 4 antimycobacterial drugs

(C) Prescribe isoniazid for prophylaxis and send the patient home to await culture results

(D) Send the patient home to await the culture results

(E) Start outpatient treatment with isoniazid and rifampin

3. When treatment is started, which drug regimen should be initiated in this patient?

(A) Amikacin, isoniazid, pyrazinamide, streptomycin

(B) Ciprofloxacin, cycloserine, isoniazid, PAS

(C) Ethambutol, isoniazid, rifabutin, streptomycin

(D) Ethambutol, pyrazinamide, rifampin, streptomycin

(E) Isoniazid, rifampin, pyrazinamide, ethambutol

4. Which statement concerning the possible use of isoniazid (INH) in this patient is false?

(A) Flushing, palpitations, sweating, and dyspnea may occur after ingestion of tyramine-containing foods

(B) Persons from Southeast Asia require lower maintenance doses of INH than most other persons in the United States

(C) She should take pyridoxine daily

(D) Symptoms of peripheral neuritis may occur during treatment

(E) The risk of this patient developing hepatitis from INH is less than 2%

5. On her release from the hospital, the patient is advised not to rely solely on oral contraceptives to avoid pregnancy because they may be less effective while she is being maintained on antimycobacterial drugs. The agent most likely to interfere with the action of oral contraceptives is

(A) Ethambutol

(B) Isoniazid

(C) Pyrazinamide

(D) Rifampin

(E) Streptomycin

6. The mechanism of high-level INH resistance of *M tuberculosis* is

(A) Change in the pathway of mycolic acid synthesis

(B) Decreased intracellular accumulation of INH

(C) Formation of drug-inactivating *N*-acetyl-transferase

(D) Mutation in the *inhA* gene

(E) Reduced expression of the *katG* gene

7. A patient with AIDS and a CD4 cell count of $100/\mu L$ has persistent fever and weight loss associated with invasive pulmonary disease that is due to *M avium* complex. Optimal management of this patient is to

(A) Select an antibiotic regimen based on drug susceptibility of the cultured organism

(B) Start treatment with INH and pyrazinamide

(C) Treat with rifabutin because it prevents the development of MAC bacteremia

(D) Treat with clarithromycin, ethambutol, and rifabutin

(E) Treat with trimethoprim-sulfamethoxazole

8. A patient with pulmonary tuberculosis resulting from an INH-susceptible strain of *M tuberculosis* (rate of INH resistance known to be < 4%) has been treated with INH, rifampin, and pyrazinamide for a total of 2 mo. If the pyrazinamide is stopped at this time, treatment should be continued with INH and rifampin for a further minimum time period of

(A) 2 mo

(B) 4 mo

(C) 6 mo

(D) 12 mo

(E) 18 mo

9. A 10-year-old boy has uncomplicated pulmonary tuberculosis. After initial hospitalization, he is now being treated at home with isoniazid, rifampin, and ethambutol. Which statement about this case is accurate?

(A) A baseline auditory function test is essential before drug treatment is initiated

(B) His mother, who takes care of him, should receive INH prophylaxis

(C) His 3-year-old sibling should not receive INH prophylaxis

(D) Potential nephrotoxicity of the prescribed drugs warrants periodic assessment of renal function

(E) The boy may develop symptoms of polyarthralgia caused by rifampin

10. This drug has been used prophylactically in contacts of children with infection caused by *Haemophilus influenzae* type B. It is also prophylactic in meningococcal and staphylococcal carrier states. Although the drug eliminates a majority of meningococci from carriers, highly resistant strains may be selected out during treatment.

(A) Ciprofloxacin

(B) Clofazimine

(C) Dapsone

(D) Rifampin

(E) Streptomycin

11. Which statement about antitubercular drugs is accurate?

(A) Antimycobacterial actions of streptomycin involve inhibition of arabinosyl transferases

(B) Cross-resistance of *M tuberculosis* to isoniazid and pyrazinamide is common

(C) Ocular toxicity of ethambutol is prevented by thiamine

(D) Pyrazinamide treatment should be discontinued immediately if hyperuricemia occurs

(E) Resistance to ethambutol involves mutations in the *emb* gene

12. Once-weekly administration of which of the following antibiotics has prophylactic activity against bacteremia caused by *M avium* complex in AIDS patients?
(A) Azithromycin
(B) Clarithromycin
(C) Isoniazid
(D) Kanamycin
(E) Rifabutin

13. Risk factors for multidrug-resistant tuberculosis include
(A) A history of treatment of tuberculosis without rifampin
(B) Recent immigration from Asia and living in an area of over 4% isoniazid resistance
(C) Recent immigration from Latin America
(D) Residence in regions where isoniazid resistance is known to exceed 4%
(E) All of the above

14. Which drug is most likely to cause loss of equilibrium and auditory damage?
(A) Amikacin
(B) Ethambutol
(C) Isoniazid
(D) Para-aminosalicylic acid
(E) Rifabutin

ANSWERS

1. Although it is sometimes possible to achieve synergistic effects against mycobacteria with drug combinations, the primary reason for their use is to delay the emergence of resistance. The answer is **A**.

2. Despite the fact that this patient does not appear to be acutely ill, she would in most cases be treated with 4 drugs that have activity against *M tuberculosis*. This is because organisms infecting patients from Southeast Asia are commonly INH resistant, and coverage must be provided with 3 other antituberculosis drugs in addition to isoniazid. This patient should be hospitalized for several reasons, including potential difficulties with compliance regarding the drug regimen and the fact that young children are in the home where she is living. The answer is **B**.

3. Sputum cultures will not be available for several weeks, and no information is available regarding drug susceptibility of the organism at this stage. For optimum coverage, the initial regimen should include INH, rifampin, pyrazinamide, and ethambutol. INH-resistant organisms are usually sensitive to both rifampin and pyrazinamide. Streptomycin is usually reserved for use in severe forms of tuberculosis or for infections known to be resistant to first-line drugs. Likewise, amikacin and ciprofloxacin are possible agents for treatment of multidrug-resistant strains of *M tuberculosis*. Cycloserine, PAS, and rifabutin are alternative second-line drugs that may be used in cases of failed response to more conventional agents. The answer is **E**.

4. Peripheral neuropathy caused by INH is due to pyridoxine deficiency. It is more common in the diabetic, malnourished, or AIDS patient and can be prevented by a daily dose of 25–50 mg of pyridoxine. INH can inhibit monoamine oxidase type A and has caused tyramine reactions. Hepatotoxicity is age dependent, with an incidence of 0.3% in patients aged 21–35 years and greater than 2% in patients older than 50 years. Patients from Pacific Rim countries do not require lower doses of INH. Fast acetylators, including Native Americans, may require higher doses of the drug than others. The answer is **B**.

5. Rifampin induces the formation of several microsomal drug-metabolizing enzymes, including cytochrome P450 isoforms. This action increases the rate of elimination of a number of drugs, including anticoagulants, ketoconazole, methadone, and steroids present in oral contraceptives. The pharmacologic activity of these drugs can be reduced in patients taking rifampin. The answer is **D**.

6. Mutations in the *katG* gene result in the underproduction of mycobacterial catalase-peroxidase, an enzyme that bioactivates INH, facilitating its interaction with its target, ketoacyl carrier protein synthetase. The result is high-level resistance to isoniazid but without cross-resistance to pyrazinamide. Mutations in the *inhA* gene result in low-level resistance, with cross-resistance to pyrazinamide. The answer is **E**.

7. Combinations of antibiotics are essential for suppression of disease caused by *M avium* complex in the AIDS patient, and treatment should be started before culture results are available. Although rifabutin is prophylactic against MAC bacteremia, when it is used as sole therapy in active disease resistant strains of the organism emerge rapidly. MAC is much less susceptible than *M tuberculosis* to conventional antimycobacterial drugs. Currently, the optimum regimen consists of clarithromycin (or azithromycin) with ethambutol and rifabutin. The answer is **D**.

8. The duration of antimycobacterial drug therapy depends on the severity and location of the infection, the drug susceptibility characteristics of the infecting organism, and the effectiveness of the individual drugs used in the combination regimens. In pulmonary tuberculosis, treatment with INH, rifampin, and pyrazinamide should be continued for a total of 6 mo, with pyrazinamide included for the first 2 mo only. If pyrazinamide is not used during the first 2 mo, INH and rifampin must be given for a total of 9 mo. The answer is **B.**

9. A baseline test of ocular (not auditory) function may be useful prior to starting ethambutol. None of the drugs prescribed are associated with nephrotoxicity. Polyarthralgia is a common adverse effect of pyrazinamide, which was not prescribed in this case. Periodic tests of liver function may be advisable in younger patients who are treated with isoniazid plus rifampin, especially if higher doses of these drugs are used. Prophylaxis with INH is advisable for all household members and very close contacts of patients with active tuberculosis, **especially** young children. The answer is **B.**

10. Resistance emerges rapidly when rifampin is used as a single agent in the treatment of bacterial infections. It is an effective prophylactic and is used as a backup drug to INH to prevent tuberculosis. However, when rifampin is used to treat the meningococcal carrier state, up to 10% of treated carriers may harbor rifampin-resistant organisms. The answer is **D.**

11. Ethambutol inhibits arabinosyl transferases. Ocular toxicity due to ethambutol is dose dependent and is usually reversible when the drug is discontinued. Thiamine is not protective. There is minimal cross-resistance between pyrazinamide and other antimycobacterial drugs. Pyrazinamide uniformly causes hyperuricemia, but this is not a reason to halt therapy even though the drug may provoke acute gouty arthritis in susceptible individuals. The answer is **E.**

12. Owing to its long elimination half-life (3–4 days), weekly administration of azithromycin has proved to be equivalent to daily administration of clarithromycin when used for prophylaxis against *M avium* complex in AIDS patients. The answer is **A.**

13. Multidrug-resistant tuberculosis (MDR-TB) is defined as resistance to 2 or more drugs. All of the risk factors listed are relevant. In the case of resistance to both INH and rifampin, initial regimens still include both drugs plus ethambutol, pyrazinamide, streptomycin (or other aminoglycoside), and a fluoroquinolone. Continuation therapy should include at least 3 drugs shown to be active in vitro against the infecting strain. The appropriate duration of therapy has not been established. The answer is **E.**

14. Ototoxicity is characteristic of the aminoglycoside antibiotics. Many multidrug-resistant strains of mycobacteria remain susceptible to amikacin, and there is no cross-resistance with streptomycin. Although disturbances of equilibrium may occur with overdosage, PAS does not cause hearing loss. The answer is **A.**

> SKILL KEEPER ANSWER:
> GENOTYPIC VARIATIONS
> IN DRUG METABOLISM
> (SEE CHAPTER 4)

Examples of genotypic variations in drug metabolism include succinylcholine (pseudocholinesterase) and isoniazid (N-acetyltransferase). Genetic polymorphisms also occur in isoforms of cytochrome P450 and contribute to variability in the rates of metabolism of phenformin, dextromethorphan, and metoprolol. Variants in the CYP2D6 isoform have been implicated in excessive responses to codeine and nortriptyline, and variants in CYP2C9 may be responsible for unusual sensitivity to the anticoagulant effects of warfarin.

Enzyme	Drugs	Clinical Consequences
Aldehyde dehydrogenase	Ethanol	Facial flushing, emesis and cardiovascular symptoms in Asians with low enzyme activity
N-acetyltransferase	Isoniazid Hydralazine, procainamide	Increased dose requirement in fast acetylators Increased risk of lupus-like syndrome in slow acetylators; possible increased cardiotoxicity with procainamide in fast acetylators
Pseudocholinesterase	Succinylcholine	Deficiences may lead to prolonged apnea

CHECKLIST

When you complete this chapter, you should be able to:

☐ List 5 special problems associated with chemotherapy of mycobacterial infections.

☐ Identify the characteristic pharmacodynamic and pharmacokinetic properties of isoniazid and rifampin.

☐ List the typical adverse effects of ethambutol, pyrazinamide, and streptomycin.

☐ Describe the standard protocols for drug management of latent tuberculosis, pulmonary tuberculosis, and multidrug-resistant tuberculosis.

☐ Identify the drugs used in leprosy and in the prophylaxis and treatment of *M avium-intracellulare* complex disease.

Antifungal Agents

Fungal infections are difficult to treat, particularly in the immunocompromised or neutropenic patient. Most fungi are resistant to conventional antimicrobial agents, and relatively few drugs are available for the treatment of systemic fungal diseases. Amphotericin B and the azoles (fluconazole, itraconazole, ketoconazole, and voriconazole) are the primary drugs used in systemic infections. They are selectively toxic to fungi because they interact with or inhibit the synthesis of ergosterol, a sterol unique to fungal cell membranes.

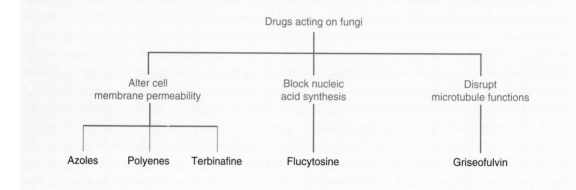

DRUGS FOR SYSTEMIC FUNGAL INFECTIONS

A. AMPHOTERICIN B

1. Classification and pharmacokinetics— Amphotericin B is a polyene antibiotic related to nystatin. Amphotericin is poorly absorbed from the gastrointestinal tract and is usually administered intravenously as a nonlipid colloidal suspension, as a lipid complex, or in a liposomal formulation. The drug is widely distributed to all tissues except the CNS. Elimination is mainly via slow hepatic metabolism; the half-life is approximately 2 weeks. A small fraction of the drug is excreted in the urine; dosage modification is necessary only in extreme renal dysfunction. Amphotericin B is not dialyzable.

2. Mechanism of action—The fungicidal action of amphotericin B is due to its effects on the permeability

and transport properties of fungal membranes. Polyenes are molecules with both hydrophilic and lipophilic characteristics (ie, they are amphipathic). They bind to **ergosterol,** a sterol specific to fungal cell membranes, and cause the formation of artificial pores (Figure 48–1). Resistance, although uncommon, can occur via a decreased level of or a structural change in membrane ergosterol.

3. Clinical uses—Amphotericin B is one of the most important drugs available for the treatment of systemic mycoses and is often used for initial induction regimens before follow-up treatment with an azole. It has the widest antifungal spectrum of any agent and remains the drug of choice, or codrug of choice, for most systemic infections caused by *Aspergillus, Blastomyces, Candida albicans, Cryptococcus, Histoplasma,* and *Mucor.* Amphotericin B is usually given by slow intravenous infusion, but in fungal meningitis intrathecal administration, although dangerous,

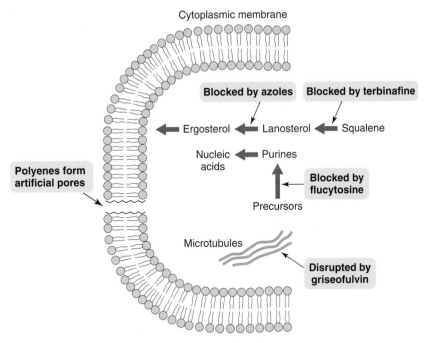

Figure 48–1. Sites of action of some antifungal drugs. The cell cytoplasmic membrane shown is that of a typical fungus. Because ergosterol is not a component of mammalian membranes, significant selective toxicity is achieved with the azole drugs.

has been used. Local administration of the drug, with minimal toxicity, has been used in treatment of mycotic corneal ulcers and keratitis.

4. Toxicity

a. Infusion related—Adverse effects related to intravenous infusion commonly include fever, chills, muscle spasms, vomiting, and a shocklike fall in blood pressure. These effects may be attenuated by a slow infusion rate and by premedication with antihistamines, antipyretics, meperidine, or glucocorticoids.

b. Dose limiting—Amphotericin B decreases the glomerular filtration rate and causes renal tubular acidosis with magnesium and potassium wasting. Anemia may result from decreases in the renal formation of erythropoietin. Although concomitant saline infusion may reduce renal damage, the nephrotoxic effects of the drug are dose limiting. Dose reduction (with lowered toxicity) is possible in some infections when amphotericin B is used with flucytosine. Liposomal formulations of amphotericin B have reduced nephrotoxic effects, possibly because of decreased binding of the drug to renal cells.

c. Neurotoxicity—Intrathecal administration of amphotericin B may cause seizures and neurologic damage.

B. FLUCYTOSINE (5-FLUOROCYTOSINE [5-FC])

1. Classification and pharmacokinetics—5-FC is a pyrimidine antimetabolite related to the anticancer drug 5-fluorouracil. It is effective orally and is distributed to most body tissues, including the CNS. The drug is eliminated intact in the urine, and the dose must be reduced in patients with renal impairment.

2. Mechanism of action—Flucytosine is accumulated in fungal cells by the action of a membrane permease and converted by cytosine deaminase to 5-FU, an inhibitor of thymidylate synthase (Figure 48–1). Selective toxicity occurs because mammalian cells have low levels of permease and deaminase. Resistance can occur rapidly if flucytosine is used alone and involves decreased activity of the fungal permeases or deaminases. When 5-FC is given with amphotericin B, or triazoles such as itraconazole, emergence of resistance is decreased and synergistic antifungal effects may occur.

3. Clinical uses—The antifungal spectrum of 5-FC is narrow; its clinical use is limited to the treatment, in combination with amphotericin B or a triazole, of infections resulting from *Cryptococcus neoformans,* possibly systemic candidal infections, and chromoblastomycosis caused by molds.

4. Toxicity—Prolonged high plasma levels of flucytosine cause reversible bone marrow depression, alopecia, and liver dysfunction.

C. Azole Antifungal Agents

1. Classification and pharmacokinetics—The azoles used for systemic mycoses include **ketoconazole,** an imidazole, and the triazoles **fluconazole, itraconazole,** and **voriconazole.** Oral bioavailability is variable (normal gastric acidity is required). Fluconazole and voriconazole are more reliably absorbed via the oral route than the other azoles. The triazoles are available in both oral and intravenous formulations. The drugs are distributed to most body tissues, but with the exception of fluconazole, drug levels achieved in the CNS are very low. Liver metabolism is responsible for the elimination of ketoconazole, itraconazole, and voriconazole. Inducers of drug-metabolizing enzymes (eg, rifampin) decrease the bioavailability of itraconazole. Fluconazole is eliminated by the kidneys, largely in unchanged form.

2. Mechanism of action—The azoles interfere with fungal cell membrane permeability by inhibiting the synthesis of ergosterol. These drugs act at the step of 14α-demethylation of lanosterol, which is catalyzed by a fungal cytochrome P450 isozyme. With increasing use of azole antifungals, especially for long-term prophylaxis in immunocompromised and neutropenic patients, resistance is occurring, possibly via changes in the sensitivity of the target enzymes.

3. Clinical uses

a. Ketoconazole—Because it has a narrow antifungal spectrum and causes more adverse effects than other azoles, ketoconazole is now rarely used for systemic mycoses. The drug is not available in parenteral form. However, ketoconazole continues to be used for chronic mucocutaneous candidiasis and is also effective against dermatophytes.

b. Fluconazole—Fluconazole is a drug of choice in esophageal and oropharyngeal candidiasis and for most infections caused by *Coccidioides.* A single oral dose usually eradicates vaginal candidiasis. Fluconazole is the drug of choice for treatment and secondary prophylaxis against cryptococcal meningitis and is an alternative drug of choice (with amphotericin B) in treatment of active disease due to *Cryptococcus neoformans.* The drug is also equivalent to amphotericin B in candidemia.

c. Itraconazole—This azole is currently the drug of choice for systemic infections caused by *Blastomyces* and *Sporothrix* and for subcutaneous chromoblastomycosis. Itraconazole is an alternative agent in the treatment of infections caused by *Aspergillus, Coccidioides, Cryptococcus,* and *Histoplasma.* In esophageal candidiasis, the drug is active against some strains resistant to fluconazole. Itraconazole is also used extensively in the treatment of dermatophytoses, especially onychomycosis.

d. Voriconazole—Voriconazole is a newer triazole with an even wider spectrum of fungal activity than itraconazole. It is a codrug of choice for treatment of invasive aspergillosis; some studies report greater efficacy than amphotericin B. Voriconzole is an alternative drug in candidemia, with activity against some fluconazole-resistant organisms, and in AIDS patients it has been used in the treatment of candidial esophagitis and stomatitis.

4. Toxicity—Adverse effects of the azoles include vomiting, diarrhea, rash, and sometimes hepatotoxicity, especially in patients with preexisting liver dysfunction. Ketoconazole is a notorious inhibitor of hepatic cytochrome P450 isozymes and may increase the plasma levels of many other drugs, including cyclosporine, oral hypoglycemics, phenytoin, and warfarin. Inhibition of cytochrome P450 isoforms by ketoconazole interferes with the synthesis of adrenal and gonadal steroids and may lead to gynecomastia, menstrual irregularities, and infertility. The other azoles are more selective inhibitors of fungal cytochrome P450. Although they are less likely than ketoconazole to cause endocrine dysfunction, their inhibitory effects on liver drug-metabolizing enzymes have resulted in drug interactions. Voriconazole causes immediate but transient visual disturbances, including blurring of vision of unknown cause in more than 30% of patients. Based on animal studies voriconzole is a class D drug in terms of pregnancy risk.

> **SKILL KEEPER: INHIBITORS OF CYTOCHROMES P450 (SEE CHAPTERS 4 AND 61)**
>
> *Ketoconazole has the unenviable reputation of association with multiple drug interactions because of its inhibition of cytochromes P450 involved in drug metabolism.*
>
> 1. *How many drugs can you identify that have their metabolism via such enzymes inhibited by ketoconazole?*
>
> 2. *How many other drugs that inhibit hepatic cytochromes P450 can you recall?*
>
> The Skill Keeper Answers appear at the end of the chapter.

D. Echinocandins

1. Classification and pharmacokinetics—Caspofungin is an echinocandin, the first of a novel class of antifungal agents. Other echinocandins include anidulafungin and micafungin. Used intravenously, the drugs distribute widely to the tissues and are eliminated largely via hepatic metabolism. Caspofungin has a half-life of 9–12 h. The half-life of micafungin is slightly longer and that of anidulafungin is 24–48 h.

2. Mechanism of action—The echinocandins have a unique fungicidal action, inhibiting the synthesis of β(1–2)glycan, a critical component of fungal cell walls.

3. Clinical uses—Caspofungin is used for disseminated and mucocutaneous *Candida* infections and for salvage therapy in the management of invasive aspergillosis in patients who fail to respond to amphotericin B. Anidulafungin is used for esophageal and invasive candidiasis. Micafungin is used for mucocutaneous candidiasis and for prophylaxis of *Candida* infections in bone marrow transplant patients.

4. Toxicity—Infusion-related effects of caspofungin include headache, gastrointestinal distress, fever, rash, and flushing (histamine release). Micafungin also causes histamine release and elevates blood levels of the immunosuppressant drugs cyclosporine and sirolimus. Combined use of echinocandins with cyclosporine may elevate liver transaminases.

SYSTEMIC DRUGS FOR SUPERFICIAL FUNGAL INFECTIONS

A. GRISEOFULVIN

1. Pharmacokinetics—Oral absorption of griseofulvin depends on the physical state of the drug—ultra-microsize formulations, which have finer crystals or particles, are more effectively absorbed—and is aided by high-fat foods. The drug is distributed to the stratum corneum, where it binds to keratin. Biliary excretion is responsible for its elimination.

2. Mechanism of action—Griseofulvin interferes with microtubule function in dermatophytes (Figure 48–1) and may also inhibit the synthesis and polymerization of nucleic acids. Sensitive dermatophytes take up the drug by an energy-dependent mechanism, and resistance can occur via decrease in this transport. Griseofulvin is fungistatic.

3. Clinical uses and toxicity—Griseofulvin is not active topically. The oral formulation of the drug is indicated for dermatophytoses of the skin and hair, but it has been largely replaced by terbinafine and the azoles. Adverse effects include headaches, mental confusion, gastrointestinal irritation, photosensitivity, and changes in liver function. Griseofulvin should not be used in patients with porphyria. Griseofulvin decreases the bioavailability of warfarin, resulting in decreased anticoagulant effect, and it also causes disulfiram-like reactions with ethanol.

B. TERBINAFINE

1. Mechanism of action—Terbinafine inhibits a fungal enzyme, squalene epoxidase. It causes accumulation of toxic levels of squalene, which can interfere with ergosterol synthesis. Terbinafine is fungicidal.

2. Clinical uses and toxicity—Terbinafine is available in both oral and topical forms. Like griseofulvin, terbinafine accumulates in keratin, but it is much more effective than griseofulvin in onychomycosis. Adverse effects include gastrointestinal upsets, rash, headache, and taste disturbances. Terbinafine does not inhibit cytochrome P450.

C. AZOLES

The azoles other than voriconazole are commonly used orally for the treatment of dermatophytoses. Pulse or intermittent dosing with itraconazole is as effective in onychomycoses as continuous dosing because the drug

---

KEY DRUGS		
Subclass	**Prototype**	**Other Significant Agents**
Drugs for systemic mycoses		
Polyenes	Amphotericin B	Nystatin
Azoles	Ketoconazole	Fluconazole, itraconazole, voriconazole
Pyrimidines	Flucytosine	
Echinocandins	Caspofungin	Anidulafungin, micafungin
Systemic drugs for superficial infections	Griseofulvin	Terbinafine, ketoconazole, fluconazole, itraconazole
Drugs for topical or local use	Nystatin	Miconazole, clotrimazole

persists in the nails for several months. Typically, treatment for 1 week is followed by 3 weeks without drug. Advantages of pulse dosing include a lower incidence of side effects and major cost savings.

TOPICAL DRUGS FOR SUPERFICIAL FUNGAL INFECTIONS

A number of antifungal drugs are used topically for superficial infections caused by *C albicans* and dermatophytes. **Nystatin** is a polyene antibiotic (toxicity precludes systemic use) that disrupts fungal membranes by binding to ergosterol. Nystatin is commonly used topically to suppress local *Candida* infections and has been used orally to eradicate gastrointestinal fungi in patients with impaired defense mechanisms. Other topical antifungal agents that are widely used include the azole compounds **miconazole** and **clotrimazole.**

QUESTIONS

1. Interactions between this drug and cell membrane components can result in the formation of pores lined by hydrophilic groups present in the drug molecule.
   (A) Caspofungin
   (B) Fluconazole
   (C) Griseofulvin
   (D) Nystatin
   (E) Terbinafine

2. Which statement about fluconazole is accurate?
   (A) It is a potent inducer of hepatic drug-metabolizing enzymes
   (B) It does not penetrate the blood-brain barrier
   (C) It is highly effective in treatment of aspergillosis
   (D) It inhibits demethylation of lanosterol
   (E) Oral bioavailability is less than that of ketoconazole

3–6. A 20-year-old woman with leukemia was undergoing chemotherapy with intravenous antineoplastic drugs. During treatment, she developed a systemic infection from an opportunistic pathogen. There was no erythema or edema at the catheter insertion site. A white vaginal discharge was observed. After appropriate specimens were obtained for culture, empiric antibiotic therapy was started with gentamicin, nafcillin, and ticarcillin intravenously. This regimen was maintained for 72 h, during which time the patient's condition did not improve significantly. Her throat was sore, and white plaques had appeared in her pharynx. On day 4, none of the cultures had shown any bacterial growth, but both the blood and urine cultures grew out *Candida albicans.*

3. At this point, the best course of action is to
   (A) Continue current antibiotics and start amphotericin B
   (B) Continue current antibiotics and start flucytosine
   (C) Continue current antibiotics and start griseofulvin
   (D) Stop current antibiotics and start amphotericin B
   (E) Stop current antibiotics and start ketoconazole

4. If amphotericin B is administered, the patient should be premedicated with
   (A) Diphenhydramine
   (B) Ibuprofen
   (C) Prednisone
   (D) Any or all of the above
   (E) None of the above

5. The dose-limiting toxicity of amphotericin B is
   (A) Hepatitis
   (B) Hypotension
   (C) Infusion-related adverse effects
   (D) Myelosuppression
   (E) Renal tubular acidosis

6. *Candida* is a major cause of nosocomial bloodstream infection. The opportunistic fungal infection in this patient could have been prevented by administration of
   (A) Caspofungin
   (B) Itraconazole
   (C) Ketoconazole
   (D) Nystatin
   (E) None of the above

7–8. An African-American man living on the East Coast was transferred by his employer to California for 6 mo. On his return, he complains of having influenza-like symptoms with fever and a cough. He also has red, tender nodules on his shins. His physician suspects that these symptoms are due to coccidioidomycosis contracted during his stay in California.

7. This patient should be treated immediately with
   (A) Amphotericin B
   (B) Griseofulvin
   (C) Itraconazole
   (D) Ketoconazole
   (E) None of these antifungal drugs

8. Which is the drug of choice if this patient is suffering from persistent lung lesions or disseminated disease caused by *Coccidioides immitis*?
   (A) Amphotericin B
   (B) Fluconazole
   (C) Ketoconazole
   (D) Terbinafine
   (E) Voriconazole

9. Which drug is LEAST likely to be effective in the treatment of esophageal candidiasis if it is used by the oral route?
   (A) Amphotericin B
   (B) Clotrimazole
   (C) Fluconazole
   (D) Griseofulvin
   (E) Ketoconazole

10. Which statement about flucytosine is accurate?
    (A) It is bioactivated by fungal cytosine deaminase
    (B) It does not cross the blood-brain barrier
    (C) It inhibits cytochrome P450
    (D) It is useful in esophageal candidiasis
    (E) It has a wide spectrum of antifungal activity

11. Serious cardiac effects have occurred when this drug was taken by patients using the antihistamines astemizole or terfenadine.
    (A) Amphotericin B
    (B) Griseofulvin
    (C) Ketoconazole
    (D) Nystatin
    (E) Voriconazole

12. Which drug is most appropriate for oral use in vaginal candidiasis?
    (A) Clotrimazole
    (B) Griseofulvin
    (C) Fluconazole
    (D) Flucytosine
    (E) Nystatin

13. Regarding the clinical use of liposomal formulations of amphotericin B, which statement is accurate?
    (A) Affinity of amphotericin B for these lipids is greater than affinity for ergosterol
    (B) They are less expensive to use than conventional amphotericin B
    (C) They are more effective in fungal infections because they increase tissue uptake of amphotericin B
    (D) They decrease nephrotoxicity of amphotericin B
    (E) They have a wider spectrum of antifungal activity than conventional formulations of amphotericin B

14. Which drug used intravenously for disseminated and mucocutaneous *Candida* infections is an inhibitor of the synthesis of fungal cell wall components?
    (A) Amphotericin B
    (B) Caspofungin
    (C) Clotrimazole
    (D) Itraconazole
    (E) Voriconazole

ANSWERS

1. The polyene antifungal drugs are amphipathic molecules that can interact with ergosterol in fungal cell membranes to form artificial pores. In these structures, the lipophilic groups on the drug molecule are arranged on the outside of the pore and the hydrophilic regions are located on the inside. The fungicidal action of amphotericin B and nystatin derives from this interaction, which results in leakage of intracellular constituents. The answer is **D**.

2. The azoles with activity against *Aspergillus* are itraconazole and voriconazole. Fluconazole is the best absorbed member of the azole group by the oral route and the only one that readily penetrates into cerebrospinal fluid. Fluconazole inhibits hepatic cytochrome P450. The answer is **D**.

3. The antibiotic regimen should be stopped on the grounds that the condition of the patient did not improve after 3 days of such treatment, the cultures were negative for bacteria, and the clinical picture suggested that the patient had a fungal infection. This was confirmed by blood culture. The answer is **D**.

4. Infusion-related adverse effects of amphotericin B include chills and fevers (the "shake and bake" syndrome), muscle spasms, nausea, headache, and hypotension. Antipyretics, antihistamines, and glucocorticoids have all been shown to be helpful. The administration of a 1-mg test dose of amphotericin B is sometimes useful in predicting the severity of infusion-related toxicity. The answer is **D**.

5. Renal toxicity is dose limiting with amphotericin B. Azotemia is common and sometimes severe enough to warrant dialysis. Decreases in glomerular filtration rate may be reversible, but irreversible damage can occur, presenting as renal tubular acidosis with hypokalemia and hypomagnesemia. The answer is **E**.

6. In the case of opportunistic candidal infections in the immunocompromised patient, no prophylactic drugs have been shown to be clinically effective. Prophylaxis against other fungi may be effective in some instances, including suppression of cryptococcal meningitis in AIDS patients with fluconazole. However, prophylactic use of azoles may contribute to the development of fungal resistance. The answer is **E**.

7. A travel history can be important in the diagnosis of fungal disease. If this patient has a fungal infection of the lungs, it is probably due to *C immitis,* which is endemic in dry regions of the western United States. Pulmonary symptoms of coccidioidomycosis are usually self-limiting, and drug therapy is not commonly required in an otherwise healthy patient. The presence of tender red nodules on extensor

surfaces is a good prognostic sign. Erythema nodosum is a delayed hypersensitivity response to fungal antigens. No organisms are present in the lesions, and it is not a sign of disseminated disease. The answer is **E.**

8. In progressive or disseminated forms of coccidioidomycosis, systemic antifungal drug treatment is needed. Until recently, amphotericin B was the recommended therapy, but fluconazole or itraconazole are now generally preferred. Note that the risk of dissemination is much greater in African-Americans(10% incidence) and in pregnant women during the third trimester. The answer is **B.**

9. Griseofulvin has no activity against *C albicans* and is not effective in the treatment of systemic or superficial infections caused by such organisms. "Swish and swallow" formulations of clotrimazole and nystatin have been used commonly. Most of the azoles are effective in esophageal candidiasis. The answer is **D.**

10. Flucytosine is converted via fungal cytosine deaminase to the antimetabolite fluorouracil, which causes inhibition of thymidylate synthase. Flucytosine enters the cerebrospinal fluid and has been used in combination with amphotericin B in cryptococcal meningitis. The drug has a narrow spectrum of antifungal activity and is not effective in esophageal candidiasis. The answer is **A.**

11. Cardiotoxicity may occur when ketoconazole is used by patients taking astemizole or terfenadine as a result of the ability of ketoconazole to inhibit their metabolism via hepatic cytochromes P450. The answer is **C.**

12. Clotrimazole and nystatin may be used topically (not orally) for vaginal candidiasis. The activity of griseofulvin is limited to dermatophytes. Fluconazole in a single oral dose is usually effective in vaginal candidiasis. Itraconazole is also effective. The answer is **C.**

13. Liposomal formulations of amphotericin B result in decreased accumulation of the drug in tissues, including the kidney. As a result, nephrotoxicity is decreased. With some lipid formulations, infusion-related toxicity may also be reduced. Lipid formulations do not have a wider antifungal spectrum; their daily cost ranges from 10 to 40 times more than the conventional formulation of amphotericin B. The answer is **D.**

14. With the exception of caspofungin, all of the drugs listed exert their actions on fungal cell membranes. The echinocandins are fungicidal via their inhibition of the synthesis of β(1–2)glycan, a critical component of fungal cell walls. The answer is **B.**

SKILL KEEPER ANSWERS: INHIBITORS OF CYTOCHROMES P450 (SEE CHAPTERS 4 AND 61)

1. *A sampling of commonly used drugs with cytochrome P450-mediated metabolism inhibited by ketoconazole or other azoles includes chlordiazepoxide, cisapride, cyclosporine, didanosine, fluoxetine, loratadine, lovastatin, methadone, nifedipine, phenytoin, quinidine, tacrolimus, theophylline, verapamil, warfarin, zidovudine, and zolpidem.*

2. *Other drugs that inhibit hepatic cytochromes P450 include chloramphenicol, cimetidine, clarithromycin, disulfiram, erythromycin, ethanol, grapefruit juice (contains furanocoumarins), ethinyl estradiol, fluconazole, isoniazid, itraconazole, MAO inhibitors, phenylbutazone, and secobarbital.*

CHECKLIST

When you complete this chapter, you should be able to:

☐ Describe the mechanisms of action of the azole, polyene, and echinocandin antifungal drugs.

☐ Identify the clinical uses of amphotericin B, flucytosine, individual azoles, caspofungin, griseofulvin, and terbinafine.

☐ Describe the pharmacokinetics and toxicities of amphotericin B

☐ Describe the pharmokinetics, toxicities, and drug interactions of the azoles.

☐ Identify the main topical antifungal agents.

Antiviral Chemotherapy & Prophylaxis

As obligate intracellular parasites, the replication of viruses depends on synthetic processes of the host cell. Antiviral drugs can exert their actions at several stages of viral replication including viral adsorption and penetration, nucleic acid synthesis, late protein synthesis and processing, and in the final stages of viral packaging and virion release (Figure 49–1). Most of the drugs active against herpes viruses and many agents active against HIV are antimetabolites, structurally similar to naturally occurring compounds. The selective toxicity of antiviral drugs usually depends on greater susceptibility of viral enzymes to their inhibitory actions than host cell enzymes.

One of the most important trends in viral chemotherapy, especially in the management of HIV infection, has been the introduction of combination drug therapy. This can result in greater clinical effectiveness in viral infections and can also prevent, or delay, the emergence of resistance.

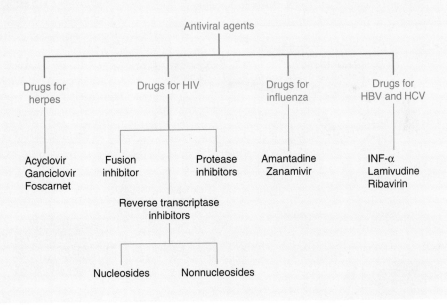

ANTIHERPES DRUGS

Most drugs active against herpes viruses are antimetabolites bioactivated via viral or host cell kinases to form compounds that inhibit viral DNA polymerases.

A. ACYCLOVIR (ACYCLOGUANOSINE)

1. **Mechanisms**—Acyclovir is a guanosine analog active against herpes simplex virus (HSV-1, HSV-2) and varicella-zoster virus (VZV). The drug is activated to form

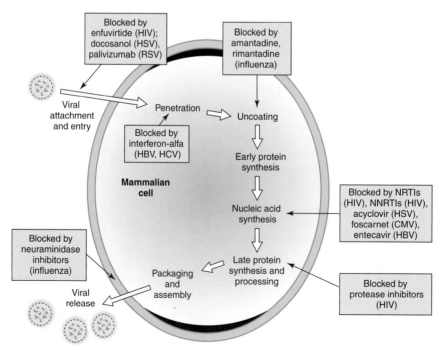

Figure 49–1. The major sites of antiviral drug action. *Note:* interferon alfas are speculated to have multiple sites of action on viral replication. (Reproduced, with permission, from Katzung BG, editor: *Basic & Clinical Pharmacology*, 10th ed. McGraw-Hill, 2007.)

acyclovir triphosphate, which interferes with viral DNA synthesis in 2 ways. It acts as a competitive substrate for DNA polymerase and it leads to chain termination following its incorporation into viral DNA (Figure 49–2). Resistance of HSV can involve changes in viral DNA polymerase. However, many resistant strains of HSV (TK⁻ strains) lack thymidine kinase, the enzyme involved in the initial *viral-specific* phosphorylation of acyclovir. Such strains are cross-resistant to famciclovir, ganciclovir, and valacyclovir.

2. Pharmacokinetics—Acyclovir can be administered by the topical, oral, and intravenous routes. Because of its short half-life, oral administration requires multiple daily doses of acyclovir. Renal excretion is the major route of elimination of acyclovir, and dosage should be reduced in patients with renal impairment.

3. Clinical uses and toxicity—Oral acyclovir is commonly used for the treatment of mucocutaneous and genital herpes lesions (Table 49–1) and for prophylaxis in AIDS and in other immunocompromised patients (eg, those undergoing organ transplantation). The oral drug is well tolerated but may cause gastrointestinal distress and headache. Intravenous administration is used for severe herpes disease, including encephalitis, and for neonatal HSV infection. Toxic effects with parenteral administration include delirium, tremor, seizures, hypotension, and nephrotoxicity. Acyclovir has no significant toxicity on the bone marrow.

4. Other drugs for HSV and VZV infections— Several newer agents have characteristics similar to acyclovir. **Valacyclovir** is a prodrug converted to acyclovir by hepatic metabolism after oral administration; it reaches plasma levels 3–5 times greater than those achieved by acyclovir. Valacyclovir also has a longer duration of action than acyclovir. **Penciclovir** undergoes activation by viral thymidine kinase, and the triphosphate form inhibits DNA polymerase but does not cause chain termination. **Famciclovir** is a prodrug converted to penciclovir by first-pass metabolism in the liver. Used orally in genital herpes and for herpes zoster, famciclovir is well tolerated and is similar to acyclovir in its pharmacokinetic properties. None of the acyclovir congeners have activity against TK⁻ strains of HSV. **Docosanol** is an aliphatic alcohol that inhibits fusion between the HSV envelope and plasma membranes. It prevents viral entry and subsequent replication. Used topically, docosanol shortens healing time.

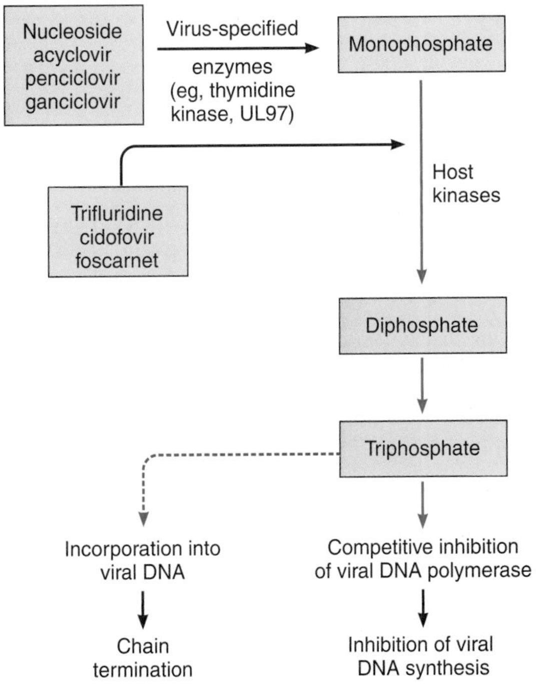

B. GANCICLOVIR

1. Mechanisms—Ganciclovir, a guanine derivative, is triphosphorylated to form a nucleotide that inhibits DNA polymerases of cytomegalovirus (CMV) and HSV and causes chain termination. The first phosphorylation step is catalyzed by virus-specific enzymes in both CMV-infected and HSV-infected cells. CMV resistance mechanisms involve mutations in the genes that code for the activating viral phosphotransferase and the viral DNA polymerases. Thymidine kinase-deficient HSV strains are resistant to ganciclovir.

2. Pharmacokinetics—Ganciclovir is usually given intravenously and penetrates well into tissues, including the eye and the CNS. The drug undergoes renal elimination in direct proportion to creatinine clearance. Oral bioavailability is less than 10%. An intraocular implant form of ganciclovir can be used in CMV retinitis. Valganciclovir, a prodrug of ganciclovir, has high oral bioavailability and has decreased the usage of intravenous forms of ganciclovir in end-organ CMV disease

3. Clinical uses and toxicity—Ganciclovir and valganciclovir are used for the prophylaxis and treatment of CMV retinitis and other CMV infections in immunocompromised patients. Systemic toxic effects include leukopenia, thrombocytopenia, mucositis, hepatic dysfunction, and seizures. The drugs may cause severe neutropenia when used with zidovudine or other myelosuppressive agents.

Figure 49–2. Mechanism of action of antiherpes agents. (Reproduced, with permission, from Katzung BG, editor: *Basic & Clinical Pharmacology*, 10th ed. McGraw-Hill, 2007.)

Table 49-1. Important antiviral drugs.

Virus	Primary Drugs	Alternative or Adjunctive Drugs
CMV	Ganciclovir, valganciclovir	Cidofovir, foscarnet, fomiversin
HSV, VZV	Acyclovir	Cidofovir, foscarnet, vidarabine
HBV	IFN-α, lamivudine	Adefovir dipivoxil, entecavir
HCV	IFN-α	Ribavirin
Influenza A	Oseltamivir	Amantadine, rimantadine, zanamivir
Influenza B	Oseltamivir	Zanamivir

[a]Anti-HSV drugs similar to acyclovir include famciclovir, penciclovir, and valacyclovir.

C. CIDOFOVIR

1. Mechanisms and pharmacokinetics—Cidofovir is activated exclusively by host cell kinases and the active diphosphate inhibits DNA polymerases of HSV, CMV, adenovirus, and papillomavirus (HPV). Because phosphorylation does not require viral kinase, cidofovir is active against many acyclovir and ganciclovir-resistant strains. Resistance is due to mutations in the DNA polymerase gene. The drug is given intravenously and undergoes renal elimination. Dosage should be adjusted in proportion to creatinine clearance and full hydration maintained.

2. Clinical uses and toxicity—Cidofovir is effective in CMV retinitis, in mucocutaneous HSV infections, including those resistant to acyclovir, and in genital warts. Nephrotoxicity is the major dose-limiting toxicity of cidofovir, additive with other nephrotoxic drugs including amphotericin B and aminoglycoside antibiotics. Pretreatment with probenicid decreases active tubular secretion and reduces nephrotoxicity.

D. FOSCARNET

1. Mechanisms—Foscarnet is a phosphonoformate derivative that does not require phosphorylation for antiviral activity. Although it is not an antimetabolite, foscarnet inhibits viral RNA polymerase, DNA polymerase, and HIV reverse transcriptase. Resistance involves point mutations in the DNA polymerase gene.

2. Pharmacokinetics—Foscarnet is given intravenously and penetrates well into tissues, including the CNS. The drug undergoes renal elimination in direct proportion to creatinine clearance.

3. Clinical uses and toxicity—The drug is an alternative for prophylaxis and treatment of CMV infections, including CMV retinitis, and has activity against ganciclovir-resistant strains of this virus. Foscarnet inhibits herpes DNA polymerase in acyclovir-resistant strains that are thymidine kinase deficient and may suppress such resistant herpetic infections in patients with AIDS. Adverse effects are severe and include nephrotoxicity (30% incidence) with disturbances in electrolyte balance (especially hypocalcemia), genitourinary ulceration, and CNS effects (headache, hallucinations, seizures).

E. OTHER ANTIHERPES DRUGS

1. Vidarabine—Vidarabine is an adenine analog and has activity against HSV, VZV, and CMV. Its use for systemic infections is limited by rapid metabolic inactivation and marked toxic potential. Vidarabine is used topically for herpes keratitis but has no effect on genital lesions. Toxic effects with systemic use include gastrointestinal irritation, paresthesias, tremor, convulsions, and hepatic dysfunction. Vidarabine is teratogenic in animals.

2. Idoxuridine and trifluridine—These pyrimidine analogs are used topically in herpes keratitis (HSV-1). They are too toxic for systemic use.

3. Fomivirsen—Fomivirsen is an antisense oligonucleotide that binds to mRNA of CMV, inhibiting early protein synthesis. The drug is injected intravitreally for treatment of CMV retinitis. Cross-resistance between fomivirsen and other anti-CMV agents has not been observed. Concurrent systemic anti-CMV therapy is recommended to protect against extraocular and contralateral retinal CMV disease. Fomiversen causes iritis, vitreitis, increased intraocular pressure and changes in vision.

ANTI-HIV DRUGS

The primary drugs effective against HIV are antimetabolite inhibitors of viral reverse transcriptase and inhibitors of viral aspartate protease (Table 49-2). The current approach to treatment of infection with HIV is the initiation of treatment with 3 or more anti-retroviral drugs, if possible, before symptoms appear. Such combinations

Table 49–2. Major antiretroviral drugs.

Subclass	Prototype	Other Significant Agents
Nucleoside reverse transcriptase inhibitors	Zidovudine	Abacavir, didanosine, emtricitabine, lamivudine, stavudine, zalcitabine, zidovudine
Nonnucleoside reverse transcriptase inhibitors	Delavirdine	Efavirenz, nevirapine, tenofovir
Protease inhibitors	Indinavir	Amprenavir, atazanavir, indinavir, lopinavir, nelfinavir, ritonavir, saquinavir
Fusion inhibitor	Enfuvirtide	

usually include reverse transcriptase inhibitors (RTIs) together with inhibitors of HIV protease (PI). Highly active antiretroviral therapy (HAART) involving drug combinations can slow or reverse the increases in viral RNA load that normally accompany progression of disease. In many AIDS patients, HAART slows or reverses the decline in CD4 cells and decreases the incidence of opportunistic infections.

Drug management of HIV infection is subject to change. Updated recommendations can be obtained at the following websites: ATIS, http://www.hivatis.org, and NPIN, http://www.cdcnpin.org.

A. Nucleoside Reverse Transcriptase Inhibitors (NRTIs)

To convert their RNA into dsDNA, retroviruses require virally encoded RNA-dependent DNA polymerase (reverse transcriptase). Mammalian RNA and DNA polymerases are sufficiently distinct to permit a selective inhibition of the viral reverse transcriptase.

Most NRTIs are prodrugs converted by host cell kinases to triphosphates, which not only competitively inhibit binding of natural nucleotides to the dNTP-binding site of reverse transcriptase but also act as chain terminators via their insertion into the growing DNA chain. Because NRTIs lack a 3′-hydroxyl group on the ribose ring, attachment of the next nucleotide is impossible. Resistance emerges rapidly if NRTIs are used as single agents via mutations in the *pol* gene; cross-resistance occurs but is not complete.

1. Abacavir—Abacavir is a guanosine analog with good oral bioavailability and an intracellular half-life of 12–24 h. HIV resistance requires several concomitant mutations and tends to develop slowly. Hypersensitivity reactions, occasionally fatal, occur in 5% of HIV patients.

2. Didanosine (ddI)—Oral bioavailability of ddI is reduced by food and by chelating agents. The drug is eliminated by the kidney, and the dose must be reduced in patients with renal dysfunction. Pancreatitis is dose limiting and occurs more frequently in alcoholic patients and those with hypertriglyceridemia. Other adverse effects include peripheral neuropathy, diarrhea, hepatic dysfunction, hyperuricemia, and CNS effects.

3. Emtricitabine—Good oral bioavailability and renal elimination with long half-life permits once-daily dosing of emtricitabine. Because of propylene glycol in the oral solution, the drug is contraindicated in pregnant patients, young children, and patients with hepatic or renal dysfunction. Common adverse effects of the drug include asthenia, gastrointestinal distress, headache, and hyperpigmentation of the palms, soles, or both.

4. Lamivudine (3TC)—Lamivudine is 80% bioavailable by the oral route and is eliminated almost exclusively by the kidney. In addition to its use in HAART regimens for HIV, lamivudine is also effective in hepatitis B infections. Dosage adjustment is needed in patients with renal insufficiency. Adverse effects of lamivudine are usually mild and include gastrointestinal distress, headache, insomnia, and fatigue.

5. Stavudine (d4T)—Stavudine has good oral bioavailability and penetrates most tissues, including the CNS. Dosage adjustment is needed in renal insufficiency. Peripheral neuropathy is dose limiting and increases with co-administration of didanosine or zalcitabine. Lactic acidosis with hepatic steatosis occurs more frequently than with other NRTIs.

6. Tenofovir—Although it is a nucleotide, tenofovir acts like NRTIs to competitively inhibit reverse transcriptase and cause chain termination after incorporation into DNA. Oral bioavailability of tenofovir is in the range of 25–40%, the intracellular half-life is more than 60 h, and the drug undergoes renal elimination. Tenofovir may impede the renal excretion of acyclovir and ganciclovir. Adverse effects include gastrointestinal distress, asthenia, and headache; rare cases of acute renal failure and Fanconi's syndrome have been reported.

7. Zalcitabine (ddC)—Zalcitabine has high oral bioavailability. Dosage adjustment is needed in patients with renal insufficiency, and nephrotoxic drugs (eg, amphotericin B, aminoglycosides) increase toxic potential. Dose-limiting peripheral neuropathy is the major adverse effect of ddC. Pancreatitis, esophageal ulceration, stomatitis, and arthralgias may also occur.

8. Zidovudine (ZDV)—Formerly called azidothymidine (AZT), zidovudine is active orally and is distributed to most tissues, including the CNS. Elimination of the drug involves both hepatic metabolism to glucuronides and renal excretion. Dosage reduction is necessary in uremic patients and those with cirrhosis. The primary toxicity of ZDV is bone marrow suppression (additive with other myelosuppressive drugs) leading to anemia and neutropenia, which may require transfusions. Gastrointestinal distress, thrombocytopenia, headaches, myalgia, acute cholestatic hepatitis, agitation, and insomnia may also occur. Drugs that may increase plasma levels of zidovudine include azole antifungals and protease inhibitors. Rifampin increases the clearance of zidovudine.

9. NRTIs and lactic acidosis—The use of NRTI agents, alone or in combination with other antiretroviral agents, may cause lactic acidemia and severe hepatomegaly with steatosis. Risk factors include obesity, prolonged treatment with NRTIs, and preexisting liver dysfunction. Consideration should be given to suspension of NRTI treatment in patients who develop elevated aminotransferase levels.

B. NONNUCLEOSIDE REVERSE TRANSCRIPTASE INHIBITORS (NNRTIs)

NNRTIs bind to a site on reverse transcriptase different from the binding site of NRTIs. Nonnucleoside drugs do not require phosphorylation to be active and do not compete with nucleoside triphosphates. There is no cross-resistance with NRTIs. Resistance from mutations in the *pol* gene occur very rapidly if these agents are used as monotherapy.

1. Delavirdine—Drug interactions are a major problem with delavirdine, which is metabolized by both CYP3A4 and CYP2D6. Its blood levels are decreased by antacids, ddI, phenytoin, rifampin, and nelfinavir. Conversely, the blood levels of delavirdine are increased by azole antifungals and macrolide antibiotics. Delavirdine increases plasma levels of several benzodiazepines, nifedipine, protease inhibitors, quinidine, and warfarin. Delavirdine causes skin rash in up to 20% of patients, and the drug should be avoided in pregnancy because it is teratogenic in animals.

2. Efavirenz—Efavirenz can be given once daily because of its long half-life. Fatty foods may enhance its oral bioavailability. Efavirenz is metabolized by hepatic cytochromes P450 and is frequently involved in drug interactions. Toxicity of efavirenz includes CNS dysfunction, skin rash, and elevations of plasma cholesterol. The drug should be avoided in pregnancy, particularly in the first trimester, because fetal abnormalities have been reported in animals at doses similar to those used in humans.

3. Nevirapine—Nevirapine has good oral bioavailability, penetrates most tissues (including the CNS), has a half-life > 24 h, and is metabolized by the hepatic CYP3A isoform. The drug is used in combination regimens and is effective in preventing HIV vertical transmission when given as single doses to mothers at the onset of labor and to the neonate. Hypersensitivity reactions with nevirapine include a rash, which occurs in 15–20% of patients, especially females. Stevens-Johnson syndrome and a life-threatening toxic epidermal necrolysis have also been reported. Nevirapine blood levels are increased by cimetidine and macrolide antibiotics and decreased by enzyme inducers such as rifampin.

C. PROTEASE INHIBITORS

The assembly of infectious HIV virions is dependent on an aspartate protease (HIV-1 protease) encoded by the pol gene. This viral enzyme cleaves precursor polyproteins to form the final structural proteins of the mature virion core. The HIV protease inhibitors are designer drugs based on molecular characterization of the active site of the viral enzyme. Resistance is mediated via multiple point mutations in the pol gene; the extent of cross-resistance is variable depending on the specific protease inhibitor (PI). PIs have important clinical use in AIDS, most commonly in combinations with reverse transcriptase inhibitors as components of HAART. All of the PIs are substrates and inhibitors of CYP3A4, with ritonavir having the most pronounced inhibitory effect. The PIs are implicated in many drug-drug interactions with other antiretroviral agents and with commonly used medications.

1. Amprenavir and fosamprenavir—Oral absorption of amprenavir is impeded by fatty foods. The drug formulation contains propylene glycol and should not be used in children or in pregnancy. Fosamprenavir is a prodrug with superior oral bioavailability. Amprenavir undergoes hepatic metabolism and is both an inhibitor and an inducer of CYP3A4. The drug causes gastrointestinal distress, paresthesias, and rash, the latter sometimes severe enough to warrant drug discontinuation. Cross-allergenicity may occur with sulfonamides.

2. Atazanavir—This is a newer PI with a pharmacokinetic profile that permits once-daily dosing. Oral absorption of atazanavir requires an acidic environment—antacid ingestion should be separated by 12 h. The drug penetrates cerebrospinal and seminal fluids and undergoes biliary elimination. Adverse effects include gastrointestinal distress, peripheral neuropathy, skin rash, and hyperbilirubinemia. Prolongation of the QTc interval may occur at high doses. Unlike most PIs, atazanavir does not appear to be associated with dyslipidemias, fat redistribution, or a metabolic syndrome. However, it is a potent inhibitor of CYP3A and CYP2C9.

3. Indinavir—Oral bioavailability of indinavir is good except in the presence of food. Clearance is mainly via the liver, with about 10% renal excretion. Adverse effects include nausea, diarrhea, thrombocytopenia, hyperbilirubinemia, and nephrolithiasis. To reduce renal damage, it is important to maintain good hydration. Insulin resistance may be more common with indinavir than other PIs. Indinavir is a substrate for and an inhibitor of the cytochrome P450 isoform CYP3A4 and is implicated in drug interactions. Serum levels of indinavir are increased by azole antifungals and decreased by rifamycins. Indinavir increases the serum levels of antihistamines, benzodiazepines, and rifampin.

4. Lopinavir/ritonavir—In this combination a subtherapeutic dose of ritonavir acts as a pharmacokinetic enhancer by inhibiting the CYP3A-mediated metabolism of lopinavir. Patient compliance is improved due to lower pill burden, and the combination is usually well tolerated.

5. Nelfinavir—This PI is characterized by increased oral absorption in the presence of food, hepatic metabolism via CYP3A, and a short half-life. As an inhibitor of drug metabolism, nelfinavir has been involved in many drug interactions. Adverse effects include diarrhea, which can be dose limiting. The drug has the most favorable safety profile of the PIs in pregnancy.

6. Ritonavir—Oral bioavailability is good, and the drug should be taken with meals. Clearance is mainly via the liver, and dosage reduction is necessary in patients with hepatic impairment. The most common adverse effects of ritonavir are gastrointestinal irritation and a bitter taste. Paresthesias and elevations of hepatic aminotransferases and triglycerides in the plasma also occur. Drugs that increase the activity of the cytochrome P450 isoform CYP3A4 (anticonvulsants, rifamycins) reduce serum levels of ritonavir, and drugs that inhibit this enzyme (azole antifungals, cimetidine, erythromycin) elevate serum levels of the antiviral drug. Ritonavir inhibits the metabolism of a wide range of drugs, including erythromycin, dronabinol, ketoconazole, prednisone, rifampin, and saquinavir.

Subtherapeutic doses of ritonavir inhibit the CYP3A-mediated metabolism of other PIs (eg, indinavir, lopinavir, saquinavir); this is the rationale for PI combinations that include ritonavir because it permits the use of lower doses of the other PI.

7. Saquinavir—Original formulations of saquinavir had low and erratic oral bioavailability. Reformulation for once-daily dosing in combination with low-dose ritonavir has improved efficacy, with decreased gastrointestinal side effects. The drug undergoes extensive first-pass metabolism and functions as both a substrate and inhibitor of CYP3A4. Adverse effects of saquinavir include nausea, diarrhea, dyspepsia, and rhinitis. Saquinavir plasma levels are increased by azole antifungals,

clarithromycin, grapefruit juice, indinavir, and ritonavir. Drugs that induce CYP3A4 decrease plasma levels of saquinavir.

8. Effects on carbohydrate and lipid metabolism—The use of PIs in HAART drug combinations has led to the development of disorders in carbohydrate and lipid metabolism. It has been suggested that this is due to the inhibition of lipid-regulating proteins, which have active sites with structural homology to that of HIV protease. The syndrome includes hyperglycemia and insulin resistance or hyperlipidemia, with altered body fat distribution. Buffalo hump, gynecomastia, and truncal obesity may occur with facial and peripheral lipodystrophy. The syndrome has been observed with PIs used in HAART regimens, with an incidence of 30–50% and a median onset time of approximately 1 year duration of treatment.

D. FUSION INHIBITOR

1. Enfuvirtide—Enfuvirtide is a synthetic 36-amino-acid peptide. The drug binds to the gp41 subunit of the viral envelope glycoprotein, preventing the conformational changes required for the fusion of the viral and cellular membranes. There is no cross-resistance with other anti-HIV drugs, but resistance may occur via mutations in the *env* gene. Enfuvirtide is administered subcutaneously in combination with other anti-HIV agents in previously drug-treated patients with persistent HIV-1 replication despite ongoing therapy. Its metabolism via hydrolysis does not involve the cytochrome P450 system. Injection site reactions and hypersensitivity may occur. An increased incidence of bacterial pneumonia has been reported.

ANTI-INFLUENZA AGENTS

A. AMANTADINE AND RIMANTADINE

1. Mechanisms—Amantadine and rimantadine inhibit an early step in replication of the influenza A (but not influenza B) virus (Figure 49–1). They prevent "uncoating" by binding to a protein M2. This protein functions as a proton ion channel required at the onset of infection to permit acidification of the virus core, which in turn activates viral RNA transcriptase. Amantadine-resistant influenza A virus mutants are now common.

2. Clinical uses and toxicity—These drugs are prophylactic against influenza A virus infection and can reduce the duration of symptoms if given within 48 h after contact. However, amantadine-resistant influenza A virus mutants including H3N2 strains causing seasonal influenza in the United States have increased dramatically in the past 2–3 years. Fortunately, there is no cross-resistance to the neuraminidase inhibitors. Toxic effects of these agents include gastrointestinal irritation, dizziness, ataxia, and slurred speech. Rimantadine's activity is no greater than that of amantadine, but it has a longer half-life and requires no dosage adjustment in renal failure.

B. Oseltamivir and Zanamivir

1. Mechanisms—These drugs are inhibitors of neuraminidases produced by influenza A and B. These viral enzymes cleave sialic acid residues from viral proteins and surface proteins of infected cells. They function to promote virion release and to prevent clumping of newly released virions. By interfering with these actions, neuraminidase inhibitors impede viral spread. Decreased susceptibility to the drugs is associated with mutations in viral neuraminidase, but worldwide resistance remains rare.

2. Clinical use and toxicity—Oseltamivir is a prodrug used orally, activated in the gut and the liver. Zanamivir is administered intranasally. Both drugs decrease the time to alleviation of influenza symptoms and are more effective if used within 24 h after onset of symptoms. Taken prophylactically, oseltamivir significantly decreases the incidence of influenza. Gastrointestinal symptoms may occur with oseltamivir; zanamivir may cause cough and throat discomfort and has induced bronchospasm in asthmatic patients.

AGENTS USED IN VIRAL HEPATITIS

The agents available for use in the treatment of infections caused by hepatitis B virus (HBV) and hepatitis C virus (HCV) are suppressive rather than curative. They include interferon-α (IFN-α), lamivudine, ribavirin, adefovir, and entecavir.

A. IFN-α

1. Mechanisms—IFN-α is a cytokine that acts through host cell surface receptors increasing the activity of Janus kinases (JAKS). These enzymes phosphorylate signal transducers and activators of transcription (STATS) to increase the formation of antiviral proteins. The selective antiviral action of IFN-α is primarily due to activation of a host cell ribonuclease that preferentially degrades viral mRNA. IFN-α also promotes formation of natural killer cells that destroy infected liver cells.

2. Pharmacokinetics—There are several forms of IFN-α with minor differences in amino acid composition. Absorption from intramuscular or subcutaneous injection is slow; elimination of IFN-α is mainly via proteolytic hydrolysis in the kidney. Conventional forms of IFN-α are usually administered daily or 3 times a week. Pegylated forms of IFN-α conjugated to polyethylene glycol can be administered once a week.

3. Clinical uses—Interferon-α is used in chronic HBV as an individual agent or in combination with lamivudine. When used in combinations with ribavirin, the progression of acute HCV infection to chronic HCV is reduced. Pegylated IFN-α together with ribavirin is superior to standard forms of IFN-α in chronic HCV. Other uses of IFN-α include treatment of Kaposi's sarcoma, papillomatosis, and topically for genital warts. Interferons also prevent dissemination of herpes zoster in cancer patients and reduce CMV shedding after renal transplantation.

4. Toxicity—Toxic effects of IFN-α include gastrointestinal irritation, a flulike syndrome, neutropenia, profound fatigue and myalgia, alopecia, reversible hearing loss, thyroid dysfunction, mental confusion, and severe depression.

B. Adefovir Dipivoxil

1. Mechanisms—Adefovir dipivoxil is the prodrug of adefovir which, following its phosphorylation by cellular kinases, competitively inhibits HBV DNA polymerase and results in chain termination after incorporation into the viral DNA. HBV resistance to adefovir, though uncommon, has recently been reported. There is no cross-resistance with lamivudine.

2. Pharmacokinetics and clinical use—Adefovir has good oral bioavailability unaffected by foods. The drug is eliminated by the kidney, and dose reductions are required in renal dysfunction.

Adefovir suppresses HBV replication and improves liver histology and fibrosis. However, serum HBV DNA reappears after cessation of therapy. Adefovir has activity against lamivudine-resistant strains of HBV.

3. Toxicity—Nephrotoxicity is dose limiting. Lactic acidosis and severe hepatomegaly with steatosis may also occur.

C. Lamivudine

This nucleoside inhibitor of HIV reverse transcriptase (see prior discussion) is active in chronic HBV infection. Lamivudine has a longer intracellular half-life in HBV-infected cells than in HIV-infected cells (see prior discussion) and thus can be used in lower doses for hepatitis than for HIV infection. Used as monotherapy, the drug rapidly suppresses HBV replication and is remarkably nontoxic. However, co-infection with HIV may increase the risk of pancreatitis. Lamivudine–resistant HBV mutants emerge at a rate of about 20% per year if the drug is used alone. On reappearance of detectable levels of HBV DNA, patients should be switched to IFN-α or adefovir.

D. Entecavir

Entecavir is a guanosine nucleoside that inhibits HBV DNA polymerase. Effective orally, the drug has an intracellular half-life of > 12 h and undergoes renal elimination in part via active tubular secretion. Clinical efficacy is similar to that of lamivudine, and there is cross-resistance between the 2 drugs. The drug causes headache, dizziness, fatigue, and nausea.

E. RIBAVIRIN

1. Mechanisms—Ribavirin inhibits the replication of a wide range of DNA and RNA viruses, including influenza A and B, parainfluenza, respiratory syncytial virus (RSV), paramyxoviruses, HCV, and HIV. Although the precise antiviral mechanism of ribavirin is not known, the drug inhibits guanosine triphosphate formation, prevents capping of viral mRNA, and can block RNA-dependent RNA polymerases.

2. Pharmacokinetics and clinical uses—Ribavirin is effective orally (avoid antacids) and is also available in intravenous and aerosolic forms. It is eliminated by the kidney, necessitating dose reductions in renal dysfunction. Ribavirin is used adjunctively with IFN-α in chronic HCV infection in patients with compensated liver disease. Monotherapy with ribavirin alone is not effective. Early intravenous administration of ribavirin decreases mortality in viral hemorrhagic fevers. Despite its alleged activity against RSV, ribavirin has been shown to have no benefit in treatment of RSV infections, although it is still recommended by some authorities in immunocompromised children.

3. Toxicity—Systemic use results in dose-dependent hemolytic anemia. Aerosolic ribavirin may cause conjunctival and bronchial irritation. Ribavirin is a known human teratogen, absolutely contraindicated in pregnancy.

QUESTIONS

1. Which statement about the mechanisms of action of antiviral drugs is accurate?
   (A) Cidofovir has no requirement for activation by phosphorylation
   (B) Ganciclovir inhibits viral DNA polymerase but does not cause chain termination
   (C) Increased activity of host cell ribonucleases that degrade viral mRNA is one of the antiviral actions of interferon-α
   (D) The initial step in activation of foscarnet in HSV-infected cells is its phosphorylation by viral thymidine kinase
   (E) The reverse transcriptase of HIV is 30–50 times more sensitive to inhibition by indinavir than host cell DNA polymerases

2–3. A 30-year-old male patient who is HIV positive and symptomatic has a CD4 count of 300/mcL and a viral RNA load of 5000 copies/mL. His treatment involves a 3-drug antiviral regimen consisting of zidovudine, didanosine, and ritonavir. Because of weight loss, he is taking dronabinol. Nystatin had been used for oral candidiasis, but for the past week the patient has been taking ketoconazole. Verapamil has been prescribed since he suffers from angina of effort. He now complains

of anorexia, nausea and vomiting, and abdominal pain. His abdomen is tender in the epigastric area. Laboratory results reveal an amylase activity of 220 units/L, and a preliminary diagnosis is made of acute pancreatitis.

2. If this patient has acute pancreatitis, the drug most likely to be responsible is
   (A) Didanosine
   (B) Dronabinol
   (C) Ketoconazole
   (D) Saquinavir
   (E) Zidovudine

3. In the further treatment of this patient, the drug causing the pancreatitis should be withdrawn and replaced by
   (A) Atazanavir
   (B) Cidofovir
   (C) Foscarnet
   (D) Lamivudine
   (E) Ribavirin

4. Which statement about antiviral agents is accurate?
   (A) Dosage modification of nevirapine is required in renal insufficiency.
   (B) Interferons prevent dissemination of herpes zoster in cancer patients
   (C) Oral use of valacyclovir necessitates multiple daily doses due to the short half-life of the drug
   (D) Peripheral neuropathy is the major dose-limiting toxic effect of ganciclovir
   (E) Vidarabine is safe to use in a pregnant patient if applied topically

5. In an accidental needlestick, an unknown quantity of blood from an AIDS patient is injected into a nurse. The most recent laboratory report on the AIDS patient shows a CD4 count of 20/μL and a viral RNA load of greater than 10^7 copies/mL. The most appropriate course of action regarding treatment of the nurse is to
   (A) Administer single doses of acyclovir and zidovudine
   (B) Administer full doses of zidovudine for 2 weeks
   (C) Monitor the nurse's blood to determine whether HIV transmission has occurred
   (D) Treat with full doses of zidovudine for 4 weeks
   (E) Treat with zidovudine plus lamivudine for 4 weeks

6–7. A patient with AIDS has a CD4 count of 45/μL. He is being maintained on a 3-drug regimen of indinavir, didanosine, and zidovudine. For prophylaxis against opportunistic infections, he is also receiving cidofovir, fluconazole, rifabutin, and trimethoprim-sulfamethoxazole.

6. The drug most likely to suppress herpetic infections and provide prophylaxis against CMV retinitis in this patient is
   (A) Cidofovir
   (B) Fluconazole
   (C) Indinavir
   (D) Rifabutin
   (E) Trimethoprim-sulfamethoxazole

7. The dose of indinavir in this patient may need to be increased above normal. This is because
   (A) Cidofovir increases the renal clearance of other drugs
   (B) Indinavir has to be taken with meals
   (C) Rifabutin increases liver drug-metabolizing enzymes
   (D) Sulfamethoxazole displaces indinavir from plasma proteins
   (E) Fluconazole slows gastric emptying

8. Which drug is most likely to cause additive anemia and neutropenia if administered to an AIDS patient taking zidovudine?
   (A) Acyclovir
   (B) Amantadine
   (C) Ganciclovir
   (D) Pentamidine
   (E) Stavudine

9. A 27-year-old nursing mother is diagnosed as suffering from genital herpes. She has a history of this viral infection. Previously she responded to a drug used topically. Apart from her current problem, she is in good health. Which drug to be used orally is most likely to be prescribed at this time?
   (A) Acyclovir
   (B) Amantadine
   (C) Foscarnet
   (D) Ritonavir
   (E) Trifluridine

10. Oral formulations of this drug should not be used in a pregnant AIDS patient because they contain propylene glycol. One of the characteristic side effects of the drug is hyperpigmentation on the palms of the hand and soles of the feet, especially in African-American patients. Which drug is referred to here?
    (A) Amprenavir
    (B) Efavirenz
    (C) Emtricitabine
    (D) Enfuvirtide
    (E) Zalcitabine

11. Which drugs bind to a viral envelope protein preventing the conformational changes required for the fusion of viral and cellular membranes?
    (A) Abacavir
    (B) Adenavir
    (C) Enfuvirtide
    (D) Oseltamivir
    (E) Ribavirin

12. Regarding interferon-α, which statement is false?
    (A) At the start of treatment, most patients experience flu-like symptoms
    (B) Indications include treatment of genital warts
    (C) It is used in the management of hepatitis B and C
    (D) Lamivudine interferes with its activity against hepatitis B
    (E) Toxicity includes bone marrow suppression

13. More than 90% of this drug is excreted in the urine in intact form. Because its urinary solubility is low, patients should be well hydrated to prevent nephrotoxicity. Which drug is described?
    (A) Acyclovir
    (B) Amantadine
    (C) Indinavir
    (D) Zanamivir
    (E) Zidovudine

14. Used in the prophylaxis and treatment of infection caused by influenza viruses, this drug inhibits the release of mature virions from infected cells.
    (A) Amantadine
    (B) Efavirenz
    (C) Oseltamivir
    (D) Rimantadine
    (E) Saquinavir

15. Which statement about stavudine is accurate?
    (A) Bone marrow suppression is dose limiting
    (B) It causes marked neurotoxicity
    (C) It inhibits HIV protease
    (D) It is a nonnucleoside reverse transcriptase inhibitor
    (E) Resistance occurs via mutations in the gene that codes for thymidine kinase

ANSWERS

1. Cidofovir is activated by host cell kinases. Ganciclovir, like acyclovir, inhibits viral DNA polymerase and causes chain termination. However, foscarnet inhibits viral polymerases without requiring bioactivation. Indinavir is an inhibitor of HIV protease and has no significant effect on reverse transcriptase. The answer is **C.**

2. Gastrointestinal problems occur with most antiviral drugs used in the HIV-positive patient, and acute pancreatitis has been reported for several reverse transcriptase inhibitors. However, didanosine is the drug most likely to be responsible because its most characteristic adverse effect is a dose-limiting acute

pancreatitis. Other risk factors that are relative contraindications to didanosine are advanced AIDS, hypertriglyceridemia, and alcoholism. The answer is **A**.

3. Symptomatic AIDS patients should be treated with a HAART regimen irrespective of a relatively high CD4 count or a relatively low HIV RNA load. Use of a second protease inhibitor (eg, atazanavir) with a single reverse transcriptase inhibitor is unlikely to be as effective as regimens that include 2 reverse transcriptase inhibitors. Because didanosine must be discontinued, lamivudine would be the best choice for replacement in this case. The answer is **D**.

4. The elimination of nevirapine involves hepatic metabolism via CYP3A4. Valacylovir has a much longer half-life than acyclovir, and its use does not necessitate multiple daily doses. Systemic absorption follows topical use of vidarabine, and the drug is potentially teratogenic. The adverse effects of ganciclovir are similar to those caused by radiation therapy and include myelosuppression, gastrointestinal distress, and mucositis. The answer is **B**.

5. The viral RNA titer in the blood from the AIDS patient in this case is very high, and this needlestick must be considered as a high risk situation. Although full doses of zidovudine for 4 weeks has been shown to have prophylactic value, in high-risk situations combination regimens are favored. Optimal prophylaxis in this case might best be provided by the combination of zidovudine with lamivudine (basic regimen), and many authorities would advise the further addition of a protease inhibitor (expanded regimen). The answer is **E**.

6. Ganciclovir (not listed) has been the most commonly used drug for prevention and treatment of CMV infections in the immunocompromised patient. Cidofovir is also very effective in CMV retinitis and has good activity against many strains of HSV, including those resistant to acyclovir. The answer is **A**.

7. Drug interactions can be severe in the immunocompromised patient because many of the drugs administered can influence the pharmacokinetic properties of other drugs. Rifabutin acts as an inducer of several isoforms of hepatic cytochrome P450 though less so than rifampin. This action may result in an increased clearance of other drugs, including indinavir. The answer is **C**.

8. Like zidovudine, ganciclovir is myelosuppressant, and more than 40% of patients who are treated with the drug as a single agent develop granulocytopenia or thrombocytopenia. When the 2 drugs are coadministered, there is a much higher incidence

of anemia and neutropenia. Colony-stimulating factors may be needed if the 2 drugs must be given together. None of the other drugs listed have significant hematotoxicity. The answer is **C**.

9. Three of the drugs listed (acyclovir, foscarnet, trifluridine) are active against strains of herpes simplex virus. Foscarnet is not used in genital infections (HSV-2) because clinical efficacy has not been established, it has poor oral bioavailability, and the drug causes many toxic effects. Trifluridine is used topically but only for herpes keratoconjunctivitis (HSV-1). The answer is **A**.

10. Three of the drugs listed should be avoided, or used with extreme caution, in the pregnant patient. Oral formulations of amprenavir and emtricitabine both contain propylene glycol, a potentially toxic compound. Efavirenz has caused fetal abnormalities in pregnant monkeys. However, one of the distinctive adverse effects of emtricitabine is hyperpigmentation. The answer is **C**.

11. Enfuvirtide is a novel synthetic peptide that binds to the gp41 subunit of the HIV viral envelope glycoprotein, preventing the conformational changes required for penetration of the virus through host cell membranes. The answer is **C**.

12. Lamivudine is used in monotherapy of HBV infections and does not oppose the beneficial effects of interferon-α when both agents are used together in the treatment of hepatitis B. The answer is **D**.

13. Acyclovir is eliminated in the urine by glomerular filtration and by active tubular secretion, which is inhibited by probenecid. Nephrotoxic effects, including hematuria and crystalluria, are enhanced in patients who are dehydrated or who have preexisting renal dysfunction. Adequate hydration is equally important in the case of indinavir because it causes nephrolithiasis. However, more than 80% of a dose of indinavir is eliminated via hepatic metabolism. The answer is **A**.

14. Oseltamivir and zanamivir (not listed) are inhibitors of neuraminidase produced by influenza A and B. They prevent the trimming of sialic acid residues from viral proteins, which interferes with virion release and facilitates their clumping and adhesion to host cells that are already infected. The answer is **C**.

15. Stavudine (d4T) is a nucleoside reverse transcriptase inhibitor. Although it has only minor hematotoxic potential, the drug is markedly neurotoxic, causing dose-limiting peripheral neuropathy. Resistance occurs via mutations in the *pol* gene, which encodes for several proteins including reverse transcriptase. The answer is **B**.

CHECKLIST

When you complete this chapter, you should be able to:

☐ Identify the main steps in viral replication that are targets for antiviral drug action.

☐ Describe the mechanisms of action of antiherpes drugs and the mechanisms of HSV and CMV resistance.

☐ List the characteristic pharmacokinetic properties and toxic effects of acyclovir, ganciclovir, cidofovir, and foscarnet.

☐ Describe the mechanisms of anti-HIV action of zidovudine, indinavir, and enfuvirtide.

☐ Match a specific anti-retroviral drug with each of the following: hyperpigmentation, neutropenia, pancreatitis, peripheral neuropathy, inhibition of P450, severe hypersensitivity reaction, injection site reactions, to be avoided in pregnancy.

☐ Identify the significant characteristics of 4 drugs active against HBV and HCV.

☐ Identify the significant characteristics of an anti-influenza drug acting at the stage of viral uncoating and another acting at the stage of viral release.

Miscellaneous Antimicrobial Agents & Urinary Antiseptics

50

This chapter includes miscellaneous agents that have antibacterial activity, urinary tract and other antiseptics, and disinfectants.

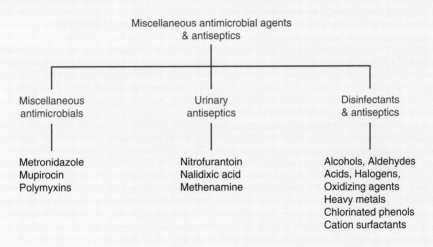

MISCELLANEOUS ANTIMICROBIAL AGENTS

A. METRONIDAZOLE

1. Mechanisms—Metronidazole is an imidazole derivative with activity against protozoa and bacteria. The drug undergoes a reductive bioactivation of its nitro group by ferredoxin (present in anaerobic parasites) to form reactive cytotoxic products that interfere with nucleic acid synthesis.

2. Pharmacokinetics—Metronidazole is effective orally and is distributed widely to tissues, achieving cerebrospinal fluid (CSF) levels similar to those in the blood. The drug can also be given intravenously and is available in topical formulations. Elimination of metronidazole requires hepatic metabolism, and dosage reduction may be needed in patients with liver dysfunction.

3. Clinical use—As an antibacterial agent, metronidazole has greatest activity against *Bacteroides* and *Clostridium*. It is the drug of choice for treatment of pseudomembranous colitis resulting from *C difficile* and is effective in anaerobic or mixed intra-abdominal infections and in brain abscess. Metronidazole is also used for infections involving *Gardnerella vaginalis* and in regimens for the eradication of *Helicobacter pylori* in gastric ulcers. As an antiprotozoal drug, metronidazole (or a structurally related drug, **tinidazole**) is the drug of choice in trichomoniasis, giardiasis, and the treatment of intestinal amebiasis and amebic hepatic abscess.

HIGH-YIELD TERMS TO LEARN

Antiseptic	An agent used to inhibit bacterial growth in vitro and in vivo
Disinfectant	An agent used to kill microorganisms in an inanimate environment
Sterilization	Procedures that kill microorganisms on instruments and dressings; methods include autoclaving, dry heat, and exposure to ethylene oxide
Chlorine demand	The amount of chlorine bound to organic matter in water and thus unavailable for antimicrobial activity

---

4. Toxicity—Adverse effects include gastrointestinal irritation, headache, and dark coloration of urine. More serious toxicity includes leukopenia, dizziness, and ataxia. Opportunistic fungal infections may occur during treatment with metronidazole. Drug interactions with metronidazole include a disulfiram-like reaction with ethanol and potentiation of coumarin anticoagulant effects. Although it is not contraindicated in pregnancy, the drug should be used with caution.

B. MUPIROCIN

1. Mechanisms—Mupirocin is a fermentation product of *Pseudomonas fluorescens* and is unrelated to any other antimicrobial drug. It acts on gram-positive cocci and inhibits protein synthesis by specifically binding to isoleucyl-tRNA synthetase.

2. Pharmacokinetics and clinical use—Mupirocin is used topically and is not absorbed. This drug is indicated for impetigo caused by staphylococci (including methicillin-resistant strains), beta-hemolytic streptococci, and *Streptococcus pyogenes*. It is also used intranasally to eliminate staphylococcal carriage by patients and medical personnel.

3. Toxicity—Local itching and burning sensations are common. Mupirocin may also cause rash, erythema, and contact dermatitis.

C. POLYMYXINS

1. Mechanisms—The polymyxins are polypeptides that are bactericidal against gram-negative bacteria. These drugs interact with a specific lipopolysaccharide component of the outer cell membrane that is also a binding site for calcium. Membrane lipid structure is distorted, with an increase in permeability to polar molecules, resulting in marked changes in cell metabolism.

2. Clinical use—Because of toxicity, the clinical applications of the polymyxins are limited to topical therapy of resistant gram-negative infections, including those caused by *Enterobacter* and *Pseudomonas*. These drugs are occasionally administered into infected cavities (eg, the joints and the pleural and peritoneal cavities).

3. Toxicity—If absorbed into the systemic circulation, adverse effects include neurotoxicity (paresthesias, dizziness, ataxia) and acute renal tubular necrosis (hematuria, proteinuria, nitrogen retention).

URINARY ANTISEPTICS

Urinary antiseptics are oral drugs that are rapidly excreted into the urine and act there to suppress bacteriuria. The drugs lack systemic antibacterial effects but may be toxic. Urinary antiseptics are often administered with acidifying agents, because low pH is an independent inhibitor of bacterial growth in urine.

A. NITROFURANTOIN

This drug is active against many urinary tract pathogens (but not *Proteus* or *Pseudomonas*), and resistance emerges slowly. Single daily doses of the drug can prevent recurrent urinary tract infections. The drug is active orally and is excreted in the urine via filtration and secretion; toxic levels may occur in the blood of patients with renal dysfunction. Adverse effects of nitrofurantoin include gastrointestinal irritation, skin rashes, phototoxicity, neuropathies, and hemolysis in patients with glucose-6-phosphate dehydrogenase (G6PD) deficiency.

B. NALIDIXIC ACID

This quinolone drug acts against many gram-negative organisms (but not *Proteus* or *Pseudomonas*) by mechanisms that may involve acidification or inhibition of DNA gyrase. Resistance emerges rapidly. The drug is active orally and is excreted in the urine partly unchanged and partly as the inactive glucuronide. Toxic effects include gastrointestinal irritation, glycosuria, skin rashes, phototoxicity, visual disturbances, and CNS stimulation.

C. METHENAMINE

Methenamine mandelate and methenamine hippurate combine urine acidification with the release of the antibacterial compound formaldehyde at pH levels below 5.5. These drugs are not usually active against *Proteus* because those organisms alkalinize the urine. Insoluble complexes form between formaldehyde and sulfonamides, and the drugs should not be used together.

DISINFECTANTS, ANTISEPTICS, & STERILANTS

Although the terms are often used interchangeably, a **disinfectant** is a compound that is used to kill microorganisms in an inanimate environment, whereas an **antiseptic** is one that is used to inhibit bacterial growth both in vitro and in contact with the surfaces of living tissues. Disinfectants and antiseptics do not have selective toxicity. Most antiseptics delay wound healing. **Sterilants** kill both vegetative cells and spores when applied to materials for appropriate times and temperatures.

A. ALCOHOLS, ALDEHYDES, AND ACIDS

Ethanol (70%) and **isopropanol** (70–90%) are effective skin antiseptics because they denature microbial proteins. **Formaldehyde,** which also denatures proteins, is too irritating for topical use but is a disinfectant for instruments. **Acetic acid** (1%) is used in surgical dressings and has activity against gram-negative bacteria, including *Pseudomonas,* when used as a urinary irrigant and in the external ear. **Salicylic acid** and **undecylenic acid** are useful in the treatment of dermatophyte infections.

B. HALOGENS

Iodine tincture is an effective antiseptic for intact skin and, although it can cause dermatitis, is commonly used in preparing the skin before taking blood samples. Iodine complexed with povidone (**povidone-iodine**) is widely used, particularly as a preoperative skin antiseptic, but solutions can become contaminated with aerobic gram-negative bacteria.

Hypochlorous acid, formed when **chlorine** dissolves in water, is antimicrobial. This is the basis for the use of chlorine and **halazone** in water purification. Organic matter binds chlorine, thus preventing antimicrobial actions. In a given water sample, this process is referred to as the **chlorine demand** because the chlorine-binding capacity of the organic material must be exceeded before bacterial killing is accomplished. Many preparations of chlorine for water purification do not eradicate all bacteria or entamoeba cysts.

Sodium hypochlorite is the active component in household bleach, a 1:10 dilution of which is recommended by the Centers for Disease Control and Prevention for the disinfection of blood spills that may contain HIV or hepatitis B virus (HBV).

C. OXIDIZING AGENTS

Hydrogen peroxide exerts a short-lived antimicrobial action through the release of molecular oxygen. The agent is used as a mouthwash, for cleansing wounds, and for disinfection of contact lenses. **Potassium permanganate** is an effective bactericidal agent but has the disadvantage of causing persistent brown stains on skin and clothing.

KEY DRUGS

Class	Prototype	Other Significant Agents
Antimicrobials		
Nitroimidazole	Metronidazole	Tinidazole
Pseudomonic acid	Mupirocin	
Peptide	Polymixin B	
Urinary tract antiseptics		
Quinolones	Nalidixic acid	Cinoxacin
Methenamine salts	Methenamine mandelate	
Nitrofurans	Nitrofurantoin	
Disinfectants and antiseptics		
Alcohols, aldehydes, and acids	Ethanol, formaldehyde	Isopropanol, glutaraldehyde, salicylic acid
Halogens	Iodine, chlorine	Povidone-iodide, halazone, sodium hypochlorite (bleach)
Heavy metals	Silver nitrate, mercuric bichloride	Silver sulfadiazine, nitromersol, thimerosal
Chlorinated phenols	Hexachlorophene	Chlorhexidine, triclocarban
Cationic surfactants	Benzalkonium chloride	Cetylpyridinium chloride

D. Heavy Metals

Mercury and **silver** precipitate proteins and inactivate sulfhydryl groups of enzymes but are used rarely because of toxicity. Organic mercurials such as **nitromersol** and **thimerosal** frequently cause hypersensitivity reactions but continue to be used as preservatives for vaccines, antitoxins, and immune sera. **Merbromin** is a weak antiseptic and stains tissues a bright red color. In the past **silver nitrate** was commonly used for prevention of neonatal gonococcal ophthalmia, but it has been largely replaced by topical antibiotics. **Silver sulfadiazine** (a sulfonamide) is used to decrease bacterial colonization in burns.

E. Chlorinated Phenols

Owing to its toxicity, **phenol** itself is used only as a disinfectant of inanimate objects. Mixtures of phenolic derivatives are used in antiseptics but can cause skin irritation. **Hexachlorophene** has been widely used in surgical scrub routines and in deodorant soaps, where it forms antibacterial deposits on the skin, decreasing the population of resident bacteria. Repeated use on the skin in infants can lead to absorption of the drug, resulting in CNS white matter degeneration. Antiseptic soaps may also contain other chlorinated phenols such as **triclocarban** and **chlorhexidine.** Chlorhexidine is mainly active against gram-positive cocci and is commonly used in hospital scrub routines to cleanse skin sites. All antiseptic soaps may cause allergies or photosensitization.

Lindane (gamma benzene hexachloride) is used to treat infestations with mites or lice and also as an agricultural insecticide. The agent can be absorbed through the skin; if excessive amounts are applied, toxic effects, including blood dyscrasias and convulsions, may occur.

F. Cationic Surfactants

Benzalkonium chloride and **cetylpyridinium chloride** are used as disinfectants of surgical instruments and surfaces such as floors and bench tops. Because they are effective against most bacteria and fungi and are not irritating, they are also used as antiseptics. However, when used on the skin, the antimicrobial action of these agents is antagonized by soaps and multivalent cations. The CDC has recommended that benzalkonium chloride and similar quaternary compounds *not* be used as antiseptics because outbreaks of infection have resulted from growth of gram-negative bacteria (eg, *Pseudomonas*) in such antiseptic solutions.

QUESTIONS

1. Infections caused by gram-negative bacilli have occurred when this agent has been used as a skin antiseptic.
   (A) Acetic acid
   (B) Benzalkonium chloride
   (C) Hexachlorophene
   (D) Merbromin
   (E) Thimerosal

2–3. A young woman is brought to a hospital emergency department with intense abdominal pain of 2 days' duration. The pain has spread to the right lower quadrant and is accompanied by nausea, vomiting, and fever. She arrives in the emergency department with a blood pressure of 85/45, pulse 120/min, and temperature 40°C. Her abdomen has a boardlike rigidity with diffuse pain to palpation. Laboratory values include the following: WBC 20,000/μL and creatinine 1.5 mg/dL. After abdominal x-ray films are taken, a preliminary diagnosis of abdominal sepsis is made, possibly resulting from bowel perforation. After appropriate samples are sent to the laboratory for culture, the patient is hospitalized, and antimicrobial therapy is started with intravenous ampicillin and gentamicin.

2. Regarding the treatment of this patient, which statement is accurate?
   (A) A drug active against anaerobes should be included in the antibiotic regimen
   (B) A Gram stain of the blood would provide positive identification of the specific organism involved in this infection
   (C) Cultures are pointless because this is probably a mixed infection
   (D) Empiric antimicrobial therapy of abdominal sepsis should always include a third-generation cephalosporin
   (E) The combination of ampicillin and gentamicin provides good coverage for all likely pathogens

3. If the antibiotic regimen in this patient is modified to include metronidazole, which statement is accurate?
   (A) Ampicillin should be excluded from the regimen
   (B) Coverage will be extended to methicillin-resistant staphylococci
   (C) Gentamicin should be excluded from the regimen
   (D) Metronidazole should not be administered intravenously
   (E) The patient should be monitored for candidiasis

4. Which compound is used topically to treat scabies and pediculosis?
   (A) Lindane
   (B) Mupirocin
   (C) Nitrofurazone
   (D) Polymyxin B
   (E) Silver sulfadiazine

5. Methenamine salts are used as urinary antiseptics. The reason they lack systemic antibacterial action is that they are

(A) Converted to formaldehyde only at low urinary pH
(B) Metabolized rapidly by hepatic drug-metabolizing enzymes
(C) More than 98% bound to plasma proteins
(D) Not absorbed into the systemic circulation after oral ingestion
(E) Substrates for active tubular secretion

6. Which statement about the actions of antimicrobial agents is LEAST accurate?
(A) Polymyxins act as cationic detergents to disrupt bacterial cell membranes
(B) Resistance to nitrofurantoin emerges rapidly, and there is cross-resistance with sulfonamides
(C) Salicylic acid has useful antidermatophyte activity when applied topically
(D) Neonatal gonococcal ophthalmia can be prevented by silver nitrate
(E) Daptomycin has activity against strains of staphylococci resistant to vancomycin

7. Which antiseptic *promotes* wound healing?
(A) Cetylpyridium chloride
(B) Chlorhexidine
(C) Hexachlorophene
(D) Iodine
(E) None of the above

8. A 22-year-old man with gonorrhea is to be treated with cefixime and will need another drug to provide coverage for possible urethritis caused by *C trachomatis*. Which drug is unlikely to be effective in nongonococcal urethritis?
(A) Azithromycin
(B) Ciprofloxacin
(C) Erythromycin
(D) Nitrofurantoin
(E) Tetracycline

9. A patient with AIDS has an extremely high viral RNA titer. While blood is being drawn from this patient, the syringe is accidentally dropped, contaminating the floor, which is made of porous material. The best way to deal with this is to
(A) Clean the floor with a 10% solution of household bleach
(B) Clean the floor with soap and water
(C) Completely replace the contaminated part of the floor
(D) Neutralize the spill with a solution of potassium permanganate
(E) Seal the room and decontaminate with ethylene oxide

DIRECTIONS: 10–15. The matching questions in this section consist of a list of lettered options followed by several numbered items. For each numbered item, select the ONE lettered option that is most closely associated with it.
(A) Benzalkonium chloride
(B) Chlorhexidine
(C) Formaldehyde
(D) Halazone
(E) Hexachlorophene
(F) Methenamine
(G) Metronidazole
(H) Nitrofurantoin
(I) Polymyxin B

10. This compound is used in tablet form to purify drinking water. If a large quantity of organic material is present, cysts of *Entamoeba histolytica* may not be eradicated.

11. Daily use of this substituted phenol results in a bacteriostatic deposit on the skin. The compound may be absorbed and has caused neurotoxic effects in neonates when used as an antistaphylococcal agent.

12. Neuropathies are more likely to occur with this agent when it is used in patients with renal dysfunction. The drug may cause acute hemolysis in patients with glucose-6-phosphate dehydrogenase (G6PD) deficiency.

13. This agent is commonly incorporated into soaps used for skin antisepsis and surgical scrub procedures. The compound has minimal activity against *Pseudomonas* and *Serratia*.

14. A urinary antiseptic, this agent is not effective in the treatment of urinary tract infections caused by *Proteus*. Mutual antagonism may occur if this drug is used concomitantly with sulfonamides.

15. Consumption of ethanol together with this drug will cause nausea, vomiting, abdominal cramps, flushing, and headache in some patients.

ANSWERS

1. *Pseudomonas* and other gram-negative bacteria have caused infections after the use of cationic surfactants, partly because they form a film on the skin under which microorganisms can survive. In addition, some gram-negative bacilli are able to grow in solutions containing benzalkonium salts. Bacterial growth may also occur in solutions of povidone-iodine. The answer is **B.**

2. Abdominal sepsis is commonly a mixed infection; the most likely pathogens are *Bacteroides fragilis*, *Enterobacteriaceae*, and *Enterococcus faecalis*. An antibiotic regimen that includes only ampicillin and

gentamicin will not control *B fragilis.* Empiric treatment in this case should include a drug active against this pathogen (eg, metronidazole, cefoxitin, cefotetan, or clindamycin). The answer is **A.**

3. Fungal superinfections, especially from *Candida albicans,* occur quite frequently during treatment with metronidazole. In most cases of abdominal sepsis, metronidazole would be given by slow intravenous infusion. Both ampicillin and gentamicin should be maintained until the infection is controlled, at which time surgery is indicated. Metronidazole has no activity against aerobes. The combination of ampicillin, gentamicin, and metronidazole does not provide coverage for methicillin-resistant staphylococci. The answer is **E.**

4. Of the agents listed, only lindane is an effective scabicide and pediculicide. There is some concern about the systemic absorption of topically applied lindane, which may cause neurotoxicity. Accidental ingestion in children has caused seizures. The answer is **A.**

5. Below pH 5.5, methenamine releases formaldehyde, which is antibacterial. This pH is achieved in the urine but nowhere else in the body. Ascorbic acid is sometimes given with methenamine salts to ensure a low urinary pH. The answer is **A.**

6. Resistance emerges very slowly when nitrofurantoin is used as a urinary antiseptic. There is no cross-resistance between the drug and other drugs used in the treatment of bacterial infections of the urinary tract. The answer is **B.**

7. No antiseptic in current use is able to promote wound healing, and most agents do the opposite. In general, cleansing of abrasions and superficial wounds with soap and water is just as effective as and less damaging than the application of topical antiseptics. The answer is **E.**

8. Urinary tract infections resulting from *C trachomatis* are likely to respond to all of the drugs listed except nitrofurantoin. However, nitrofurantoin is effective against many bacterial urinary tract pathogens with the exception of *Pseudomonas aeruginosa* and strains of *Proteus.* The answer is **D.**

9. Household bleach contains sodium hypochlorite. A 1:10 dilution of bleach is effective for disinfection of a direct blood spill on a porous surface. In addition to inactivating HIV, sodium hypochlorite solutions have disinfectant activity against other viruses, including hepatitis B virus. The answer is **A.**

10. The addition of 4–8 mg of halazone per liter will sterilize most water samples in about 30 min but will not kill cysts of *Entamoeba histolytica.* The answer is **D.**

11. Repeated bathing of newborns with hexachlorophene to prevent staphylococcal colonization may permit systemic absorption, which leads to neurotoxic effects (eg, spongiform degeneration of white matter). The answer is **E.**

12. Acute hemolytic reactions in G6PD deficiency occur with drugs that are oxidizing agents, including antimalarials, nalidixic acid, sulfonamides, and the nitrofurans. Severe polyneuropathies, with both motor and sensory nerve degeneration, may occur with nitrofurantoin. These reactions are more likely to occur in patients with renal dysfunction. The answer is **H.**

13. Chlorhexidine is a biguanide that disrupts bacterial cytoplasmic membranes, especially of gram-positive organisms. The agent is less effective against *Pseudomonas* and *Serratia.* Hospital uses include hand-washing, wound cleansing, and preparation of skin sites for operative procedures. The answer is **B.**

14. The activity of methenamine as a urinary antiseptic is mainly due to the release of formaldehyde at acidic pH. Sulfonamides may form insoluble complexes with formaldehyde, resulting in mutual antagonism. *Proteus* organisms alkalinize the urine, preventing the release of formaldehyde. The answer is **F.**

15. Metronidazole inhibits aldehyde dehydrogenase and may cause a disulfiram-like reaction in patients who consume alcoholic beverages while taking the drug. The answer is **G.**

CHECKLIST

When you complete this chapter, you should be able to:

☐ Identify the clinical uses of metronidazole and its characteristic pharmacokinetics and toxicities.

☐ List the clinical uses of mupirocin and polymyxins.

☐ Identify the major urinary antiseptic and their characteristic adverse effects.

☐ List the agents used as antiseptics and disinfectants and point out their limitations.

Clinical Use of Antimicrobials

51

A. Empiric Antimicrobial Therapy

Empiric antimicrobial therapy is begun before a specific pathogen has been identified and is based on the presumption of an infection that requires immediate drug treatment. Before initiation of such therapy, accepted practice involves making a clinical diagnosis of microbial infection, obtaining specimens for laboratory analyses, making a microbiologic diagnosis, deciding whether treatment should precede the results of laboratory tests, and, finally, selecting the optimal drug or drugs. A variety of publications provide annually updated lists of antimicrobial drugs of choice for specific pathogens. Such lists can provide a useful guide to empiric therapy based on presumptive microbiologic diagnosis. Tables 51–1 and 51–2 show examples of empiric antimicrobial therapy based on microbiologic etiology.

B. Principles of Antimicrobial Therapy

Antimicrobial therapy in established infections is guided by several principles.

1. Susceptibility testing—The results of susceptibility testing establish the drug sensitivity of the organism. These results usually predict the **minimum inhibitory concentrations (MICs)** of a drug for comparison with anticipated blood or tissue levels. The 2 most common methods of susceptibility testing are disk diffusion (Kirby-Bauer) and broth dilution. For severe infections caused by certain bacteria (eg, gram-positive cocci, *Haemophilus influenzae*), a direct test for beta-lactamase is used to aid in the selection of an appropriate antibiotic.

2. Drug concentration in blood—The measurement of drug concentration in the blood may be appropriate when using agents with a low therapeutic index (eg, aminoglycosides, vancomycin) and when investigating poor clinical response to a drug treatment regimen.

3. Serum bactericidal titers—In certain infections in which host defenses may contribute minimally to cure, the estimation of serum bactericidal titers can confirm the appropriateness of choice of drug and dosage. Serial dilutions of serum are incubated with standardized quantities of the pathogen isolated from the patient; killing at a dilution of 1:8 is generally considered satisfactory.

4. Route of administration—Parenteral therapy is preferred in most cases of serious microbial infections. Chloramphenicol, the fluoroquinolones, and trimethoprim-sulfamethoxazole (TMP-SMX) may be effective orally.

5. Monitoring of therapeutic response—Therapeutic responses to drug therapy should be monitored clinically and microbiologically to detect the development of resistance or superinfections. The duration of drug therapy required depends on the pathogen (eg, longer courses of therapy are required for infections caused by fungi or mycobacteria), the site of infection (eg, endocarditis and osteomyelitis require longer duration of treatment), and the immunocompetence of the patient.

6. Clinical failure of antimicrobial therapy—Inadequate clinical or microbiologic response to antimicrobial therapy can result from laboratory testing errors, problems with the drug (eg, incorrect choice, poor tissue penetration, inadequate dose), the patient (poor host defenses, undrained abscesses), or the pathogen (resistance, superinfection).

C. Factors Influencing Antimicrobial Drug Use

1. Bactericidal versus bacteriostatic actions—Antibiotics classified as bacteriostatic include clindamycin, macrolides, sulfonamides, and tetracyclines. For bacteriostatic drugs, the concentrations that inhibit growth are much lower than those that kill bacteria. Antibiotics classified as bactericidal include the aminoglycosides, beta-lactams, fluoroquinolones, metronidazole, most antimycobacterial agents, streptogramins, and vancomycin. For such drugs, there is little difference between the concentrations that inhibit growth and those that kill bacteria. Bactericidal drugs are preferred for the treatment of infections in patients with impaired defense mechanisms, especially immunocompromised patients.

Some bactericidal agents (aminoglycosides, fluoroquinolones) cause **concentration-dependent** killing. Maximizing peak blood levels of such drugs increases the rate and the extent of their bactericidal effects. This is one of the factors responsible for the clinical effectiveness of high-dose, once-daily administration of aminoglycosides.

HIGH-YIELD TERMS TO LEARN

Antimicrobial prophylaxis	The use of antimicrobial drugs to decrease the risk of infection
Combination antimicrobial drug therapy	The use of 2 or more drugs together to increase efficacy more than can be accomplished with the use of a single agent
Empiric (presumptive) antimicrobial therapy	Initiation of drug treatment before identification of a specific pathogen
Minimum inhibitory concentration (MIC)	An estimate of the drug sensitivity of pathogens for comparison with anticipated levels in blood or tissues
Postantibiotic effect	Antibacterial effect that persists after drug concentration falls below the minimum inhibitory concentration
Susceptibility testing	Laboratory methods to determine the sensitivity of the isolated pathogen to antimicrobial drugs

---

Table 51–1. Examples of empiric antimicrobial therapy based on microbiologic etiology.[a]

Pathogen	Drug(s) of First Choice	Alternative Drugs
Enterococcus spp	Ampicillin +/− gentamicin	Vancomycin + gentamicin, linezolid, daptomycin, streptogramins
S aureus or *epidermidis* Methicillin-susceptible	Nafcillin	Cephalosporin, clindamycin, fluoroquinolone, imipenem
Methicillin-resistant	Vancomycin +/− gentamicin +/− rifampin	Daptomycin, doxycycline, fluoroquinolone, linezolid, streptogramins
S pneumoniae Penicillin-susceptible	Penicillin G, amoxicillin	Cephalosporin, clindamycin, fluoroquinolone, macrolide, TMP-SMX
Penicillin-resistant	Vancomycin + ceftriaxone or cefotaxime +/− rifampin	Linezolid, streptogramins, third-generation fluoroquinolone
N gonorrhoeae	Ceftriaxone	Cefixime, cefotaxime
M meningitidis	Penicillin G	Third-generation cephalosporin, chloramphenicol, fluoroquinolone
M catarrhalis	Cefuroxime, fluoroquinolone	Amoxicillin-clavulanate, doxycycline, third-generation fluoroquinolone, macrolide, TMP-SMX
C difficile	Metronidazole	Vancomycin
C trachomatis	Azithromycin or other macrolide	Doxycycline or sulfonamide
Chlamydophyla (*C pneumoniae*)	Macrolide or tetracycline	Fluoroquinolone
M pneumoniae	Macrolide or tetracycline	Fluoroquinolone
T pallidum	Penicillin G	Doxycycline or ceftriaxone

[a]Based on various sources of treatment guidelines (USA) available in June 2007.

Table 51–2. Further examples of empiric antimicrobial therapy based on microbiologic etiology.[a]

Pathogen	Drug(s) of First Choice	Alternative Drugs
Bacteroides	Metronidazole	Carbapenems, penicillins + beta-lactamase inhibitor, chloramphenicol
Campylobacter jejuni	Macrolide	Fluoroquinolone, tetracycline
Enterobacter spp	Carbapenem, cefepime	Aminoglycoside, TMP-SMX, fluoroquinolone, third-generation cephalosporin
E coli	Cephalosporin (third-generation)	Many penicillins +/– beta-lactamase inhibitor, fluoroquinolones, TMP-SMX, aminoglycosides
G vaginalis	Metronidazole	Clindamycin
K pneumoniae	Cephalosporin (third-generation)	Carbapenems, penicillins + beta-lactamase inhibitor, aminoglycosides, TMP-SMX, fluoroquinolones
P mirabilis	Ampicillin	Cephalosporins, penicillins + beta-lactamase inhibitor, aminoglycosides, TMP-SMX, fluoroquinolones
Proteus-indole positive	Cephalosporin (third-generation)	Carbapenems, penicillins + beta-lactamase inhibitor, aminoglycosides, TMP-SMX, fluoroquinolones
S typhi	Ceftriaxone or fluoroquinolone	Chloramphenicol, TMP-SMX, ampicillin
Serratia spp	Carbapenem	Aminoglycoside, third-generation cephalosporin, fluoroquinolone, TMP-SMX
Shigella spp	Fluoroquinolone	Azithromycin, TMP-SMX, ampicillin, ceftriaxone

[a]Based on various sources of treatment guidelines (USA) available in June 2007.

Other bactericidal agents (beta-lactams, vancomycin) cause **time-dependent** killing. Their killing action is independent of drug concentration and continues only while blood levels are maintained above the minimal bactericidal concentration (MBC).

Inhibition of bacterial growth that continues after antibiotic blood concentrations have fallen to low levels is called the **postantibiotic effect (PAE).** The mechanisms of PAE are unclear but may reflect the lag time required by bacteria to synthesize new enzymes and cellular components, the possible persistence of antibiotic at the target site, or an enhanced susceptibility of bacteria to phagocytic and other defense mechanisms. PAE is another factor contributory to the effectiveness of once-daily administration of aminoglycosides and may also contribute to the clinical efficacy of the fluoroquinolones.

2. Drug elimination mechanisms—Changes in hepatic and renal function—and the use of dialysis—can influence the pharmacokinetics of antimicrobials and may necessitate dosage modifications. The major mechanisms of elimination of commonly used antimicrobial drugs are shown in Table 51–3. In anuria (creatinine clearance < 5 mL/min), the elimination half-life of drugs that are eliminated by the kidney is markedly increased, usually necessitating major reductions in drug dosage. Erythromycin, clindamycin, chloramphenicol, rifampin, and ketoconazole are notable exceptions, requiring no change in dosage in renal failure. In patients with biliary dysfunction or cirrhosis, reductions in dosage may be required for drugs that undergo hepatic elimination. Dialysis, especially hemodialysis, may markedly decrease the plasma levels of many antimicrobials; supplementary doses of such drugs may be required to reestablish effective plasma levels following these procedures. Drugs that are *not* removed from the blood by hemodialysis include amphotericin B, cefonicid, cefoperazone, ceftriaxone, erythromycin, nafcillin, tetracyclines, and vancomycin.

3. Pregnancy and the neonate—Antimicrobial therapy during pregnancy and the neonatal period requires special consideration. Aminoglycosides (eg, gentamicin) may cause neurologic damage. Tetracyclines cause tooth enamel dysplasia and inhibition of bone growth. Sulfonamides, by displacing bilirubin from serum albumin, may cause kernicterus in the neonate.

Table 51–3. Elimination of commonly used antimicrobial agents.

Mode of Elimination	Drugs or Drug Groups
Renal	Acyclovir, aminoglycosides, amphotericin B, most cephalosporins, fluconazole, fluoroquinolones, penicillins, sulfonamides and tetracyclines (except doxycycline), TMP-SMX, vancomycin
Hepatic	Amphotericin B, ampicillin, cefoperazone, chloramphenicol, clindamycin, erythromycin, isoniazid, most azoles (not fluconazole), nafcillin, rifampin
Hemodialysis	Acyclovir (and most antiviral agents), aminoglycosides, cephalosporins (not cefonicid, cefoperazone, ceftriaxone), penicillins (not nafcillin), sulfonamides

Chloramphenicol may cause gray baby syndrome. Other drugs that should be used with extreme caution during pregnancy include most antiviral and antifungal agents. The fluoroquinolones are not recommended for use in pregnancy or in small children because of possible effects on growing cartilage.

4. Drug interactions—Interactions sometimes occur between antimicrobials and other drugs (see also Chapter 62). Interactions include enhanced nephrotoxicity or ototoxicity when aminoglycosides are given with loop diuretics, vancomycin, or cisplatin. Several drug interactions with sulfonamides are based on competition for plasma protein binding; these include excessive hypoglycemia with sulfonylureas and increased hypoprothrombinemia with warfarin. Disulfiram-like reactions to ethanol occur with metronidazole, with TMP-SMX, and with several cephalosporins (see Chapter 43). Erythromycin inhibits the hepatic metabolism of a number of drugs, including clozapine, lidocaine, loratadine, phenytoin, quinidine, sildenafil, theophylline, and warfarin. The azole antifungals (eg, ketoconazole) inhibit the metabolism of caffeine, carbamazepine, cyclosporine, hepatic hydroxylmethylglutaryl coenzyme A (HMG-CoA) reductase inhibitors, methadone, oral contraceptives, phenytoin, sildenafil, verapamil, and zidovudine. Rifampin, an inducer of hepatic drug-metabolizing enzymes, decreases the effects of digoxin, ketoconazole, oral contraceptives, propranolol, quinidine, several antiretroviral drugs, and warfarin.

D. ANTIMICROBIAL DRUG COMBINATIONS

Therapy with multiple antimicrobials may be indicated in the several clinical situations.

1. Emergency situations—In severe infections (eg, sepsis, meningitis), combinations of antimicrobial drugs are used empirically to suppress all of the most likely pathogens.

2. To delay resistance—The combined use of drugs is valid when the rapid emergence of resistance impairs the chances for cure. For this reason, combined drug therapy is especially important in the treatment of tuberculosis.

3. Mixed infections—Multiple organisms may be involved in some infections. For example, peritoneal infections may be caused by several pathogens (eg, anaerobes and coliforms); a combination of drugs may be required to achieve coverage. Skin infections are often due to mixed bacterial, fungal, or viral pathogens.

4. To achieve synergistic effects—The use of a drug combination against a specific pathogen may result in an effect greater than that achieved with a single drug. Examples include the use of penicillins with gentamicin in enterococcal endocarditis, the use of an extended-spectrum penicillin plus an aminoglycoside in *Pseudomonas aeruginosa* infections, and the combined use of amphotericin B and flucytosine in cryptococcal meningitis. Antibiotic combinations are also commonly used in the management of infections resulting from *S epidermidis* and penicillin-resistant pneumococci (eg, vancomycin plus rifampin)

Several mechanisms, discussed next, may account for synergism.

a. Sequential blockade—The combined use of drugs may cause inhibition of 2 or more steps in a metabolic pathway. For example, trimethoprim and sulfamethoxazole (TMP-SMX) block different steps in the formation of tetrahydrofolic acid.

b. Blockade of drug-inactivating enzymes—Clavulanic acid, sulbactam, and tazobactam inhibit penicillinases and are often combined with penicillinase-sensitive beta-lactam drugs.

c. Enhanced drug uptake—Increased permeability to aminoglycosides after exposure of certain bacteria to cell wall–inhibiting antimicrobials (eg, beta-lactams) is thought to underlie some synergistic effects.

E. ANTIMICROBIAL CHEMOPROPHYLAXIS

The general principles of antimicrobial chemoprophylaxis can be summarized as follows: (1) Prophylaxis should always be directed toward a **specific pathogen**; (2) **no resistance** should develop during the period of drug use; (3) prophylactic drug use should be of **limited duration**; (4) conventional **therapeutic doses** should be employed; and (5) prophylaxis should be used only in situations of documented **drug efficacy.**

Nonsurgical prophylaxis, mentioned in earlier chapters, includes the prevention of cytomegalovirus (CMV) and HIV infections, influenza, meningococcal infections, and tuberculosis. Although somewhat less effective, antimicrobial prophylaxis is also commonly used for animal or human bite wounds and chronic bronchitis. Severely leukopenic patients are often given prophylactic antibiotics.

Prophylaxis against postsurgical infections should be limited to procedures that are associated with infection in more than 5% of untreated cases under optimal conditions. Prophylaxis should embody the principles listed previously, with drug selection based on the most likely infecting organism and treatment initiated just before surgery and continued throughout the procedure. A first-generation cephalosporin (eg, cefazolin) is often selected. Cefoxitin or cefotetan may be used for surgical patients at risk for infection caused by anaerobic bacteria. Situations in which surgical prophylaxis is of benefit (or commonly used) include gastrointestinal procedures, vaginal hysterectomy, cesarean section, joint replacement, open fracture surgery, and dental procedures in patients with congenital heart disease or cardiac prostheses.

QUESTIONS

1–3. A hospitalized AIDS patient is receiving anti-retroviral drugs but no antimicrobial prophylaxis. He develops sepsis with fever, suspected to be caused by a gram-negative bacillus. Treatment will include antibiotics, and the drugs under consideration include aminoglycosides, cephalosporins, fluoroquinolones, and imipenem.

1. Antimicrobial treatment of this severely immune-depressed patient should NOT be initiated before
   (A) Antipyretic drugs have been given to reduce body temperature
   (B) Pathogens have been identified by the microbiology laboratory
   (C) Specimens have been taken for laboratory tests and examinations
   (D) The results of a Gram stain are available
   (E) The results of antibacterial drug susceptibility tests are available

2. If gentamicin is used systemically in the treatment of this patient, monitoring of serum drug level may be advised because the drug
   (A) Does not readily penetrate into the cerebrospinal fluid
   (B) Has a narrow therapeutic window
   (C) Is antagonized by beta-lactam antibiotics
   (D) Is hematotoxic
   (E) Is unstable in gastric acid

3. A combination of drugs might be given to this patient to provide coverage against multiple organisms or to obtain a synergistic action. Examples of antimicrobial drug synergism established at the clinical level include
   (A) Amphotericin B and flucytosine in cryptococcal meningitis
   (B) Carbenicillin and gentamicin in pseudomonal infections
   (C) Rifampin and vancomycin in enterococcal infections
   (D) Trimethoprim and sulfamethoxazole in coliform infections
   (E) All of the above

4–5. A 27-year-old pregnant patient with a history of pyelonephritis has developed a severe upper respiratory tract infection that appears to be due to a bacterial pathogen. The woman is hospitalized, and an antibacterial agent is to be selected for treatment.

4. Assuming that the physician is concerned about the effects of renal impairment on drug dosage in this patient, which drug would not require dosage modification in renal dysfunction?
   (A) Amikacin
   (B) Ciprofloxacin
   (C) Clindamycin
   (D) Trimethoprim-sulfamethoxazole
   (E) Vancomycin

5. Which antibacterial agent appears to be safe for the treatment of infections in the pregnant patient?
   (A) Azithromycin
   (B) Clarithromycin
   (C) Streptomycin
   (D) Sulfadiazine
   (E) Tetracycline

6. There is no evidence that antimicrobial prophylaxis is of established benefit in
   (A) Contacts of the index case in gonorrhea
   (B) Contacts of the index case in mycoplasmal pneumonia
   (C) Recurrent urinary tract infection
   (D) "Traveler's diarrhea"
   (E) Tuberculin converters

7. Which drug is unlikely to be of value in a bioterrorist attack that utilizes anthrax?
   (A) Cefazolin
   (B) Ciprofloxacin
   (C) Clindamycin
   (D) Doxycycline
   (E) Rifampin

8–9. A 51-year-old patient is scheduled for a vaginal hysterectomy. An antimicrobial drug will be used for prophylaxis against postoperative infection. It is proposed that cefazolin, a first-generation cephalosporin, be given intravenously at the normal therapeutic dose immediately before surgery and continued until the patient is released from the hospital.

8. Which statement about the proposed drug management of this patient is not accurate?
   (A) Nosocomial (hospital-acquired) infection will be prevented by treatment throughout the period of hospitalization
   (B) Probable pathogens do not become rapidly resistant to this drug
   (C) Prophylaxis has documented efficacy in this type of surgical procedure
   (D) This drug will not be effective against anaerobes
   (E) Without prophylaxis, the infection rate following this procedure exceeds 5% under optimal conditions

9. If the patient had been scheduled for elective colonic surgery, optimal prophylaxis against infection would be achieved by mechanical bowel preparation and the use of
   (A) Intravenous cefotetan
   (B) Intravenous third-generation cephalosporin
   (C) Oral ampicillin
   (D) Oral fluoroquinolone
   (E) Oral neomycin and erythromycin

10. Which drug increases the hepatic metabolism of other drugs?
    (A) Clarithromycin
    (B) Erythromycin
    (C) Ketoconazole
    (D) Rifampin
    (E) Ritonavir

11. Which antimicrobial drug does not require supplementation of dosage following hemodialysis?
    (A) Ampicillin
    (B) Cefazolin
    (C) Ganciclovir
    (D) Tobramycin
    (E) Vancomycin

12. The persistent suppression of bacterial growth that may occur after limited exposure to some antimicrobial drugs is called
    (A) Clinical synergy
    (B) Concentration-dependent killing
    (C) Postantibiotic effect
    (D) Sequential blockade
    (E) Time-dependent killing

13. If ampicillin and piperacillin are used in combination in the treatment of infections resulting from

Pseudomonas aeruginosa, antagonism may occur. The most likely explanation is that
(A) Ampicillin is bacteriostatic
(B) Ampicillin induces beta-lactamase production
(C) Autolytic enzymes are inhibited by piperacillin
(D) Piperacillin blocks the attachment of ampicillin to penicillin-binding proteins
(E) The 2 drugs form an insoluble complex

14. In a patient suffering from pseudomembranous colitis due to *C difficile* with established hypersensitivity to metronidazole, the most likely drug to be of clinical value is
(A) Ampicillin
(B) Chloramphenicol
(C) Clindamycin
(D) Doxycycline
(E) Vancomycin

ANSWERS

1. To delay therapy until laboratory results are available is inappropriate in serious bacterial infections, but specimens for possible microbial identification must be obtained before drugs are administered. The answer is **C**.

2. Monitoring plasma aminoglycoside levels is important because aminoglycosides have a low therapeutic index; toxicity may occur when plasma levels are only 3 to 4 times higher than minimal inhibitory concentrations. Decreases in renal function may elevate the plasma levels of aminoglycosides to toxic levels within a few hours. The answer is **B**.

3. Combinations of antimicrobial drugs are not always synergistic. However, all of the choices listed are established examples of situations where antimicrobial combinations have greater clinical efficacy than individual drugs. The answer is **E**.

4. Antimicrobial drugs that are eliminated via hepatic metabolism or biliary excretion include erythromycin, cefoperazone, clindamycin, doxycycline, isoniazid, ketoconazole, and nafcillin. The answer is **C**.

5. Several groups of antimicrobial drugs should be avoided in pregnancy, including aminoglycosides, sulfonamides, and tetracyclines. Although the macrolide azithromycin appears to be safe, studies in animals have shown that clarithromycin is potentially embryotoxic. The answer is **A**.

6. Tetracycline has been administered to subjects exposed to mycoplasmal pneumonia, but the effectiveness of such treatment has not been documented. The answer is **B**.

7. Cephalosporins have minimal activity against *Bacillus anthracis,* the causative agent in anthrax. A combination of ciprofloxacin (or doxycycline), plus clindamycin, plus rifampin is recommended for treatment of inhalational exposure to anthrax. The answer is **A.**

8. With few exceptions, the prophylactic use of antibiotics in surgery should not extend beyond the duration of the procedure. After routine surgical procedures, the risk of opportunistic infection (from disturbances in microbial flora) *increases* in a hospitalized patient if prophylaxis is prolonged; there is also more likelihood of drug toxicity. The answer is **A.**

9. Second-generation cephalosporins, including cefoxitin and cefotetan, are more active than cefazolin against bowel anaerobes such as *Bacteroides fragilis* and are sometimes used for prophylaxis in "dirty" surgical procedures. However, for elective bowel surgery, most authorities favor the oral use of neomycin together with a poorly absorbed formulation of erythromycin. In cases of bowel perforation, the use of a second- or third-generation cephalosporin is more appropriate. The answer is **E.**

10. Clarithromycin, erythromycin, ketoconazole, and ritonavir inhibit the hepatic metabolism of various drugs. Rifampin is an inducer of liver microsomal drug-metabolizing enzymes. The answer is **D.**

11. Vancomycin is not removed from the blood during hemodialysis, and no change in dosage is required. The answer is **E.**

12. Antibiotics that have a postantibiotic effect (PAE) continue to exert effects on the growth of bacteria when blood levels are lower than those that are normally thought of as the minimal inhibitory concentration. The PAE may contribute to the clinical effectiveness of antibiotics, especially in the case of bactericidal agents such as aminoglycosides and fluoroquinolones, which exert concentration-dependent killing. The answer is **C.**

13. Gram-negative rods such as *Enterobacter* and *Pseudomonas aeruginosa* have inducible beta-lactamases. Several beta-lactam antibiotics, including ampicillin, cefoxitin, and imipenem, are potent inducers of beta-lactamase production. When such inducers are used in combination with a hydrolyzable penicillin (eg, piperacillin), antagonism may result. The answer is **B.**

14. Disturbances of gut flora occur commonly during treatment with antibiotics, and pseudomembranous colitis has been associated with the use of many agents, including ampicillin and clindamycin. Vancomycin can be used for treatment of pseudomembranous colitis in patients with established hypersensitivity to metronidazole. The answer is **E.**

CHECKLIST

When you complete this chapter, you should be able to:

☐ List the steps that should be taken before the initiation of empiric antimicrobial therapy.

☐ Appreciate why susceptibility testing of isolates and the determination of antibiotic blood levels are important in the treatment of many infections.

☐ Identify the antibiotics of choice for treatment of infections resulting from *B fragilis,* atypical organisms (*Chlamydia, Mycoplasma*), enterococci, gonococci, pneumococci (including PRSP strains), staphylococci (including MRSA strains), and *Treponema pallidum.*

☐ Identify antibiotics that require major modifications of dosage in renal or hepatic dysfunction.

☐ List the reasons for use of antimicrobial drugs in combination and the probable mechanisms involved in drug synergy.

☐ Understand the principles underlying valid antimicrobial chemoprophylaxis and give examples of commonly used surgical and nonsurgical prophylaxis.

Basic Principles of Antiparasitic Chemotherapy

52

Rational approaches to antiparasite chemotherapy use the principle of **selective toxicity,** which exploits biochemical and physiologic differences between parasite and host cells. Many antiparasitic agents target enzymes that are unique to, or indispensable to, parasites; other drugs affect cellular functions common to both host and parasite cells (Table 52–1).

A. MECHANISMS INVOLVING ENZYMES UNIQUE TO PARASITES

These enzymes are not found in the host's cells.

1. Dihydropteroate synthase—Sporozoans (eg, *Plasmodium, Toxoplasma,* and *Eimeria* species) lack the ability to use exogenous folate and, therefore, possess enzymes for its synthesis; these enzymes can be inhibited by drugs. **Sulfonamides,** which are antimetabolites of para-aminobenzoic acid (PABA), inhibit dihydropteroate synthase. **Sequential blockade** can be achieved with a sulfonamide and an inhibitor of dihydrofolate reductase; such drug combinations are effective in malaria and toxoplasmosis. For example, Fansidar, a combination of sulfadoxine and pyrimethamine, is effective against some strains of chloroquine-resistant *Plasmodium falciparum* malaria (see Chapter 53).

2. Pyruvate-ferredoxin oxidoreductase—Certain anaerobic protozoans (trichomonas, entamoeba) lack mitochondria and possess a pyruvate-ferredoxin oxidoreductase of low redox potential that generates acetyl-coenzyme A via electron transport. In trichomonal flagellates, this enzyme is coupled to a hydrogenase located in hydrogenosomes. Under anaerobic conditions, electron transport results in formation of hydrogen. The system also transfers electrons from pyruvate to the nitro groups of nitroimidazoles (eg, **metronidazole**), forming cytotoxic products that inhibit growth by binding to the parasite's proteins and DNA. Pyruvate-ferredoxin oxidoreductase has no counterpart in mammalian systems. The selective toxicity of metronidazole is the basis for its effectiveness and safety in the management of amebiasis and trichomoniasis. Nitazoxanide inhibits

the pyruvate-ferredoxin oxidoreductase pathway in *Giardia lamblia* and *Cryptosporidium parvum.*

3. Nucleoside phosphotransferases—Protozoan parasites depend critically on purine salvage pathways because these organisms are unable to synthesize purine nucleotides de novo. In leishmania, purine nucleoside phosphotransferase (a salvage enzyme that transfers phosphate groups to the 5′ position of purine nucleosides) also phosphorylates purine nucleoside analogs such as **allopurinol riboside, formycin B,** and **thiopurinol riboside.** The triphosphate derivatives of these drugs may be incorporated into nucleic acids or may inhibit enzymes in purine metabolism. Toxicity is low because mammalian cells lack this salvage enzyme.

4. Trypanothione reductase—In the protozoans known as kinetoplastidans, glutathione exists largely in the form of trypanothione, a unique conjugate with spermidine. Trypanothione, via the action of a specific trypanothione reductase, plays a central role in maintaining the reduced state of intracellular thiols and is essential for the survival of such parasites. **Nifurtimox,** used in Chagas' disease, and trivalent arsenicals used in African trypanosomiasis are inhibitors of trypanothione reductase.

B. MECHANISMS INVOLVING ENZYMES INDISPENSABLE TO PARASITES

These enzymes are present in the host as well as the parasite, but they are essential only to the parasite.

1. Purine phosphoribosyl transferases—Hypoxanthine-guanine phosphoribosyltransferase (HGPRTase) is a key enzyme in purine synthesis in many parasites, including *Leishmania, Schistosoma,* and *Trypanosoma* species. **Allopurinol** is a good substrate for this enzyme in certain parasites (but not for the mammalian enzyme); the drug is metabolized to the ribotide, which is incorporated after phosphorylation into RNA forms that interfere with normal growth. Purine salvage in *Giardia* depends critically on adenine phosphoribosyltransferase and guanine phosphoribosyltransferase. Unlike mammalian forms of these enzymes, the parasitic

HIGH-YIELD TERMS TO LEARN

Glycosome	A membrane-bounded intracellular organelle in trypanosomes that contains glycolytic enzymes
Hydrogenosome	A membrane-bounded intracellular organelle in certain anaerobic protozoans that contains hydrogenase
Salvage enzymes	Nucleoside phosphotransferases involved in the salvage of purines and pyrimidines in protozoans
Sequential blockade	Actions of 2 or more drugs that interfere with sequential steps in a metabolic pathway
Suicide substrate	A chemical that forms a stable complex with an enzyme leading to its irreversible inhibition; suicide substrates are chemically related to natural enzyme substrates

enzymes do not use hypoxanthine, xanthine, or adenine as substrates and are thus amenable to inhibition by a designed inhibitor.

2. Ornithine decarboxylase—This enzyme controls the formation of the polyamine, putrescine, and appears to be more critical for the growth of certain parasites than for the growth of mammalian cells. Eflornithine is a suicide substrate of ornithine decarboxylase and has antiparasitic activity against *Trypanosoma, Plasmodium,* and *Giardia* species. In African trypansomiasis caused

Table 52–1. Identified targets and mechanisms of action of selected antiparasitic drugs.

Mechanism	Parasites	Examples of Drugs
Act on enzymes specific to parasites		
Dihydropteroate synthase	Sporozoa	Sulfonamides, sulfones
Pyruvate-ferredoxin oxidoreductase	Anaerobic protozoa	Nitroimidazoles
Nucleoside phosphotransferase	Flagellated protozoa	Allopurinol riboside
Trypanothione reductase	Kinetoplastida	Nifurtimox, melarsoprol
Act on enzymes indispensable to parasites		
Purine phosphoribosyl transferase	Protozoa	Allopurinol
Ornithine decarboxylase	Protozoa	α-Difluoromethylornithine
Glycolytic enzymes	Kinetoplastida	Glycerol plus salicylhydroxamic acid and suramin
Act on functions common to both host and parasite[a]		
Dihydrofolate reductase	Sporozoa	Pyrimethamine, trimethoprim
Thiamin transporter	Coccidia	Amprolium
Mitochondrial electron transporter	Coccidia	4-Hydroxyquinolones
Microtubules	Helminths	Benzimidazoles
Neurotransmission, muscle contraction	Helminthes and ectoparasites	Levamisole, piperazines, avermectins, milbemycins
Ergosterol demethylase	Kinetoplastida	Fluconazole

[a]Differences in the structures of regulatory macromolecules among parasites and host cells and differences in drug access may account for the selective toxicities of drugs in this subgroup.

by *T gambiense,* the irreversible inhibitory action of eflornithine transforms the organism into a nondividing form that can be eliminated by the host immune system.

3. Glycolytic enzymes—The bloodstream form of the African trypanosome *T brucei* is entirely dependent on glycolysis for generation of adenosine triphosphate (ATP). The enzymes involved are arranged in close proximity to each other in glycosomes. Glycerol-3-phosphate oxidase is a key enzyme that can be inhibited by **salicylhydroxamic acid,** bringing the parasite into an anaerobic state. The addition of glycerol inhibits the reversed glycerol kinase reaction, stops glycolysis, and results in the death of the parasite. Biogenesis of glycosomes may also be a target for antiparasitic drugs. **Suramin,** a very large polar molecule, binds to glycolytic enzymes and may prevent the incorporation of the enzymes into the glycosome.

C. Mechanisms Involving Biochemical Functions Common to Host and Parasite

Several processes that occur in both parasites and hosts are nevertheless more susceptible to inhibition in the parasite.

1. Dihydrofolate reductase—Dihydrofolate reductase (DHFR) is a classic target in antimicrobial and cancer chemotherapy. The enzyme is also a useful therapeutic target in *Plasmodium, Toxoplasma,* and *Eimeria* species. **Pyrimethamine** inhibits DHFR in all 3 species of parasites. However, in the case of *P falciparum,* point mutations in the gene that codes for DHFR have rendered the enzyme less susceptible to pyrimethamine.

2. Thiamin transporter—Carbohydrate metabolism is the primary energy source in coccidia. Inhibition of the cellular transport of thiamin by the structurally similar agent **amprolium** leads to a deficiency of this cofactor in coccidia. Amprolium has been used extensively as an effective anticoccidial agent in chickens and cattle with relatively low host toxicity.

3. Mitochondrial electron transporter—**4-Hydroxyquinoline** drugs with anticoccidial effects interact with components of the respiratory chain that are specific to *Eimeria* species and inhibit electron transport in the mitochondria of these organisms. Mitochondrial respiration in other parasites and in mammals is not inhibited by hydroxyquinolines. **Atovaquone,** a quinone, is an antimalarial drug and is also used in the treatment of *Pneumocystis carinii* infections. The primary site of action of atovaquone in *Plasmodium* is the cytochrome bc$_1$ complex, where a drug-binding site is present in cytochrome b.

4. Microtubules—The microtubules of the cytoskeleton and mitotic spindle consist of tubulin polymers. These tubulins are heterogeneous among species.

Structural features of alpha-tubulins in helminths may account for the selective toxicity of benzimidazole drugs (eg, **mebendazole**). These agents bind to microtubules in helminths to block transport processes.

5. Neurotransmission and muscle contraction—The antiparasitic effect of nicotinic agonist drugs (eg, **levamisole, pyrantel pamoate**) in nematodes is caused by stimulation of neuromuscular transmission, which leads to muscle contraction. **Piperazine** acts as a γ-aminobutyric acid (GABA) receptor agonist in nematodes, causing flaccid paralysis. Facilitation of the actions of GABA underlies the actions of **milbemycins** and **avermectins,** agents that promote release of the neurotransmitter and increase its binding to postjunctional receptors. These natural products do not cross the blood-brain barrier in mammalian hosts and are relatively nontoxic. **Praziquantel,** an antischistosomal and antitapeworm agent, stimulates Ca^{2+} entry into muscles of these parasites and causes unphysiologic contraction.

6. Lanosterol demethylase—*T cruzi* and *Leishmania* contain ergosterol as the principal sterol in plasma membranes. The **azole** antifungal agents, which are known to act by inhibiting the cytochrome P450-dependent C-14α demethylation of lanosterol in the ergosterol biosynthetic pathway, also inhibit growth of *T cruzi* and *Leishmania.* Fluconazole is used in the treatment of cutaneous leishmaniasis.

QUESTIONS

1. Certain anaerobic protozoan parasites lack mitochondria and generate energy-rich compounds, such as acetyl-CoA, by means of enzymes present in organelles called hydrogenosomes. A key enzyme involved in this process is
   (A) Cytochrome P450
   (B) Glycerol-3-phosphate oxidase
   (C) Hypoxanthine-guanine phosphoribosyltransferase
   (D) Pyruvate-ferredoxin oxidoreductase
   (E) Thymidylate synthase

2. Which compound is a good substrate for hypoxanthine-guanine phosphoribosyltransferase in trypanosomes (but not mammals) and is eventually converted into metabolites that are incorporated into RNA?
   (A) Allopurinol
   (B) Alpha-difluoromethylornithine
   (C) Glycerol
   (D) Mebendazole
   (E) Salicylhydroxamic acid

3. One chemotherapeutic strategy used to eradicate the bloodstream form of African trypanosomes is based on the absolute dependence of the organism on

(A) Cytochrome-dependent electron transfer
(B) Dihydropteroate synthesis
(C) Glycolysis
(D) Lactate dehydrogenase
(E) Mitochondrial respiration

4. Which drug enhances GABA actions on the neuromuscular junctions of nematodes and arthropods?
   (A) Glutamic acid
   (B) Ivermectin
   (C) Picrotoxin
   (D) Pyrantel pamoate
   (E) Pyrimethamine

5. Which drug is an antimetabolite that inhibits a trypanosomal enzyme involved in putrescine synthesis?
   (A) Amprolium
   (B) Eflornithine
   (C) Metronidazole
   (D) Polymyxin
   (E) Thiopurinol riboside

6. Which statement about the mechanisms of action of antiparasitic drugs is not accurate?
   (A) 4-Hydroxyquinolines inhibit phospholipase C
   (B) Mebendazole binds to tubulins to alter the transport functions of microtubules
   (C) Metronidazole is activated in the parasite to a cytotoxic product
   (D) Salicylhydroxamic acid is an inhibitor of glycerol-3-phosphate oxidase
   (E) Sulfonamides inhibit 7,8-dihydropteroate synthase

7. Which enzyme is not unique to parasites?
   (A) Dihydropteroate synthetase
   (B) Hypoxanthine-guanine phosphoribosyltransferase
   (C) Pyruvate-ferridoxin oxidoreductase
   (D) Purine nucleoside phosphotransferase
   (E) Trypanothione reductase

8. Which statement about specific antiparasitic drugs is not accurate?
   (A) Amprolium is an inhibitor of thiamin transport in *Eimeria* species
   (B) Sulfadoxine is an inhibitor of dihydropteroate synthase in the malaria parasite
   (C) Suramin binds to glycolytic enzymes and prevents their incorporation into glycosomes
   (D) The mechanism of action of diloxanide furoate in amebiasis is unknown
   (E) Thiopurinol riboside is a potent inhibitor of mitochondrial electron transfer

9. "Baghdad boil," a form of cutaneous leishmaniasis that occurs commonly in Iraq, can be treated with

(A) Albendazole
(B) Fluconazole
(C) Metronidazole
(D) Praziquantel
(E) Pyrimethamine

10. Which agent is thought to act by increasing membrane permeability to calcium in trematode and cestode muscles?
    (A) Atovaquone
    (B) Eflornithine
    (C) Praziquantel
    (D) Pyrantel pamoate
    (E) Sulfadoxine

ANSWERS

1. In *T vaginalis,* conversion of pyruvate to acetyl-CoA occurs via the actions of pyruvate-ferredoxin oxidoreductase. Metronidazole inhibits this enzyme system. The answer is **D.**

2. Allopurinol is a good substrate for HGPRTase in trypanosomes but not mammals. Recall that allopurinol is also an inhibitor of xanthine oxidase and is used in gout and cancer chemotherapy. The answer is **A.**

3. Glycolytic enzyme inhibitors (such as salicylhydroxamic acid) that inhibit glycerol-3-phosphate oxidase may be selectively toxic to African trypanosomes. The answer is **C.**

4. Several antiparasitic drugs enhance GABA neurotransmission in nematodes and arthropods and cause muscle paralysis. These drugs include piperazine, milbemycins, and avermectins (eg, ivermectin). The answer is **B.**

5. Eflornithine is a suicide inhibitor of ornithine decarboxylase. Although it also inhibits mammalian ornithine decarboxylase, eflornithine is less toxic to the host because of more rapid turnover and replacement of the irreversibly inhibited enzyme in the host than in parasites. The answer is **B.**

6. The anticoccidial 4-hydroxyquinolines inhibit mitochondrial respiration in *Eimeria* species, probably through interaction with a component between NADH oxidase and cytochrome b in the electron transport chain. The answer is **A.**

7. HGPRTase, an enzyme involved in purine salvage, is present in both parasites and mammals. Allopurinol is a suicide substrate for this enzyme in certain parasites but not human forms of the enzyme. However, as a suicide substrate for xanthine oxidase, allopurinol is an effective drug in gout! The answer is **B.**

8. Thiopurinol riboside is not an inhibitor of mitochondrial electron transport. *Leishmania* species

possess the unique salvage enzyme, purine nucleoside phosphotransferase. This enzyme phosphorylates thiopurinol riboside to form the corresponding nucleotide, which interferes with purine and nucleic acid metabolism. The answer is **E.**

9. The synthesis of ergosterol, the principle sterol in the plasma membranes of *Leishmania* and certain trypanosomal species, is inhibited by antifungal azoles such as fluconazole. The answer is **B.**

10. Praziquantel and pyrantel pamoate are anthelmintics. Pyrantel pamoate is an activator of nicotinic receptors, causing initial contraction and then paralysis of nematode muscles. Praziquantel causes initial contraction and then paralysis in cestodes and trematodes by increasing calcium permeability. The answer is **C.**

CHECKLIST

When you complete this chapter, you should be able to:

☐ Identify 4 mechanisms of agents whose targets are enzymes unique to parasites.

☐ List 3 mechanisms of drugs whose targets are enzymes indispensable to parasites but not to their hosts.

☐ Identify 6 mechanisms of drugs whose targets are biochemical functions common to host and parasites.

Antiprotozoal Drugs

53

Diseases caused by protozoans constitute a worldwide health problem. This chapter concerns the drugs used to combat malaria, amebiasis, toxoplasmosis, pneumocystosis, trypanosomiasis, and leishmaniasis.

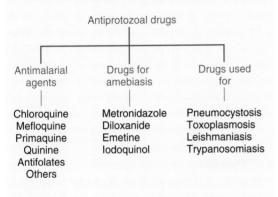

DRUGS FOR MALARIA

Malaria is one of the most common diseases worldwide and a leading cause of death. *Plasmodium* species that infect humans (*P falciparum, P malariae, P ovale, P vivax*) undergo a primary developmental stage in the liver and then parasitize erythrocytes. *P falciparum* and *P malariae* have only 1 cycle of liver cell invasion. The other species have a dormant hepatic stage responsible for recurrent infections and relapses. Primary **tissue schizonticides** (eg, primaquine) kill schizonts in the liver, whereas **blood schizonticides** (eg, chloroquine, quinine) kill these parasitic forms only in the erythrocyte. **Sporonticides** (proguanil, pyrimethamine) prevent sporogony and multiplication in the mosquito.

Drugs used for the treatment of malaria are shown in Table 53–1.

A. CHLOROQUINE

1. Classification and pharmacokinetics—Chloroquine is a 4-aminoquinoline derivative. The drug is rapidly absorbed when given orally, is widely distributed to tissues, and has an extremely large volume of distribution. Antacids may decrease oral absorption of the drug. Chloroquine is excreted largely unchanged in the urine.

2. Mechanism of action—Chloroquine accumulates in the food vacuole of plasmodia and prevents polymerization of the hemoglobin breakdown product heme into hemozoin. Intracellular accumulation of heme is toxic to the parasite. Decreased intracellular accumulation via increased activity of membrane "pumps" is a mechanism of resistance to chloroquine and other antimalarial drugs. Resistance in *P falciparum* can also result from decreased intravacuolar accumulation of chloroquine via a transporter encoded by the *pfcrt* (*P falciparum* chloroquine-resistance transporter) gene.

3. Clinical use—Chloroquine is the drug of choice for acute attacks of nonfalciparum and sensitive falciparum malaria and for chemoprophylaxis, except in regions where *P falciparum* is resistant. The drug is solely a blood schizonticide. Chloroquine and hydroxychloroquine are also used in autoimmune disorders, including rheumatoid arthritis.

4. Toxicity—At low doses, chloroquine causes gastrointestinal irritation, skin rash, and headaches. High doses may cause severe skin lesions, peripheral neuropathies, myocardial depression, retinal damage, auditory impairment, and toxic psychosis. Chloroquine may also precipitate porphyria attacks.

B. QUININE

1. Classification and pharmacokinetics—Quinine is rapidly absorbed orally and is metabolized before renal excretion. Intravenous administration of quinine is possible in severe infections.

2. Mechanism of action—Quinine complexes with double-stranded DNA to prevent strand separation, resulting in block of DNA replication and transcription to RNA. Quinine is solely a blood schizonticide.

3. Clinical use—The main use of quinine is in *P falciparum* infections resistant to chloroquine in patients who can tolerate oral treatment. Quinine is often used with doxycycline or clindamycin to shorten the duration

Table 53–1. Drugs used in the treatment of malaria.

Drug	Uses	Adverse Effects
Chloroquine	Prophylaxis and treatment in areas without resistant *P falciparum*; treatment of *P vivax* and *P ovale* malaria	GI distress, rash, headache; auditory dysfunction and retinal dysfunction (high dose)
Mefloquine	Prophylaxis and treatment in areas with resistant *P falciparum*	GI distress, rash, headache; cardiac conduction defects and neurologic symptoms (high dose)
Quinine[a]	Treatment of multidrug-resistant malaria	Cinchonism, hemolysis in G6PD deficiency, blackwater fever
Primaquine	Eradication of liver stages of *P vivax* and *P ovale*	GI distress, methemoglobinemia, hemolysis in G6PD deficiency
Antifolates	Prophylaxis and treatment of multidrug-resistant *P falciparum* malaria	GI distress, renal dysfunction, hemolysis, folate deficiency
Atovaquone-proguanil (Malarone)	Prophylaxis and treatment of multidrug-resistant *P falciparum* malaria	GI distress, headache and rash
Artesunate, artemether	Treatment of multidrug-resistant malaria	GI distress

[a]In most cases quinine is used together with doxycycline, or clindamycin, or an antifolate. Quinidine gluconate (IV) is used in severe infections or patients unable to take oral quinine.

of therapy and limit toxicity. Quinidine, the dextrorotatory stereoisomer of quinine, is used intravenously in the treatment of severe or complicated falciparum malaria. To delay emergence of resistance, quinine should not be used routinely for prophylaxis.

4. Toxicity—Quinine commonly causes **cinchonism**, symptoms of which include gastrointestinal distress, headache, vertigo, blurred vision, and tinnitus. Severe overdose results in disturbances in cardiac conduction that resemble quinidine toxicity. Hematotoxic effects occur, including hemolysis in glucose-6-phosphate dehydrogenase (G6PD)-deficient patients. **Blackwater fever** (intravascular hemolysis) is a rare and sometimes fatal complication in quinine-sensitized persons. Quinine is contraindicated in pregnancy.

C. MEFLOQUINE

1. Classification and pharmacokinetics—Mefloquine is a synthetic 4-quinoline derivative. Because of local irritation, mefloquine can only be given orally, although it is subject to variable absorption. Its mechanism of action is not known.

2. Clinical use—A first-line drug for prophylaxis in all geographical areas with chloroquine resistance and an alternative drug to quinine in acute attacks resulting from *P falciparum*. Resistance to mefloquine has emerged in regions of Southeast Asia.

3. Toxicity—Common adverse effects include gastrointestinal distress, skin rash, headache, and dizziness. At high doses, mefloquine has caused cardiac conduction defects, psychiatric disorders, neurologic symptoms, and seizures.

D. PRIMAQUINE

1. Classification and pharmacokinetics—Primaquine is a synthetic 8-aminoquinoline. Absorption is complete after oral administration and is followed by extensive metabolism.

2. Mechanism of action—Primaquine forms quinoline-quinone metabolites, which are electron-transferring redox compounds that act as cellular oxidants. The drug is a tissue schizonticide and also limits malaria transmission by acting as a gametocide.

3. Clinical use—Primaquine eradicates liver stages of *P vivax* and *P ovale* and should be used in conjunction with a blood schizonticide. Although not active alone in acute attacks of vivax and ovale malaria, a 14-day course of primaquine is standard after treatment with chloroquine.

4. Toxicity—Primaquine is usually well tolerated but may cause gastrointestinal distress, pruritus, headaches, and methemoglobinemia. More serious toxicity involves hemolysis in G6PD-deficient patients. Primaquine is contraindicated in pregnancy.

E. ANTIFOLATE DRUGS

1. Classification and pharmacokinetics—The antifolate group includes pyrimethamine, proguanil, sulfadoxine, and dapsone. All of these drugs are absorbed orally and are excreted in the urine, partly in unchanged form. Proguanil has a shorter half-life (12–16 h) than other drugs in this subclass (half-life >100 h).

2. Mechanisms of action—Sulfonamides act as antimetabolites of PABA and block folic acid synthesis in certain protozoans by inhibiting dihydropteroate synthase. Proguanil (chloroguanide) is bioactivated to cycloguanil. Pyrimethamine and cycloguanil are selective inhibitors of protozoan dihydrofolate reductases. The combination of pyrimethamine with sulfadoxine has synergistic antimalarial effects through the **sequential blockade** of 2 steps in folic acid synthesis.

3. Clinical use—The antifols are blood schizonticides that act mainly against *P falciparum*. Pyrimethamine with sulfadoxine in fixed combination (Fansidar) is used in the treatment of chloroquine-resistant forms of this species, although the onset of activity is slow. Proguanil with atovaquone in fixed combination (Malarone) is a first-line choice for chemoprophylaxis of chloroquine-resistant malaria and is also protective against mefloquine-resistant falciparum strains.

4. Toxicity—The toxic effects of sulfonamides include skin rashes, gastrointestinal distress, hemolysis, kidney damage, and drug interactions caused by competition for plasma protein binding sites. Pyrimethamine may cause folic acid deficiency when used in high doses.

F. Other Antimalarial Drugs

1. Doxycycline—This tetracycline is chemoprophylactic for travelers to geographical areas with both chloroquine- and mefloquine-resistant *P falciparum*.

2. Amodiaquine—This drug has been widely used to treat malaria in many countries because of its low cost and, in some geographical areas, effectiveness against chloroquine-resistant strains of *P falciparum*. Hematological toxicity, including agranulocytosis and aplastic anemia, has been associated with the use of amodiaquine.

3. Atovaquone—This quinone derivative, a component of Malarone (with proguanil), appears to disrupt mitochondrial electron transport in protozoa. Malarone is effective for both chemoprophylaxis and treatment of falciparum malaria. Abdominal pain and gastrointestinal effects occur at the higher doses used for treatment. Atovaquone is an alternative treatment for *P jiroveci* infection.

4. Halofantrine—Although its mechanism of action is unknown, this drug is active against erythrocytic stages of all 4 human malaria species, including chloroquine-resistant falciparum. Halofantrine is not used for chemoprophylaxis because of its potential cardiotoxicity (QT prolongation) and embryotoxicity.

5. Artesunate and artemether—These artemisinin derivatives are metabolized in the food vacuole of the parasite forming toxic free radicals. Artemisinins are blood schizonticides active against *P falciparum*, including multidrug-resistant strains. They are not used for chemoprophylaxis because of their short half-lives of 1–3 h. However, they are playing an increasingly important role in the treatment of malaria and are best used in combination with other agents. The artemisinins are the only drugs reliably effective against quinine-resistant strains. Adverse effects are mild but include nausea, vomiting, and diarrhea. Their safety in pregnancy has not been established.

G. Drugs for the Prevention of Malaria in Travelers

Chloroquine (weekly) remains an appropriate agent for prophylaxis in regions without resistant *P falciparum*, as does mefloquine (weekly) for regions with *P falciparum* resistance. In areas with multidrug-resistant malaria, the choice is either doxycycline or Malarone (atovaquone plus proguanil) daily. Primaquine is recommended for terminal prophylaxis of *P vivax* and *P ovale* infections. (For updated information, check the Centers for Disease Control and Prevention guidelines at http://www.cdc.gov).

DRUGS FOR AMEBIASIS

Tissue amebicides (**chloroquine, emetines, metronidazole**) act on organisms in the bowel wall and the liver; luminal amebicides (**diloxanide furoate, iodoquinol, paromomycin**) act only in the lumen of the bowel. The choice of a drug depends on the form of amebiasis. For asymptomatic disease, diloxanide furoate is the first choice. For mild to severe intestinal infection, metronidazole is used with a luminal agent, and this regimen is recommended in amebic liver abscess (Table 53–2). The mechanisms of amebicidal action of most drugs in this subclass are unknown.

A. Diloxanide Furoate

This drug is commonly used as the sole agent for the treatment of asymptomatic amebiasis and is also useful in mild intestinal disease when used with other drugs. Diloxanide furoate is converted in the gut to the diloxanide freebase form, which is the active amebicide. Toxic effects are mild and are usually restricted to gastrointestinal symptoms.

B. Emetines

Emetine and dehydroemetine inhibit protein synthesis by blocking ribosomal movement along messenger RNA. These drugs are used parenterally (SC or IM) as backup drugs for treatment of severe intestinal or hepatic amebiasis together with a luminal agent in hospitalized patients. The drugs may cause severe toxicity, including gastrointestinal distress, muscle weakness, and cardiovascular dysfunction (arrhythmias and congestive heart failure).

Table 53–2. Drugs used in the treatment of amebiasis.

Disease Form	Drug(s) of Choice	Alternative Drug(s)
Asymptomatic, intestinal infection	Diloxanide furoate	Iodoquinol, paromomycin
Mild to moderate intestinal infection	Metronidazole *plus* luminal agent (see above)	Tinidazole, *or* tetracycline, *or* erythromycin *plus* luminal agent
Severe intestinal infection	Metronidazole *or* tinidazole *plus* luminal agent	Tetracycline *or* emetine *or* dihydroemetine *plus* luminal agent
Hepatic abscess and other extraintestinal disease	Metronidazole *or* tinidazole *plus* luminal agent	Emetine or dihydroemetine *plus* chloroquine (for liver abscess) *plus* luminal agent

Adapted, with permission, from Katzung, BG, editor: *Basic & Clinical Pharmacology*, 10th ed. McGraw-Hill, 2007.

C. IODOQUINOL

Iodoquinol, a halogenated hydroxyquinoline, is an orally active luminal amebicide used as an alternative to diloxanide for mild-to-severe intestinal infections. Adverse gastrointestinal effects are common but usually mild. Systemic absorption after high doses may lead to thyroid enlargement and neurotoxic effects, including peripheral neuropathy and visual dysfunction.

D. METRONIDAZOLE AND TINIDAZOLE

1. Pharmacokinetics—Metronidazole and tinidazole are effective orally and distributed widely to tissues. The half-life of metronidazole is 6–8 h and that of tinidazole 12–14 h. Elimination of the drugs requires hepatic metabolism.

2. Mechanism of action—Metronidazole undergoes a reductive bioactivation of its nitro group by ferredoxin (present in anaerobic parasites) to form reactive cytotoxic products. The mechanism of tinidazole is assumed to be similar.

3. Clinical use—Metronidazole or tinidazole is the drug of choice in severe intestinal wall disease and in hepatic abscess and other extraintestinal amebic disease. Both drugs are used with a luminal amebicide. The duration of treatment required with metronidazole is longer than with tinidazole. Metronidazole is the drug of choice for trichomoniasis; tinidazole may be effective against some resistant organisms. Other clinical uses of metronidazole include treatment of giardiasis, and infections caused by *Gardnerella vaginalis* and anaerobic bacteria (*B fragilis, C difficile*). Metronidazole is also used in combination regimens for gastrointestinal ulcers associated with *H pylori*.

4. Toxicity—Adverse effects of metronidazole include gastrointestinal irritation, headache, and dark coloration of urine. Tinidazole has a similar adverse effect profile but may be better tolerated than metronidazole. More serious toxicity includes leukopenia, dizziness, and ataxia. Drug interactions with metronidazole include a disulfiram-like reaction with ethanol and potentiation of coumarin anticoagulant effects. Safety of metronidazole in pregnancy and in nursing mothers has not been established.

E. PAROMOMYCIN

This drug is an aminoglycoside antibiotic used as a luminal amebicide and may be superior to diloxanide in asymptomatic infection. Paromomycin may also have some efficacy against cryptosporidiosis in the AIDS patient. Systemic absorption may lead to headaches, dizziness, rashes, and arthralgia. Tetracyclines (eg, doxycycline) are sometimes used with a luminal amebicide in mild intestinal disease.

F. NITAZOXANIDE

This agent has activity against various protozoans (including *Entamoeba*) and helminthes. It is currently approved in the United States for treatment of gastrointestinal infections caused by *G lamblia* and *Cryptosporidium parvum*. Nitazoxanide appears to have activity against metronidazole-resistant protozoal strains.

DRUGS FOR PNEUMOCYSTOSIS & TOXOPLASMOSIS

A. PENTAMIDINE

1. Mechanism of action—Pentamidine's mechanism of action is unknown but may involve inhibition of glycolysis or interference with nucleic acid metabolism of protozoans and fungi. Preferential accumulation of the drug by susceptible parasites may account for its selective toxicity.

2. Clinical use—Aerosol pentamidine (once monthly) can be used in primary and secondary prophylaxis, although oral trimethoprim-sulfamethoxazole (TMP-SMX) is usually preferred. Daily intravenous or intramuscular administration of the drug for 21 days is needed in the treatment of active pneumocystosis in the HIV-infected patient. Pentamidine is also used in trypanosomiasis (see later discussion).

3. Toxicity—Severe adverse effects follow parenteral use, including respiratory stimulation followed by depression, hypotension resulting from peripheral vasodilation, hypoglycemia, anemia, neutropenia, hepatitis, and pancreatitis. Systemic toxicity is minimal when pentamidine is used by inhalation.

B. TMP-SMX

1. Clinical use—TMP-SMX is the first choice in prophylaxis and treatment of pneumocystis pneumonia (PCP). Prophylaxis in AIDS patients is recommended when the CD4 count drops below 200 cells/μL. Oral treatment with the double-strength formulation 3 times weekly is usually effective. The same regimen of TMP-SMX is prophylactic against toxoplasmosis and infections caused by *Isospora belli*. For treatment of active PCP, daily oral or intravenous administration of TMP-SMX is required.

2. Toxicity—Adverse effects from TMP-SMX occur in up to 50% of AIDS patients. Toxicity includes gastrointestinal distress, rash, fever, neutropenia, and thrombocytopenia. These effects may be serious enough to warrant discontinuance of TMP-SMX and substitution of alternative drugs. (See Chapter 46 for additional information on TMP-SMX.)

C. Antifols: Pyrimethamine and Sulfonamides

1. Clinical use—Combination of pyrimethamine with sulfadiazine has synergistic activity against *Toxoplasma gondii* through the **sequential blockade** of 2 steps in folic acid synthesis. Pyrimethamine plus sulfadiazine (or clindamycin) is a regimen of choice for prophylaxis against and treatment of toxoplasmosis. For treatment of active toxoplasmosis, the drug combination is given daily for 3–4 weeks, with folinic acid to offset hematologic toxicity. For patients allergic to sulfonamides, clindamycin can be used in combination with pyrimethamine. For *Toxoplasma* encephalitis in AIDS, high-dose treatment with pyrimethamine plus sulfadiazine (or clindamycin) must be maintained for at least 6 weeks.

2. Toxicity—High doses of pyrimethamine plus sulfadiazine are associated with gastric irritation, glossitis, neurologic symptoms (headache, insomnia, tremors, seizures), and hematotoxicity (megaloblastic anemia, thrombocytopenia). Antibiotic-associated colitis may occur during treatment with clindamycin.

D. Atovaquone

1. Mechanism and pharmacokinetics—Atovaquone inhibits mitochondrial electron transport and probably folate metabolism. Used orally, it is poorly absorbed and should be given with food to maximize bioavailability. Most of the drug is eliminated in the feces in unchanged form.

2. Clinical use and toxicity—Atovaquone is approved for use in mild to moderate pneumocystis pneumonia. It is less effective than TMP-SMX or pentamidine but is better tolerated. As noted, it is also used in combination with proguanil (as Malarone) for chemoprophylaxis and treatment of chloroquine-resistant malaria. Common adverse effects include rash, cough, nausea, vomiting, diarrhea, fever, and abnormal liver function tests. The drug should be avoided in patients with a history of cardiac conduction defects, psychiatric disorders, or seizures.

E. Miscellaneous Agents

Other alternative drug regimens for the treatment of pneumocystis pneumonia include trimethoprim plus dapsone, primaquine plus clindamycin, and trimetrexate plus leucovorin.

DRUGS FOR TRYPANOSOMIASIS

A. Pentamidine

Pentamidine is commonly used in the hemolymphatic stages of disease caused by *Trypanosoma gambiense* and *T rhodesiense*. Because it does not cross the blood-brain barrier, pentamidine is not used in later stages of trypanosomiasis. Other clinical uses include pneumocystosis and treatment of the kala azar form of leishmaniasis (Table 53–3).

B. Melarsoprol

This drug is an organic arsenical that inhibits enzyme sulfhydryl groups. Because it enters the CNS, melarsoprol is the drug of choice in African sleeping sickness. However, treatment failures do occur, possibly because of resistance. Melarsoprol is given parenterally because it causes gastrointestinal irritation; it may also cause a reactive encephalopathy that can be fatal.

C. Nifurtimox

This drug is a nitrofurazone derivative that inhibits the parasite-unique enzyme trypanothione reductase. Nifurtimox is the drug of choice in American trypanosomiasis, an alternative agent in African forms of the disease, and has also been effective in mucocutaneous leishmaniasis. The drug causes severe toxicity, including allergies, gastrointestinal irritation, and CNS effects.

D. Suramin

This polyanionic compound is a drug of choice for the early hemolymphatic stages of African trypanosomiasis (before CNS involvement). It is also an alternative to ivermectin in the treatment of onchocerciasis (see Chapter 54). Suramin is used parenterally and causes skin rashes, gastrointestinal distress, and neurologic complications.

E. Eflornithine

This agent, a suicide substrate of ornithine decarboxylase, is effective in some forms of African trypanosomiasis. It is available for both oral and intravenous use and penetrates

Table 53–3. Drugs used in the treatment of other protozoal infections.

Drug	Indications
Melarsoprol	Mucocutaneous forms of trypanosomiasis and the late CNS stage (African sleeping sickness)
Metronidazole	Drug of choice for infections caused by *Giardia lamblia* and *Trichomonas vaginalis*
Nifurtimox	Trypanosomiasis caused by *T cruzi*
Pentamidine	Hemolymphatic stage of trypanosomiasis and for *Pneumocystis jiroveci* infections
Pyrimethamine plus clindamycin or sulfadiazine plus folinic acid	Drug combinations used in treatment of toxoplasmosis
Sodium stibogluconate	Treatment of leishmaniasis (all stages)
Suramin	Drug of choice for hemolymphatic stage of trypanosomiasis (*T brucei gambiense*, *T rhodesiense*)
Trimethoprim-sulfamethoxazole	Drug combination of choice in *Pneumocystis jiroveci* infections

into the CNS. It causes gastrointestinal irritation and hematotoxicity; seizures have occurred in overdose.

DRUGS FOR LEISHMANIASIS

Leishmania, parasitic protozoa transmitted by flesh-eating flies, cause various diseases ranging from cutaneous or mucocutaneous lesions to splenic and hepatic enlargement with fever. **Sodium stibogluconate** (pentavalent antimony), the primary drug in all forms of the disease, appears to kill the parasite by inhibition of glycolysis or effects on nucleic acid metabolism. Stibogluconate must be administered parenterally and is potentially cardiotoxic (QTc prolongation). Alternative agents include pentamidine or miltefosine (for visceral leishmaniasis), fluconazole or metronidazole (for cutaneous lesions), and amphotericin B (for mucocutaneous leishmaniasis).

QUESTIONS

1. Which statement about antiprotozoal drugs is accurate?
   (A) A combination of primaquine and clindamycin is an alternative drug regimen for *Pneumocystis jiroveci* pneumonia
   (B) Chloroquine is an inhibitor of plasmodial dihydrofolate reductase
   (C) Mefloquine destroys secondary exoerythrocytic schizonts
   (D) Primaquine is a blood schizonticide and does not affect secondary tissue schizonts
   (E) Proguanil complexes with double-stranded DNA, blocking replication

2. Which antimalarial drug causes a dose-dependent toxic state that includes flushed and sweaty skin, dizziness, nausea, diarrhea, tinnitus, blurred vision, and impaired hearing?
   (A) Amodiaquine
   (B) Primaquine
   (C) Pyrimethamine
   (D) Quinine
   (E) Sulfadoxine

3. Plasmodial resistance to chloroquine is due to
   (A) Change in receptor structure
   (B) Decreased accumulation of the drug in the food vacuole
   (C) Increase in the activity of DNA repair mechanisms
   (D) Induction of drug-inactivating enzymes
   (E) Increased synthesis of dihydrofolate reductase

4–6. A traveler in a geographical region where chloroquine-resistant *P falciparum* is endemic used a drug for prophylaxis but nevertheless developed a severe attack of *P vivax* malaria.

4. The drug taken for chemoprophylaxis was probably
   (A) Atovaquone
   (B) Mefloquine
   (C) Metronidazole
   (D) Primaquine
   (E) Quinine

5. Which drug should be used for oral treatment of the acute attack of *P vivax* malaria?
   (A) Chloroquine
   (B) Mefloquine
   (C) Primaquine
   (D) Pyrimethamine-sulfadoxine
   (E) Quinidine

6. Which drug should be given later to eradicate schizonts and latent hypnozoites in the patient's liver?
(A) Artemisinin
(B) Doxycycline
(C) Primaquine
(D) Proguanil
(E) Sulfadoxine

7–8. A male patient presents with lower abdominal discomfort, flatulence, and occasional diarrhea. A diagnosis of intestinal amebiasis is made, and *E histolytica* is identified in his diarrheal stools. An oral drug is prescribed, which reduces his intestinal symptoms. Later he presents with severe dysentery, right upper quadrant pain, weight loss, fever, and an enlarged liver. Amebic liver abscess is diagnosed, and the patient is hospitalized. He has a recent history of drug treatment for a tachyarrhythmia.

7. The preferred treatment that he *should* have received for the initial symptoms (which were indicative of mild to moderate disease) is
(A) Diloxanide furoate
(B) Emetine
(C) Metronidazole
(D) Metronidazole plus diloxanide furoate
(E) Paromomycin

8. The drug regimen most likely to be effective in treating severe extraintestinal disease in this patient is
(A) Chloroquine
(B) Diloxanide furoate plus iodoquinol
(C) Emetine plus diloxanide furoate plus chloroquine
(D) Metronidazole plus diloxanide furoate
(E) Pentamidine followed by mefloquine

9. This drug is the antimalarial agent most commonly associated with causing an acute hemolytic reaction in patients with glucose-6-phosphate dehydrogenase deficiency.
(A) Chloroquine
(B) Clindamycin
(C) Mefloquine
(D) Primaquine
(E) Quinine

10. After a backpacking trip in the mountains, a 24-year-old man develops diarrhea. He acknowledges drinking stream water without purification, and you suspect he is showing symptoms of giardiasis. Because you know that laboratory detection of cysts or trophozoites in the feces can be difficult, you decide to treat the patient empirically with
(A) Chloroquine
(B) Emetine
(C) Metronidazole
(D) Pentamidine
(E) TMP-SMX

11. This drug can clear trypanosomes from the blood and lymph nodes and is active in the late CNS stages of African sleeping sickness.
(A) Emetine
(B) Melarsoprol
(C) Nifurtimox
(D) Pentamidine
(E) Suramin

12. Metronidazole is not effective in the treatment of
(A) Amebiasis
(B) Infections resulting from *Bacteroides fragilis*
(C) Pneumocystosis
(D) Pseudomembranous colitis
(E) Trichomoniasis

13. Which drug is recommended as the agent of choice for oral treatment of uncomplicated malaria caused by chloroquine-resistant *P falciparum* strains?
(A) Atovaquone
(B) Iodoquinol
(C) Primaquine
(D) Proguanil
(E) Quinine

ANSWERS

1. Proguanil (not choroquine) is an inhibitor of dihydrofolate reductase. Primaquine (not mefloquine) is the drug that destroys secondary exoerythrocytic schizonts. The answer is **A**.

2. These dose-related symptoms are characteristic adverse effects of alkaloids (eg, quinine, quinidine) derived from the bark of the cinchona tree and are termed cinchonism. The answer is **D**.

3. Resistance to chloroquine in *P falciparum* can result from decreased accumulation of the drug in the food vacuole caused by the activity of a transporter system encoded by the *pfcrt* gene. The answer is **B**.

4. Mefloquine is a recommended drug for prophylaxis in regions of the world where chloroquine-resistant *P falciparum* is endemic. One dose of mefloquine weekly starting before travel and continuing until 4 weeks after leaving the region is the preferred regimen. Doxycycline is an alternative drug for this indication, as is atovaquone plus proguanil (Malarone). The answer is **B**.

5. Chloroquine is the drug of choice for the oral treatment of an acute attack of malaria caused by *P vivax* but will not eradicate exoerythrocytic forms of the parasite. The answer is **A**.

6. Primaquine is the only antimalarial drug that reliably acts on tissue schizonts in liver cells. Starting about day 4 after an acute attack, primaquine should be given daily for 2 weeks. The answer is **C**.

7. Metronidazole plus a luminal amebicide is the treatment of choice in mild to moderate amebic colitis. Diloxanide furoate (or iodoquinol) can be used as the sole agent in asymptomatic intestinal infection. The answer is **D**.

8. Metronidazole given for 10 days (or tinidazole for 5 days) plus a luminal agent is effective in most cases of hepatic abscess and has the dual advantage of being both amebicidal and active against anaerobic bacteria. Although active in amebic hepatic abscess, treatment with emetine is contraindicated in patients with a history of cardiac disease. The answer is **D**.

9. Primaquine is the prototypical drug that induces hemolysis in persons deficient in glucose-6-phosphate dehydrogenase. It may also occur, less frequently, during treatment with chloroquine or quinine. The answer is **D**.

10. Giardiasis is a common intestinal protozoan infection caused by *Giardia lamblia*. A large number of infections result from fecal contamination of food or water. Metronidazole is often the drug of choice, but tinidazole is equally effective. The answer is **C**.

11. In the advanced stages of African sleeping sickness, melarsoprol is the drug of choice because, unlike pentamidine or suramin, it effectively enters the CNS. Nifurtimox is the most commonly used drug for Chagas' disease. The answer is **B**.

12. Metronidazole is the drug of first choice for all of the conditions listed except pneumocystosis. The answer is **C**.

13. Quinine sulfate is the standard drug for oral treatment of acute attacks of malaria caused by chloroquine-resistant *P falciparum*. It should be used in combination with another antimalarial drug such as doxycycline, clindamycin, or pyrimethamine plus sulfadiazine. The answer is **E**.

CHECKLIST

When you complete this chapter, you should be able to:

☐ Name the major antimalarial drugs. Know which are used for chemoprophylaxis, which are effective in chloroquine resistance, and which are exoerythrocytic schizonticides.

☐ Identify the characteristic adverse effects of the major antimalarial drugs.

☐ Describe the clinical uses and adverse effects of metronidazole.

☐ Be able to identify the intestinal amebicides and backup drugs to metronidazole for amebiasis.

☐ Identify the drugs used for prophylaxis and treatment of pneumocystosis and toxoplasmosis and know their characteristic toxic effects.

☐ Identify the major drugs used for trypanosomiasis and leishmaniasis and know their characteristic toxic effects.

Anthelmintic Drugs

54

Anthelmintic drugs have diverse chemical structures, mechanisms of action, and properties. Most were discovered by empiric screening methods; many act against specific parasites, and few are devoid of significant toxicity to host cells. In addition to the direct toxicity of the drugs, reactions to dead and dying parasites may cause serious toxicity in patients. In the text that follows, the drugs are divided into 3 groups on the basis of the type of helminth primarily affected (nematodes, trematodes, and cestodes). The drugs of choice and alternative agents for selected important helmintic infections are listed in Table 54–1.

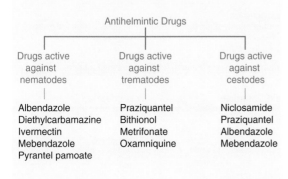

DRUGS THAT ACT AGAINST NEMATODES

The medically important intestinal nematodes responsive to drug therapy include *Enterobius vermicularis* (pinworm), *Trichuris trichiura* (whipworm), *Ascaris lumbricoides* (roundworm), *Ancyclostoma* and *Necator* species (hookworms), and *Strongyloides stercoralis* (threadworm). More than 1 billion persons worldwide are estimated to be infected by intestinal nematodes.

Pinworm infections are common throughout the United States, and hookworm and threadworm are endemic in the southern United States.

Tissue nematodes responsive to drug therapy include *Ancyclostoma* species, which cause cutaneous larva migrans. Species of *Dracunculus, Onchocerca, Toxocara,* and *Wuchereria bancrofti* (the cause of filariasis) are all responsive to drug treatment. The number of persons worldwide estimated to be infected by tissue nematodes exceeds 0.5 billion.

A. Albendazole

1. Mechanisms—The mechanism of action of albendazole is unclear. The drug blocks glucose uptake in both larval and adult parasites, which leads to decreased formation of adenosine triphosphate (ATP) and subsequent parasite immobilization. The actions of albendazole may also include inhibition of microtubule assembly, as has been described for mebendazole and thiabendazole.

2. Clinical use—Albendazole has a wide anthelmintic spectrum. It is a primary drug for ascariasis, hookworm, pinworm, and whipworm infections and an alternative drug for treatment of threadworm infections, filariasis, and both visceral and cutaneous larva migrans. Albendazole is also used in hydatid disease and is active against the pork tapeworm in the larval stage (cysticercosis).

3. Toxicity—Albendazole has few toxic effects during short courses of therapy. However, a reversible leukopenia, alopecia, and elevation of liver function enzymes can occur with more prolonged use. Long-term animal toxicity studies have described bone marrow suppression and fetal toxicity. The safety of the drug in pregnancy and in young children has not been established.

B. Diethylcarbamazine

1. Mechanisms—Diethylcarbamazine immobilizes microfilariae by an unknown mechanism, increasing their susceptibility to host defense mechanisms.

2. Clinical use—Diethylcarbamazine is the drug of choice for a few filarial infections including eye worm disease (loa loa) and is an alternative drug for elephantiasis.

Table 54–1. Drugs for the treatment of helmintic infections.

Infecting Organism	Drugs of Choice	Alternative Drugs
Nematodes		
Ascaris lumbricoides (roundworm)	Albendazole *or* mebendazole *or* pyrantel pamoate	Piperazine
Necator americanus and *Ancylostoma duodenale* (hookworm)	Pyrantel pamoate *or* albendazole *or* mebendazole	
Trichuris trichiura (whipworm)	Albendazole *or* mebendazole	Pyrantel pamoate
Strongyloides stercoralis (threadworm)	Ivermectin	Albendazole, mebendazole
Enterobius vermicularis (pinworm)	Mebendazole *or* pyrantel pamoate	Albendazole
Trichinella spiralis (trichinosis)	Mebendazole (+/– corticosteroids)	Albendazole
Cutaneous larva migrans	Albendazole or ivermectin	
Wuchereria bancrofti and *Brugia malayi* (filariasis)	Diethylcarbamazine	Ivermectin
Onchocerca volvulus (onchocerciasis)	Ivermectin	
Trematodes (flukes)		
Schistosoma haematobium	Praziquantel	Metrifonate
Schistosoma mansoni	Praziquantel	Oxamniquine
Schistosoma japonicum	Praziquantel	
Paragonimus westermani	Praziquantel	
Fasciola hepatica (sheep liver fluke)	Bithional or triclabendazole	
Fasciolopsis buski (large intestinal fluke)	Praziquantel or niclosamide	
Cestodes (tapeworms)		
Taenia saginata (beef tapeworm)	Praziquantel or niclosamide	Mebendazole
Taenia solium (pork tapeworm)	Praziquantel or niclosamide	
Cysticercosis (pork tapeworm larval stage)	Albendazole	Praziquantel
Diphyllobothrium latum (fish tapeworm)	Praziquantel or niclosamide	
Echinococcus granulosus (hydatid disease)	Albendazole	

The drug undergoes renal elimination and its half-life is increased significantly by urinary alkalinization.

3. Toxicity—Adverse effects include headache, malaise, weakness, and anorexia. Reactions to proteins released by dying filariae include fever, rashes, ocular damage, joint and muscle pain, and lymphangitis. In onchocerciasis, the **Mazzotti reaction** includes most of these symptoms as well as hypotension, pyrexia, respiratory distress, and prostration.

C. IVERMECTIN

1. Mechanisms—Ivermectin intensifies γ-aminobutyric acid (GABA)-mediated neurotransmission in nematodes and causes immobilization of parasites, facilitating their removal by the reticuloendothelial system. Selective toxicity results because in humans GABA is a neurotransmitter only in the CNS, and ivermectin does not cross the blood-brain barrier.

2. Clinical use

Ivermectin is the drug of choice for onchocerciasis, cutaneous larva migrans, strongyloidiasis, and some forms of filariasis.

3. Toxicity

Single-dose oral treatment in onchocerciasis results in Mazzotti reactions, including fever, headache, dizziness, rashes, pruritus, tachycardia, hypotension, and pain in joints, muscles, and lymph glands. These symptoms are usually of short duration, and most can be controlled with antihistamines and nonsteroidal anti-inflammatory drugs. Ivermectin should not be used in pregnancy.

D. MEBENDAZOLE

1. Mechanism—Mebendazole acts by selectively inhibiting microtubule synthesis and glucose uptake in nematodes.

2. Clinical use—Mebendazole is a primary drug for treatment of ascariasis and for pinworm and whipworm infections. Mebendazole has also been used as a backup drug in visceral larval migrans. Less than 10% of the drug is absorbed systemically after oral use, and this portion is metabolized rapidly by hepatic enzymes. Plasma levels may be decreased by carbamazepine or phenytoin and increased by cimetidine.

3. Toxicity—Mebendazole toxicity is usually limited to gastrointestinal irritation, but at high doses agranulocytopenia and alopecia have occurred. The drug is teratogenic in animals and therefore contraindicated in pregnancy.

E. PIPERAZINE

1. Mechanism—Piperazine paralyzes ascaris by acting as an agonist at GABA receptors. The paralyzed roundworms are expelled live by normal peristalsis.

2. Clinical use—Piperazine is an alternative drug for ascariasis.

3. Toxicity—Mild gastrointestinal irritation is the most common side effect. Piperazine should not be used in patients with seizure disorders.

F. PYRANTEL PAMOATE

1. Mechanism—Pyrantel pamoate stimulates nicotinic receptors present at neuromuscular junctions of nematodes. Contraction of muscles occurs, followed by a depolarization-induced paralysis. The drug has no actions on flukes or tapeworms.

2. Clinical use—Pyrantel pamoate has wide activity against nematodes, killing adult worms in the colon but not the eggs. It is a drug of choice for hookworm and roundworm infections and an alternative drug for pinworms. The drug is poorly absorbed when given orally.

3. Toxicity—Adverse effects are minor but include gastrointestinal distress, headache, and weakness.

G. THIABENDAZOLE

1. Mechanism—Thiabendazole is a structural congener of mebendazole and has a similar action on microtubules.

2. Clinical use—Because of its adverse effects, thiabendazole is an alternative drug in strongyloidiasis and trichinosis (adult worms). Thiabendazole is rapidly absorbed from the gut and is metabolized by liver enzymes. The drug has anti-inflammatory and immunorestorative actions in the host.

3. Toxicity—Thiabendazole's toxic effects include gastrointestinal irritation, headache, dizziness, drowsiness, leukopenia, hematuria, and allergic reactions, including intrahepatic cholestasis. Reactions caused by dying parasites include fever, chills, lymphadenopathy, and skin rash.

 SKILL KEEPER: ANTIMICROBIAL CHEMOTHERAPY IN PREGNANCY

Mebendazole is widely used for the treatment of nematode infections but is contraindicated in the pregnant patient because of possible embryotoxicity. Think back over the drugs used for the treatment of bacterial, fungal, protozoal, and viral infections.

1. *Which drugs are associated with a greater risk compared with benefit in pregnancy?*

2. *Which drugs are nominally contraindicated in pregnancy but might be used if the benefit was judged to outweigh the risk?*

The Skill Keeper Answers appear at the end of the chapter.

DRUGS THAT ACT AGAINST TREMATODES

The medically important trematodes include *Schistosoma* species (blood flukes, estimated to affect more than 150 million persons worldwide), *Clonorchis sinensis* (liver fluke, endemic in Southeast Asia), and *Paragonimus westermani* (lung fluke, endemic to both Asia and the Indian subcontinent). With few exceptions, fluke infections respond well to praziquantel.

A. PRAZIQUANTEL

1. Mechanism—Praziquantel increases membrane permeability to calcium, causing marked contraction initially and then paralysis of trematode and cestode muscles; this is followed by vacuolization and parasite death.

2. Clinical use—Praziquantel has a wide anthelmintic spectrum that includes activity in both trematode and cestode infections. It is the drug of choice in schistosomiasis (all species), clonorchiasis, and paragonimiasis and for infections caused by small and large intestinal flukes. The drug is active against immature and adult schistosomal forms. Praziquantel is also 1 of 2 drugs of choice (with niclosamide) for infections caused by cestodes (all common tapeworms) and an alternative agent in the treatment of cysticercosis.

3. Pharmacokinetics—Absorption from the gut is rapid, and the drug is metabolized by the liver to inactive products.

4. Toxicity—Common adverse effects include headache, dizziness, drowsiness, malaise, and, less frequently, gastrointestinal irritation, skin rash, and fever. Neurologic effects can occur in the treatment of neurocysticercosis, including intracranial hypertension and seizures. Corticosteroid therapy reduces the risk of the more serious reactions. Praziquantel is contraindicated in ocular cysticercosis.

B. BITHIONOL

1. Clinical use—Bithionol is the drug of choice for treatment of fascioliasis (sheep liver fluke) and an alternative agent in paragonimiasis. The mechanism of action of the drug is unknown. Bithionol is orally effective and is eliminated in the urine.

2. Toxicity—Common adverse effects include nausea and vomiting, diarrhea and abdominal cramps, dizziness, headache, and phototoxicity. Less frequently, pyrexia, tinnitus, proteinuria, and leukopenia may occur.

C. METRIFONATE

Metrifonate is an organophosphate prodrug that is converted in the body to the cholinesterase inhibitor dichlorvos. The active metabolite acts solely against *Schistosoma haematobium* (the cause of bilharziasis). Toxic effects occur from excess cholinergic stimulation.

D. OXAMNIQUINE

Oxamniquine is effective solely in *Schistosoma mansoni* infections (intestinal bilharziasis), acting on male immature forms and adult schistosomal forms. Dizziness is a common adverse effect; headache, gastrointestinal irritation, and pruritus may also occur. Reactions to dying parasites include eosinophilia, urticaria, and pulmonary infiltrates. It is not advisable to use the drug in pregnancy or in patients with a history of seizure disorders.

DRUGS THAT ACT AGAINST CESTODES (TAPEWORMS)

The 4 medically important cestodes are *Taenia saginata* (beef tapeworm), *Taenia solium* (pork tapeworm, which

can cause cysticerci in the brain and the eyes), *Diphyllobothrium latum* (fish tapeworm), and *Echinococcus granulosus* (dog tapeworm, which can cause hydatid cysts in the liver, lungs, and brain). The primary drugs for treatment of cestode infections are praziquantel (see prior discussion) and niclosamide.

A. NICLOSAMIDE

1. Mechanism—Niclosamide may act by uncoupling oxidative phosphorylation or by activating ATPases.

2. Clinical use—Niclosamide is 1 of 2 drugs of choice (with praziquantel) for infections caused by beef, pork, and fish tapeworm infections. However, it is not effective in cysticercosis (for which albendazole or praziquantel is used) or hydatid disease caused by *Echinococcus granulosus* (for which albendazole is used). Scoleces and cestode segments are killed, but ova are not. Niclosamide is effective in the treatment of infections from small and large intestinal flukes.

3. Toxicity—Toxic effects are usually mild but include gastrointestinal distress, headache, rash, and fever. Some of these effects may result from systemic absorption of antigens from disintegrating parasites.

QUESTIONS

1. Which drug causes muscle paralysis in nematodes by enhancing the actions of the inhibitory transmitter GABA?
   (A) Albendazole
   (B) Diethylcarbamazine
   (C) Ivermectin
   (D) Mebendazole
   (E) Pyrantel pamoate

2. A patient is to be treated with niclosamide. Which parasite is susceptible to this drug?
   (A) *Ascaris lumbricoides*
   (B) *Echinococcus granulosus*
   (C) *Enterobius vermicularis*
   (D) *Necator americanus*
   (E) *Taenia solium*

3. A missionary from Chicago is sent to work in a geographic region of a Central American country where *Onchocerca volvulus* is endemic. Infections resulting from this tissue nematode (onchocerciasis) are a cause of "river blindness," because microfilariae migrate through subcutaneous tissues and concentrate in the eyes. Which drug should be used prophylactically to prevent onchocerciasis?
   (A) Bithionol
   (B) Diethylcarbamazine
   (C) Ivermectin
   (D) Oxamniquine
   (E) Suramin

4. A nonindigenous individual who develops onchocerciasis in an endemic region and receives drug treatment is likely to experience the Mazzotti reaction. Which statement concerning this reaction is accurate?
   (A) Characteristic symptoms include hematuria, leukopenia, and allergic reactions, including intrahepatic cholestasis
   (B) Extensive fluid replacement is essential
   (C) Symptoms are more intense in indigenous adults than expatriate adults
   (D) The reaction is due to drug toxicity
   (E) The reaction is due to killing of microfilariae

5. Which statement about pyrantel pamoate is accurate?
   (A) It acts as an agonist at GABA receptors
   (B) It is equivalent in efficacy to niclosamide in the treatment of tapeworm infections
   (C) Its hepatotoxicity is dose limiting
   (D) It is synergistic with praziquantel in fluke infections
   (E) The drug kills adult worms in the colon but not the eggs

6. A student studying medicine at a Caribbean university develops fever, chills, and diarrhea resulting from *S mansoni,* and oxamniquine is prescribed. Which statements about the proposed therapy is accurate?
   (A) If the patient has a history of seizure disorders, hospitalization is recommended during treatment
   (B) It is not effective in late stages of the disease
   (C) Oxamniquine is safe to use in pregnancy
   (D) The drug is effective in other forms of schistosomiasis
   (E) The drug blocks GABA receptors in trematodes

7. A 22-year-old Korean male has recently moved to Minnesota. He has symptoms of clonorchiasis (anorexia, upper abdominal pain, eosinophilia), presumably contracted in his homeland, where the Oriental liver fluke is endemic. He also has symptoms of diphyllobothriasis (abdominal discomfort, diarrhea, megaloblastic anemia), probably caused by consumption of raw fish from lakes near the Canadian border. Which drug is most likely to be effective in the treatment of both clonorchiasis and diphyllobothriasis in this patient?
   (A) Albendazole
   (B) Ivermectin
   (C) Levamisole
   (D) Niclosamide
   (E) Praziquantel

8. Which helmintic infection does not respond to treatment with praziquantel?
   (A) Hydatid disease
   (B) Opisthorchiasis
   (C) Paragonimiasis
   (D) Pork tapeworm infection
   (E) Schistosomiasis

9-10. A sheepherder who lives most of the year in the mountains of eastern Nevada is hospitalized with liver cysts (hydatid disease) attributed to infection with *Echinococcus granulosus,* the dog tapeworm. He refuses to undergo surgery for removal of the cysts.

9. Which drug is most likely to be of some help in this situation?
   (A) Albendazole
   (B) Ivermectin
   (C) Niclosamide
   (D) Oxamniquine
   (E) Suramin

10. Since the patient will have to undergo drug treatment for many months, he should be monitored for toxicity to the
   (A) Gonads
   (B) Kidney
   (C) Liver
   (D) Peripheral nerves
   (E) Retina

11. Which adverse effect occurs with the use of mebendazole during intestinal nematode therapy?
   (A) Cholestatic jaundice
   (B) Corneal opacities
   (C) Mazzotti reactions
   (D) Peripheral neuropathy
   (E) None of the above

12. A malnourished 12-year-old child who lives in a rural area of the southern United States presents with weakness, fever, cough, abdominal pain, and eosinophilia. His mother tells you that she has seen long, thin worms in the child's stools, sometimes with blood. A presumptive diagnosis of ascariasis is confirmed by the presence of the ova of *A lumbricoides* in the stools. However, microscopy also reveals that the stools contain the eggs of *Necator americanus.* The drug most likely to be effective in the treatment of this child is
   (A) Diethylcarbamazine
   (B) Ivermectin
   (C) Mebendazole
   (D) Niclosamide
   (E) Praziquantel

ANSWERS

1. Ivermectin and piperazine (not listed in the question) both cause muscle paralysis in nematodes by acting through GABA receptors. Pyrantel pamoate relaxes muscles by blocking nicotinic receptors.

Diethylcarbamazine also causes muscle relaxation, but the mechanism is unknown. The answer is **C**.

2. Niclosamide is not active against nematodes but does have activity in certain intestinal fluke infections. It is considered a drug of choice to treat common tapeworm infections because it is usually effective in a single dose. It is minimally absorbed from the gastrointestinal tract and causes few side effects. The answer is **E**.

3. Ivermectin prevents onchocerciasis and is the drug of choice in the individual and mass treatment of the disease. The only other drugs active against *Onchocerca volvulus* are suramin and diethylcarbamazine (not listed). They are no longer recommended for onchocerciasis because they are less effective and more toxic than ivermectin. The answer is **C**.

4. The Mazzotti reaction is due to the killing action of ivermectin on microfilariae, and its intensity correlates with skin microfilaria load. It is not a drug toxicity. Symptoms include headache, weakness, rash, muscle aches, hypotension, and peripheral edema. It occurs more frequently and with greater severity in nonindigenous persons than in the indigenous inhabitants of endemic areas. The answer is **E**.

5. Pyrantel pamoate, an activator of nicotinic receptors, is equivalent to albendazole and mebendazole in the treatment of common nematode infections. The drug causes only mild gastrointestinal side effects and it is not hepatotoxic. It is not effective in the treatment of infections caused by cestodes or flukes. The answer is **E**.

6. Oxamniquine may cause seizures, especially in persons with a history of convulsive disorders. Such persons should be hospitalized or treated with praziquantel. Oxamniquine is effective in all stages of disease caused by *S mansoni*, including advanced hepatosplenomegaly. It has been used extensively for mass treatment. The drug is not effective in other schistosomal diseases, and it is contraindicated in pregnancy. The answer is **A**.

7. Praziquantel is a primary drug for treatment of infections caused by the Oriental liver fluke and by the fish tapeworm. Both types of infection are transmitted mainly via the consumption of raw fish. Niclosamide is also a primary drug for fish tapeworm infections but it is not active against *Clonorchis sinensis*. Albendazole is not effective in fish tapeworm infections but is useful in the pork tapeworm larval stage (cysticercosis). The answer is **E**.

8. Praziquantel has a wide spectrum of activity that includes many cestodes and trematodes. However, in hydatid disease the drug has marginal efficacy because it does not affect the inner germinal membrane of *Echinococcus granulosus* present in hydatid cysts. The answer is **A**.

9. The optimal treatment of hydatid cysts is their surgical removal. Albendazole has been used—at high doses for 3 mo or longer, combined with drainage—for liver hydatid cysts. However, the cure rate, judged by shrinkage or disappearance of cysts, is less than 40%. The answer is **A**.

10. Elevations of aminotransferase occur most frequently (15–20% incidence) during long-term therapy with albendazole. Jaundice has been reported, and patients may also suffer from alopecia and mild leukopenia. The answer is **C**.

11. Doses of mebendazole required for intestinal nematode therapy are almost free of adverse effects even in the malnourished or debilitated patient. Gastrointestinal distress may occur in children with ascariasis who are heavily parasitized, together with a slight headache or dizziness. The answer is **E**.

SKILL KEEPER ANSWERS: ANTIMICROBIAL CHEMOTHERAPY IN PREGNANCY

1. *In the United States a drug is designated (by the FDA) as Pregnancy Risk Category **X** if the risk of its use in pregnancy is judged to be greater than any possible benefit. Such drugs have been established to cause fetal abnormalities or miscarriage in humans. This category includes the antiviral agent ribavirin and the antimalarial drug quinine. Clomiphene, ergots, ethionamide, HMG-CoA reductase inhibitors, isotretinoin, misoprostol, Premarin, and thalidomide are also category **X** drugs.*

2. *For drugs in FDA Pregnancy Risk Category **D**, there is evidence of human risk, but their potential benefit may outweigh such risk. In other words, they are not absolutely contraindicated in pregnancy. These include aminoglycosides (eg, gentamicin) and tetracyclines. Although they are not category **D** drugs, fluoroquinolones are not approved by the FDA for use in pregnancy, and many other drugs should be used with caution or avoided if alternatives are available.*

12. Mebendazole is effective against both nematodes causing infection in this child. Albendazole and pyrantel pamoate (not listed in this question) are also primary drugs for the treatment of combined infections due to hookworm and roundworm. The answer is **C.**

CHECKLIST

When you complete this chapter, you should be able to:

☐ List the clinical uses and the adverse effects of albendazole/mebendazole, diethylcarbamazepine, ivermectin, and pyrantel pamoate.

☐ Name the anthelmintic drug (or drugs) that (1) facilitate the actions of GABA, (2) increase calcium permeability in muscle, (3) activate nicotinic receptors, and (4) disrupt microtubule function.

☐ Describe the clinical uses and adverse effects of both praziquantel and niclosamide.

Cancer Chemotherapy

55

Cancer chemotherapy remains an intriguing area of pharmacology. On the one hand, use of anticancer drugs produces high rates of cure of diseases that, without chemotherapy, result in extremely high mortality rates (eg, acute lymphocytic leukemia in children, testicular cancer, Hodgkin's lymphoma). On the other hand, some types of cancer are barely affected by currently available drugs. Furthermore, as a group, the anticancer drugs are more toxic than any other pharmaceutic agents, and thus their benefit must be carefully weighed against their risks. Many of the available drugs are cytotoxic agents that act on all dividing cells, cancerous or normal. The ultimate goal in cancer chemotherapy is to use advances in cell biology to develop drugs that selectively target specific cancer cells. A few such agents are in clinical use, and many more are in development.

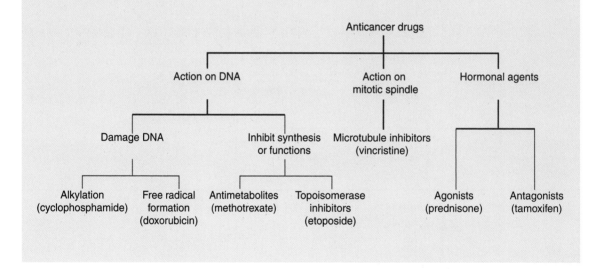

CANCER CELL CYCLE KINETICS

A. Cell Cycle Kinetics

Cancer cell population kinetics and the cancer cell cycle are important determinants of the actions and clinical uses of anticancer drugs. Some anticancer drugs act specifically on tumor cells undergoing cycling (cell cycle-specific [CCS] drugs), and others (cell cycle-nonspecific [CCNS] drugs) kill tumor cells in both cycling and resting phases of the cell cycle. CCS drugs are usually most active in a specific phase of the cell cycle (Figure 55–1). CCS drugs are particularly effective when a large proportion of the tumor cells are proliferating (ie, when the growth fraction is high).

HIGH-YIELD TERMS TO LEARN

Cell cycle-nonspecific (CCNS) drug	An anticancer agent that acts on tumor stem cells when they are traversing the cell cycle and when they are in the resting phase
Cell cycle-specific (CCS) drug	An anticancer agent that acts selectively on tumor stem cells when they are traversing the cell cycle and not when they are in the G_0 phase
Growth fraction	The proportion of cells in a tumor population that are actively dividing
Log-kill hypothesis	A concept used in cancer chemotherapy to mean that anticancer drugs kill a fixed proportion of a tumor cell population, not a fixed number of tumor cells. For example, a 1-log-kill will decrease a tumor cell population by one order of magnitude (ie, 90% of the cells will be eradicated)
Myelosuppressant	A drug that suppresses the formation of mature blood cells such as erythrocytes, leukocytes, and platelets. This effect is also known as "bone marrow suppression"
Oncogene	A mutant form of a normal gene that is found in naturally occurring tumors and which, when expressed in noncancerous cells, causes them to behave like cancer cells
Rescue therapy	The administration of endogenous metabolites to counteract the effects of anticancer drugs on normal (nonneoplastic) cells
Vesicant	A drug that causes blisters on contact with tissues. Such drugs can be particularly damaging to veins if administered in high concentrations into small vessels. The alkylating agent mechlorethamine is an example

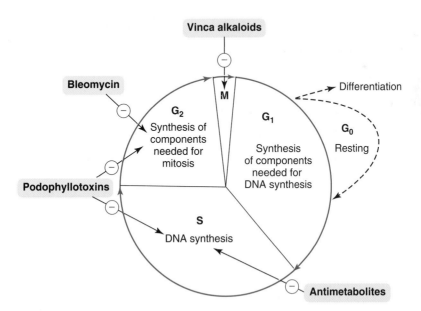

Figure 55–1. Phases of the cell cycle that are susceptible to the actions of cell cycle-specific (CCS) drugs. All dividing cells—normal and neoplastic—must traverse these cell cycle phases before and during cell division. Tumor cells are usually most responsive to specific drugs (or drug groups) in the phases indicated. Cell cycle-nonspecific (CCNS) drugs act on tumor cells while they are actively cycling and while they are in the resting phase (G_0). (Adapted, with permission, from Katzung BG, editor: *Basic & Clinical Pharmacology,* 7th ed. Originally published by Appleton & Lange. Copyright © 1998 by The McGraw-Hill Companies, Inc.)

B. THE LOG-KILL HYPOTHESIS

Cytotoxic drugs act with first-order kinetics. That is, a given dose kills a constant *proportion* of a cell population rather than a constant *number* of cells. The log-kill hypothesis proposes that the magnitude of tumor cell kill by anticancer drugs is a logarithmic function. For example, a 3-log-kill dose of an effective drug will reduce a cancer cell population of 10^{12} cells to 10^9 (a total kill of 999×10^9 cells); the same dose would reduce a starting population of 10^6 cells to 10^3 cells (a kill of 999×10^3 cells). In both cases, the dose reduces the numbers of cells by 3 orders of magnitude, or "3 logs."

C. RESISTANCE TO ANTICANCER DRUGS

Drug resistance is a major problem in cancer chemotherapy. Mechanisms of resistance include the following:

1. Increased DNA repair—An increased rate of DNA repair in tumor cells can be responsible for resistance and is particularly important for alkylating agents and cisplatin.

2. Formation of trapping agents—Some tumor cells increase their production of thiol trapping agents (eg, glutathione), which interact with anticancer drugs that form reactive electrophilic species. This mechanism of resistance is seen with the alkylating agent bleomycin, cisplatin, and the anthracyclines.

3. Changes in target enzymes—Changes in the drug sensitivity of a target enzyme, dihydrofolate reductase, and increased synthesis of the enzyme are mechanisms of resistance of tumor cells to methotrexate.

4. Decreased activation of prodrugs—Resistance to the purine antimetabolites (mercaptopurine, thioguanine) and the pyrimidine antimetabolites (cytarabine, fluorouracil) can result from a decrease in the activity of the tumor cell enzymes needed to convert these prodrugs to their cytotoxic metabolites.

5. Inactivation of anticancer drugs—Increased activity of enzymes capable of inactivating anticancer drugs is a mechanism of tumor cell resistance to most of the purine and pyrimidine antimetabolites.

6. Decreased drug accumulation—This form of multidrug resistance involves the increased expression of a normal gene (the *MDR1* gene) for a cell surface glycoprotein (P-glycoprotein). This transport molecule is involved in the accelerated efflux of many anticancer drugs in resistant cells.

ALKYLATING AGENTS

The alkylating agents include nitrogen mustards (**chlorambucil, cyclophosphamide, mechlorethamine**), nitrosoureas (**carmustine, lomustine**), and alkylsulfonates (**busulfan**). Other drugs that act in part as alkylating agents include **cisplatin, dacarbazine,** and **procarbazine.**

The alkylating agents are CCNS drugs. They form reactive molecular species that alkylate nucleophilic groups on DNA bases, particularly the N-7 position of guanine. This leads to cross-linking of bases, abnormal base pairing, and DNA strand breakage. Tumor cell resistance to the drugs occurs through increased DNA repair, decreased drug permeability, and the production of trapping agents such as thiols.

A. CYCLOPHOSPHAMIDE

1. Pharmacokinetics—Hepatic cytochrome P450-mediated biotransformation of cyclophosphamide is needed for antitumor activity. One of the breakdown products is **acrolein.**

2. Clinical use—Uses of cyclophosphamide include non-Hodgkin's lymphoma, breast and ovarian cancers, and neuroblastoma.

3. Toxicity—Gastrointestinal distress, myelosuppression, and alopecia are expected adverse effects. Hemorrhagic cystitis resulting from the formation of acrolein may be decreased by vigorous hydration and by use of mercaptoethanesulfonate (**mesna**). Cyclophosphamide may also cause cardiac dysfunction, pulmonary toxicity, and a syndrome of inappropriate antidiuretic hormone (ADH) secretion.

B. MECHLORETHAMINE

1. Mechanism and pharmacokinetics—Mechlorethamine spontaneously converts in the body to a reactive cytotoxic product.

2. Clinical use—Mechlorethamine is best known for use in regimens for Hodgkin's lymphoma.

3. Toxicity—Gastrointestinal distress, myelosuppression, alopecia, and sterility are common. Mechlorethamine has marked vesicant actions.

C. PLATINUM ANALOGS (CISPLATIN, CARBOPLATIN, OXALIPLATIN)

1. Pharmacokinetics—Cisplatin is used intravenously; the drug distributes to most tissues and is cleared in unchanged form by the kidney.

2. Clinical use—Cisplatin is commonly used as a component of regimens for testicular carcinoma and for cancers of the bladder, lung, and ovary. Carboplatin has similar uses. Oxaliplatin is used in advanced colon cancer.

3. Toxicity—Cisplatin causes gastrointestinal distress and mild hematotoxicity and is neurotoxic (peripheral neuritis and acoustic nerve damage) and nephrotoxic. Renal damage may be reduced by the use of mannitol with forced hydration. Carboplatin is less nephrotoxic than cisplatin and is less likely to cause tinnitus and hearing loss, but it has greater myelosuppressant actions. Oxaliplatin causes dose-limiting neurotoxicity.

D. Procarbazine

1. Mechanisms—Procarbazine is a reactive agent that forms hydrogen peroxide, which generates free radicals that cause DNA strand scission.

2. Pharmacokinetics—Procarbazine is orally active and penetrates into most tissues, including the cerebrospinal fluid. It is eliminated via hepatic metabolism.

3. Clinical use—The primary use of the drug is as a component of regimens for Hodgkin's lymphoma.

4. Toxicity—Procarbazine is a myelosuppressant and causes gastrointestinal irritation, CNS dysfunction, peripheral neuropathy, and skin reactions. Procarbazine inhibits many enzymes, including monoamine oxidase (MAO) and those involved in hepatic drug metabolism. Disulfiram-like reactions have occurred with ethanol. The drug is leukemogenic.

E. Other Alkylating Agents

Busulfan is sometimes used in chronic myelogenous leukemia. It causes adrenal insufficiency, pulmonary fibrosis, and skin pigmentation. Carmustine (BCNU) and lomustine (CCNU) are highly lipid-soluble drugs used as adjuncts in the management of brain tumors. Dacarbazine is used in regimens for Hodgkin's lymphoma. It causes alopecia, skin rash, gastrointestinal distress, myelosuppression, phototoxicity, and a flulike syndrome.

ANTIMETABOLITES

The antimetabolites are structurally similar to endogenous compounds and are antagonists of folic acid (**methotrexate**), purines (**mercaptopurine, thioguanine**), or pyrimidines (**fluorouracil, cytarabine, gemcitabine**). Antimetabolites are CCS drugs acting primarily in the S phase of the cell cycle. Their sites of action on DNA synthetic pathways are shown in Figure 55–2. In addition to their cytotoxic effects on neoplastic cells, the antimetabolites also have immunosuppressant actions. Some of the uses of the antimetabolites in neoplastic disease are listed in Table 55–1.

A. Methotrexate

1. Mechanisms of action and resistance—Methotrexate is a substrate for and inhibitor of dihydrofolate reductase. This action leads to a decrease in the synthesis of thymidylate, purine nucleotides, and amino acids and thus interferes with nucleic acid and protein metabolism. The formation of polyglutamate derivatives of methotrexate appears to be important for cytotoxic actions. Tumor cell resistance mechanisms include decreased drug accumulation, changes in the drug sensitivity or activity of dihydrofolate reductase, and decreased formation of polyglutamates.

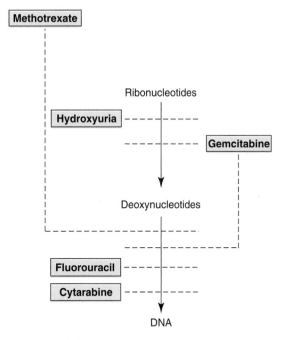

Figure 55–2. Sites of action of antimetabolites on DNA synthetic pathways.

2. Pharmacokinetics—Oral and intravenous administration of methotrexate affords good tissue distribution except to the CNS. Methotrexate is not metabolized, and its clearance is dependent on renal function. Adequate hydration is needed to prevent crystallization in renal tubules.

3. Clinical use—Methotrexate is effective in choriocarcinoma, acute leukemias, non-Hodgkin's and cutaneous T-cell lymphomas, and breast cancer. Methotrexate is used also in rheumatoid arthritis psoriasis (Chapter 36) and ectopic pregnancy and is an abortifacient.

4. Toxicity—Common adverse effects include bone marrow suppression and toxic effects on the skin and gastrointestinal mucosa (mucositis). The toxic effects of methotrexate on normal cells may be reduced by administration of folinic acid (leucovorin); this strategy is called **"leucovorin rescue."** Long-term use of methotrexate has led to hepatotoxicity and to pulmonary infiltrates and fibrosis. Salicylates, NSAIDs, sulfonamides, and sulfonylureas enhance the toxicity of methotrexate.

B. Mercaptopurine (6-MP) and Thioguanine (6-TG)

1. Mechanisms of action and resistance—Mercaptopurine and thioguanine are purine antimetabolites. Both drugs are activated by hypoxanthine-guanine

Table 55–1. Selected examples of cancer chemotherapy.

Diagnosis	Current Drug Therapy of Choice
Acute lymphocytic leukemia	Induction: vincristine plus prednisone Remission maintenance: mercaptopurine, methotrexate, and cyclophosphamide
Acute myelogenous leukemia	Cytarabine and mitoxantrone, or daunorubicin, or idarubicin
Breast carcinoma	Adjuvant combination chemotherapy with cytotoxic agents, hormonal therapy with tamoxifen or an aromatase inhibitor (eg, anastrozole), trastuzumab
Chronic myelogenous leukemia	Imatinib, busulfan, or interferon
Colon carcinoma	Fluorouracil plus leucovorin plus oxaliplatin
Hodgkin's lymphoma	ABVD regimen: doxorubicin (Adriamycin) plus bleomycin plus vincristine plus dacarbazine plus prednisone
Non-Hodgkin's lymphoma	Cyclophosphamide, doxorubicin, vincristine, prednisone
Ovarian carcinoma	Paclitaxel and cisplatin or carboplatin
Pancreatic carcinoma	Gemcitabine
Prostate carcinoma	Leuprolide and androgen receptor antagonist (eg, flutamide)
Lung carcinoma	Cisplatin plus paclitaxel or docetaxel
Testicular carcinoma	PEB regimen: cisplatin (Platinol), etoposide, and bleomycin

Modified and reproduced, with permission, from Katzung BG, editor: *Basic & Clinical Pharmacology*, 10th ed. McGraw-Hill, 2007.

phosphoribosyltransferases (HGPRTases) to toxic nucleotides that inhibit several enzymes involved in purine metabolism. Resistant tumor cells have a decreased activity of HGPRTase, or they may increase their production of alkaline phosphatases that inactivate the toxic nucleotides.

2. Pharmacokinetics—Mercaptopurine and thioguanine have low oral bioavailability because of first-pass metabolism by hepatic enzymes. The metabolism of 6-MP by xanthine oxidase is inhibited by allopurinol.

3. Clinical use—Purine antimetabolites are used mainly in the acute leukemias and chronic myelocytic leukemia.

4. Toxicity—Bone marrow suppression is dose limiting, but hepatic dysfunction (cholestasis, jaundice, necrosis) also occurs.

C. FLUOROURACIL (5-FU)

1. Mechanisms—Fluorouracil is converted in cells to 5-fluoro-2′-deoxyuridine-5′-monophosphate (5-FdUMP), which inhibits thymidylate synthase and leads to "thymineless death" of cells. Tumor cell resistance mechanisms include decreased activation of 5-FU, increased thymidylate synthase activity, and reduced drug sensitivity of this enzyme.

2. Pharmacokinetics—When given intravenously, fluorouracil is widely distributed, including into the cerebrospinal fluid. Elimination is mainly by metabolism.

3. Clinical use—Fluorouracil is used in bladder, breast, colon, head and neck, liver, and ovarian cancers. The drug can be used topically for keratoses and superficial basal cell carcinoma.

4. Toxicity—Gastrointestinal distress, myelosuppression, and alopecia are common.

D. CYTARABINE (ARA-C)

1. Mechanisms of action and resistance—Cytarabine (cytosine arabinoside) is a pyrimidine antimetabolite. The drug is activated by kinases to AraCTP, an inhibitor of DNA polymerases. Of all the antimetabolites, cytarabine is the most specific for the S phase of the cell cycle. Resistance to cytarabine can occur as a result of its decreased uptake or its decreased conversion to AraCTP.

E. GEMCITABINE

1. Mechanisms—Gemcitabine is a deoxycytidine analog that is converted into the active diphosphate and triphosphate nucleotide form. Gemcitabine diphosphate appears to inhibit ribonucleotide reductase and thereby diminish the pool of deoxyribonucleoside triphosphates required for DNA synthesis. Gemcitabine triphosphate can be incorporated into DNA, where it causes chain termination.

2. Pharmacokinetics—Elimination is mainly by metabolism.

3. Clinical use—Gemcitabine was initially approved for pancreatic cancer and now is used widely in the treatment of non-small cell lung cancer, bladder cancer, and non-Hodgkin's lymphoma.

4. Toxicity—Primarily myelosuppression occurs, mainly as neutropenia. Pulmonary toxicity has been observed.

PLANT ALKALOIDS

The most important of these CCS drugs are the vinca alkaloids (**vinblastine, vincristine, vinorelbine**), the podophyllotoxins (**etoposide, teniposide**), the camptothecins (**topotecan, irinotecan**), and the taxanes (**paclitaxel, docetaxel**).

A. VINBLASTINE, VINCRISTINE, AND VINORELBINE

1. Mechanisms—The vinca alkaloids block the formation of the mitotic spindle by preventing the assembly of tubulin dimers into microtubules. They act primarily in the M phase of the cancer cell cycle. Resistance can occur from increased efflux of the drugs from tumor cells via the membrane drug transporter.

2. Pharmacokinetics—These drugs must be given parenterally. They penetrate most tissues except the cerebrospinal fluid. They are cleared mainly via biliary excretion.

3. Clinical use—Vincristine is used in acute leukemias, lymphomas, Wilms' tumor, and choriocarcinoma. Vinblastine is used for lymphomas, neuroblastoma, testicular carcinoma, and Kaposi's sarcoma. Vinorelbine is used in non-small cell lung cancer and in breast cancer.

4. Toxicity—Vinblastine and vinorelbine cause gastrointestinal distress, alopecia, and bone marrow suppression. Vincristine does not cause serious myelosuppression but has neurotoxic actions and may cause areflexia, peripheral neuritis, and paralytic ileus.

B. ETOPOSIDE AND TENIPOSIDE

1. Mechanisms—Etoposide increases degradation of DNA, possibly via interaction with topoisomerase II, and also inhibits mitochondrial electron transport. The drug is most active in the late S and early G_2 phases of the cell cycle. Teniposide is an analog with very similar pharmacologic characteristics.

2. Pharmacokinetics—Etoposide is well absorbed after oral administration and distributes to most body tissues. Elimination of etoposide is mainly via the kidneys, and

dose reductions should be made in patients with renal impairment.

3. Clinical use—These agents are used in combination drug regimens for therapy of lung (small cell), prostate, and testicular carcinoma.

4. Toxicity—Etoposide and teniposide are gastrointestinal irritants and cause alopecia and bone marrow suppression.

C. TOPOTECAN AND IRINOTECAN

1. Mechanisms—These agents inhibit topoisomerase I: They damage DNA by inhibiting an enzyme that cuts and relegates single DNA strands during normal DNA repair processes.

2. Pharmacokinetics—Irinotecan is a prodrug that is converted in the liver into an active metabolite. Topotecan is eliminated renally, whereas irinotecan and its metabolite are eliminated in the bile and feces.

3. Clinical use—Topotecan is used as a second-line therapy for advanced ovarian cancer and for small cell lung cancer. Irinotecan is used for metastatic colorectal cancer.

4. Toxicity—Myelosuppression and diarrhea are the 2 most common toxicities.

D. PACLITAXEL AND DOCETAXEL

1. Mechanisms—Paclitaxel and docetaxel interfere with the mitotic spindle. They act differently from vinca alkaloids as they prevent microtubule *disassembly* into tubulin monomers.

2. Pharmacokinetics—Paclitaxel and docetaxel are given intravenously.

3. Clinical use—The taxanes are used in advanced breast and ovarian cancers.

4. Toxicity—Paclitaxel causes neutropenia, thrombocytopenia, a high incidence of peripheral neuropathy, and possible hypersensitivity reactions during infusion. Docetaxel causes neurotoxicity and bone marrow depression.

ANTIBIOTICS

This category of antineoplastic drugs is made up of several structurally dissimilar agents, including **doxorubicin, daunorubicin, bleomycin, dactinomycin, and mitomycin.**

A. DOXORUBICIN AND DAUNORUBICIN

1. Mechanisms—These anthracyclines intercalate between base pairs, inhibit topoisomerase II, and generate free radicals. They block the synthesis of RNA and DNA and cause DNA strand scission. Membrane disruption also occurs. Anthracyclines are CCNS drugs.

2. Pharmacokinetics—Doxorubicin and daunorubicin must be given intravenously. They are metabolized in the liver, and the products are excreted in the bile and the urine.

3. Clinical use—Doxorubicin is used in Hodgkin's lymphoma, myelomas, sarcomas, and breast, endometrial, lung, ovarian, and thyroid cancers. The main use of daunorubicin is in the treatment of acute leukemias. Idarubicin, a newer anthracycline, is approved for use in acute myelogenous leukemia.

4. Toxicity—These drugs cause bone marrow suppression, gastrointestinal distress, and severe alopecia. Their most distinctive adverse effect is cardiotoxicity, which includes initial electrocardiographic abnormalities (with the possibility of arrhythmias) and slowly developing cardiomyopathy and congestive heart failure. **Dexrazoxane,** an inhibitor of iron-mediated free radical generation, may protect against cardiotoxicity. Liposomal formulations of doxorubicin may be less cardiotoxic.

B. BLEOMYCIN

1. Mechanisms—Bleomycin is a mixture of glycopeptides that generates free radicals, which bind to DNA, cause strand breaks, and inhibit DNA synthesis. Bleomycin is a CCS drug active in the G_2 phase of the tumor cell cycle.

2. Pharmacokinetics—Bleomycin must be given parenterally. It is inactivated by tissue aminopeptidases, but some renal clearance of intact drug also occurs.

3. Clinical use—Bleomycin is a component of drug regimens for Hodgkin's lymphoma and testicular cancer. It is also used for treatment of lymphomas and for squamous cell carcinomas.

4. Toxicity—The toxicity profile of bleomycin includes pulmonary dysfunction (pneumonitis, fibrosis), which develops slowly and is dose limiting. Hypersensitivity reactions (chills, fever, anaphylaxis) are common, as are mucocutaneous reactions (alopecia, blister formation, hyperkeratosis).

C. DACTINOMYCIN

1. Mechanisms and pharmacokinetics—Dactinomycin is a CCNS drug that binds to double-stranded DNA and inhibits DNA-dependent RNA synthesis. Dactinomycin must be given parenterally, and both intact drug and metabolites are excreted in the bile.

2. Clinical use—Dactinomycin is used in melanoma and Wilms' tumor.

3. Toxicity—This drug causes bone marrow suppression, skin reactions, and gastrointestinal irritation.

D. MITOMYCIN

1. Mechanisms and pharmacokinetics—Mitomycin is a CCNS drug that is metabolized by liver enzymes to form an alkylating agent that cross-links DNA. Mitomycin is given intravenously and is rapidly cleared via hepatic metabolism.

2. Clinical use—Mitomycin acts against hypoxic tumor cells and is used in combination regimens for adenocarcinomas of the cervix, stomach, pancreas, and lung.

3. Toxicity—Mitomycin causes severe myelosuppression and is toxic to the heart, liver, lung, and kidney.

HORMONAL ANTICANCER AGENTS

A. GLUCOCORTICOIDS

Prednisone is the most commonly used glucocorticoid in cancer chemotherapy and is widely used in combination therapy for leukemias and lymphomas. Toxicity is described in Chapter 39.

SKILL KEEPER: MANAGEMENT OF ANTICANCER DRUG HEMATOTOXICITY (SEE CHAPTER 33)

Bone marrow suppression is a characteristic toxicity of most cytotoxic anticancer drugs. What agents are available for the treatment of anemia and neutropenia, and for platelet restoration in patients undergoing cancer chemotherapy? The Skill Keeper Answer appears at the end of the chapter.

B. GONADAL HORMONE ANTAGONISTS

Tamoxifen, a selective estrogen receptor modulator (see Chapter 40), blocks the binding of estrogen to receptors of estrogen-sensitive cancer cells in breast tissue. The drug is used in receptor-positive breast carcinoma and has been shown to have a preventive effect in women at high risk for breast cancer. Because it has agonist activity in the endometrium, tamoxifen increases the risk of endometrial hyperplasia and neoplasia. Other adverse effects include nausea and vomiting, hot flushes, vaginal bleeding, and venous thrombosis. **Toremifene** is a newer estrogen receptor antagonist used in advanced breast cancer. **Flutamide** is an androgen receptor antagonist used in prostatic carcinoma (see Chapter 40). Adverse effects include gynecomastia, hot flushes, and hepatic dysfunction.

C. GONADOTROPIN-RELEASING HORMONE ANALOGS

Leuprolide, goserelin, and **nafarelin** are GnRH agonists, effective in prostatic carcinoma. When administered in constant doses so as to maintain stable blood levels, they *inhibit* release of pituitary luteinizing hormone (LH) and follicle-stimulating hormone (FSH). Leuprolide may cause bone pain, gynecomastia, hematuria, impotence, and testicular atrophy (see Chapters 37 and 40).

D. Aromatase Inhibitors

Anastrozole and letrozole inhibit aromatase, the enzyme that catalyzes the conversion of androstenedione (an androgenic precursor) to estrone (an estrogenic hormone). Both drugs are used in advanced breast cancer. Toxicity includes nausea, diarrhea, hot flushes, bone and back pain, dyspnea, and peripheral edema.

OTHER ANTICANCER AGENTS

A. Asparaginase

Asparaginase is an enzyme that depletes serum asparagine; it is used in the treatment of T-cell auxotrophic cancers (leukemia and lymphomas) that require exogenous asparagine for growth. Asparaginase is given intravenously and may cause severe hypersensitivity reactions, acute pancreatitis, and bleeding.

B. Imatinib

Imatinib is an example of a selective anticancer drug whose development was guided by knowledge of a specific oncogene. It inhibits the tyrosine kinase activity of the protein product of the Bcr-Abl oncogene that is commonly expressed in chronic myelogenous leukemia (CML). In addition to its activity in CML, imatinib is effective for treatment of gastrointestinal stromal tumors that express the c-*kit* tyrosine kinase, which is also inhibited. Resistance may occur from mutation of the Bcr-Abl gene. Toxicity of imatinib includes diarrhea, myalgia, and fluid retention.

C. Interferons

The interferons are endogenous glycoproteins with antineoplastic, immunosuppressive, and antiviral actions. Alpha-interferons (see Chapter 56) are effective against a number of neoplasms, including hairy cell leukemia, the early stage of CML, and T-cell lymphomas. Toxic effects of the interferons include myelosuppression and neurologic dysfunction.

D. Rituximab

Rituximab is a monoclonal antibody that binds to a surface protein in non-Hodgkin's lymphoma cells and

Table 55–2. Selected examples of anticancer drug toxicity.

Drug	Toxicity
Bleomycin	Pneumonitis, pulmonary fibrosis, alopecia
Cisplatin	Nephrotoxicity, ototoxicity, bone marrow suppression
Cyclophosphamide	Bone marrow suppression, hemorrhagic cystitis (consider mesna), alopecia
Doxorubicin	Bone marrow suppression, cardiotoxicity (often delayed, consider dexrazoxane)
Etoposide	Bone marrow suppression, alopecia
Fluorouracil	Bone marrow suppression, oral and gastrointestinal ulcers, diarrhea
Gemcitabine	Bone marrow suppression, pulmonary toxicity
Mercaptopurine	Bone marrow suppression, cholestasis, oral and gastrointestinal ulcers, pancreatitis
Methotrexate	Bone marrow suppression, oral and gastrointestinal ulcers, hepatoxicity, pulmonary dysfunction
Paclitaxel	Bone marrow suppression, peripheral neuropathy, alopecia
Rituximab	Bone marrow suppression, fever, chills, hypersensitivity reactions
Topotecan	Bone marrow suppression, diarrhea
Trastuzumab	Fever, chills, rash, cardiac dysfunction
Vinblastine	Bone marrow suppression, alopecia, muscle pain
Vincristine	Peripheral neuropathy, paralytic ileus

induces complement-mediated lysis, direct cytotoxicity, and induction of apoptosis. It is currently used with conventional anticancer drugs (eg, cyclophosphamide plus vincristine plus prednisone) in low-grade lymphomas. Rituximab use is associated with hypersensitivity reactions and myelosuppression.

E. Growth Factor Receptor Inhibitors

Trastuzumab, a monoclonal antibody, recognizes a surface protein in breast cancer cells that overexpress the HER-2/*neu* receptor for epidermal growth factor. Acute toxicity of this antibody includes nausea and vomiting,

chills, fevers, and headache. Trastuzumab may cause cardiac dysfunction, including congestive heart failure.

Several drugs inhibit the epidermal growth factor receptor (EGFR), which is distinct from the Her-2/*neu* receptor for epidermal growth factor that is targeted by trastuzumab. The EGFR regulates signaling pathways involved in cellular proliferation, invasion and metastasis, and angiogenesis. It is also implicated in inhibiting the cytotoxic activity of some anticancer drugs and radiation therapy. **Cetuximab** is a monoclonal antibody directed to the extracellular domain of the EGFR. It is used in combination with irinotecan and oxaliplatin for

---

KEY DRUGS

Subclass	Prototype	Other Significant Agents
Alkylating agent		
Nitrogen mustards	Cyclophosphamide	Mechlorethamine
Alkylsulfonates	Busulfan	
Platinum complex	Cisplatin	Carboplatin
Triazenes	Dacarbazine	
Hydrazines	Procarbazine	
Antimetabolites		
Folate analogs	Methotrexate	
Purine analogs	Mercaptopurine	Thioguanine
Pyrimidine analogs	Fluorouracil	Cytarabine, gemcitabine
Plant alkaloids		
Vinca alkaloids	Vinblastine	Vincristine
Podophyllotoxins	Etoposide	Teniposide
Camptothecins	Topotecan	Irinotecan
Other	Paclitaxel	Docetaxel
Antibiotics		
Anthracyclines	Doxorubicin	Daunorubicin
Bleomycins	Bleomycin	
Actinomycins	Dactinomycin	
Mitomycins	Mitomycin	
Hormones		
Adrenocorticoids	Prednisone	Hydrocortisone
Antiestrogens		
Receptor blockers	Tamoxifen	Toremifene
Aromatase inhibitors	Anastrozole	Letrozole
Antiandrogens	Flutamide	Bicalutamide
Gonadotropin-releasing hormone agonists	Leuprolide	Goserelin, nafarelin
Monoclonal antibodies	Rituximab, trastuzumab	
Tyrosine kinase inhibitor	Imatinib	
Growth factor inhibitors	Cetuximab Gefitinib Bevacizumab	Erlotinib

metastatic colon cancer and is used in combination with radiation for head and neck cancer. Its primary toxicity is skin rash and a hypersensitivity infusion reaction. **Gefitinib** and **erlotinib** are small molecule inhibitors of the EGFR's tyrosine kinase domain. Both are used as second-line agents for non-small cell lung cancer, and erlotinib is also used in combination therapy of advanced pancreatic cancer. Rash and diarrhea are the main toxicities.

Bevacizumab is a monoclonal antibody that binds to vascular endothelial growth factor (VEGF) and prevents it from interacting with VEGF receptors. VEGF plays a critical role in the angiogenesis required for tumor metastasis. Bevacizumab is approved for treatment of metastatic colorectal cancer. Adverse effects include hypertension, arterial thrombosis, impaired wound healing, gastrointestinal perforation, and proteinuria.

STRATEGIES IN CANCER CHEMOTHERAPY

A. PRINCIPLES OF COMBINATION THERAPY

Chemotherapy with combinations of anticancer drugs usually increases log kill markedly and in some cases synergistic effects are achieved. Combinations are often cytotoxic to a heterogeneous population of cancer cells and may prevent development of resistant clones. Drug combinations using CCS and CCNS drugs may be cytotoxic to both dividing and resting cancer cells. The following principles are important for selecting appropriate drugs to use in combination chemotherapy:

(1) Each drug should be active when used alone against the particular cancer.

(2) The drugs should have different mechanisms of action.

(3) Cross-resistance between drugs should be minimal.

(4) The drugs should have different toxic effects (Table 55–2).

B. RESCUE THERAPY

Toxic effects of anticancer drugs can sometimes be alleviated by rescue strategy. For example, high doses of methotrexate may be given for 36–48 h and terminated before severe toxicity occurs to cells of the gastrointestinal tract and bone marrow. **Leucovorin,** a form of tetrahydrofolate that is accumulated more readily by normal than by neoplastic cells, is then administered. This results in rescue of the normal cells because leucovorin bypasses the dihydrofolate reductase step in folic acid synthesis. Mercaptoethanesulfonate (**mesna**) "traps" acrolein released from cyclophosphamide and thus reduces the incidence of hemorrhagic cystitis. **Dexrazoxane** inhibits free radical formation and affords protection against the cardiac toxicity of anthracyclines (eg, doxorubicin).

QUESTIONS

1–3. A 32-year-old woman underwent segmental mastectomy for a breast tumor of 3 cm diameter. Lymph node sampling revealed 2 involved nodes. Because chemotherapy is of established value in her situation, she underwent postoperative treatment with antineoplastic drugs. The FAC-V regimen was used, consisting of fluorouracil, doxorubicin (Adriamycin), and cyclophosphamide, plus vincristine. Six cycles 1 mo apart of this chemotherapy regimen were planned. Adjunctive drugs included tamoxifen because the tumor cells were hormone receptor positive.

1. The mechanism of anticancer action of cellular metabolites of fluorouracil is
   (A) Cross-linking of double-stranded DNA
   (B) Inhibition of DNA-dependent RNA synthesis
   (C) Interference with the activity of topoisomerases I
   (D) Irreversible inhibition of thymidylate synthase
   (E) Selective inhibition of DNA polymerases

2. The chemotherapy undertaken by this patient caused acute hemorrhagic cystitis. The drug that was responsible for this toxicity was
   (A) Cyclophosphamide
   (B) Doxorubicin
   (C) Fluorouracil
   (D) Tamoxifen
   (E) Vincristine

3. Between drug cycles 3 and 4, the patient was found to have a high resting pulse rate. A noninvasive radionuclide scan revealed evidence of cardiotoxicity, and a change in the drug regimen was suggested for the next cycle of treatment. The drug that is most likely responsible for the cardiac toxicity is
   (A) Cyclophosphamide
   (B) Doxorubicin
   (C) Fluorouracil
   (D) Tamoxifen
   (E) Vincristine

4. A cell cycle-specific anticancer drug that acts mainly in the M phase of the cell cycle is
   (A) Bleomycin
   (B) Cisplatin
   (C) Etoposide
   (D) Methotrexate
   (E) Paclitaxel

5. An adult patient is being treated for acute leukemia with a combination of anticancer drugs that includes cyclophosphamide, mercaptopurine, methotrexate, vincristine, and prednisone. He is also using ondansetron for emesis, a chlorhexidine mouthwash to reduce mucositis, and laxatives. The patient complains of "pins and needle" sensations in

the extremities and muscle weakness. He is not able to execute a deep knee bend or get up out of a chair without using his arm muscles. He is also very constipated. If these problems are related to the chemotherapy, the most likely causative agent is
(A) Cyclophosphamide
(B) Mercaptopurine
(C) Methotrexate
(D) Prednisone
(E) Vincristine

6. A drug that is used in combination therapy of testicular carcinoma and is associated with nephrotoxicity is
(A) Bleomycin
(B) Cisplatin
(C) Etoposide
(D) Leuprolide
(E) Vinblastine

7. A cancer cell that is resistant to the effects of both vincristine and methotrexate probably has developed the resistance as a result of
(A) Changes in the properties of a target enzyme
(B) Decreased activity of an activating enzyme
(C) Increased expression of a P-glycoprotein transporter
(D) Increased production of drug-trapping molecules
(E) Increase in proteins that are involved in DNA repair

8–9. A 23-year-old man with Hodgkin's lymphoma was treated unsuccessfully with the MOPP regimen (mechlorethamine, vincristine, prednisone, procarbazine). He subsequently underwent a successful course of therapy with the ABVD regimen (doxorubicin, bleomycin, vinblastine, dacarbazine).

8. Which of the following classes of anticancer drugs used in the treatment of this patient is cell cycle specific (CCS) and is used in both the MOPP and ABVD regimens?
(A) Alkylating agents
(B) Antibiotics
(C) Antimetabolites
(D) Glucocorticoids
(E) Plant alkaloids

9. During the second course of drug treatment (ABVD regimen), this patient developed dyspnea, a nonproductive cough, and intermittent fever. Chest x-ray film revealed pulmonary infiltration. If these problems are due to the anticancer drugs to which he has been exposed, the most likely causative agent is
(A) Bleomycin
(B) Dacarbazine

(C) Doxorubicin
(D) Prednisone
(E) Vinblastine

10. All of the following agents have been used in drug regimens for the treatment of breast carcinoma. Which one has specific activity in a subset of female breast cancers?
(A) Cyclophosphamide
(B) Doxorubicin
(C) Fluoxymesterone
(D) Methotrexate
(E) Trastuzumab

DIRECTIONS: 11–13. For each numbered item, select the ONE lettered option from the following list that is most closely associated with it. Each lettered option may be selected once, more than once, or not at all.
(A) Bleomycin
(B) Cytarabine
(C) Dacarbazine
(D) Doxorubicin
(E) Etoposide
(F) Flutamide
(G) Fluorouracil
(H) Leuprolide
(I) Mechlorethamine
(J) Mercaptopurine
(K) Methotrexate
(L) Paclitaxel
(M) Procarbazine
(N) Tamoxifen
(O) Vincristine

11. If allopurinol is used adjunctively in cancer chemotherapy to offset hyperuricemia, the dosage of this anticancer drug should be reduced to 25% of normal.

12. This drug is used in combination therapy for testicular carcinoma. It is a CCS drug that acts in the late S and early G_0 phases of the tumor cell cycle via interactions with topoisomerase II.

13. This antimetabolite inhibits DNA polymerase and is one of the most active drugs in leukemias. Although myelosuppression is dose limiting, the drug may also cause cerebellar dysfunction, including ataxia and dysarthria.

ANSWERS

1. Fluorouracil (5-FU) undergoes metabolism to form 5-fluoro-2′-deoxyuridine 5′-phosphate (5-dUMP). This metabolite forms a covalently bound ternary complex with thymidylate synthase and its coenzyme N-methylenetetrahydrofolate. The synthesis of

thymine nucleotides is blocked, DNA synthesis is inhibited, and a "thymineless death" of cells results. The answer is **D**.

2. Acrolein, a toxic metabolite of cyclophosphamide that is concentrated in the urine, is associated with hemorrhagic cystitis. Mesna, a sulfur-containing substance that also concentrates in urine, can be administered in an attempt to prevent this complication. The answer is **A**.

3. A high resting pulse rate is one of the first signs of cardiotoxicity resulting from anthracyclines, which can include arrhythmias, cardiomyopathies, and congestive heart failure. The risk of cardiotoxicity depends on cumulative dosage, so doxorubicin should be discontinued. The answer is **B**.

4. The taxanes, paclitaxel and docetaxel, interfere with the separation of chromosomes during mitosis because of their effects on microtubules. The answer is **E**.

5. Neuropathy is a toxic side effect of vincristine. In its mildest form paresthesias occur, but it progresses to significant muscle weakness, initially in the quadriceps muscle group. Constipation is the most common symptom of autonomic neuropathy. The answer is **E**.

6. Nephrotoxicity is a characteristic toxicity of cisplatin. Renal toxicity can be reduced by slow intravenous infusion, maintenance of good hydration, and administration of mannitol to maximize urine flow. For testicular cancer, cisplatin is used in combination with etoposide and bleomycin. The answer is **B**.

7. The P-glycoprotein family of transporters moves foreign molecules out of cells. Cancer cells acquire resistance to multiple drugs that act through different mechanisms by increasing the expressions of genes encoding these transporters. The answer is **C**.

8. The cell cycle-specific drugs used in standard treatment protocols for Hodgkin's lymphoma are bleomycin and the vinca alkaloids. Vinblastine is used in the ABVD regimen, and vincristine (Oncovin) is used in the MOPP regimen. The answer is **E**.

9. The anticancer drug most commonly associated with pulmonary toxicity is bleomycin. The answer is **A**.

10. Each of the drugs listed has been used in drug regimens for breast cancer, but only trastuzumab has specificity in its actions. The drug is a monoclonal antibody to a surface protein in breast cancer cells that overexpress the HER-2 protein. Consequently, trastuzumab has value in a specific subset of breast cancers. The answer is **E**.

11. Allopurinol, a xanthine oxidase inhibitor, is given to control the hyperuricemia that occurs as a result of large cell kills in the successful drug therapy of malignant diseases. The antimetabolite mercaptopurine is metabolized by xanthine oxidase and, in the presence of an inhibitor of this enzyme (eg, allopurinol), toxic levels of the drug may be reached rapidly. The answer is **J**.

12. Bleomycin, etoposide, and vinblastine are all CCS drugs used for the treatment of testicular carcinoma. Bleomycin is an antibiotic, not a plant alkaloid. Vinblastine is a spindle poison that acts in the M phase of the cell cycle. The answer is **E**.

13. The pyrimidine antimetabolite cytarabine (Ara-C) is commonly used in drug regimens for the acute leukemias. Cytarabine is dose limited by hematotoxicity. Cerebellar dysfunction may also occur with Ara-C, especially if the drug is used at high doses. The answer is **B**.

SKILL KEEPER ANSWER: MANAGEMENT OF ANTICANCER DRUG HEMATOTOXICITY (SEE CHAPTER 33)

Recombinant DNA technology has provided several agents that have value in the management of hematotoxicity caused by anticancer drugs. Erythropoietin stimulates red cell formation by interaction with receptors on erythroid progenitors in bone marrow. Myeloid growth factors filgrastim (G-CSF) and sargramostim (GM-CSF) stimulate the production and function of neutrophils. Megakaryocyte growth factor oprelvekin (IL-11) stimulates the growth of platelet progenitors.

CHECKLIST

When you complete this chapter, you should be able to:

☐ Describe the relevance of cell cycle kinetics to the modes of action and clinical uses of anticancer drugs.

☐ Identify the major subclasses of anticancer drugs and describe the mechanisms of action of the main drugs in each subclass

☐ List the mechanisms by which tumor cells develop drug resistance.

☐ Name 3 anticancer drugs that are "cell cycle specific" and act at different phases of the cell cycle.

☐ Identify a distinctive "characteristic" toxicity for each of the following anticancer drugs: bleomycin, cisplatin, cyclophosphamide, doxorubicin, and vincristine.

☐ Describe the rationale underlying strategies of combination drug chemotherapy and rescue therapies.

Immunopharmacology 56

Although the immune system is essential for protection against pathogens, in certain instances its powerful destructive mechanisms do more harm than good. Examples include hypersensitivity reactions, autoimmune disorders, and rejection reactions to transplanted tissues. Drugs that suppress immune mechanisms play an important role in treating these conditions. In other situations, drugs that potentiate the immune response provide benefit.

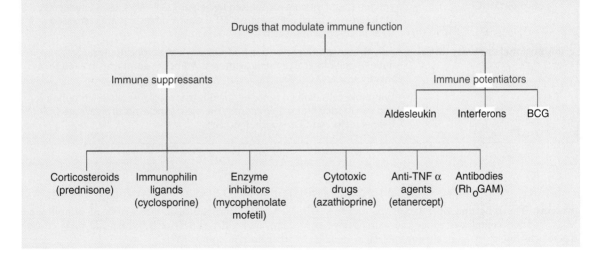

IMMUNE MECHANISMS

A. OVERVIEW

Employing the concerted actions of complement components, lysozyme, macrophages, and neutrophils, the *innate* immune system initiates the defense against pathogens and antigenic insult. If the innate response is inadequate, the *adaptive* immune response is mobilized. This culminates in the activation of T lymphocytes, the effectors of **cell-mediated immunity,** and the production of antibodies, by activated B lymphocytes, the effectors of **humoral immunity.** The subsets of lymphocytes that mediate different parts of the immune response can be identified by specific cell surface components or **clusters of differentiation (CDs).** For

example, helper T cells bear the CD4 protein complex, whereas cytotoxic T lymphocytes express the CD8 protein complex. Clusters of differentiation also can be used to characterize other types of hematopoietic cells, including precursors of granulocytes, megakaryocytes, and erythrocytes (see Chapter 33).

B. ANTIGEN RECOGNITION AND PROCESSING

This critical inaugural step in the adaptive immune response involves **antigen-presenting cells (APCs),** which process antigens into small peptides that can be recognized by T-cell receptors (TCRs) on the surface of T helper (TH) cells (Figure 56–1). The most important antigen-presenting cell surface molecules are the **major histocompatibility complex (MHC) class I and II**

HIGH-YIELD TERMS TO LEARN

Antigen-presenting cells (APCs)	Dendritic and Langerhans cells, macrophages, and B lymphocytes involved in the processing of proteins into cell surface forms recognizable by lymphoid cells
B cells	Lymphoid cells derived from the bone marrow that mediate humoral immunity through the formation of antibodies
Clusters of differentiation (CDs)	Specific cell surface constituents identified by number (eg, CD1, CD2)
Cytokines	Polypeptide modulators of cellular functions, including interferons, interleukins, and growth-stimulating factors
Immunophilins	A family of cytoplasmic proteins that bind to the immunosuppressants cyclosporine, tacrolimus, and sirolimus and assist these drugs in inhibiting T- and B-cell function. Cyclophilin binds cyclosporine, whereas FK-binding protein (FKBP) binds tacrolimus and sirolimus
Major histocompatibility complex (MHC)	Cell surface molecules that bind antigen fragments and, when bound to antigen fragments, are recognized by helper T cells. MHC class I molecules are expressed by all cells, whereas MHC class II molecules are expressed by antigen-presenting cells
Monoclonal antibody (MAb)	An antibody produced by a hybridoma clone that specifically targets an antigen of biological or medical interest. MAbs are employed in a range of therapeutic areas
T cells	Lymphoid cells derived from the thymus that mediate cellular immunity and can modify humoral immunity. The main subclasses of T cells are CD4 (helper) cells and CD8 (suppressor) cells

---

proteins. The activation of T_H cells by the class II MHC-peptide complex requires the participation of specific costimulatory and adhesion molecules in addition to activation of TCRs.

C. Cell-Mediated Immunity

Activated T_H cells secrete interleukin-2 (IL-2), a cytokine that causes proliferation and activation of 2 subsets of T helper cells, T_H1 and T_H2 (Figure 56–1). T_H1 cells orchestrate cell-mediated immunity and delayed hypersensitivity reactions. They produce interferon (IFN)-γ, IL-2, and tumor necrosis factor (TNF)-β. These cytokines activate macrophages, cytotoxic T lymphocytes (CTLs), and **natural killer (NK)** cells. Activated CTLs recognize processed peptides that are bound to class I MHC molecules on the surface of virus-infected or tumor cells. The CTLs induce target cell death via lytic enzyme and nitric oxide production and by stimulation of apoptosis pathways in the target cells. CTLs also play a role in autoimmune diseases by reacting against normal tissues, such as the synovium in rheumatoid arthritis and myelin in multiple sclerosis. NK cells kill both virus-infected and neoplastic cells.

They are also the main precursors of lymphokine-activated killer (LAK) cells, which are toxic to cells that do not express MHC.

D. Humoral Immunity

The **B lymphoid cells,** which are capable of differentiating into antibody-forming cells, mediate humoral immunity. The humoral response is triggered when B lymphocytes bind antigen via their surface immunoglobulins. The antigens are internalized, processed into peptides, bound to MHC class II molecules and presented on the B cell surface. When T-cell receptors on T_H2 cells are activated by the of MHC II-peptide complex, they release interleukins (IL-4, IL-5, IL-6). These cytokines induce B-lymphocyte proliferation and differentiation into memory B cells and antibody-secreting plasma cells (Figure 56–1). Antibodies produced by plasma cells bind to antigens on the surface of pathogens and trigger the precipitation of viruses and the destruction of bacteria by phagocytic cells or lysis by the complement system.

The proliferation and differentiation of both B and T lymphocytes is under the control of a complex interplay

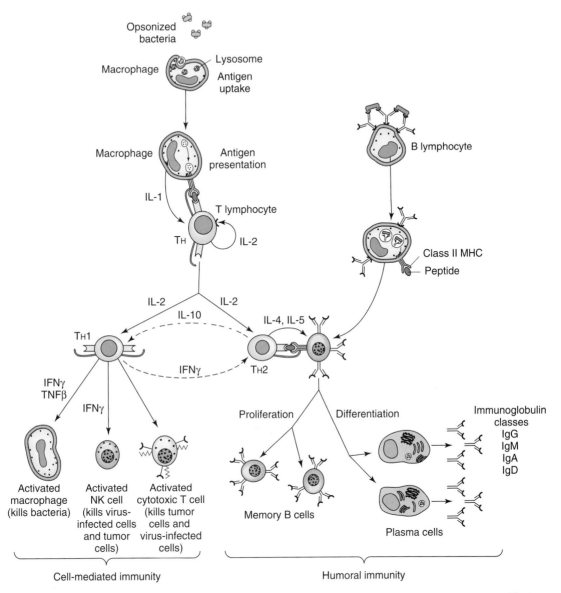

Figure 56-1. Scheme of cell-mediated and humoral immune responses. An immune response is initiated by internalization and processing of antigen by an antigen-presenting cell such as a macrophage. The class II MHC-peptide complex is recognized by the TCR on T helper cells, resulting in T-cell activation. Activated TH cells secrete cytokines such as IL-2, which cause proliferation and activation of CTLs, and TH1 and TH2 cell subsets. TH1 cells also produce IFN-γ and TNF-β, which activate macrophages and NK cells. A humoral response is triggered when B lymphocytes bind antigen via their surface immunoglobulins. They are then induced by TH2-derived cytokines (eg, IL-4, IL-5) to proliferate and differentiate into memory cells and antibody-secreting plasma cells. (Modified and reproduced, with permission, from Katzung BG, editor: *Basic & Clinical Pharmacology*, 10th ed. McGraw-Hill, 2007.)

between the cytokines (Table 56–1) and other endogenous molecules, including leukotrienes, and prostaglandins. For example, IL-10 and IFN-γ downregulate TH1 and TH2 responses, respectively (Figure 56–1).

E. ABNORMAL IMMUNE RESPONSES

Abnormal immune responses include hypersensitivity, autoimmunity, and immunodeficiency states. Immediate hypersensitivity is usually antibody mediated and

Table 56–1. Cytokines that modulate immune responses.

Cytokine	Characteristic Properties
Interferon-α (IFN-α)	Activates NK cells, antiviral, oncostatic
Interferon-β (IFN-β)	Activates NK cells, antiviral, oncostatic
Interferon-γ (IFN-γ)	Activates TH1, NK, cytotoxic T cells, and macrophages; antiviral, oncostatic
Interleukin-1 (IL-1)	T-cell activation, B-cell proliferation
Interleukin-2 (IL-2)	T-cell proliferation, activation of TH1, NK, and LAK cells
Interleukin-11 (IL-11)	B-cell differentiation (megakaryocyte proliferation, see Chapter 33)
Tumor necrosis factor-α (TNF-α)	Proinflammatory, macrophage activation, oncostatic
Tumor necrosis factor-β (TNF-β)	Proinflammatory, chemotactic, oncostatic
Granulocyte colony-stimulating factor (G-CSF)	Granulocyte production (see Chapter 33)
Granulocyte-macrophage colony-stimulating factor (GM-CSF)	Granulocyte, monocyte, eosinophil production (see Chapter 33)
Macrophage colony-stimulating factor (M-CSF)	Monocyte production, macrophage activation

Modified and reproduced, with permission, from Katzung BG, editor: *Basic & Clinical Pharmacology,* 10th ed. McGraw-Hill, 2007.

includes anaphylaxis and hemolytic disease of the newborn. Delayed hypersensitivity, associated with extensive tissue damage, is cell mediated. Autoimmunity arises from self-reactive lymphocytes that react to one's own molecules, or self-antigens. Examples of autoimmune diseases that are amenable to drug treatment include rheumatoid arthritis and systemic lupus erythematosus. Immunodeficiency states can be genetically acquired (eg, DiGeorge syndrome) or can result from extrinsic factors (eg, HIV infection).

IMMUNOSUPPRESSIVE AGENTS

A. CORTICOSTEROIDS

1. Mechanism of action—Glucocorticoids act at multiple cellular sites to cause broad effects on inflammatory and immune processes (see Chapter 39). At the biochemical level, their actions on gene expression decrease the synthesis of prostaglandins, leukotrienes, cytokines, and other signaling molecules that participate in immune responses (eg, platelet activating factor). At the cellular level, the glucocorticoids inhibit the proliferation of T lymphocytes (suppressing cellular immunity) and, to a lesser degree, dampen humoral immunity. At doses used for immunosuppression, the glucocorticoids are cytotoxic to certain subsets of T cells. Continuous therapy lowers IgG levels by increasing catabolism of this class of immunoglobulins.

2. Clinical use—Glucocorticoids are used alone or in combination with other agents in a wide variety of medical conditions that have an underlying undesirable immunologic reaction (see Chapter 39). Their ability to induce apoptosis in immune cells makes them useful for the treatment of several types of cancer (see Chapter 55). Corticosteroids are also used to suppress immunologic reactions in patients who undergo organ transplantation.

3. Toxicity—Predictable adverse effects include adrenal suppression, growth inhibition, muscle wasting, osteoporosis, salt retention, glucose intolerance, and possible psychoses (see Chapter 39).

B. CYCLOSPORINE, TACROLIMUS, AND SIROLIMUS

1. Mechanism of action—These immunosuppressants interfere with T-cell function by binding to **immunophilins,** small cytoplasmic proteins that play critical roles in T-cell responses to TCR activation and to cytokines. **Cyclosporine** binds to cyclophilin and **tacrolimus** binds to FK-binding protein (FKBP). Both complexes inhibit **calcineurin,** a cytoplasmic phosphatase. Calcineurin regulates the ability of the nuclear factor of activated T cells (NF-AT) to translocate to the nucleus and increase the production of cytokines. Cyclophilin and tacrolimus both inhibit the production of cytokines that normally occurs in response to TCR activation. **Sirolimus** also binds to FKBP. However, it inhibits the response of T cells to cytokines without affecting cytokine production. Sirolimus is a potent inhibitor of B-cell proliferation, antibody production, and mononuclear cell responses to colony-stimulating factors.

2. Clinical uses and pharmacokinetics—Use of these immunosuppressants is a major factor in the success of solid organ transplantation. Cyclosporine is used in solid organ transplantation and in graft-versus-host (GVH) disease. Tacrolimus is used in solid organ and stem cell transplantation and for GVH disease. Sirolimus is used alone or in combination with cyclosporine in solid organ transplantation and is being investigated for use in GVH disease. These agents, particularly cyclosporine, are also used in some autoimmune diseases, including rheumatoid arthritis, uveitis, psoriasis, asthma, and type 1 diabetes.

Cyclosporine and tacrolimus are available as oral or intravenous agents, while sirolimus is only available as an oral drug. Because cyclosporine exhibits erratic bioavailability, serum levels should be monitored. The drug undergoes slow hepatic metabolism by the cytochrome P450 system and has a long half-life. Its metabolism is affected by a host of other drugs.

3. Toxicity—Cyclosporine and tacrolimus have similar toxicity profiles. The most frequent adverse effects are renal dysfunction, hypertension, and neurotoxicity. They can also cause hyperglycemia, hyperlipidemia, and cholelithiasis. Sirolimus is more likely than the other agents to cause hypertriglyceridemia, hepatotoxicity, diarrhea, and myelosuppression.

C. Mycophenolate Mofetil

1. Mechanism of action—This drug is rapidly converted into mycophenolic acid, which inhibits inosine monophosphate dehydrogenase, an enzyme in the de novo pathway of purine synthesis. This action suppresses both B- and T-lymphocyte activation. Lymphocytes are particularly susceptible to inhibitors of the de novo pathway because they lack the enzymes necessary for the alternative salvage pathway for purine synthesis.

2. Clinical use—The drug has been used successfully as a sole agent in kidney, liver, and heart transplants. In renal transplants, its use with low-dose cyclosporine has reduced cyclosporine-induced nephrotoxicity.

3. Toxicity—This drug can cause gastrointestinal disturbances and myelosuppression, especially neutropenia.

D. Azathioprine

1. Mechanism of action—This prodrug is transformed to the antimetabolite mercaptopurine, which on further metabolic conversion inhibits enzymes involved in purine metabolism. Azathioprine is cytotoxic in the early phase of lymphoid cell proliferation and has a greater effect on the activity of T cells than B cells.

2. Clinical use—Azathioprine is used in autoimmune diseases (eg, systemic lupus erythematosus, rheumatoid arthritis) and for immunosuppression in renal homografts. The drug has minimal effects on established graft rejections.

3. Toxicity—The major toxic effect is bone marrow suppression, but gastrointestinal irritation, skin rashes, and liver dysfunction also occur. The use of azathioprine is associated with an increased incidence of cancer. The active metabolite of azathioprine, mercaptopurine, is metabolized by xanthine oxidase, and toxic effects may be increased by concomitant administration of allopurinol, a drug used for prevention of gout.

E. Cyclophosphamide

1. Mechanism of action—This orally active prodrug is transformed by liver enzymes to an alkylating agent that is cytotoxic to proliferating lymphoid cells. The drug has a greater effect on B cells than T lymphocytes and will inhibit an established immune response. Other cytotoxic drugs that similarly suppress proliferating lymphoid cells, and are sometimes used as immunosuppressants, include **cytarabine, dactinomycin, methotrexate,** and **vincristine** (see Chapter 55).

2. Clinical use—Cyclophosphamide is effective in autoimmune diseases (including hemolytic anemia), antibody-induced red cell aplasia, bone marrow transplants, and possibly other organ transplant procedures.

3. Toxicity—The large doses of the drug that are usually needed for immunosuppression cause pancytopenia, gastrointestinal distress, hemorrhagic cystitis, and alopecia. Cyclophosphamide (and other alkylating agents) may cause sterility.

F. Newer Immunosuppressants

1. Etanercept—This chimeric protein is a recombinant form of the human TNF receptor. The agent sequesters TNF-α, a proinflammatory cytokine, and thereby decreases formation of interleukins and adhesion molecules involved in leukocyte activation. Etanercept is used in rheumatoid arthritis and psoriatic arthritis and is being investigated in other inflammatory diseases. Injection site reactions and hypersensitivity may occur. Infliximab and adalimumab are monoclonal antibodies that also block the actions of TNF-α (see later discussion). All of these agents increase the risk of serious infection and lymphoma.

2. Leflunomide—This drug inhibits pyrimidine synthesis and arrests lymphocytes in the G₁ phase of the cell cycle. Leflunomide is used in rheumatoid arthritis. The drug can cause liver damage, renal impairment, and teratogenic effects and may cause cardiovascular effects (angina, tachycardia).

3. Thalidomide—This sedative drug, notorious for its teratogenic effects, has complex immune effects that include suppression of TNF production, increased IL-10, reduced neutrophil phagocytosis, altered adhesion molecule expression, and enhanced cell-mediated immunity. Thalidomide is used for some forms of leprosy reactions, for immunologic diseases (eg, systemic lupus), and as an anticancer drug. It is also effective in treating aphthous ulcers and the wasting syndrome in AIDS patients.

4. Alefacept—This engineered protein blocks the CD2 receptor found on the surface of T cells. The natural ligand for the CD2 receptor is lymphocyte-associated antigen 3 (LFA-3), a 55- to 70-kd protein expressed on the surface of many cells. Alefacept contains the CD2-binding region of LFA-3 fused to a human IgG Fc region. It inhibits T-cell activation and is approved for treatment of psoriasis. Treatment also causes a dose-dependent reduction in circulating T cells, so T-cell counts must be monitored in patients treated with the drug.

ANTIBODIES AS IMMUNOSUPPRESSANTS

A. ANTILYMPHOCYTE GLOBULIN AND ANTITHYMOCYTE GLOBULIN

1. Mechanism of action—Two types of antisera directed against lymphocytes are available. Antilymphocyte globulin (ALG) and antithymocyte globulin (ATG) are produced in horses or sheep by immunization against human thymus cells. Antibodies in these preparations bind to T cells involved in antigen recognition and initiate their destruction by serum complement. These antibodies selectively block cellular immunity rather than antibody formation, which accounts for their ability to suppress organ graft rejection, a cell-mediated process.

2. Clinical use—ALG and ATG are used before bone marrow transplantation to prevent the GVH reaction. They are also used in combination with cyclosporine or cytotoxic drugs (or both) for maintenance after bone marrow, heart, and renal transplantations.

3. Toxicity—Because humoral immunity may remain intact, injection of antilymphocyte globulin (ALG) or antithrombocyte globulin (ATG) can cause hypersensitivity reactions, including serum sickness and anaphylaxis. Pain and erythema occur at injection sites, and lymphoma has been noted as a late complication.

B. RH$_o$(D) IMMUNE GLOBULIN

1. Mechanism of action—Rh$_o$GAM is a human IgG preparation that contains antibodies against red cell Rh$_o$(D) antigens. Administration of this antibody to Rh$_o$(D)-negative, D^u-negative mothers at time of antigen exposure (ie, birth of an Rh$_o$(D)-positive, D^u-positive child) blocks the primary immune response to the foreign cells.

2. Clinical use—Rh$_o$(D) immune globulin is used for prevention of Rh hemolytic disease of the newborn. In women treated with Rh$_o$(D) immune globulin, maternal antibodies to Rh-positive cells are not produced in subsequent pregnancies, and hemolytic disease of the neonate is averted.

C. MONOCLONAL ANTIBODIES

Monoclonal antibodies (MAbs) have the potential advantage of high specificity because they can be developed for interaction with a single molecule. "Humanization" of murine monoclonal antibodies has reduced the likelihood of formation of neutralizing antibodies and of immune reactions. Characteristics of some therapeutic MAbs are shown in Table 56–2.

1. Muromonab-CD3—This MAb binds to the CD3 antigen on the surface of human thymocytes and mature T cells. It blocks the killing action of cytotoxic T cells and probably interferes with other T-cell functions. Muromonab-CD3 is used to manage renal transplant rejection crises. First-dose effects include fever, chills, dyspnea, and pulmonary edema. Hypersensitivity reactions may also occur.

2. Daclizumab—Daclizumab is a highly specific MAb that binds to the alpha subunit of the IL-2 receptor displayed on the surface of T cells and prevents activation by IL-2. It is used in combination with other immunosuppressants to prevent renal transplant rejection. In contrast to cyclosporine, tacrolimus, or cytotoxic immunosuppressants, the adverse effects of daclizumab are equivalent to those of placebo. **Basiliximab** is a chimeric human mouse IgG with an action that is equivalent to that of daclizumab.

3. Infliximab—This humanized MAb has a mechanism similar to that of etanercept because it is targeted against TNF-α. Infliximab induces remissions in treatment-resistant Crohn's disease. In combination with methotrexate, infliximab improves symptoms in patients with rheumatoid arthritis. It also is effective in the treatment of ulcerative colitis, ankylosing spondylitis, and psoriatic arthritis. Infusion reactions and an increased rate of infection may occur. **Adalimumab** is a completely human IgG monoclonal antibody that binds to TNF-α and is approved for treatment of rheumatoid arthritis.

IMMUNOMODULATING AGENTS

Agents that stimulate immune responses represent a newer area in immunopharmacology with the potential for important therapeutic uses, including the treatment of immune deficiency diseases, chronic infectious diseases, and cancer.

A. ALDESLEUKIN

Aldesleukin is recombinant **interleukin-2 (IL-2)**, an endogenous lymphokine that promotes the production

Table 56–2. Characteristics of selected monoclonal antibodies (MAbs).

MAb	Characteristics and Clinical Uses
Abciximab	Antagonist of glycoprotein IIb1/IIIa receptor, preventing cross-linking reaction in platelet aggregation. Used post-angioplasty and in acute coronary syndromes
Daclizumab	Binds to the alpha subunit of the IL-2 receptor, preventing lymphocyte activation. Used in renal transplants
Infliximab	Antibody targeted against TNF-α. Used in Crohn's disease and rheumatoid arthritis
Muromonab	Antibody to the T3 (CD3) antigen on thymocytes. Used in acute renal allograft rejection
Palivizumab	Antibody to surface protein of RSV. Used for prophylaxis and treatment of respiratory syncytial viral infection
Rituximab	Binds to the CD20 antigen on B lymphocytes and recruits immune effector functions to mediate lysis. Used in B-cell non-Hodgkin's lymphoma
Trastuzumab	Binds to the HER-2 protein on the surface of tumor cells. Cytotoxic for breast tumors that overexpress HER-2 protein

of cytotoxic T cells and activates natural killer cells (Table 56–1). Aldesleukin is indicated for the adjunctive treatment of renal cell carcinoma and malignant melanoma. It is investigational for possible efficacy in restoring immune function in AIDS and other immune deficiency disorders.

B. INTERFERONS

Interferon-α-2a inhibits cell proliferation and is used in hairy cell leukemia, chronic myelogenous leukemia, malignant melanoma, Kaposi's sarcoma, and hepatitis B and C. **Interferon-β-1b** has some beneficial effects in relapsing multiple sclerosis. **Interferon-γ-1b** has greater immune-enhancing actions than the other interferons and appears to act by increasing the synthesis of TNF. The recombinant form is used to decrease the incidence and severity of infections in patients with chronic granulomatous disease.

C. BCG (BACILLE CALMETTE-GUÉRIN)

BCG is used in some countries for immunization against tuberculosis and also as an immunostimulant in the treatment of superficial bladder cancer. Its efficacy may be due to its activation of macrophages and the resulting enhancement of immune responses.

MECHANISMS OF DRUG ALLERGY

Immunologic reactions to drugs can fall into any of the 4 categories of hypersensitivity reactions.

A. TYPE I (IMMEDIATE) DRUG ALLERGY

This form of drug allergy involves **IgE**-mediated reactions to animal and plant stings and pollens as well as drugs. Such reactions include anaphylaxis, urticaria, and angioedema. When linked to carrier proteins, small

drug molecules can act as haptens and initiate B-cell proliferation and formation of IgE antibodies. These antibodies bind to Fc receptors on tissue mast cells and blood basophils. On subsequent exposure, the antigenic drug cross-links the IgE antibodies on the surface of mast cells and basophils and triggers release of mediators of vascular responses and tissue injury, including histamine, kinins, prostaglandins, and leukotrienes. Drugs that commonly cause type I reactions include penicillins and sulfonamides.

SKILL KEEPER: ANAPHYLAXIS AND SYMPATHOMIMETIC DRUGS (SEE CHAPTERS 6 AND 9)

In severe anaphylactic reactions, the life-threatening events commonly involve airway obstruction, laryngeal edema, and vascular collapse resulting from peripheral vasodilation and reduction in blood volume. Hypoxemia can contribute to cardiac events, including arrhythmias and myocardial infarction. Drugs used to treat anaphylaxis mainly target the receptors used by neurotransmitters of the sympathetic nervous system.

1. *Why is epinephrine used in anaphylaxis instead of norepinephrine?*

2. *What other sympathomimetic drugs might be useful in the treatment of anaphylaxis?*

The Skill Keeper Answers appear at the end of the chapter.

KEY DRUGS

Subclass	Prototypes	Other Significant Agents
Glucocorticoids	Prednisone	
Antibiotics	Cyclosporine	Tacrolimus, sirolimus
Cytotoxic drugs	Azathioprine, cyclophosphamide	Mercaptopurine, cytarabine, dactinomycin, methotrexate
Enzyme inhibitors	Mycophenolate mofetil, leflunomide	
Anti-TNF-α agents	Etanercept, infliximab Thalidomide	Adalimumab
Immune potentiators Cytokines	Aldesleukin Interferon-β-1b	Interferon-γ-1b
Vaccine	BCG vaccine	

B. Type II Drug Allergy

Type II allergy involves IgG or IgM antibodies that are bound to circulating blood cells. On reexposure to the antigen, complement-dependent cell lysis occurs. Type II reactions include autoimmune syndromes such as hemolytic anemia from methyldopa, systemic lupus erythematosus from hydralazine or procainamide, thrombocytopenic purpura from quinidine, and agranulocytosis from exposure to many drugs.

C. Type III Drug Allergy

Type III hypersensitivity is a complex type of drug allergy reaction that involves complement-fixing IgM or IgG antibodies and, possibly, IgE antibodies. Drug-induced serum sickness and vasculitis are examples of type III reactions; Stevens-Johnson syndrome (associated with sulfonamide therapy) may also result from type III mechanisms.

D. Type IV Drug Allergy

Type IV allergy is a cell-mediated reaction that can occur from topical application of drugs. It results in contact dermatitis.

E. Modification of Drug Allergies

Drugs that modify allergic responses to other drugs or toxins act at several steps of the immune mechanism. For example, corticosteroids inhibit lymphoid cell proliferation and reduce tissue injury and edema. However, most drugs that are useful in type I reactions (eg, epinephrine, theophylline, dopamine) block mediator release or act as physiologic antagonists of the mediators.

QUESTIONS

1. An immune cell that recognizes foreign peptides bound to MHC class II molecules on the surface of APC cells, secretes interleukin-2, and initiates the cell-mediated immunity reaction responsible for host-versus-graft reactions is a
   (A) B lymphocyte
   (B) Cytotoxic T lymphocyte
   (C) Dendritic cell
   (D) Macrophage
   (E) TH lymphocyte

2. Cyclosporine is effective in organ transplantation. The immunosuppressant action of the drug appears to be due to
   (A) Activation of natural killer (NK) cells
   (B) Blockade of tissue responses to inflammatory mediators
   (C) Increased catabolism of IgG antibodies
   (D) Inhibition of the gene transcription of interleukins
   (E) Interference with antigen recognition

3. A widely used drug that suppresses cellular immunity, inhibits prostaglandin and leukotriene synthesis, and increases the catabolism of IgG antibodies is
   (A) Cyclophosphamide
   (B) Cyclosporine
   (C) Infliximab
   (D) Mercaptopurine
   (E) Prednisone

4. Leukocyte-activated killer cells (LAKs) are cytotoxic across MHC barriers and can even kill cells

that do not express MHC. An agent that activates LAKs is
(A) Aldesleukin
(B) Cyclosporine
(C) Etanercept
(D) Leflunomide
(E) Thalidomide

5. An agent that is used to prevent the primary immune response of an Rh-negative mother to an Rh-positive newborn is
(A) Cyclosporine
(B) Cyclophosphamide
(C) Methotrexate
(D) Rh$_o$(D) immune globulin
(E) Tacrolimus

6. Tumor necrosis factor-α appears to play an important role in autoimmunity and inflammatory diseases. A humanized monoclonal antibody that binds to TNF-α and inhibits its action is
(A) Etanercept
(B) Infliximab
(C) Muromonab-CD3
(D) Sirolimus
(E) Thalidomide

7–8. A patient was treated for a bacterial infection with a parenteral penicillin. Within a few minutes of the penicillin injection, he developed severe bronchoconstriction, laryngeal edema, and hypotension. Because of the rapid administration of epinephrine, the patient survived. Unfortunately, a year later he was treated with an antipsychotic drug and developed agranulocytosis.

7. The type of drug reaction that was caused by the penicillin is
(A) An autoimmune syndrome
(B) A cell-mediated reaction
(C) A type II drug allergy
(D) Mediated by IgE
(E) Serum sickness

8. The type of drug reaction that was caused by the antipsychotic drug is
(A) A type III drug reaction
(B) A type IV drug reaction
(C) Delayed-type hypersensitivity
(D) Mediated by IgG or IgM antibodies
(E) The Stevens-Johnson syndrome

9. An immunosuppressant that suppresses both B and T lymphocytes via inhibition of de novo synthesis of purines is
(A) Cyclophosphamide
(B) Methotrexate
(C) Mycophenolate mofetil

(D) Prednisone
(E) Tacrolimus

10. Recombinant interleukin-2 has proved useful in the treatment of
(A) Graft-versus-host disease in patients with hematopoietic stem cell transplantation
(B) Psoriasis
(C) Renal cell carcinoma
(D) Rheumatoid arthritis
(E) Superficial bladder carcinoma

11. Although sirolimus and cyclosporine have similar immunosuppressant effects, their toxicity profiles differ. Sirolimus is more likely than cyclosporine to cause
(A) An anaphylactic reaction
(B) Hypertension
(C) Osteoporosis
(D) Renal insufficiency
(E) Thrombocytopenia

12. An immune modulator that increases phagocytosis by macrophages in patients with chronic granulomatous disease is
(A) Aldesleukin
(B) Interferon-γ
(C) Lymphocyte immune globulin
(D) Prednisone
(E) Trastuzumab

ANSWERS

1. T$_H$ lymphocytes recognize foreign antigens presented by APC cells and, once activated, secrete cytokines that drive cell-mediated immunity (see Figure 56–1). The answer is **E**.

2. Cyclosporine inhibits calcineurin, a serine phosphatase that is needed for activation of T-cell-specific transcription factors. Gene transcription of IL-2, IL-3, and interferon-γ is inhibited. The answer is **D**.

3. The corticosteroid prednisone is used extensively as an immunosuppressant in autoimmune diseases and organ transplantation. Glucocorticoids have multiple actions, including those described. The answer is **E**.

4. Aldesleukin (IL-2) and several other interleukins activate natural killer cells (NK cells) and LAK cells. The investigational use of aldesleukin in AIDS patients is partly based on the fact that lymphocytes from such individuals produce significantly less IL-2 than lymphocytes from healthy controls. The answer is **A**.

5. Rh$_o$(D) immune globulin contains antibodies against Rh$_o$(D) antigens. Administration to an Rh-negative mother within 72 h after the birth of an Rh-positive

infant prevents Rh hemolytic disease of the newborn in subsequent pregnancies. The answer is **D**.

6. Infliximab is a humanized monoclonal antibody that binds to TNF-α. Etanercept also binds to TNF-α, but it is a chimeric protein containing a portion of the human TNF-α receptor linked to the Fc region of a human IgG. Thalidomide is a small molecule that appears to inhibit production of TNF-α. The answer is **B**.

7. The patient experienced an anaphylactic response to the penicillin. This is a type I (immediate) drug reaction, mediated by IgE antibodies. The answer is **D**.

8. Agranulocytosis (and systemic lupus erythematosus) are autoimmune syndromes that can be drug induced. They are type II reactions involving IgM and IgG antibodies that bind to circulating blood cells. The patient was probably treated with clozapine for his psychosis (see clozapine toxicity, Chapter 29). The answer is **D**.

9. Mycophenolic acid, formed from mycophenolate mofetil, inhibits inosine monophosphate dehydrogenase, the rate-limiting enzyme in the de novo pathway of purine synthesis. This action suppresses both B- and T-lymphocyte activation. Mycophenolate mofetil is used both individually and in combination with cyclosporine in organ transplants. The answer is **C**.

10. Interleukin-2 is a cytokine that stimulates T-cell proliferation and activates TH1, NK, and LAK cells. It has shown efficacy in renal cell carcinoma and malignant melanoma, 2 cancers that respond poorly to conventional cytotoxic anticancer drugs. The answer is **C**.

11. Cyclosporine and tacrolimus both are associated with renal toxicity and hypertension. In contrast, sirolimus appears to spare the kidney and instead is more likely to cause gastrointestinal disturbance, hypertriglyceridemia, and myelosuppression,

especially in the form of thrombocytopenia. The answer is **E**.

12. Interferon-γ is approved for use in chronic granulomatous disease, a condition that results from phagocyte deficiency. The agent markedly reduces the frequency of recurrent infections. The answer is **B**.

SKILL KEEPER ANSWERS: ANAPHYLAXIS AND SYMPATHOMIMETIC DRUGS (SEE CHAPTERS 6 AND 9)

1. *Epinephrine activates all adrenoceptors, whereas norepinephrine has minimal agonist activity at β_2 adrenoceptors. This difference is important in anaphylaxis because β_2 adrenoceptor activation is needed to provide a bronchodilatory effect that will oppose the anaphylaxis-induced airway obstruction. The α_1 adrenoceptor agonist effect of epinephrine opposes the anaphylaxis-induced vasodilation and, to some extent, the vascular leak (administration of fluid is also a cornerstone of the treatment of anaphylaxis), whereas the β_1 adrenoceptor agonist effect helps maintain cardiac output.*

2. *If bronchospasm is predominant, then administration by inhalation of a β_2 selective agonist like albuterol—or intravenous administration of theophylline—may be useful. If cardiovascular collapse is predominant, then vasopressor drugs may be helpful; these include α adrenoceptor agonists such as phenylephrine and β_1 adrenoceptor agonists such as dobutamine or dopamine.*

CHECKLIST

When you complete this chapter, you should be able to:

☐ Describe the primary features of cell-mediated and humoral immunity.

☐ Name 7 immunosuppressants and, for each, describe the mechanism of action, clinical uses, and toxicities.

☐ Describe the mechanisms of action, clinical uses, and toxicities of antibodies used as immunosuppressants.

☐ Identify the major cytokines and other immunomodulating agents and know their clinical applications.

☐ Describe the different types of allergic reactions to drugs.

PART IX
Toxicology

Environmental and Occupational Toxicology

57

Toxicology is the branch of pharmacology that encompasses the deleterious effects of chemicals on biologic systems. A number of chemicals in the environment (eg, atmosphere, home, workplace) pose important health hazards.

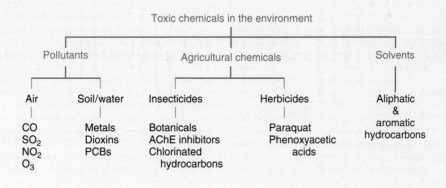

AIR POLLUTANTS

A. CLASSIFICATION AND PROTOTYPES

The major air pollutants in industrialized countries include carbon monoxide (which accounts for about 50% of the total amount of air pollutants), sulfur oxides (18%), hydrocarbons (12%), particulate matter (eg, smoke particles, 10%), and nitrogen oxides (6%). Air pollution appears to be a contributing factor in bronchitis, obstructive pulmonary disease, and lung cancer.

B. CARBON MONOXIDE

CO is an odorless, colorless gas that competes avidly with oxygen for hemoglobin. The affinity of CO for

HIGH-YIELD TERMS TO LEARN	
Bioaccumulation	The increasing concentration of a substance in the environment as the result of environmental persistence and physical properties (eg, lipid solubility) that leads to accumulation in biologic tissues
Environmental toxicology	The area of toxicology that deals with the effects of agents found in the environment; regulated by the Environmental Protection Agency (EPA) in the United States
Occupational toxicology	The area of toxicology that deals with the toxic effects of chemicals found in the workplace; regulated by the Occupational Safety and Health Administration (OSHA) in the United States
Threshold limit value	The amount of exposure to a given agent that is deemed safe for a stated time period. It is higher for shorter periods than for longer periods

hemoglobin is more than 200-fold greater than that of oxygen. The threshold limit value of CO for an 8-h work day is 25 parts per million (ppm); in heavy traffic, the concentration of CO may exceed 100 ppm.

1. Effects—Carbon monoxide causes tissue hypoxia. Headache is one of the first symptoms, followed by confusion, decreased visual acuity, tachycardia, syncope, coma, convulsions, and death. Collapse and syncope occur when approximately 40% of hemoglobin has been converted to carboxyhemoglobin. These adverse effects may be aggravated by heavy labor, high ambient temperature, and high altitude. Prolonged hypoxia can result in residual irreversible damage to the brain and the myocardium.

2. Treatment—Removal of the source of carbon monoxide and 100% oxygen are the main features of treatment. Hyperbaric oxygen accelerates the clearance of carbon monoxide.

C. Sulfur Dioxide

SO_2 is a colorless, irritating gas formed from the combustion of fossil fuels.

1. Effects—SO_2 forms sulfurous acid on contact with moist mucous membranes; this acid is responsible for most of the pathologic effects. Conjunctival and bronchial irritation (especially in individuals with asthma) are the primary signs of exposure. Five to 10 ppm in the air is enough to cause severe bronchospasm. Heavy exposure may lead to delayed pulmonary edema. Chronic low-level exposure may aggravate cardiopulmonary disease.

2. Treatment—Removal from exposure and relief of irritation and inflammation comprise the major treatment.

D. Nitrogen Oxides

Nitrogen dioxide (NO_2), a brownish irritant gas, is the principal member of this group. It is formed in fires and in silage on farms.

1. Effects—NO_2 causes deep lung irritation and pulmonary edema. Farm workers exposed to high concentrations of the gas within enclosed silos may die rapidly of acute pulmonary edema. Irritation of the eyes, nose, and throat is common.

2. Treatment—No specific treatment is available. Measures to reduce inflammation and pulmonary edema are important.

E. Ozone

O_3 is a bluish irritant gas produced in air and water purification devices and in electrical fields.

1. Effects—Exposure to 0.01–0.1 ppm may cause irritation and dryness of the mucous membranes. Pulmonary function may be impaired at higher concentrations. Chronic exposure leads to bronchitis, bronchiolitis, pulmonary fibrosis, and emphysema.

2. Treatment—No specific treatment is available. Measures that reduce inflammation and pulmonary edema are emphasized.

ENVIRONMENTAL POLLUTANTS

The chemical compounds that contribute to environmental pollution include the heavy metals discussed in Chapter 58, the dioxins, and the polychlorinated biphenyls.

A. Dioxins

1. Source—The polychlorinated dibenzo-*p*-dioxins (PCDDs) are a large group of related compounds of which the most important is 2,3,7,8-tetrachlorodibenzo-*p*-dioxin (TCDD). The dioxins have no commercial uses. They have appeared in the environment as unwanted by-products of the chemical industry. PCDDs are chemically stable and highly resistant to environmental degradation.

2. Effects—In laboratory animals, exposure to TCDD has multiple effects, including a wasting syndrome, hepatotoxicity, immune dysfunction, teratogenicity, and cancer. In humans, the most common signs of toxicity are dermatitis and chloracne. However, epidemiologic evidence suggests that the dioxins may have carcinogenic effects in humans, perhaps increasing the risk of non-Hodgkin's lymphoma.

B. POLYCHLORINATED BIPHENYLS (PCBs)

1. Source—The polychlorinated biphenyls were used extensively in manufacturing electrical equipment until their potential for environmental damage was recognized. PCBs are among the most stable organic compounds known. They are poorly metabolized and lipophilic. They are, therefore, highly persistent in the environment and accumulate in the food chain.

2. Effects—In workers exposed to PCBs, the most common effect is dermatotoxicity (acne, erythema, folliculitis, hyperkeratosis). Less frequently, mild increases in plasma triglycerides and elevated liver enzymes have been observed. Some data suggest a link between teratogenicity and ingestion during pregnancy of cooking oils containing PCBs and other polychlorinated compounds.

SKILL KEEPER: SAFETY OF NEW DRUGS (SEE CHAPTER 5)

The FDA requires evidence of relative safety of a new drug before its clinical evaluation. If a new drug is destined for chronic systemic administration, what animal toxicity testing is required? The Skill Keeper Answer appears at the end of the chapter.

INSECTICIDES

A. CLASSIFICATION AND PROTOTYPES

The 3 major classes of insecticides are the chlorinated hydrocarbons (DDT and its analogs), acetylcholinesterase inhibitors (carbamates, organophosphates), and the botanical agents (nicotine, rotenone, pyrethrum alkaloids).

B. CHLORINATED HYDROCARBONS

These agents are persistent, very poorly metabolized, lipophilic chemicals that exhibit significant bioaccumulation.

1. Effects—Chlorinated hydrocarbons block physiologic inactivation in the sodium channels of nerve membranes and cause uncontrolled firing of action potentials. Tremor is usually the first sign of acute toxicity and may progress to seizures. Chronic exposure of animals to these insecticides is tumorigenic. The toxicologic impact

of long-term exposure in humans is unclear. No relationship has been shown in humans between the risk of breast cancer and serum levels of DDT metabolites.

2. Treatment—No specific treatment is available for the acute toxicity caused by chlorinated hydrocarbons. Because of their extremely long half-lives in organisms and in the environment (years), their use in North America and Europe has been curtailed.

C. CHOLINESTERASE INHIBITORS

The carbamates (eg, aldicarb, carbaryl) and organophosphates (eg, dichlorvos, malathion, parathion) are effective insecticides with short environmental half-lives. These inexpensive insecticides are heavily used in agriculture.

1. Effects—As described in Chapter 7, cholinesterase inhibitors increase muscarinic and nicotinic activity. The signs and symptoms include pinpoint pupils, sweating, salivation, bronchoconstriction, vomiting and diarrhea, CNS stimulation followed by depression, and muscle fasciculations, weakness, and paralysis. The most common cause of death is respiratory failure. Chronic exposure to some organophosphates (not carbamates) has resulted in a delayed neurotoxicity with axonal degeneration.

2. Treatment—Atropine is used in large doses to control muscarinic excess; pralidoxime is used to regenerate cholinesterase. Mechanical ventilation may be necessary.

D. BOTANICAL INSECTICIDES

1. Nicotine—Nicotine has the same effects on nicotinic cholinoceptors in insects as in mammals and probably kills by the same mechanism (ie, excitation followed by paralysis of ganglionic, CNS, and neuromuscular transmission). Treatment is supportive.

2. Rotenone—This plant alkaloid insecticide causes gastrointestinal distress when ingested and conjunctivitis and dermatitis after direct contact with exposed body surfaces. Treatment is symptomatic.

3. Pyrethrum—The most common toxic effect of this mixture of plant alkaloids is contact dermatitis. Ingestion or inhalation of large quantities may cause CNS excitation (including seizures) and peripheral neurotoxicity. Treatment is symptomatic, with anticonvulsants if necessary.

HERBICIDES

A. PARAQUAT

Paraquat is used extensively to kill weeds on farms and for highway maintenance.

1. Effects—The compound is relatively nontoxic unless ingested. After ingestion, the initial effect is gastrointestinal irritation with hematemesis and bloody stools.

Within a few days, signs of pulmonary impairment occur and are usually progressive, resulting in severe pulmonary fibrosis and, often, death.

2. Treatment—No antidote is available; the best supportive treatment, including gastric lavage and dialysis, still results in less than 50% survival after ingestion of as little as 5 mL.

B. PHENOXYACETIC ACIDS

The 2 most important members of this group are 2,4-dichlorophenoxyacetic acid (2,4-D) and 2,4,5-trichlorophenoxyacetic acid (2,4,5-T). During the manufacturing process, dioxin contaminants are produced.

1. Effects—Large doses of 2,4-D or 2,4,5-T cause muscle hypotonia and coma. Long-term exposure has been associated with an increased risk of non-Hodgkin's lymphoma.

SOLVENTS

Solvents used in industry and to clean clothing are a major source of direct exposure to hydrocarbons and also contribute to air pollution.

A. ALIPHATIC HYDROCARBONS

This group includes halogenated solvents such as carbon tetrachloride, chloroform, and trichloroethylene.

1. Effects—Solvents are potent CNS depressants. The acute effects of excessive exposure are nausea, vertigo, locomotor disturbances, headache, and coma. Chronic exposure leads to hepatic dysfunction and nephrotoxicity. Long-term exposure to tetrachloroethylene—or to trichloroethane—has caused peripheral neuropathy.

2. Treatment—Removal from exposure is the only specific treatment available. Serious CNS depression must be treated with support of vital signs (see Chapter 59).

B. AROMATIC HYDROCARBONS

Benzene and toluene are important aromatic hydrocarbons.

1. Effects—Acute exposure leads to CNS depression with ataxia and coma. Long-term exposure to benzene is associated with hematotoxicity (thrombocytopenia, leukopenia, aplastic anemia), and the compound may be leukemogenic.

2. Treatment—Removal from exposure is the only specific way to reduce toxicity. CNS depression is managed by support of vital signs.

QUESTIONS

1. The light brownish color of smog often apparent in a major metropolitan area on a hot summer day is mainly due to
   - (A) Carbon monoxide
   - (B) Hydrocarbons
   - (C) Ozone
   - (D) Nitrogen dioxide
   - (E) Sulfur dioxide

2. You are stuck in traffic in New York City in summer for 3 or 4 h and you begin to get a headache, a feeling of tightness in the temporal region, and an increased pulse rate. The most likely cause of these effects is inhalation of
   - (A) Carbon monoxide
   - (B) Nicotine
   - (C) Nitrogen dioxide
   - (D) Ozone
   - (E) Sulfur dioxide

3. Toxicity that stems from exposure to parathion is treated with
   - (A) Antiseizure drugs
   - (B) Atropine and pralidoxime
   - (C) Hemodialysis
   - (D) Hyperbaric oxygen
   - (E) Measures to reduce pulmonary edema

4. A compound that is toxic to bone marrow cells in the early stages of development and that may also be leukemogenic is
   - (A) Benzene
   - (B) Carbon monoxide
   - (C) DDT
   - (D) Pyrethrum
   - (E) Sarin

5. A compound or group of compounds that damages the skin and whose use in manufacturing has largely been eliminated because of extensive persistence in the environment and bioaccumulation is
   - (A) Aromatic hydrocarbons such as benzene
   - (B) Dichlorvos
   - (C) Phenoxyacetic acids such as 2,4-dichlorophenoxyacetic acid
   - (D) Polychlorinated biphenyls (PCBs)
   - (E) 2,3,7,8-tetrachlorodibenzo-*p*-dioxin (TCDD)

6. An employee of a company engaged in clearing vegetation from county roadsides accidentally ingested a small quantity of a herbicidal solution that contained paraquat. Within 2 h, he was admitted to the emergency department of a nearby hospital. Which of the following best describes his probable signs and symptoms in the emergency department?
   - (A) Diarrhea, vomiting, sweating, and profound skeletal muscle weakness
   - (B) Dizziness, nausea, agitation, and hyperreflexia
   - (C) Dyspnea, pulmonary dysfunction, and elevated body temperature

(D) Gastrointestinal irritation with hematemesis and bloody stools

(E) Hypotension, tachycardia, and respiratory impairment

7. Chemical warfare agents that had been manufactured in the 1950s were being stored at a military installation. Several civilian workers at the facility began to feel unwell, with symptoms that included dyspnea, abdominal cramps, and diarrhea. They also had copious nasal and tracheobronchial secretions. Which type of toxic compound is most likely to be the cause of these effects?

(A) Aliphatic hydrocarbons

(B) Botulinum toxins

(C) Nitrogen mustards

(D) Organophosphates

(E) Rotenones

DIRECTIONS: 8–10. The matching questions in this section consist of a list of lettered options followed by several numbered items. For each numbered item, select the ONE lettered option that is most closely associated with it. Each lettered option may be selected once, more than once, or not at all.

(A) Aldicarb

(B) Benzene

(C) Carbon monoxide

(D) Carbon dioxide

(E) DDT

(F) Dioxin

(G) Malathion

(H) Nitrogen dioxide

(I) Paraquat

(J) Pyrethrum

(K) Rotenone

(L) Sulfur dioxide

(M) Tetrachloroethylene

(N) Toluene

8. Asthma is often exacerbated in patients exposed to this reducing agent when concentrations in the air are as low as 1–2 ppm. It is formed mainly from combustion of fossil fuels.

9. Acute exposure to this *aliphatic* hydrocarbon solvent causes CNS depression; chronic exposure has led to impairment of memory and peripheral neuropathy.

10. This compound is a potential environmental hazard that is formed as a contaminating by-product in the manufacture of herbicides.

ANSWERS

1. Smog color is derived in part from suspended particulate matter. When smog is light brown, the color derives from nitrogen oxides. All of the other air pollutants listed are colorless. The answer is **D.**

2. The symptoms described are those of carbon monoxide inhalation. The answer is **A.**

3. Organophosphate poisoning is treated with the muscarinic receptor antagonist atropine and pralidoxime, which regenerates cholinesterase. The answer is **B.**

4. The aromatic hydrocarbon benzene is used as a solvent in industry. Long-term exposure appears to be associated with increased risk of leukemia. The answer is **A.**

5. The polychlorinated biphenyls (PCBs) are dermatotoxic drugs that persist in the environment and accumulate in living organisms. PCBs have been banned from manufacture in the United States since 1979. However, many electrical transformers still retain traces of them. The answer is **D.**

6. Paraquat is highly corrosive to the gastrointestinal tract. Oral ingestion of the herbicide leads to marked gastrointestinal irritation, hematemesis, and usually blood in the stools. Gastric lavage with activated charcoal should be performed repeatedly to remove unabsorbed paraquat from the stomach. Signs of pulmonary impairment do not appear for several days and are usually progressive, resulting in severe pulmonary fibrosis and, often, death. The answer is **D.**

7. Highly potent organophosphate inhibitors of acetylcholinesterase (eg, sarin, tabun) have been developed for chemical warfare purposes. Their storage represents a potential toxicologic hazard. It is important to recognize the signs and symptoms of excess acetylcholine (DUMBBELSS; see Chapter 7), which include those described. The answer is **D.**

SKILL KEEPER ANSWER:
SAFETY OF NEW DRUGS
(SEE CHAPTER 5)

Acute toxicity studies in 2 animal species are required by the FDA for all new drugs before their use in humans. Subacute and chronic toxicity studies are required for drugs that are intended for chronic systemic use. Toxicity testing in animals usually involves the determination of lethal dose, monitoring of blood, hepatic, renal, and respiratory functions, gross and histopathologic examination of tissues, and tests of reproductive effects and potential carcinogenicity.

8. Sulfur dioxide is a reducing agent that forms sulfurous acid on contact with moist surfaces. This is responsible for irritant effects on mucous membranes of the eye, the oropharyngeal cavity, and the respiratory tract. People with cardiac disease or asthma and the elderly are especially sensitive to sulfur dioxide. Nitrogen dioxide causes similar problems, but it is an oxidizing agent formed from fires and in silage on farms. The answer is **L.**

9. Three hydrocarbon solvents are listed: benzene, tetrachloroethylene, and toluene. Each can cause CNS effects such as headache, fatigue, and loss of appetite. However, benzene and toluene are *aromatic* hydrocarbons. The answer is **M.**

10. Dioxin is a contaminant formed in the manufacture of herbicides, including 2,4-D and 2,4,5-T ("agent orange"). The answer is **F.**

CHECKLIST

When you complete this chapter, you should be able to:

☐ List the major air pollutants and their clinical effects.

☐ Describe the signs and symptoms of carbon monoxide poisoning.

☐ Identify the major organ system toxicities of common solvents.

☐ Describe the signs, symptoms, and treatment of toxicity resulting from cholinesterase inhibitor insecticides.

☐ Identify the toxic effects of chlorinated hydrocarbons and botanical insecticides.

☐ List 2 important herbicides and their major toxicities.

☐ Appreciate the toxicologic significance of environmental pollution resulting from dioxins and polychlorinated biphenyls (PCBs).

Heavy Metals

The heavy metals discussed in this chapter—lead, arsenic, mercury, and iron—frequently cause toxicity in humans. The toxicity profiles of metals differ, but most of their effects appear to result from interaction with sulfhydryl groups of enzymes and regulatory proteins. Chelators are organic compounds with 2 or more electronegative groups that form stable covalent-coordinate bonds with cationic metal atoms. These stable complexes lack the toxicity of the free metals and often are excreted readily. The chelators are used as antidotes in the treatment of heavy metal poisoning.

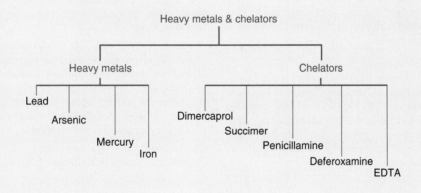

TOXICOLOGY OF HEAVY METALS

A. LEAD

Lead serves no useful purpose in the body and instead can damage the hematopoietic tissues, liver, nervous system, kidneys, gastrointestinal tract, and reproductive system (Table 58–1). Lead is a major environmental hazard because it is present in the air and water throughout the world.

1. Acute lead poisoning—Due to the ban over 20 years ago of lead in gasoline and bans of other industrial products that previously contained lead, acute inorganic lead poisoning is no longer common in the United States. It can occur rarely from industrial exposures (usually via the inhalation of dust) and in children who have ingested large quantities of chips or flakes from surfaces in older houses covered with lead-containing paint. The primary signs of this syndrome are acute abdominal colic and CNS changes, including, particularly in children, acute encephalopathy. The mortality rate is high in lead encephalopathy, and prompt chelation therapy is mandatory.

2. Chronic lead poisoning—Chronic inorganic lead poisoning (plumbism) is much more common than the acute form. Signs include peripheral neuropathy (wrist-drop is characteristic), anorexia, anemia, tremor, weight loss, and gastrointestinal symptoms. Treatment involves removal from the source of exposure, and chelation therapy, usually with oral succimer in outpatients and with parenteral agents (eg, edetate with or without dimercaprol) in more severe cases. Chronic lead poisoning in children presents as growth retardation, neurocognitive

---

HIGH-YIELD TERMS TO LEARN

Chelating agent	A molecule with 2 or more electronegative groups that can form stable coordinate complexes with multivalent cationic metal atoms
Erethism	Syndrome resulting from mercury poisoning characterized by insomnia, memory loss, excitability, and delirium
Pica	The ingestion of nonfood substances; in the present context, pica refers to ingestion of lead-based paint fragments by small children
Plumbism	A range of toxic syndromes due to chronic lead poisoning that may vary as a function of blood or tissue levels and patient age

---

deficits, and developmental delay. Succimer is generally used in such children. In workers exposed to lead, prophylaxis with oral chelating agents is contraindicated because some evidence suggests that lead absorption may be enhanced by the presence of chelators. In contrast, high dietary calcium is indicated because it impedes lead absorption.

3. Organic lead poisoning—Now rare, poisoning by organic lead was usually due to tetraethyl lead or tetramethyl lead contained in "antiknock" gasoline additives, which are no longer used. This form of lead is readily absorbed through the skin and lungs. The primary signs of intoxication include hallucinations, headache, irritability, convulsions, and coma. Treatment consists of decontamination and seizure control.

B. ARSENIC

This element is widely used in industrial processes and is also an environmental pollutant released during the burning of coal. Although it exists in both trivalent and pentavalent forms, its toxicity is entirely due to the trivalent form.

1. Acute arsenic poisoning—Acute arsenic poisoning results in severe gastrointestinal discomfort, vomiting, "ricewater" stools, and capillary damage with dehydration and shock. A sweet, garlicky odor may be detected in the breath and the stools. Treatment consists of supportive therapy to replace water and electrolytes and chelation therapy with dimercaprol.

2. Chronic arsenic poisoning—Chronic arsenic intoxication causes skin changes, hair loss, bone marrow

---

Table 58–1. Important characteristics of the toxicology of arsenic, iron, lead, and mercury.

Metal	Form Entering Body	Route of Absorption	Target Organs for Toxicity	Treatment[a]
Lead	Inorganic lead oxides and salts	Gastrointestinal, respiratory, skin (minor)	Hematopoietic system, CNS, kidneys	Dimercaprol, EDTA, succimer, unithiol
	Tetraethyl lead	Skin (major), gastrointestinal	CNS	Seizure control, supportive
Arsenic	Inorganic arsenic salts	All mucous surfaces	Capillaries, gastrointestinal tract, hematopoietic system	Dimercaprol, unithiol, succimer, penicillamine
	Arsine gas	Inhalation	Erythrocytes	Supportive
Mercury	Elemental	Inhalation	CNS, kidneys	Succimer, unithiol
	Inorganic salts	Gastrointestinal	Kidneys, gastrointestinal tract	Succimer, unithiol, penicillamine, dimercaprol
	Organic mercurials	Gastrointestinal	CNS	Supportive
Iron	Ferrous sulfate	Gastrointestinal	Gastrointestinal, CNS, blood	Deferoxamine

[a]In all cases, removal of the individual from the source of toxicity is the first requirement of management.

depression and anemia, and chronic nausea and gastrointestinal disturbances. Dimercaprol therapy appears to be of value. Arsenic is a known human carcinogen.

3. Arsine gas—Arsine gas (AsH_3), an occupational hazard, is formed during the refinement and processing of certain metals and is used in the semiconductor industry. Arsine causes a unique form of toxicity characterized by massive hemolysis. Pigment overload from red cell breakdown can cause renal failure. Treatment is supportive.

C. MERCURY

The main source of inorganic mercury as a toxic hazard is through the use of mercury-containing materials in dental laboratories and in the manufacture of wood preservatives, insecticides, and batteries. Organic mercury compounds are used as seed dressings (treatments to prevent fungal and bacterial infection of seed and to improve the seed's dispersion and adhesiveness) and fungicides.

1. Acute mercury poisoning—Acute mercury poisoning usually occurs through inhalation of inorganic elemental mercury. It causes chest pain, shortness of breath, nausea and vomiting, kidney damage, gastroenteritis, and CNS damage. In addition to intensive supportive care, prompt chelation with oral succimer or with intramuscular dimercaprol is essential. Acute ingestion of mercuric chloride causes a severe, life-threatening hemorrhagic gastroenteritis followed by renal failure.

2. Chronic mercury poisoning—Chronic mercury poisoning may occur with inorganic or organic mercury. Poisoning from inhalation of mercury vapor presents as a diffuse set of symptoms involving the gums and teeth, gastrointestinal disturbances, and neurologic and behavioral changes (erethism). Chronic mercury intoxication has been treated with succimer and unithiol, but their efficacy has not been established. Dimercaprol may redistribute mercury to the CNS and should not be used in chronic exposure to elemental mercury.

3. Organic mercury poisoning—Intoxication with organic mercury compounds was first recognized in connection with an epidemic of neurologic and psychiatric disease in the village of Minamata, Japan, that was first noticed in the 1950s. The outbreak was a result of consumption of fish containing a high content of methylmercury, which was produced by bacteria in seawater from mercury in the effluent of a nearby vinyl plastics manufacturing plant. Similar epidemics have resulted from the consumption of grain that was intended for use as seed and treated with fungicidal organic mercury compounds. Treatment with chelators has been tried, but the benefits are uncertain.

D. IRON

Acute poisoning from the ingestion of ferrous sulfate tablets occurs quite frequently in small children, although the incidence of poisonings dropped dramatically in the United States after iron supplements were required to be packed in unit-dose packing. The initial symptoms of iron poisoning include vomiting, gastrointestinal bleeding, lethargy, and gray cyanosis. These can be followed by signs of severe gastrointestinal necrosis, pneumonitis, jaundice, seizures, and coma. Deferoxamine is the chelating agent of choice. Chronic excessive intake of iron can lead to hemosiderosis or hemochromatosis (see Chapter 33).

SKILL KEEPER: IRON DEFICIENCY (SEE CHAPTER 33)

Iron is the essential metallic element of heme, the molecule responsible for the bulk of oxygen transport in the blood.

1. *How is the iron content of the body regulated?*

2. *How is iron deficiency diagnosed and treated?*

The Skill Keeper Answers appear at the end of the chapter.

CHELATORS

Chelators used clinically include dimercaprol (BAL), succimer, unithiol, penicillamine, edetate (EDTA), and deferoxamine. Variations among these agents in their affinities for specific metals govern their clinical applications (Table 58–1).

A. DIMERCAPROL

Dimercaprol (2,3-dimercaptopropanol; BAL [British antilewisite]) is a **bidentate** chelator; that is, a chelator that forms 2 bonds with the metal ion, preventing the metal's binding to tissue proteins and permitting its rapid excretion.

1. Clinical use—Dimercaprol is used in acute arsenic and mercury poisoning and, in combination with EDTA, for lead poisoning. It is an oily liquid that must be given parenterally.

2. Toxicity—Dimercaprol causes a high incidence of adverse effects, possibly because it is highly lipophilic and readily enters cells. Its toxicity includes transient hypertension, tachycardia, headache, nausea and vomiting, paresthesias, and fever (especially in children). It may cause pain and hematomas at the injection site. Long-term use is associated with thrombocytopenia and increased prothrombin time.

B. SUCCIMER

Succimer (2,3-dimercaptosuccinic acid; DMSA) is a water-soluble bidentate congener of dimercaprol.

1. Clinical use—Succimer is used for the oral treatment of lead toxicity in children and adults. It is as effective as parenteral EDTA in reducing blood lead concentration. Succimer is also effective in arsenic and mercury poisoning, if given within a few hours of exposure.

2. Toxicity—Although succimer appears to be less toxic than dimercaprol, gastrointestinal distress, CNS effects, skin rash, and elevation of liver enzymes may occur.

C. Unithiol

A water-soluble derivative of dimercaprol, unithiol can be administered orally or intravenously.

1. Clinical use—Intravenous unithiol is used in the initial treatment of severe acute poisoning by inorganic mercury or arsenic. Oral unithiol is an alternative to succimer in the treatment of lead intoxication.

2. Toxicity—Unithiol causes a low incidence of dermatological reactions, usually mild. Vasodilation and hypotension may occur with rapid intravenous infusion.

D. Penicillamine

Penicillamine, a derivative of penicillin, is another bidentate chelator.

1. Clinical use—The major uses of penicillamine are in the treatment of copper poisoning and Wilson's disease. It is sometimes used as adjunctive therapy in gold, arsenic, and lead intoxication and in rheumatoid arthritis. The agent is water soluble, well absorbed from the gastrointestinal tract, and excreted unchanged.

2. Toxicity—Adverse effects are common and may be severe. They include nephrotoxicity with proteinuria, pancytopenia, and autoimmune dysfunction, including lupus erythematosus and hemolytic anemia.

E. Ethylenedinitrilotetraacetic Acid (EDTA)

EDTA (edetate) is an efficient polydentate chelator of many divalent cations, including calcium, and trivalent cations.

1. Clinical use—The primary use of EDTA is in the treatment of lead poisoning. Because the agent is highly polar, it is given parenterally. To prevent dangerous hypocalcemia, EDTA is usually given as the calcium disodium salt.

2. Toxicity—The most important adverse effect of the agent is nephrotoxicity, including renal tubular necrosis. This risk can be reduced by adequate hydration and restricting treatment with EDTA to 5 days or less. Electrocardiographic changes can occur at high doses.

F. Deferoxamine and Deferasirox

Deferoxamine is a polydentate bacterial product that has an extremely high and selective affinity for iron and a much lower affinity for aluminum. Fortunately, the drug competes poorly for heme iron in hemoglobin and cytochromes. Deferasirox is a new tridentate chelator with selectively high affinity for iron.

1. Clinical use—Deferoxamine is used parenterally in the treatment of acute iron intoxication and in the treatment of iron overload caused by blood transfusions in patients with diseases such as thalassemia or myelodysplastic syndrome (see Chapter 33). Deferasirox is an oral drug approved for treatment of iron overload.

2. Toxicity—Skin reactions (blushing, erythema, urticaria) may occur. With long-term use, neurotoxicity (eg, retinal degeneration), hepatic and renal dysfunction, and severe coagulopathies have been reported. Rapid intravenous administration of deferoxamine can cause histamine release and hypotensive shock.

QUESTIONS

1. A small child is brought to a hospital emergency department suffering from severe gastrointestinal distress and abdominal colic. If this patient has severe acute lead poisoning with signs and symptoms of encephalopathy, treatment should be instituted immediately with
   (A) Acetylcysteine
   (B) Deferoxamine
   (C) EDTA
   (D) Penicillamine
   (E) Succimer

2. A young woman employed as a dental laboratory technician complains of conjunctivitis, skin irritation, and hair loss. On examination, she has perforation of the nasal septum and a "milk and roses" complexion. These signs and symptoms are most likely due to
   (A) Acute mercury poisoning
   (B) Chronic inorganic arsenic poisoning
   (C) Chronic mercury poisoning
   (D) Excessive use of supplementary iron tablets
   (E) Lead poisoning

3. A patient complains of chronic headache, fatigue, loss of appetite, and constipation. He has slight weakness of the extensor muscles in the upper limbs. Based on the laboratory data in the table on the top of the next page, the most reasonable diagnosis is chronic poisoning caused by
   (A) Arsenic
   (B) Hexane
   (C) Inorganic lead
   (D) Iron
   (E) Mercuric chloride

Test	Result in Patient	Normal
Hemoglobin	<13 g/dL	>14 g/dL
Urinary coproporphyrin	>80 mcg/100 mg creatinine	<10 mcg/100 mg creatinine
Urinary aminolevulinic acid	>2 mg/100 mg creatinine	<0.5 mg/100 mg creatinine

4. In the treatment of acute inorganic arsenic poisoning, the most likely drug to be used is
(A) Deferoxamine
(B) Dimercaprol
(C) EDTA
(D) Penicillamine
(E) Succimer

5. A 24-year-old man was employed in the supply department of a company that manufactures semiconductors. After an accident at the plant, he presented with nausea and vomiting, headache, hypotension, and shivering. Laboratory analyses showed hemoglobinuria and a plasma free hemoglobin level greater than 1.4 g/dL. This young man was probably exposed to
(A) Arsine
(B) Inorganic arsenic
(C) Mercury vapor
(D) Methylmercury
(E) Tetraethyl lead

6. A 2-year-old child was brought to the emergency department 1 h after ingestion of tablets he had managed to obtain from a bottle on top of the refrigerator. His symptoms included marked gastrointestinal distress, vomiting (with hematemesis), and epigastric pain. Metabolic acidosis and leukocytosis were also present. This patient is most likely to have ingested tablets containing
(A) Acetaminophen
(B) Aspirin
(C) Diphenhydramine
(D) Iron
(E) Vitamin C

DIRECTIONS: 7–10. The matching questions in this section consist of a list of lettered options followed by several numbered items. For each numbered item, select the ONE lettered option that is most closely associated with it. Each lettered option may be selected once, more than once, or not at all.
(A) Arsine
(B) Deferoxamine
(C) Dimercaprol
(D) Edetate calcium disodium
(E) Inorganic mercury
(F) Iron

(G) Methylmercury
(H) Mercury vapor
(I) Penicillamine
(J) Succimer
(K) Tetraethyl lead
(L) Trivalent arsenic

7. This toxic compound can be produced in seawater by the action of bacteria and algae. It is also synthesized chemically for commercial use as a fungicide.

8. This agent has been reported to cause lupus erythematosus and hemolytic anemia.

9. High doses of this agent can cause histamine release and extreme vasodilation.

10. Gingivitis, discolored gums, and loose teeth are common symptoms of chronic exposure to this agent.

ANSWERS

1. Encephalopathy in severe lead poisoning is a medical emergency. Of the drugs listed, intravenous EDTA is the most effective chelating agent. Oral succimer is used in children with mild to moderate lead poisoning and may be initiated 4–5 days after the parenteral use of EDTA or dimercaprol in severe poisoning. The answer is **C.**

2. The "milk and roses" complexion, which results from vasodilation and anemia, is a characteristic of chronic inorganic arsenic poisoning, whereas patients with lead poisoning often have a gray pallor. Other signs and symptoms of arsenic poisoning include gastrointestinal distress, hyperpigmentation, and white lines on the nails. We hope you were not led astray by her employment. The answer is **B.**

3. Of the agents listed, lead is most likely to cause a decrease in heme biosynthesis. The urinary concentrations of lead before and after EDTA treatment can confirm the diagnosis. The answer is **C.**

4. The treatment of choice in acute arsenic poisoning is intramuscular dimercaprol. Although succimer is less toxic, it is only available in an oral formulation, and its absorption may be impaired by the severe gastroenteritis that occurs in acute arsenic poisoning. The answer is **B.**

5. From the signs and symptoms alone, a diagnosis of arsine gas poisoning cannot be made. However, clues to the cause of poisoning are often provided by a patient's occupation. The laboratory reports suggest marked hemolysis. Arsine gas binds to hemoglobin and decreases erythrocyte glutathione levels, causing membrane fragility and resulting hemolysis. The answer is **A.**

6. This question emphasizes that the ingestion of iron tablets is a relatively common cause of accidental poisoning in young children. The signs and symptoms described usually occur in the first 6 h after ingestion. In a child of body weight 22 lb, the ingestion of 600 mg can cause severe, perhaps lethal, toxicity. The answer is **D.**

7. Methylmercury is used as a fungicide to prevent mold growth in seed grain. The answer is **G.**

8. Autoimmune diseases such as lupus erythematosus and hemolytic anemia have occurred during the treatment of Wilson's disease with penicillamine. The answer is **I.**

9. Deferoxamine can cause shock if given by rapid intravenous infusion. The answer is **B.**

10. Oral and gastrointestinal complaints are common in chronic mercury poisoning, and tremor involving the fingers and arms is often present. The answer is **E.**

SKILL KEEPER ANSWERS: IRON DEFICIENCY (SEE CHAPTER 33)

1. *Regulation of body iron occurs through modulation of its intestinal absorption. Ferrous iron is absorbed and oxidized in mucosal cells to the ferric form. Ferric iron can be stored in mucosal cells bound to ferritin or may be distributed throughout the body bound to transferrin. Most of the iron in the body is present in hemoglobin. Small quantities of iron are eliminated in sweat, saliva, and the exfoliation of skin and mucosal cells.*

2. *Iron deficiency can be diagnosed from red blood cell changes, including microcytic size and decreased hemoglobin content, and from measurement of serum and bone marrow iron stores. Iron deficiency anemia is treated by dietary ferrous iron supplements or, in severe cases, parenteral use of iron dextran.*

CHECKLIST

When you complete this chapter, you should be able to:

☐ Describe the general mechanism of metal chelation.

☐ Identify the clinically useful chelators and know their indications and their adverse effects.

☐ Describe the major clinical features and treatment of acute and chronic lead poisoning.

☐ Describe the major clinical features and treatment of arsenic poisoning.

☐ Describe the major clinical features and treatment of inorganic and organic mercury poisoning.

☐ Describe the major clinical features and treatment of iron poisoning.

Management of the Poisoned Patient

59

Toxic substances include therapeutic agents as well as agricultural and industrial chemicals that have no medical applications. Most chemicals are capable of causing toxic effects when given in excessive dosage; even for therapeutic drugs, the difference between a therapeutic action and a toxic one is most often a matter of dose. Many toxic effects of therapeutic agents have been discussed in previous chapters. Common toxic syndromes associated with major drug groups are summarized in this chapter. This chapter also reviews the principles of management of the poisoned patient.

TOXICOKINETICS, TOXICODYNAMICS, & CAUSE OF DEATH

A. TOXICOKINETICS

This term denotes the disposition of poisons in the body (ie, their pharmacokinetics). Knowledge of a toxin's absorption, distribution, and elimination permits assessment of the value of procedures designed to remove it from the skin or gastrointestinal tract. For example, drugs with large apparent volumes of distribution, such as antidepressants and antimalarials, are not amenable to dialysis procedures for drug removal. Drugs with low volumes of distribution, including lithium, phenytoin, and salicylates, are more readily removed by dialysis and diuresis procedures. In some cases, renal elimination of weak acids can be accelerated by urinary alkalinization, while renal elimination of some weak bases can be accelerated by urinary acidification. The clearance of drugs may be different at toxic concentrations than at therapeutic concentrations. For example, in overdoses of phenytoin or salicylates, the capacity of the liver to metabolize the drugs is usually exceeded, and elimination changes from first-order (constant half-life) to zero-order (variable half-life) kinetics.

B. TOXICODYNAMICS

Toxicodynamics denotes the injurious effects of toxins (pharmacodynamic effects). A knowledge of toxicodynamics can be useful in the diagnosis and management of poisoning. For example, hypertension and tachycardia are typically seen in overdoses with amphetamines, cocaine, and antimuscarinic drugs. Hypotension with bradycardia occurs with overdoses of calcium channel blockers, β-blockers, and sedative-hypnotics. Hypotension with tachycardia occurs with tricyclic antidepressants, phenothiazines, and theophylline. Hyperthermia is most frequently a result of overdose of drugs with antimuscarinic actions, the salicylates, or sympathomimetics. Hypothermia is more likely to occur with toxic doses of ethanol and other CNS depressants. Increased respiratory rate is often a feature of overdose with carbon monoxide, salicylates, and other drugs that cause metabolic acidosis or cellular asphyxia. Overdoses of agents that depress the heart are likely to affect the functions of all organ systems that are critically dependent on blood flow, including brain, liver, and kidney. Note that restoration of blood pressure after a period of hypotension may increase the tissue distribution of a toxin, which can result in waxing and waning of signs and symptoms.

C. CAUSE OF DEATH IN INTOXICATED PATIENTS

The most common causes of death from drug overdose in the United States reflect the drug groups most often selected for abuse or for suicide. Sedative-hypnotics and opioids cause respiratory depression, coma, aspiration of gastric contents, and other respiratory malfunctions. Drugs such as cocaine, PCP, tricyclic antidepressants, and theophylline cause seizures, which may lead to vomiting and aspiration of gastric contents and to postictal respiratory depression. Tricyclic antidepressants and cardiac glycosides cause dangerous and frequently lethal arrhythmias. Severe hypotension can occur with any of these drugs. A few intoxicants directly damage the liver and kidney. These include acetaminophen, mushroom poisons of the *Amanita phalloides* type, certain inhalants, and some heavy metals. The metals are discussed in Chapter 58.

HIGH-YIELD TERMS TO LEARN	
ABCDs	Mnemonic for the treatment of a poisoned patient that stands for **A**irway, **B**reathing, **C**irculation and **D**extrose or **D**econtamination
Anion gap	The difference between the serum concentrations of the major cations (Na^+, K^+) and anions (HCO_3^-, Cl^-); an elevated anion gap indicates the presence of extra anions and is most commonly caused by metabolic acidosis
Antidote	A substance that counteracts the effect of a poison
Decontamination	Efforts to remove unabsorbed poison from the skin or gastrointestinal tract
Osmolar gap	The difference between the measured serum osmolality and the osmolality that is calculated from serum concentrations of sodium, glucose and BUN; ethanol and other alcohols can cause an osmolar gap

MANAGEMENT OF THE POISONED PATIENT

Management of the poisoned patient consists of maintenance of vital functions, identification of the toxic substance, decontamination procedures, enhancement of elimination, and, in a few instances, the use of a specific antidote.

A. VITAL FUNCTIONS

The most important aspect of treatment of a poisoned patient is maintenance of vital functions, as indicated by the mnemonic "ABCDs." The most commonly endangered or impaired vital function is respiration. Therefore, an open and protected airway (A) must be established first and effective ventilation (B for breathing) must be ensured. The circulation (C) should be evaluated and supported as needed. The cardiac rhythm should be determined, and if ventricular fibrillation is present, it must be corrected at once. The blood pressure should be measured but rarely needs immediate treatment except in cases of traumatic hemorrhage. Because of the danger of brain damage from hypoglycemia, intravenous 50% dextrose (D) should be given to comatose patients immediately after blood has been drawn for laboratory tests and before laboratory results have been obtained. Thiamine should be administered to prevent Wernicke's syndrome in patients with suspected alcoholism or malnourishment. In patients with signs of respiratory or CNS depression, intravenous naloxone will offset possible toxic effects of opioid analgesic overdose.

B. IDENTIFICATION OF POISONS

Many intoxicants cause a characteristic syndrome of clinical and laboratory changes. Table 59–1 summarizes toxic syndromes associated with major drug groups and the key interventions called for. The toxic features of selected individual agents are listed in Table 59–2.

When the toxic agent cannot be directly examined and identified, the clinician must rely on indirect means to identify the type of intoxication and the progress of therapy. In addition to the history and physical examination, certain laboratory examinations may be useful. A few intoxicants can be directly identified in the blood or urine, especially when information in the history narrows the search. In the more common situation of a comatose patient unable to provide a history, general tests for replacement of anions or osmotic equivalents in the blood (anion gap, osmolar gap) may be useful. A few intoxicants can be identified or strongly suspected on the basis of electrocardiographic or radiologic findings.

1. Osmolar gap—The osmolar gap is the difference between the measured serum osmolarity (measured by the freezing point depression method) and the osmolarity predicted by measured serum concentrations of sodium glucose and BUN:

$$\text{Gap} = \text{Osm (measured)} - [(2 \times Na^+ \text{ [meq/L]}) + (\text{Glucose [mg/dL]} \div 18) + (\text{BUN[mg/dL]} \div 3)]$$

This gap is normally zero. A significant gap is produced by high serum concentrations of intoxicants of low molecular weight such as ethanol, methanol, and ethylene glycol.

2. Anion gap—The anion gap is the difference between the sum of the measured serum concentrations of the 2 primary cations, sodium and potassium, and the sum of the measured serum concentrations of the 2 primary anions, chloride and bicarbonate:

$$\text{Anion gap} = (Na^+ + K^+) - (HCO_3^- + Cl^-)$$

This gap is normally 12–16 mEq/L. A significant increase can be produced by diabetic ketoacidosis, renal

Table 59–1. Toxic syndromes caused by major drug groups.

Drug Group	Clinical Features	Key Interventions
Antimuscarinic drugs	Delirium, hallucinations, seizures, coma, tachycardia, hypertension, hyperthermia, mydriasis, decreased bowel sounds, urinary retention	Control hyperthermia; physostigmine may be helpful, but not for tricyclic OD
Cholinomimetic drugs (carbamate or organo-phosphate inhibitors of acetylcholinesterase)	Anxiety, agitation, seizures, coma, bradycardia or tachycardia, pinpoint pupils, salivation, sweating, hyperactive bowel, muscle fasciculations, then paralysis	Support respiration. Treat with atropine and pralidoxime. Decontaminate
Opioids (eg, heroin, morphine, methadone)	Lethargy, sedation, coma, bradycardia, hypotension, hypoventilation, pinpoint pupils, cool skin, decreased bowel sounds, flaccid muscles	Provide airway and respiratory support. Give naloxone as required
Salicylates	Confusion, lethargy, coma, seizures, hyperventilation, hyperthermia, dehydration, hypokalemia, anion gap metabolic acidosis	Correct acidosis and fluid and electrolyte imbalance. Alkaline diuresis or hemodialysis to aid elimination
Sedative-hypnotics (barbiturates, benzodiazepines, ethanol)	Disinhibition initially, later lethargy, stupor, coma. Nystagmus is common, decreased muscle tone, hypothermia. Small pupils, hypotension, and decreased bowel sounds in severe OD	Provide airway and respiratory support. Avoid fluid overload. Consider flumazenil for benzodiazepine OD
Stimulants (amphetamines, cocaine, phencyclidine)	Agitation, anxiety, seizures. Hypertension, tachycardia, arrhythmias. Mydriasis, vertical and horizontal nystagmus with PCP. Skin warm and sweaty, hyperthermia, increased muscle tone, possible rhabdomyolysis	Control seizures, hypertension, and hyperthermia
Tricyclic antidepressants	Antimuscarinic effects (see above). The "3 C's" of coma, convulsions, cardiac toxicity (QRS prolongation, arrhythmias, hypotension)	Control seizures. Correct acidosis and cardiotoxicity with ventilation, sodium bicarbonate, and norepinephrine (for hypotension). Control hyperthermia

Modified and reproduced, with permission, from Katzung BG, editor: *Basic & Clinical Pharmacology,* 10th ed. McGraw-Hill, 2007.

failure, or drug-induced metabolic acidosis. Drugs that cause an anion gap include cyanide, ethanol, ethylene glycol, ibuprofen, isoniazid, iron, methanol, phenelzine, salicylates, tranylcypromine, valproic acid, and verapamil.

3. Serum potassium—Myocardial function is critically dependent on serum potassium level. Drugs that cause hyperkalemia include β adrenoceptor blockers, digitalis (in suicidal overdose), fluoride, lithium, and potassium-sparing diuretics. Drugs associated with hypokalemia include barium, β adrenoceptor agonists, methylxanthines, most diuretics, and toluene.

C. DECONTAMINATION

Decontamination is the removal of any unabsorbed poison from the skin or gastrointestinal tract. In the case of ingested noncorrosive toxins, this may involve inducing vomiting (emesis) by means of **syrup of ipecac** if the patient is conscious. (*Fluid extract* of ipecac should not be used because it contains cardiotoxic alkaloids.) In unconscious patients, emesis will lead to aspiration into the respiratory tree and must be avoided. **Gastric lavage** with a large-bore tube can be used to remove noncorrosive drugs from the stomach of a comatose patient if the airway has been protected with a cuffed endotracheal tube. **Activated charcoal,** given orally or by stomach tube, may be very effective in adsorbing any remaining drug. Toxins that can be removed by multiple treatments with activated charcoal include amitriptyline, barbiturates, carbamazepine, digitalis glycosides, phencyclidine, propoxyphene, theophylline, tricyclic antidepressants, and valproic acid. In the case of topical

Table 59–2. Toxic features of specific agents.

Agent	Toxic Features
Acetaminophen	Mild anorexia, nausea, vomiting, delayed jaundice, hepatic and renal failure
Antifreeze (ethylene glycol)	Renal failure, crystals in urine, anion and osmolar gap, initial CNS excitation; eye examination normal
Botulism	Dysphagia, dysarthria, ptosis, ophthalmoplegia, muscle weakness; incubation period 12–36 h
Carbon monoxide	Coma, metabolic acidosis, retinal hemorrhages
Cyanide	Bitter almond odor, seizures, coma, abnormal ECG
Iron	Bloody diarrhea, coma, radiopaque material in gut (seen on x-ray), high leukocyte count, hyperglycemia
Lead	Abdominal pain, hypertension, seizures, muscle weakness, metallic taste, anorexia, encephalopathy, delayed motor neuropathy, changes in renal and reproductive function
LSD	Hallucinations, dilated pupils, hypertension
Mercury	Acute renal failure, tremor, salivation, gingivitis, colitis, erethism (fits of crying, irrational behavior), nephrotic syndrome
Methanol	Rapid respiration, visual symptoms, osmolar gap, severe metabolic acidosis
Mushrooms (*Amanita phalloides* type)	Severe nausea and vomiting 8 h after ingestion; delayed hepatic and renal failure
Phencyclidine (PCP)	Coma with eyes open, horizontal and vertical nystagmus, hyperacusis

exposure (insecticides, solvents), the clothing should be removed and the patient washed to remove any chemical still present on the skin. Medical personnel must be careful not to contaminate themselves during this procedure.

D. Enhancement of Elimination

Enhancement of elimination is possible for a number of toxins, including manipulation of urine pH to accelerate renal excretion of weak acids and bases. For example, alkaline diuresis is effective in toxicity caused by fluoride, isoniazid, fluoroquinolones, phenobarbital, and salicylates. Urinary acidification may be useful in toxicity caused by weak bases, including amphetamines, nicotine, and phencyclidine, but care must be taken to avoid acidosis and renal failure in rhabdomyolysis. Hemodialysis (HD) or hemoperfusion (HP) enhances the elimination of many toxic compounds, including carbamazepine (HP), ethylene glycol (HD), lithium (HD), methanol (HD), procainamide (HD or HP), quinidine, salicylates (HD), theophylline (HD or HP), and valproic acid (HD). Cathartics (laxatives) such as sorbitol (70%) can decrease absorption and hasten removal of toxins from the gastrointestinal tract. Whole bowel irrigation with a balanced polyethylene-glycol

electrolyte solution can enhance gut decontamination of iron tablets, enteric-coated pills, and illicit drug-filled packets.

E. Antidotes

Antidotes exist for a few poisons (Table 59–3). Since the duration of action of most antidotes is shorter than that of the intoxicant, the antidotes may need to be given repeatedly. The use of chelating agents for metal poisoning is discussed in Chapter 58.

SKILL KEEPER: CYANIDE
POISONING (SEE
CHAPTERS 11 AND 12)

Cyanide forms a stable complex with the ferric ion of cytochrome oxidase enzymes and inhibits cellular respiration. What is the connection between the management of cyanide poisoning and the drugs amyl nitrite and nitroprusside? The Skill Keeper Answer appears at the end of the chapter.

Table 59–3. Important antidotes.

Antidote	Poison(s)
Acetylcysteine	Acetaminophen; best given within 8–10 h of overdose
Atropine	Cholinesterase inhibitors
Bicarbonate, sodium	Membrane-depressant cardiotoxic drugs (eg, quinidine, tricyclic antidepressants)
Calcium	Fluoride; calcium channel blockers
Deferoxamine	Iron salts
Digoxin antibodies	Digoxin and related cardiac glycoside
Esmolol	Caffeine, theophylline, metaproterenol
Ethanol	Methanol, ethylene glycol
Flumazenil	Benzodiazepines, zolpidem
Fomepizole	Methanol, ethylene glycol
Glucagon	Beta adrenoceptor blockers
Naloxone	Opioid analgesics
Oxygen	Carbon monoxide
Physostigmine	"Suggested" for muscarinic receptor blockers, NOT tricyclics
Pralidoxime	Organophosphate cholinesterase inhibitors

Modified and reproduced, with permission, from Katzung BG, editor: *Basic & Clinical Pharmacology,* 10th ed. McGraw-Hill, 2007.

F. SNAKEBITE

The most common dangerous snake in the United States is the rattlesnake. Although snakebites are common (several thousand per year in the Unites States), severe envenomation is infrequent.

1. Effects—Snake venom contains many enzymes and tissue toxins that produce local tissue necrosis, vascular damage, thrombosis, hemorrhage, and neural injury.

2. Treatment—It is now well documented that once-popular remedies such as incision and suction, ice packs, and tourniquets are usually more deleterious than helpful. The most important prehospital therapy is to minimize movement of the bitten part to limit the spread of the venom in the tissues. Effective therapy consists of adequate dosage with antivenin. Because antivenins are prepared in horses, serum sickness frequently follows and may also require therapy.

QUESTIONS

1–3. A 2-year-old girl presented with lethargy, increased respiratory rate, and an elevated temperature that appeared to result from a drug poisoning. Laboratory testing revealed the following serum concentrations: glucose, 36 mg/dL; Na^+, 148 mEq/L; K^+, 5 mEq/L; Cl^-, 111 mEq/L; HCO_3^-, 12 mEq/L; BUN, 21 mg/dL; osmolality, 300 mOsm/L.

1. The anion gap in this patient is
   - **(A)** −60 mEq/L
   - **(B)** −20 mEq/L
   - **(C)** +5 mEq/L
   - **(D)** +30 mEq/L
   - **(E)** +304 mEq/L

2. The osmolar gap in this patient is
   - **(A)** −40 mOsm/L
   - **(B)** −5 mOsm/L
   - **(C)** +15 mOsm/L
   - **(D)** +60 mOsm/L
   - **(E)** +305 mOsm/L

3. The patent's signs, symptoms, and laboratory values are MOST consistent with an overdose of
   - **(A)** Acetaminophen
   - **(B)** Aspirin
   - **(C)** Ethylene glycol
   - **(D)** Lead
   - **(E)** Phencyclidine

4. An 18-month-old boy presented in a semiconscious state with profound hypotension and bradycardia

after ingesting a number of his grandmother's metoprolol tablets.

In this case, an appropriate antidote is
(A) Adenosine
(B) Dobutamine
(C) Glucagon
(D) Naloxone
(E) Physostigmine

5. A patient is brought to the emergency department suffering from nausea, vomiting, and abdominal pain. He has muscle weakness, which seems to be progressing downward from the head and neck. The patient has difficulty talking clearly and has ptosis and ophthalmoplegia. The most likely cause of these symptoms is
(A) Accidental ingestion of paraquat
(B) An overdose of phenobarbital
(C) Excessive consumption of ethanol
(D) Food poisoning
(E) Organophosphate poisoning

6. Which drug is MOST likely to cause hypotension, seizures, and cardiac arrhythmia when taken in overdose?
(A) Acetaminophen
(B) Diazepam
(C) Ethylene glycol
(D) Morphine
(E) Tricyclic antidepressant

7. A patient with heart failure has accidentally taken an overdose of digoxin. The blood concentration of the drug is 8 times the threshold for toxicity. Pharmacokinetic parameters for digoxin include a clearance of 7 L/h and an elimination half-life of 56 h. If no procedures are instituted to decontaminate this patient, the time taken to reach a safe level of digoxin will be approximately
(A) 3.5 days
(B) 7 days
(C) 14 days
(D) 28 days
(E) 56 days

8–9. A patient is brought to the emergency department having taken an overdose (unknown quantity) of a sustained-release preparation of theophylline by oral administration 2 h previously. He has marked gastrointestinal distress with vomiting and is agitated, hyperreflexic, and hypotensive.

8. The plasma level of theophylline measured immediately upon hospitalization was 80 mg/L. If the oral bioavailability of theophylline is 98%, the clearance is 50 mL/min, volume of distribution is

35 L, and the elimination half-life is 7.5 h, the amount ingested must have been at least
(A) 0.3 g
(B) 0.6 g
(C) 1.6 g
(D) 2.8 g
(E) 8.0 g

9. A short-acting antidote that can reduce this patient's tachycardia is
(A) Acetylcysteine
(B) Deferoxamine
(C) Esmolol
(D) Fomepizole
(E) Pralidoxime

10. A contraindication to the use of gastric lavage for the removal of drugs from the stomach of victim of poisoning is
(A) An overdose of iron pills
(B) An unconscious patient
(C) Ingestion of a corrosive
(D) Overdose with a sustained-release formulation

DIRECTIONS: 11–13. The matching questions in this section consist of a list of lettered options followed by several numbered items. For each numbered item, select the ONE lettered option that is most closely associated with it.
(A) Acetaminophen
(B) Acetylsalicylic acid
(C) Benzene
(D) Carbon monoxide
(E) Heroin
(F) Hydrogen sulfide
(G) Iron
(H) Lead
(I) Methanol
(J) Physostigmine
(K) Sodium cyanide
(L) Theophylline
(M) Triazolam

11. The best antidote for overdose of this substance is atropine.

12. Acetylcysteine should be administered to a patient who overdoses on this drug.

13. The ingestion of this chemical is best managed by fomepizole.

ANSWERS

1. Anion gap is calculated by subtracting measured serum anions (bicarbonate plus chloride) from cations (potassium plus sodium). Increases in anion

gap above normal are due to the presence of unmeasured anions that accompany acidosis. The gap in this case is 30 mEq/L, a value that is well in excess of the normal gap (12–16 mEq/L). The answer is **D.**

2. The osmolar gap is the difference between the measured serum osmolality and the osmolarity calculated from the serum sodium, glucose, and BUN concentrations according to the equation above. In this case, the measured osmolality is 300 mOsm/L, while the calculated osmolality is 305 mOsm/L; the difference is −5 mOsm/L. The answer is **B.**

3. Of the drugs listed, the 2 that are likely to cause an anion gap are aspirin and ethylene glycol. However, if the child had ingested ethylene glycol, she would be expected to exhibit a significant osmolar gap. The anion gap, lethargy, tachypnea, and hyperthermia are all consistent with aspirin poisoning. The answer is **B.**

4. The pancreatic hormone glucagon (see Chapter 41) stimulates heart rate and contractility through cardiac glucagon receptors that are coupled to adenylyl cyclase and the cAMP signaling pathway. This ability to increase cardiac cAMP without requiring access to β receptors make it valuable in the treatment of β-blocker overdose. The answer is **C.**

5. Foodborne botulism (resulting from *C botulinum*) may lead to a symmetric descending paralysis that results in respiratory failure. Patients are initially alert but may suffer from dysarthria and dysphagia. Ptosis and ophthalmoplegia are also characteristic symptoms. The answer is **D.**

6. Tricyclic antidepressants are extremely toxic in overdose because of their effects in the CNS and cardiovascular systems. In addition to hypotension, seizures, and cardiac arrhythmias, the tricyclics have strong antimuscarinic effects. The answer is **E.**

7. Estimations of the time period required for drug or toxin elimination may be of value in the management of the poisoned patient. If no procedures were used to hasten the elimination of digoxin in this patient, the time taken to reach a safe plasma level of the drug (12.5% of the measured level) is 3 half-lives, or approximately 7 days. The answer is **B.**

8. Estimations of the quantity of a drug or toxin ingested may be of value in the management of the poisoned patient. Applying toxicokinetic principles, a rough estimate of ingested dose of theophylline could be made by multiplying the peak plasma level of the drug (80 mg/L) by its volume of distribution (35 L) to give a value of 2800 mg, or 2.8 g. Because only about one fourth of a half-life has passed since ingestion, the amount eliminated since that time will be rather small. The answer is **D.**

9. The short-acting β-blocker esmolol helps reverse the tachycardia and possibly the vasodilation associated with an overdose of theophylline. The answer is **C.**

10. Neither gastric lavage nor syrup of ipecac should be used in patients who have ingested a corrosive because of the risk of esophageal damage. Gastric lavage can be used in a comatose patient if the airway has been protected with a cuffed endotracheal tube. The answer is **C.**

11. Atropine is the primary antidote for poisoning by inhibitors of acetylcholinesterase, including carbamate (eg, physostigmine) and organophosphate insecticides (eg, malathion). Pralidoxime may be administered concomitantly with atropine to regenerate inactivated enzyme in poisoning due to insecticides. The answer is **J.**

12. Hepatotoxicity resulting from overdose of acetaminophen (more likely in alcoholic patients) is due to the formation of a toxic metabolite. Early administration of acetylcysteine can be protective. The answer is **A.**

13. By inhibiting alcohol dehydrogenase, fomepizole prevents conversion of methanol to the toxic compounds formaldehyde and formic acid. The answer is **I.**

SKILL KEEPER ANSWER: CYANIDE POISONING (SEE CHAPTERS 11 AND 12)

The cyanide antidote kit contains amyl nitrite, sodium nitrite, and sodium thiosulfate. The nitrites convert hemoglobin to methemoglobin, which has a higher affinity for the cyanide ion (forming cyanmethemoglobin) than cytochrome oxidase. Subsequent treatment with sodium thiosulfate results in the formation of methemoglobin and thiocyanate ions.

Nitroprusside is often considered the drug of choice in severe hypertension. Prolonged use of nitroprusside may result in toxicity caused by the release of cyanide and subsequent conversion to thiocyanate ions.

CHECKLIST

When you complete this chapter, you should be able to:

☐ Describe the steps involved in the management of the poisoned patient, including the emergency treatment of a comatose patient.

☐ Identify toxic syndromes associated with overdose of major drug groups and of individual agents frequently involved in poisoning.

☐ Outline the methods employed for identification of toxic compounds, including descriptive signs and symptoms and laboratory methods.

☐ Describe the methods available for decontamination of poisoned patients and for increasing the elimination of toxic compounds.

☐ Identify the antidotes available for management of the poisoned patient.

PART X
Special Topics

Drugs Used in Gastrointestinal Disorders

The gastrointestinal tract serves many important functions: digestive, excretory, endocrine, exocrine, and so on. These functions are the targets of several important classes of drugs. Some of these drugs have been discussed previously. This chapter mentions them and discusses in more detail others that do not fall into the classes of agents described previously.

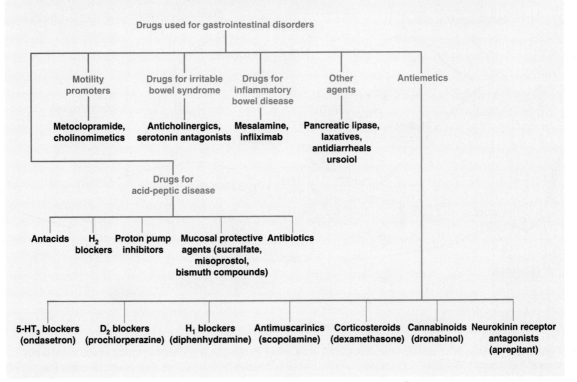

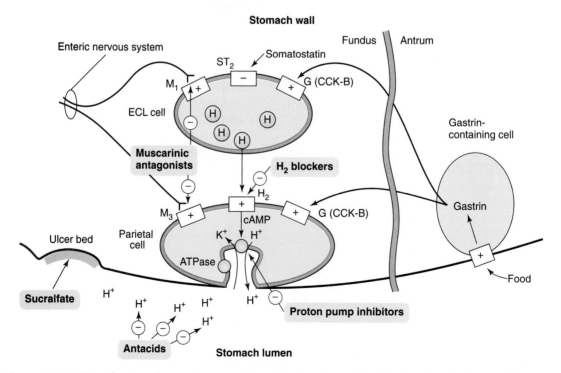

Figure 60–1. Sites of action of some drugs used in peptic ulcer disease. The site of action of misoprostol is not shown; it is thought to reduce acid secretion and increase protective factors such as mucus and bicarbonate. (Modified and reproduced, with permission, from Katzung BG, editor: *Basic & Clinical Pharmacology*, 10th ed. McGraw-Hill, 2007.)

A. Drugs Used in Acid-Peptic Disease

Ulceration and erosion of the lining of the upper portion of the gastrointestinal tract are common problems that manifest as gastroesophageal reflux (GERD), gastric and duodenal peptic ulcers, and stress-related mucosal injury. Drugs used in acid-peptic disease (Figure 60–1) reduce intragastric acidity and promote mucosal defense (or in the case of peptic ulcers, eradicate the bacterium *Helicobacter pylori*, which is detectable in over 80% of patients with duodenal ulcers).

1. Antacids—Antacids are weak bases that neutralize stomach acid by reacting with protons in the lumen of the gut and may also stimulate the protective functions of the gastric mucosa. When used regularly in the large doses needed to significantly raise the stomach pH, antacids reduce the recurrence rate of peptic ulcers.

The antacids differ mainly in their absorption and effects on stool consistency. The most popular antacids in use in the United States are **magnesium hydroxide** ($Mg[OH]_2$) and **aluminum hydroxide** ($Al[OH]_3$). Neither of these weak bases is significantly absorbed from the bowel. Magnesium hydroxide has a strong laxative effect, whereas aluminum hydroxide has a constipating action. These drugs are available as single-ingredient products and as combined preparations. Calcium carbonate and sodium bicarbonate are also weak bases, but they differ from aluminum and magnesium hydroxides in being absorbed from the gut. Because of their systemic effects, calcium and bicarbonate salts are less popular as antacids.

2. H$_2$-Receptor antagonists—**Cimetidine** and other H$_2$ antagonists (ranitidine, famotidine, and nizatidine) inhibit stomach acid production. They are effective in the treatment of GERD, peptic ulcer disease, and nonulcer dyspepsia and in the prevention of stress-related gastritis in seriously ill patients. Although they are still used widely, their clinical use is being supplanted by the more effective and equally safe proton pump inhibitors. The H$_2$ antagonists are described in detail in Chapter 16.

3. Proton pump inhibitors—**Omeprazole** and other proton pump inhibitors (esomeprazole, lansoprazole, pantoprazole, and rabeprazole) are lipophilic weak bases that diffuse into the parietal cell canaliculi, where they become protonated and concentrated >1000 fold. There they undergo conversion to compounds that irreversibly inactivate the parietal cell H^+/K^+ ATPase, the transporter that is primarily responsible for producing stomach acid. Oral formulations of these drugs are enteric coated to prevent acid inactivation in the stomach. After absorption in the intestine, they are rapidly metabolized in the liver, with half-lives of 1–2 h. However, their durations of action are approximately 24 h, and they may require 3–4 days of treatment to achieve their full effectiveness.

Proton pump inhibitors are more effective than H$_2$ antagonists for GERD and peptic ulcer and equally effective in the treatment of nonulcer dyspepsia and the prevention of stress-related mucosal bleeding. They are also useful in the treatment of Zollinger-Ellison syndrome. Adverse effects of proton pump inhibitors occur infrequently and include diarrhea, abdominal pain, and headache. Chronic treatment with proton pump inhibitors may result in hypergastrinemia. However, there is no documentation that the use of these drugs increases the incidence of carcinoid or colon cancer. Proton pump inhibitors may decrease the oral bioavailability of vitamin B$_{12}$ and certain drugs that require acidity for their gastrointestinal absorption (eg, digoxin, ketoconazole). Patients taking proton pump inhibitors may have a small increase in the risk of respiratory and enteric infections.

4. Sucralfate—Sucralfate, an aluminum sucrose sulfate, is a small, poorly soluble molecule that polymerizes in the acid environment of the stomach. The polymer binds to injured tissue and forms a protective coating over ulcer beds. Sucralfate accelerates the healing of peptic ulcers and reduces the recurrence rate. Unfortunately, sucralfate must be taken 4 times daily. Sucralfate is too insoluble to have significant systemic effects when taken by the oral route; toxicity is very low.

5. Misoprostol—Misoprostol, an analog of PGE$_1$, increases mucosal protection and inhibits acid secretion. It is effective in reducing the risk of ulcers in users of nonsteroidal anti-inflammatory drugs (NSAIDs) but is not widely used because of the need for multiple daily dosing and poorly tolerated adverse effects (gastrointestinal upset and diarrhea). Misoprostol is discussed in detail in Chapter 18.

6. Colloidal bismuth—Bismuth has multiple actions, including formation of a protective coating on ulcerated tissue, stimulation of mucosal protective mechanisms, direct antimicrobial effects, and sequestration of enterotoxins. Bismuth subsalicylate, a nonprescription formulation of bismuth and salicylate sold in the United States, reduces stool frequency and liquidity in infectious diarrhea. Bismuth causes black stools.

7. Antibiotics—Chronic infection with *H pylori* is present in the great majority of patients with recurrent non-NSAID-induced peptic ulcers. Eradication of this organism greatly reduces the rate of recurrence of ulcer in these patients. The regimens of choice consist of a proton pump inhibitor plus a course of bismuth (Pepto-Bismol), tetracycline, and metronidazole or a course of amoxicillin plus clarithromycin.

B. Drugs That Promote Upper Gastrointestinal Motility

Prokinetic drugs that stimulate upper gastrointestinal motility are helpful for gastroparesis and for postsurgical gastric emptying delay. Their ability to increase lower esophageal sphincter pressures also makes them useful for some patients with GERD. In the past cholinomimetic agonists such as bethanechol were used for GERD and gastroparesis, but the availability of less toxic agents has supplanted their use. The acetylcholinesterase inhibitor neostigmine is still used for the treatment of hospitalized patients with acute large bowel distention. The cholinomimetics are discussed in Chapter 7.

In the enteric nervous system, dopamine serves an inhibitory function by inhibiting cholinergic stimulation of smooth muscle contraction. **Metoclopramide** is a D_2 dopamine receptor antagonist that promotes gastrointestinal motility. The D_2 receptor blocking action of metoclopramide in the area postrema is also of value in preventing emesis after surgical anesthesia and emesis induced by cancer chemotherapeutic drugs. When used chronically, metoclopramide can cause symptoms of parkinsonism, other extrapyramidal effects, and hyperprolactinemia.

C. DRUGS WITH ANTIEMETIC ACTIONS

A variety of drugs are valuable in the prevention and treatment of vomiting, especially cancer chemotherapy-induced vomiting. In addition to **metoclopramide** and other D_2 dopamine receptor antagonists, useful antiemetic drugs are the **5-HT$_3$** antagonists (Chapter 16); drugs with **H$_1$ histamine blocking** activity (Chapter 16), including **diphenhydramine** and several **phenothiazines** (Chapter 29); **antimuscarinic drugs** such as **scopolamine** (Chapter 8); the corticosteroid **dexamethasone** (Chapter 39); and the cannabinoid receptor agonists **dronabinol** and nabilone (Chapter 32). The 5-HT$_3$ antagonists, **ondansetron, granisetron, dolasetron,** and **palonosetron,** are particularly useful in preventing nausea and vomiting after general anesthesia and in patients receiving cancer chemotherapy. **Aprepitant** a new antiemetic drug is an antagonist of the neurokinin 1 (NK$_1$) receptor, a receptor in the area postrema of the CNS that is activated by substance P and other tachykinins (see Chapter 17). Aprepitant is approved for use in combination with other antiemetics for prevention of the nausea and vomiting associated with highly emetogenic chemotherapeutic regimens. Aprepitant can cause fatigue, dizziness, and diarrhea. As a substrate and an inhibitor of CYP3A4, aprepitant will participate in many drug interactions.

D. DRUGS USED FOR IRRITABLE BOWEL SYNDROME

Irritable bowel syndrome (IBS) is associated with relapsing episodes of abdominal discomfort (pain, bloating, distention, or cramps) plus diarrhea or constipation (or both). The pharmacologic strategy is tailored to patients' symptoms and includes antidiarrheal agents and laxatives, and for the treatment of abdominal pain, low doses of tricyclic antidepressants (Chapter 30). The anticholinergic drugs dicyclomine and hyoscyamine are used as antispasmodics to relieve abdominal pain; however, their efficacy has not been convincingly demonstrated. **Alosetron**, a potent 5-HT$_3$ *antagonist,* is approved for treatment of women with severe IBS with diarrhea. Alosetron can cause constipation, including rare complications of severe constipation that have required hospitalization or surgery, and with rare cases of ischemic colitis. For this reason, its use is restricted. It is not known whether the less potent 5-HT$_3$ receptor antagonists that are used as antiemetics (such as ondansetron) have efficacy in IBS. **Tegaserod**, a partial agonist of 5-HT$_4$ receptors, promotes gastric emptying and enhances small and large bowel transit without an effect upon esophageal motility, and also increases stool liquidity by increasing chloride secretion in the colon. Tegaserod was approved in the United States for short-term treatment of women with IBS with constipation and for treatment of other causes of chronic constipation. However, it has recently been discontinued because of an increased risk of cardiovascular events.

E. DRUGS USED IN INFLAMMATORY BOWEL DISEASE

Drugs used in the treatment of ulcerative colitis and Crohn's disease include glucocorticoids (Chapters 39 and 56), immunosuppressive antimetabolites (eg, azathioprine, 6-mercaptopurine, methotrexate; Chapters 55 and 56), infliximab (an anti-TNF-α monoclonal antibody, Chapter 56), and aminosalicylates (eg, sulfasalazine, balsalazide, mesalamine). The aminosalicylates are not absorbed significantly after oral administration. In the small intestine, they release 5-aminosalicylic acid (5-ASA), which inhibits the synthesis of both prostaglandins and inflammatory leukotrienes. Sulfasalazine (a combination of 5-ASA and sulfapyridine) has a high incidence of adverse effects, attributable to the systemic absorption of the sulfapyridine moiety. These effects are dose related and include nausea, gastrointestinal upset, headaches, arthralgias, myalgias, bone marrow suppression, malaise, and severe hypersensitivity reactions. Other aminosalicylates, which do not contain sulfapyridine, are well tolerated.

SKILL KEEPER: 5-HT
AGONISTS AND ANTAGONISTS
(SEE CHAPTERS 16 AND 30)

List the various 5-HT receptor agonists and antagonists in current use. Describe their clinical applications. The Skill Keeper Answer appears at the end of the chapter.

KEY DRUGS

Subclass	Prototypes	Other Significant Agents
Drugs for acid-peptic disease		
Antacids	Aluminum hydroxide, magnesium hydroxide	Calcium carbonate
H_2 receptor antagonists	Cimetidine	Famotidine, nizatidine, ranitidine
Proton pump inhibitors	Omeprazole	Esomeprazole, lansoprazole, pantoprazole, rabeprazole
Mucosal protective agents	Sucralfate Misoprostol Bismuth subsalicylate	
Antibiotics for *H pylori* infection	Tetracycline, metronidazole, amoxicillin, clarithromycin	
Prokinetic drugs	Metoclopramide	Bethanechol, neostigmine
Antiemetics		
$5\text{-}HT_3$ receptor antagonists	Ondansetron	Granisetron, dolasetron, palonosetron
D_2 receptor antagonists	Metoclopramide, prochlorperazine	Promethazine, droperidol
H_1 receptor antagonists	Diphenhydramine	Dimenhydrinate, meclizine
Muscarinic receptor antagonists	Scopolamine	
Corticosteroids	Dexamethasone	
Cannabinoids	Dronabinol	Nabilone
NK_1 receptor antagonist	Aprepitant	
Antidiarrheal drugs	Loperamide	Diphenoxylate
Laxatives	See Table 60–1	
Drugs for IBS		
$5\text{-}HT_3$ receptor antagonist (for IBS with diarrhea)	Alosetron	
$5\text{-}HT_4$ receptor agonist (for IBS with constipation)	Tegaserod	
Drugs for IBD		
Aminosalicylates	Mesalamine	Sulfasalazine, olsalazine, balsalazide
Other anti-inflammatory and immunosuppressant drugs	Prednisone Azathioprine Methotrexate Infliximab	Prednisolone 6-Mercaptopurine
Pancreatic enzyme supplements	Pancreatin	Pancrelipase
Bile acid therapy for gallstones	Ursodiol	

F. Pancreatic Enzyme Replacements

Steatorrhea, a condition of decreased fat absorption coupled with an increase in stool fat excretion, results from inadequate pancreatic secretion of lipase. The abnormality of fat absorption can be significantly relieved by oral administration of pancreatic lipase (**pancreatin** or **pancrelipase**) obtained from pigs. Pancreatic lipase is inactivated at a pH below 4.0; the enzyme should be taken as enteric-coated capsules unless the pH is raised with antacids or drugs that reduce acid secretion.

G. Laxatives

Laxatives increase the probability of a bowel movement by several mechanisms: an irritant or stimulant action on the bowel wall; a bulk-forming action on the stool that evokes reflex contraction of the bowel; a softening action on hard or impacted stool; and a lubricating action that eases passage of stool through the rectum. Examples of drugs that act by these mechanisms are listed in Table 60–1.

H. Antidiarrheal Agents

The most effective antidiarrheal drugs are the opioids and derivatives of opioids that have been selected for maximal antidiarrheal and minimal CNS effect. Of the latter group, the most important are **diphenoxylate** and **loperamide,** meperidine analogs with very weak analgesic effects. **Difenoxin,** the active metabolite of diphenoxylate, is also available as a prescription medication. Diphenoxylate is formulated with antimuscarinic alkaloids (eg, atropine) to reduce the likelihood of abuse; loperamide is formulated alone.

I. Drugs That Inhibit the Formation of Gallstones

The formation of cholesterol gallstones can be inhibited by several drugs, although none are dramatically effective. Such drugs include the bile acid derivatives

Table 60–1. The major laxative mechanisms and some representative laxative drugs.

Mechanism	Examples
Bulk-forming	Psyllium, methylcellulose, polycarbophil
Stool-softening	Docusate, glycerin, mineral oil
Osmotic	Magnesium oxide, sorbitol, lactulose, polyethylene glycol
Stimulant	Aloe, senna, cascara, castor oil
5-HT$_4$ receptor agonist	Tegaserod

chenodiol and **ursodiol.** Chenodiol appears to reduce the secretion of bile acids by the liver, whereas the mechanism of action of ursodiol is unknown.

QUESTIONS

1. A 55-year-old woman with insulin-dependent diabetes of 40 years' duration complains of severe bloating and abdominal distress, especially after meals. Evaluation is consistent with diabetic gastroparesis. The prokinetic drug you would be most likely to recommend is
   (A) Alosetron
   (B) Cimetidine
   (C) Loperamide
   (D) Metoclopramide
   (E) Sucralfate

2. A patient who is taking verapamil for hypertension and angina has become constipated. Which of the following drugs is an osmotic laxative that could be used to treat the patient's constipation?
   (A) Aluminum hydroxide
   (B) Diphenoxylate
   (C) Magnesium hydroxide
   (D) Metoclopramide
   (E) Mineral oil

3. Which drug accumulates in parietal cell canaliculi and undergoes conversion to a derivative that irreversibly inhibits H$^+$/K$^+$ ATPase?
   (A) Cimetidine
   (B) Diphenoxylate
   (C) Esomeprazole
   (D) Metoclopramide
   (E) Sulfasalazine

4. Which drug is most likely to be useful in the treatment of inflammatory bowel disease?
   (A) Diphenhydramine
   (B) Diphenoxylate
   (C) Mesalamine
   (D) Ondansetron
   (E) Ursodiol

5. Which drug is most appropriate for the treatment of a patient who presents with Zollinger-Ellison syndrome resulting from a gastrinoma?
   (A) Aprepitant
   (B) Metoclopramide
   (C) Omeprazole
   (D) Ondansetron
   (E) Ranitidine

6. A 34-year-old woman has irritable bowel syndrome with diarrhea that is not responsive to conventional therapies. Despite the small risk of severe constipation

and ischemic colitis, the patient decides to begin therapy with alosetron, a drug that acts as a
(A) 5-HT$_3$ receptor antagonist
(B) 5-HT$_4$ receptor agonist
(C) D$_2$ receptor antagonist
(D) NK$_1$ receptor antagonist
(E) Muscarinic receptor antagonist

7. On your way to an examination, you experience the vulnerable feeling that an attack of diarrhea is imminent. If you stopped at a drugstore, which one of the following antidiarrheal drugs could you buy without a prescription even though it is related chemically to the strong opioid-analgesic meperidine?
(A) Aluminum hydroxide
(B) Diphenoxylate
(C) Loperamide
(D) Magnesium hydroxide
(E) Metoclopramide

8. A 45-year-old man with a duodenal ulcer was treated with a combination of drugs intended to heal the mucosal damage and to eradicate *Helicobacter pylori*. An antibacterial drug that is used commonly to eradicate intestinal *Helicobacter pylori* is
(A) Cefazolin
(B) Ciprofloxacin
(C) Clarithromycin
(D) Clindamycin
(E) Vancomycin

9. A patient is receiving highly emetogenic chemotherapy for metastatic carcinoma. To prevent chemotherapy-induced nausea and vomiting, she is likely to be treated with
(A) Levodopa
(B) Methotrexate
(C) Misoprostol
(D) Ondansetron
(E) Sucralfate

DIRECTIONS: 10–12. The following matching questions consist of a list of lettered options followed by several numbered items. For each numbered item, select the ONE option that is most closely associated with it.
(A) Aluminum hydroxide
(B) Balsalazide
(C) Castor oil
(D) Cimetidine
(E) Dexamethasone
(F) Methotrexate
(G) Metoclopramide
(H) Mineral oil
(I) Omeprazole
(J) Ondansetron

(K) Pancrelipase
(L) Sucralfate

10. Management of steatorrhea is best accomplished by the use of this agent.

11. This is a small molecule that polymerizes in stomach acid and coats the ulcer bed, resulting in accelerated healing and reduction of symptoms.

12. Extrapyramidal dysfunction, including tardive dyskinesia, has occurred with chronic administration of this drug.

ANSWERS

1. Of the drugs listed, only metoclopramide is considered a prokinetic agent (ie, one that increases propulsive motility in the gut). The answer is **D.**

2. A laxative that mildly stimulates the gut would be most suitable in a patient taking a smooth muscle relaxant drug such as verapamil. By holding water in the intestine, magnesium hydroxide provides additional bulk and stimulates increased contractions. The answer is **C.**

3. Esomeprazole, the (S) isomer of omeprazole, is a prodrug converting spontaneously in the parietal cell canaliculus to a sulfonamide that irreversibly inactivates the proton pump. The answer is **C.**

4. Mesalamine is a form of aminosalicylate that releases 5-aminosalicyclic acid in the large intestine and thereby provides a local anti-inflammatory effect that is useful in inflammatory bowel disease. The answer is **C.**

5. In patients with gastrinomas, acid hypersecretion causes gastrointestinal ulceration and malabsorption. High doses of H$_2$ antagonists usually result in suboptimal acid suppression. With proton pump inhibitors, excellent acid suppression can be achieved. The answer is **C.**

6. Serotonin plays a major regulatory role in the enteric nervous system, and the potent 5-HT$_3$ receptor antagonist alosetron has shown efficacy in treating women with IBS that is accompanied by diarrhea. The answer is **A.**

7. Aluminum hydroxide is constipating but is not related chemically to meperidine; magnesium hydroxide is a strong laxative. The 2 antidiarrheal drugs that are structurally related to opioids are diphenoxylate and loperamide. Loperamide is available over-the-counter; diphenoxylate is mixed with atropine alkaloids, and the product (Lomotil, others) requires a prescription. The answer is **C.**

8. The macrolide antibiotic clarithromycin is commonly used in antibiotic regimens designed to treat duodenal ulcers caused by *H pylori*. The other antibiotics that are used include amoxicillin, tetracycline, and metronidazole. Bismuth also has an antibacterial action. The answer is **C**.

9. The 5-HT$_3$ receptor antagonists are highly effective at preventing chemotherapy-induced nausea and vomiting, which can be a dose-limiting toxicity of anticancer drugs. The answer is **D**.

10. Steatorrhea is due to decreased fat absorption as a result of inadequate pancreatic secretion of lipase. The answer is **K**.

11. Sucralfate is a small molecule that polymerizes in stomach acid and forms a protective coat over the ulcer bed. The answer is **L**.

12. Metoclopramide is an antagonist at dopamine receptors in the CNS and has caused extrapyramidal and endocrine dysfunctions similar to those associated with the use of the older antipsychotic drugs (eg, haloperidol). The answer is **G**.

SKILL KEEPER ANSWER:
5-HT AGONISTS & ANTAGONISTS
(SEE CHAPTERS 16 AND 30)

The only serotonin agonists in common use are the 5-HT$_{1D}$-selective agonists such as sumatriptan and its congeners (see Chapter 16) that are used in migraine. Ergot alkaloids are partial agonists at several 5-HT receptors and are also used in migraine and other conditions. Several valuable antidepressants are inhibitors of the serotonin reuptake pump in neurons (see Chapter 30). Serotonin antagonists include 5-HT$_2$ blockers such as ketanserin (also an α-blocker), cyproheptadine (also an H$_1$ blocker), phenoxybenzamine (also an α-blocker), and several of the atypical antipsychotic drugs (eg, olanzapine, aripiprazole; see Chapter 29), which have high affinity for HT$_{2A}$ receptors. Ketanserin is not available in the United States but is used for hypertension in some countries. Cyproheptadine is used for pruritus and sometimes for carcinoid tumor. Phenoxybenzamine is used for carcinoid tumor as well as for pheochromocytoma. 5-HT$_3$ receptors are blocked by ondansetron and its congeners. These drugs are extremely useful in preventing postoperative and cancer chemotherapy-induced nausea and vomiting.

CHECKLIST

When you complete this chapter, you should be able to:

☐ Identify 5 different groups of drugs used in peptic ulcer disease.

☐ Describe the mechanism of action of omeprazole and related drugs.

☐ List 7 different drugs used in the prevention of chemotherapy- or radiation-induced emesis and identify the receptors with which they interact.

☐ Describe the mechanism of action, clinical uses, and adverse effects of metoclopramide.

☐ Identify 2 drugs commonly used as antidiarrheal agents and 4 drugs with different mechanisms that are used as laxatives.

☐ Identify drugs used in the management of inflammatory bowel disease and irritable bowel syndrome.

Botanical Medications & Nutritional Supplements

61

Botanical or "herbal" medications are available without prescription and, unlike over-the-counter medications, are considered to be nutritional supplements rather than drugs. These substances are marketed in the United States without FDA or other governmental review of efficacy or safety, and with little government oversight of purity, variations in potency, or the chemical identities of constituents. Purified nonherbal nutritional supplements such as dehydroepiandrosterone (DHEA) and melatonin are also used widely by the general public in pursuit of "alternative medicine." In the case of many herbal products and nutritional supplements, evidence from controlled clinical studies for their medical effectiveness is incomplete or nonexistent. A summary of the intended uses of some herbal products and nutritional supplements is presented in Table 61–1.

BOTANICAL SUBSTANCES

A. Echinacea

1. **Nature**—Leaves and roots of echinacea species (eg, *E purpurea*) contain flavonoids, polyacetylenes, and caffeoyl conjugates.

2. **Pharmacology**—In vitro studies have shown that echinacea has cytokine activation (increased interleukins and tumor necrosis factor) and anti-inflammatory properties. Older reviews and clinical trials reporting favorable results for the use of freshly pressed juice of the aerial parts of *E purpurea* in reducing cold symptoms have not been borne out with more recent trials investigating preparations of *E angustifolia*.

3. **Toxicity and drug interactions**—Unpleasant taste and gastrointestinal effects may occur, sometimes with dizziness or headache. Some preparations have a high alcohol content, but no drug interactions have been reported.

B. Ephedra (Ma Huang)

1. **Nature**—Ma huang is one of many names given to various plants of the genus *Ephedra*, the major chemical constituents of which are ephedrine and pseudoephedrine (see Chapter 9). Ephedrine is a prescription drug in the United States; pseudoephedrine is available in over-the-counter decongestants. In the United States, the FDA has banned the marketing of dietary supplements containing ephedrine alkaloids, which are considered to pose an unreasonable cardiovascular risk. The ban is not applicable to Chinese herbal remedies.

2. **Pharmacology**—The actions of ephedra products are those of ephedrine and pseudoephedrine, which are indirect-acting sympathomimetics that release norepinephrine from sympathetic nerve endings (See Chapter 9). In addition to nasal decongestion, the established clinical use of ephedrine is as a pressor agent. Ephedra herbal products are commonly used for treatment of respiratory dysfunction, including bronchitis and asthma, and as mild CNS stimulants. In Chinese medicine, ephedra products are also used for relief of cold and flu symptoms, for diuresis, and for bone or joint pain. Dietary supplements containing ephedrine alkaloids have been widely promoted for weight loss and for enhancement of athletic performance.

3. **Toxicity and drug interactions**—Toxic effects are those of ephedrine and include dizziness, insomnia, anorexia, flushing, palpitations, tachycardia, and urinary retention. In high doses, ephedra can cause a marked increase in blood pressure, cardiac arrhythmias, and a toxic psychosis. Contraindications are those for ephedrine and include anxiety states, bulimia, cardiac arrhythmias, diabetes, heart failure, hypertension, glaucoma, hyperthyroidism, and pregnancy. As a weak base, renal elimination of ephedrine in overdose can be facilitated by urinary acidification.

C. Garlic

1. **Nature**—Garlic (*Allium sativum*) contains organic thiosulfinates that can form allicin (responsible for the characteristic odor) via enzymes activated by disruption of the garlic bulb.

HIGH-YIELD TERMS TO LEARN

Alternative medicine	Treatments that are *not* generally recognized by the medical community as standard or conventional medical approaches
Controlled clinical trial	A clinical trial that compares a group of subjects who are receiving a treatment with a closely match group of individuals who are not receiving a treatment. Chapter 5 describes clinical trials in more detail
Herbal medication	Plants or plant extracts that people use to improve their health
Nutritional supplement	A substance that is added to the diet to improve health and which usually contains dietary ingredients such as vitamins, minerals, amino acids, and enzymes
Placebo	An inactive "dummy" medication made to resemble the investigational formulation as much as possible

2. Pharmacology—In vitro studies show that allicin inhibits hepatic hydroxymethylglutaryl coenzyme A (HMG-CoA) reductase and angiotensin-converting enzyme (ACE), blocks platelet aggregation, increases nitric oxide (NO), is fibrinolytic, has antimicrobial activity, and reduces carcinogen activation. Although several clinical trials have shown significant reduction in cholesterol and blood pressure, others, including a recent well-controlled study in adults with moderately elevated cholesterol, failed to show a significant effect. Preliminary clinical studies in patients with atherosclerosis suggest that garlic ingestion can significantly reduce plaque volume.

3. Toxicity and drug interactions—Nausea, hypotension, and allergic reactions may occur. Possible antiplatelet action warrants caution in patients receiving anticoagulants or conventional antiplatelet drugs.

D. GINKGO

1. Nature—Prepared from the leaves of *Ginkgo biloba,* ginkgo contains flavone glycosides and terpenoids.

2. Pharmacology—In in vitro studies, ginkgo exhibits antioxidant and radical-scavenging effects and increases NO formation. Animal studies have revealed reduced blood viscosity and changes in CNS neurotransmitters.

Table 61–1. Common intended uses of some botanical or nutritional supplements.

Botanical or Nutritional Supplement	Common Intended Use
Echinacea	Decrease duration and intensity of cold symptoms
Ephedra (Ma huang)	Treatment of respiratory ailments such as bronchitis and asthma, and as a CNS stimulant
Garlic	For cholesterol lowering and atherosclerosis
Ginkgo	Treatment of intermittent claudication, and cerebral insufficiency and dementia
Ginseng	Improvement of physical and mental performance
Milk thistle	Limitation of hepatic injury and as an antidote to *Amanita* mushroom poisoning
Saw palmetto	Improvement in symptoms of benign prostatic hyperplasia
St. John's wort	Treatment of mild to moderate depression
Coenzyme Q10	Improvement of ischemic heart disease and for Parkinson's disease
Glucosamine	Reduction of pain associated with osteoarthritis
Melatonin	Decrease jet lag symptoms and as a sleep aid

At the clinical level, ginkgo may have value in intermittent claudication, and its use as a pretreatment may reduce markers of oxidative stress associated with coronary artery bypass surgery. Several studies show a mild benefit of ginkgo in patients with cognitive impairment and dementia. Ongoing trials are investigating ginkgo as a prophylactic agent for Alzheimer's dementia.

3. Toxicity and drug interactions—Gastrointestinal effects, anxiety, insomnia, and headache occur. Possible antiplatelet action suggests caution in patients receiving anticoagulants or antiplatelet drugs. Ginkgo may be epileptogenic and should be avoided in persons with a history of seizure disorders.

E. GINSENG

1. Nature—Most ginseng products are derived from plants of the genus *Panax* that contain multiple triterpenoid saponin glycosides (ginsenosides). Siberian or Brazilian ginseng does not contain these chemicals.

2. Pharmacology—Ginseng is purported to improve mental and physical performance, but the clinical evidence for such effects is limited. A small clinical trial suggested the possibility of some value in type 2 diabetes, and newer trials have shown some immunomodulating benefits.

3. Toxicity and drug interactions—Estrogenic effects include mastalgia and vaginal bleeding. Insomnia, nervousness, and hypertension have been reported. Ginseng should be used cautiously in patients receiving anticoagulant, antihypertensive, hypoglycemic, or psychiatric medications.

F. MILK THISTLE

1. Nature—Milk thistle is derived from the fruit and seeds of *Silybum marianum,* which contain flavonolignans such as silymarin.

2. Pharmacology—In vitro studies show that milk thistle reduces lipid peroxidation, scavenges free radicals, enhances superoxide dismutase, inhibits formation of leukotrienes, and increases hepatocyte RNA polymerase activity. In animal models, milk thistle protects against liver injury caused by alcohol, acetaminophen, and *Amanita* mushrooms. The outcomes of clinical trials in patients with liver disease caused by alcohol have been mixed. In viral hepatitis and liver injury caused by *Amanita* mushrooms, results of clinical trials have been mainly favorable. A commercial preparation of silybin (an isomer of silymarin) is available in some countries as an antidote to *Amanita phalloides* mushroom poisoning.

3. Toxicity and drug interactions—Other than loose stools, milk thistle does not cause significant toxicity and there are no reports of drug interactions.

G. ST. JOHN'S WORT

1. Nature—St. John's wort is made from dried flowers of *Hypericum perforatum,* which contains the active constituents hypericin and hyperforin.

2. Pharmacology—In vitro studies with hyperforin have shown decreased activity of serotonergic reuptake systems. In animals, chronic treatment with commercial extracts led to down-regulation of adrenoceptors and up-regulation of 5-HT receptors. Some (but not all) clinical trials of the extract in patients with mild to moderate depression have shown efficacy that is greater than placebo and, in some trials, similar to those of prescription antidepressants for mild or moderate depression. Hypericin, when photoactivated, may have antiviral and anticancer effects.

3. Toxicity and drug interactions—Mild gastrointestinal side effects occur and photosensitization has been reported. St. John's wort should be avoided in patients using SSRIs or monoamine oxidase (MAO) inhibitors and in those with a history of bipolar or psychotic disorder. Constituents in St. John's wort induce the formation of cytochrome P450 isoforms and P-glycoprotein drug transporters. Decreases in effectiveness of birth control pills, cyclosporine, digoxin, HIV protease inhibitors, and warfarin have been reported in patients who regularly use St. John's wort.

H. SAW PALMETTO

1. Nature—Saw palmetto is derived from the berries of *Serenoa repens* or *Sabal serrulata* and contains phytosterols, aliphatic alcohols, polyprenes, and flavonoids.

2. Pharmacology—In vitro studies have shown inhibition of 5α-reductase and antagonistic effects at androgen receptors. Clinical trials of saw palmetto in benign prostatic hyperplasia (BPH) have been mixed. Some have shown improvement in urologic function and in urinary flow. Others, including a recent well-controlled, double-blind 1-year study in moderate to severe BPH, have shown no significant effects on symptoms or objective measures.

3. Toxicity and drug interactions—Abdominal pain with gastrointestinal distress, decreased libido, headache, and hypertension occur; overall incidence was less than 3%.

SKILL KEEPER: DRUGS FROM PLANT SOURCES

Many conventional drugs, strictly regulated by governmental agencies such as the FDA, originated from plant sources. How many of these compounds can you identify? The Skill Keeper Answer appears at the end of the chapter.

PURIFIED NUTRITIONAL SUBSTANCES

A. Coenzyme Q10

1. Nature—Coenzyme Q10, also known as ubiquinone, is a benzoquinone that serves as a cofactor in the mitochondrial electron transport chain and, in its reduced form of ubiquinol, serves as in important antioxidant. After ingestion, the reduced form predominates in the circulation.

2. Pharmacology—Coenzyme Q10 may have a small degree of efficacy in reducing systolic and diastolic blood pressure and in treating coronary artery disease and chronic stable angina, but it does not appear to be useful as adjunctive therapy of heart failure. Coenzyme Q10 has been reported to slow the progression of early Parkinson's disease and may reduce the frequency of migraine headaches.

3. Toxicity—Coenzyme Q10 is well tolerated. The most frequent adverse effect is gastrointestinal disturbances. Rare effects include rash, thrombocytopenia, irritability, dizziness, and headache.

B. Glucosamine

1. Nature—Glucosamine is an amino sugar that serves as the precursor of nitrogen-containing sugars, including the glycosaminoglycans that are a major constituent of connective tissue, including the cartilage in joints.

2. Pharmacology—Glucosamine is primarily used for pain associated with osteoarthritis. The many clinical trials examining the use of oral or intra-articular glucosamine have produced mixed results. Although some early trials and a meta-analysis found a beneficial effect in osteoarthritis, a recent large placebo-controlled, double-blind trial failed to find a benefit for glucosamine in treating osteoarthritis.

3. Toxicity—Glucosamine can occasionally cause diarrhea and nausea but otherwise is well tolerated. Because glucosamine is commercially prepared from crustaceans, there is some concern about cross-allergenicity in people with shellfish allergy.

C. Melatonin

1. Nature—Melatonin is a serotonin derivative produced mainly in the pineal gland. It appears to regulate sleep–wake cycles, and its release coincides with darkness (9 PM to 4 AM). Other purported activities include contraception, prevention of aging, protection against oxidative stress, and the treatment of cancer, major depression, and HIV infection.

2. Pharmacology—Melatonin has been used extensively for jet lag and as an alternative to prescription drugs for insomnia. In jet lag, clinical studies have shown subjective improvements in mood, more rapid recovery times, and reductions in daytime fatigue.

Melatonin improves sleep onset, duration, and quality when given to patients with sleep disorders.

3. Toxicity—Sedation and next-day drowsiness and headache have been reported. Melatonin can suppress the midcycle surge of luteinizing hormone (LH) and should not be used in pregnancy or in women attempting to conceive. Because it can decrease prolactin levels, melatonin should not be used by nursing mothers. In healthy men chronic melatonin use decreases sperm quality.

QUESTIONS

1. You have accidentally ingested mushrooms identified as *Amanita phalloides*. Which herbal substance is most likely to protect against hepatic dysfunction?
   (A) Echinacea
   (B) Ginkgo
   (C) Melatonin
   (D) Milk thistle
   (E) Saw palmetto

2. There may be a link between this important endogenous antioxidant and Parkinson's disease because patients with Parkinson's disease have been reported to have reduced serum levels of the reduced form of this compound, and there is some evidence that its use as a supplement slows the progression of early Parkinson's disease. The supplement is
   (A) Coenzyme Q10
   (B) Glucosamine
   (C) Melatonin
   (D) Tyrosine
   (E) Vitamin E

3. Which drug has a biochemical effect that most closely resembles the proposed mechanism of action of the psychoactive constituent(s) of St. John's wort?
   (A) Alprazolam
   (B) Fluoxetine
   (C) Levodopa
   (D) Methylphenidate
   (E) Selegiline

4. An alternative medicine that is commonly used to treat the urinary symptoms associated with benign prostatic hyperplasia (BPH) is
   (A) Echinacea
   (B) Ephedra
   (C) Ginseng
   (D) Milk thistle
   (E) Saw palmetto

5. Which of the following is a derivative of serotonin that may have value in managing symptoms of jet lag?
   (A) Ephedra
   (B) Garlic

(C) Ginseng
(D) Glucosamine
(E) Melatonin

6. Which compound enhances immune function in vitro and is commonly used to decrease the symptoms of the common cold?
(A) Echinacea
(B) Ginkgo
(C) Garlic
(D) Melatonin
(E) Milk thistle

7. Rejection of heart transplants has occurred in patients being treated with standard doses of cyclosporine when they also used
(A) Echinacea
(B) Ginkgo
(C) Milk thistle
(D) St. John's wort
(E) Saw palmetto

8. In 2003, a study published in the *Annals of Internal Medicine* found that this botanical substance accounted for more than 60% of adverse events associated with dietary supplements used in the United States. The "herbal" in question, which is used to aid weight loss and promote sports performance, is
(A) Echinacea
(B) Ephedra
(C) Ginkgo
(D) Ginseng
(E) Saw palmetto

9. A popular supplement whose purported efficacy in osteoarthritis is believed to be due to its role as a precursor to the glycosaminoglycans that form joint cartilage is
(A) Coenzyme Q10
(B) Dehydroepiandrosterone (DHEA)
(C) Glycosamine
(D) Nicotinic acid
(E) Melatonin

10. Couples who are attempting to conceive a child should avoid chronic use of
(A) Echinacea
(B) Ephedra
(C) Ginkgo
(D) Ginseng
(E) Melatonin

ANSWERS

1. Milk thistle contains compounds that may have cytoprotective actions against liver toxins, including those present in *Amanita* mushrooms. The answer is **D**.

2. The reduced form of coenzyme Q10 serves as an important antioxidant and may have benefit in early Parkinson's disease. The answer is **A**.

3. Extracts of the flowers of St. John's wort contain chemicals with possible antidepressant activity. In vitro studies have shown that these chemicals interfere with the neuronal reuptake of amine neurotransmitters in a fashion similar to the proposed mechanism of antidepressant actions of tricyclic antidepressants and SSRIs such as fluoxetine. The answer is **B**.

4. Saw palmetto, a complex extract from the berries of *Serenoa repens* or *Sabal serrulata,* is widely believed to improve the symptoms of BPH. The answer is **E**.

5. Garlic might get you a row of seats to yourself, but the compound that will help in jet lag is melatonin. The answer is **E**.

6. The freshly pressed juice of the aerial parts of *Echinacea purpurea* is purported to reduce the symptoms of the common cold and the time of recovery if ingested within 24 h of onset. The answer is **A**.

7. St. John's wort induces the formation of hepatic enzymes that metabolize cyclosporine, and its use can decrease the effectiveness of the immunosuppressant drug in organ and tissue transplantation. The answer is **D**.

8. Concern about the risks of using products containing ephedra during heavy workouts or in diet programs that stress the cardiovascular system has led to a ban on such nutritional supplements in the United States. The answer is **B**.

9. The amino sugar glucosamine, a building block for glycosaminoglycans, has become popular among people with osteoarthritis of the knee. The answer is **C**.

10. Chronic use of melatonin appears to suppress LH secretion in women and to decrease sperm quality in men. The answer is **E**.

SKILL KEEPER ANSWER: DRUGS FROM PLANT SOURCES

The clinical application of drugs that originated from plant sources has contributed greatly to conventional medicine. Such compounds include aspirin, atropine, cocaine, codeine, colchicine, digoxin, ephedrine, etoposide, methysergide, morphine, nicotine, physostigmine, pilocarpine, quinidine, quinine, reserpine, scopolamine, taxanes (eg, paclitaxel), tubocurarine, vinblastine, and vincristine.

CHECKLIST

When you complete this chapter, you should be able to:

☐ Contrast the regulations in the United States of botanicals and nutritional supplements with those of therapeutic drugs with regard to efficacy and safety.

☐ List several of the most widely used botanical products and describe their purported medical uses, adverse effects, and potential for drug interactions.

☐ Describe the proposed medical uses and adverse effects of several purified nutritional supplements.

Drug Interactions

62

Drug interactions occur when one drug modifies the actions of another drug in the body. Drug interactions can result from pharmacokinetic alterations, pharmacodynamic changes, or a combination of both. Interactions between drugs in vitro (eg, precipitation when mixed in solutions for intravenous administration) are usually classified as *drug incompatibilities,* not drug interactions.

Although hundreds of drug interactions have been documented, relatively few are of enough clinical significance to constitute a contraindication to simultaneous use or to require a change in dosage. Some of these are listed in Table 62–1. In patients taking many drugs, however, the likelihood of significant drug interactions is increased. Elderly patients have a high incidence of drug interactions because they often have age-related changes in drug clearance and commonly take multiple medications.

PHARMACOKINETIC INTERACTIONS

A. INTERACTIONS BASED ON ABSORPTION

Absorption from the gastrointestinal tract may be influenced by agents that bind drugs (eg, resins, antacids, calcium-containing foods), by agents that increase or decrease gastrointestinal motility (eg, metoclopramide or antimuscarinics, respectively), and by drugs that alter the P-glycoprotein transporter in the wall of the intestine. Concomitant use of antacids can decrease gastrointestinal absorption of digoxin, ketoconazole, quinolone antibiotics, and tetracyclines. In contrast, erythromycin appears to increase oral bioavailability of digoxin in some patients, probably by reducing gut flora that degrade digoxin. Compounds in grapefruit juice and some drugs inhibit the P-glycoprotein drug transporter in the intestinal epithelium and may increase the net absorption of drugs that are normally expelled by the transporter. Absorption from subcutaneous sites can be slowed predictably by vasoconstrictors given simultaneously (eg, local anesthetics and epinephrine) and by cardiac depressants that decrease tissue perfusion (eg, β-blockers).

B. INTERACTIONS BASED ON DISTRIBUTION AND BINDING

Distribution of a drug can be altered by other drugs that compete for binding sites on plasma proteins. For example, antibacterial sulfonamides can displace methotrexate, phenytoin, sulfonylureas, and warfarin from binding sites on albumin. However, it is difficult to document many clinically significant interactions of this type, and they seem to be the exception rather than the rule. The ability of quinidine to raise the blood levels of digoxin was originally attributed to displacement from tissue binding sites but probably involves a reduction in the clearance of digoxin. Changes in drug distribution can occur if one agent alters the size of the physical compartment in which another drug distributes. For example, diuretics, by reducing total body water, can increase plasma levels of aminoglycosides and lithium, possibly enhancing drug toxicities.

C. INTERACTIONS BASED ON METABOLIC CLEARANCE

Drug interactions of this type are well documented and have considerable clinical significance. The metabolism of many drugs can be increased by other agents that induce hepatic drug-metabolizing enzymes, especially cytochrome P450 isozymes. Induction of drug-metabolizing enzymes occurs predictably with the chronic administration of **barbiturates, carbamazepine, ethanol, phenytoin,** or **rifampin.** Conversely, the metabolism of some drugs may be decreased by other drugs that inhibit drug-metabolizing enzymes. Such inhibitors of drug-metabolizing enzymes include **cimetidine, disulfiram, erythromycin, furanocoumarins** (in grapefruit juice), **ketoconazole, propoxyphene, quinidine, ritonavir,** and **sulfonamides.** The CYP3A4 isozyme of cytochrome P450, the dominant form in the human liver, is particularly sensitive to such inhibitory actions.

Drugs that reduce hepatic blood flow (eg, **propranolol**) may reduce the clearance of other drugs metabolized in the liver, especially those subject to flow-limited hepatic clearance such as morphine and verapamil.

A modified form of an interaction based on metabolic clearance results from the ability of some drugs to

HIGH-YIELD TERMS TO LEARN	
Addition	The effect of 2 drugs given together is equal to the sum of the responses to the same doses given separately
Antagonism	The effect of 2 drugs given together is less than the sum of the responses to the same doses given separately
Pharmacodynamic interaction	A change in the pharmacodynamics of 1 drug caused by the interacting drug (eg, additive action of 2 drugs having similar effects)
Pharmacokinetic interaction	A change in the pharmacokinetics of 1 drug caused by the interacting drug (eg, an inducer of hepatic enzymes)
Synergism	The effect of 2 drugs given together is greater than the sum of the 2 responses when they are given separately

SKILL KEEPER: WARFARIN (SEE CHAPTER 34)

When describing pharmacokinetic drug interactions, the anticoagulant warfarin inevitably springs to mind. This is because warfarin has such a narrow therapeutic window and because its metabolism depends upon CYP450 activity. How does this important anticoagulant work, how is its action monitored, and if a drug interaction leads to an excessive effect, how is its action reversed? The Skill Keeper Answer appears at the end of the chapter.

increase the stores of endogenous substances by blocking their metabolism. These endogenous compounds may subsequently be released by other exogenous drugs, resulting in an unexpected action. The best documented reaction of this type is the sensitization of patients taking **MAO inhibitors** to indirectly acting sympathomimetics (eg, amphetamine, phenylpropanolamine). Such patients may suffer a severe hypertensive reaction in response to ordinary doses of cold remedies, decongestants, and appetite suppressants.

D. INTERACTIONS BASED ON RENAL FUNCTION

Excretion of drugs by the kidney can be changed by drugs that reduce renal blood flow (eg, β-blockers) or inhibit specific renal transport mechanisms (eg, the action of aspirin on uric acid secretion in the S_2 segment of the proximal tubule). Drugs that alter urinary pH can alter the ionization state of drugs that are weak

acids or weak bases, leading to changes in renal tubular reabsorption.

PHARMACODYNAMIC INTERACTIONS

A. INTERACTIONS BASED ON OPPOSING ACTIONS OR EFFECTS

Antagonism, the simplest type of drug interaction, is often predictable. For example, antagonism of the bronchodilating effects of β_2 adrenoceptor activators used in asthma is to be anticipated if a β-blocker is given for another condition. Likewise, the action of a catecholamine on heart rate (via β adrenoceptor activation) is antagonized by an inhibitor of acetylcholinesterase that acts through ACh (via muscarinic receptors). Antagonism by mixed agonist–antagonist drugs (eg, pentazocine) or by partial agonists (eg, pindolol) is not as easily predicted but should be expected when such drugs are used with pure agonists. Some drug antagonisms do not appear to be based on receptor interactions. For example, nonsteroidal anti-inflammatory drugs (NSAIDs) may decrease the antihypertensive action of ACE inhibitors by reducing renal elimination of sodium.

B. INTERACTIONS BASED ON ADDITIVE EFFECTS

Additive interaction describes the algebraic summing of the effects of 2 drugs. The 2 drugs may or may not act on the same receptor to produce such effects. The combined use of tricyclic antidepressants with diphenhydramine or promethazine predictably causes excessive atropine-like effects because all of these drugs have significant muscarinic receptor-blocking actions. Tricyclic antidepressants may increase the pressor responses to sympathomimetics by interference with amine transporter systems.

Table 62–1. Some important drug interactions.

Drug Causing the Interaction	Drugs Affected	Comment
Alcohol	CNS depressants	Additive CNS depression, sedation, ataxia, increased risk of accidents
	Acetaminophen	Increased formation of hepatotoxic metabolites of acetaminophen
Aminoglycosides	Loop diuretics	Enhanced ototoxicity
Antacids	Digoxin, iron supplements, fluoroquinolones, ketoconazole, tetracyclines, thyroxine	Decreased gut absorption due either to reaction with the drug affected or reduced gut acidity
Antibiotics	Estrogens, including oral contraceptives	Many antibiotics lower estrogen levels and reduce contraceptive effectiveness
Antihistamines (H$_1$-blockers)	Antimuscarinics, sedatives	Additive effects with the drugs affected
Antimuscarinic drugs	Drugs absorbed from the small intestine	Slowed onset of effect because stomach emptying is delayed
Barbiturates, especially phenobarbital	Azoles, calcium channel blockers, cyclosporine, propranolol, protease inhibitors, quinidine, steroids, warfarin, and many other drugs metabolized in the liver	Increased clearance of the affected drugs due to enzyme induction, possibly leading to decreases in drug effectiveness
Beta-blockers	Insulin	Masking of symptoms of hypoglycemia
	Prazosin	Increased "first-dose" syncope
Bile acid-binding resins	Acetaminophen, digitalis, thiazides, thyroxine	Reduced absorption of the affected drug
Carbamazepine	Cyclosporine, doxycycline, estrogen, haloperidol, theophylline, warfarin	Reduced effect of other drugs because of induction of metabolism
Cimetidine	Benzodiazepines, lidocaine, phenytoin, propranolol, quinidine, theophylline, warfarin	Increased effect of other drugs due to inhibition of hepatic metabolism
Disulfiram metronidazole, certain cephalosporins	Ethanol	Increased hangover effect of ethanol because aldehyde dehydrogenase is blocked
Erythromycin	Carbamazepine, cisapride, quinidine, sildenafil, theophylline	Risk of toxicity due to inhibition of metabolism of these drugs
Furanocoumarins (grapefruit juice)	Aprazolam, atorvastatin, cyclosporine, midazolam triazolam	Increased effect of other drugs due to inhibition of hepatic metabolism
Ketoconazole and other azoles	Benzodiazepines, cisapride cyclosporine, fluoxetine, lovastatin, omeprazole, quinidine, tolbutamide, warfarin	Risk of toxicity due to inhibition of metabolism of these drugs
MAO inhibitors	Catecholamine releasers (amphetamine, ephedrine)	Increased NE in sympathetic nerve endings released by the interacting drugs
	Tyramine-containing foods and beverages	Hypertensive crisis
Nonsteroidal anti-inflammatory drugs	Anticoagulants	Increased bleeding tendency because of reduced platelet aggregation
	ACE inhibitors	Decreased antihypertensive efficacy of ACE inhibitor
	Loop diuretics, thiazides	Reduced diuretic efficacy

(continued)

Table 62–1. Some important drug interactions. (*continued*)

Drug Causing the Interaction	Drugs Affected	Comment
Phenytoin	Doxycycline, methadone, quinidine, steroids, verapamil	Increased metabolism of other drugs due to enzyme induction; decreased efficacy
Quinidine	Digoxin	Increased digoxin levels due to decreased clearance; displacement may play a role
Rifampin	Azole antifungal drugs, corticosteroids, methadone, theophylline, tolbutamide	Decreased efficacy of these drugs due to induction of hepatic P450 isozymes
Ritonavir	Benzodiazepines, cyclosporine, diltiazem, dronabinol, HMG-CoA reductase inhibitors, lidocaine, metaprolol, other HIV protease inhibitors, propoxyphene, selective serotonin reuptake inhibitors	Decreased metabolism of other drugs; increased effects may lead to toxicity
Salicylates	Corticosteroids	Additive toxicity of gastric mucosa
	Heparin, warfarin	Increased bleeding tendency
	Methotrexate	Decreased clearance, causing greater methotrexate toxicity
	Sulfinpyrazone	Decreased uricosuric effect
Selective serotonin reuptake inhibitors	MAO inhibitors, meperidine, tricyclic antidepressants, St. John's wort	Serotonin syndrome hypertension, tachycardia, muscle rigidity, hyperthermia, seizures
Thiazides	Digitalis	Increased risk of digitalis toxicity because thiazides diminish potassium stores
	Lithium	Increased plasma levels of lithium due to decreased total body water
Warfarin	Amiodarone, cimetidine, disulfiram, erythromycin, fluconazole, lovastatin, metronidazole	Increased anticoagulant effect via inhibition of warfarin metabolism
	Anabolic steroids, aspirin, NSAIDs, quinidine, thyroxine	Increased anticoagulant effects via pharmacodynamic mechanisms
	Barbiturates, carbamazepine, phenytoin, rifabutin, rifampin, St. John's wort	Decreased anticoagulant effect due to increased clearance of warfarin via induction of hepatic P450 isozymes

One of the most common and important drug interactions is the additive depression of CNS function caused by concomitant administration of sedatives, hypnotics, and opioids with each other or associated with the consumption of ethanol. In such cases, multiple receptor systems in the brain are presumed to be involved. Similarly, the patient with moderate to severe hypertension maintained on one drug is at risk of excessive lowering of blood pressure if another drug with a different site of action is added at high dosage. This interaction is the basis for the use of "stepped-care" therapy in hypertension because it permits the use of lower, less toxic doses. Additive effects of anticoagulant drugs can lead to bleeding complications. In the case of warfarin, the potential for such adverse effects is enhanced by aspirin (via an antiplatelet action), quinidine (additive hypoprothrombinemia), thrombolytics (via plasminogen activation), and the thyroid hormones (via enhanced clotting factor catabolism).

Supra-additive interactions and potentiation appear to be much less common than antagonism and the simple additive interactions described previously. Supra-additive (synergistic) interaction is said to occur if the result of interaction is greater than the sum of the drugs

Table 62–2. Selected interactions of herbals with other drugs.

Herbal Medication	Other Drugs	Interaction
Dong quai	Warfarin	Increased anticoagulant effect of warfarin; bleeding
Garlic, ginkgo	Anticoagulants, antiplatelet agents	Increased risk of bleeding
Ginseng	Antidepressants	Increased antidepressant effect, mania
Kava	Sedative-hypnotics	Additive sedation
Liquorice root	Aldosterone, antihypertensive drugs	Liquorice root extract (not candy) increases salt retention; hypertension
Ma huang, other ephedra preparations	Sympathomimetics	Ephedrine in ma huang is additive with other sympathomimetics; hypertension, stroke
St. John's wort	Oral contraceptives, cyclosporine digoxin, HIV protease inhibitors, warfarin	Increased metabolism of drug, decreased efficacy
	Antidepressants	Increased antidepressant effect; secrotonin syndrome with selective serotonin reuptake inhibitors

used alone; the best example is the therapeutic synergism of certain antibiotic combinations such as sulfonamides and dihydrofolic acid reductase inhibitors such as trimethoprim. Potentiation is said to occur when a drug's effect is increased by another agent that has no such effect. The best example of this type of interaction is the therapeutic interaction of beta-lactamase inhibitors such as clavulanic acid with beta-lactamase-susceptible penicillins.

INTERACTIONS OF HERBAL MEDICATIONS WITH OTHER DRUGS

Because of the marked increase in use of herbal medications, more interactions of these agents with purified drugs are being reported. Some of the reported or suspected interactions are listed in Table 62–2. Several herbals listed are known to enhance the actions of anticoagulants. Many other herbs, or edible plants, also contain compounds with anticoagulant or antiplatelet potential, including anise, arnica, capsicum, celery, chamomile, clove, feverfew, garlic, ginger, horseradish, meadowsweet, onion, passion flower, turmeric, and wild lettuce.

QUESTIONS

1. Which drug increases the plasma concentration of digoxin by a pharmacokinetic mechanism?
   (A) Captopril
   (B) Hydrochlorothiazide
   (C) Lidocaine
   (D) Quinidine
   (E) Sulfasalazine

2. A 55-year-old patient currently receiving a drug for a psychiatric condition is to be started on diuretic therapy for mild heart failure. Consideration should be given to the fact that thiazides are known to reduce the excretion of
   (A) Diazepam
   (B) Fluoxetine
   (C) Imipramine
   (D) Lithium
   (E) Trifluoperazine

3. A hypertensive patient has been using nifedipine for some time without untoward effects. If he experiences a rapidly developing enhancement of the antihypertensive effect of the drug, it could be due to
   (A) Concomitant use of antacids
   (B) Foods containing tyramine
   (C) Furanocoumarins in grapefruit juice
   (D) Induction of drug metabolism
   (E) Over-the-counter decongestants

4. A patient suffering from a depressive disorder is being treated with imipramine. If he uses diphenhydramine for allergic rhinitis, a drug interaction is likely to occur because
   (A) Both drugs block muscarinic receptors
   (B) Both drugs block reuptake of norepinephrine released from sympathetic nerve endings
   (C) Diphenhydramine inhibits imipramine metabolism
   (D) Imipramine inhibits the metabolism of diphenhydramine
   (E) The drugs compete with each other for renal elimination

5. If phenelzine is administered to a patient taking fluoxetine, the most likely result is
   (A) A decrease in the plasma levels of fluoxetine
   (B) Antagonism of the antidepressant action of fluoxetine
   (C) Agitation, muscle rigidity, hyperthermia, seizures
   (D) Decreased metabolism of fluoxetine
   (E) Priapism

6. Which antibiotic is a potent inducer of hepatic drug-metabolizing enzymes?
   (A) Ciprofloxacin
   (B) Cyclosporine
   (C) Erythromycin
   (D) Rifampin
   (E) Tetracycline

7. The antihypertensive effects of captopril can be antagonized (reduced) by
   (A) Angiotensin II receptor blockers
   (B) Loop diuretics
   (C) NSAIDs
   (D) Sulfonylurea hypoglycemics
   (E) Thiazides

8. Which drug has resulted in severe hematotoxicity when administered to a patient being treated with azathioprine?
   (A) Allopurinol
   (B) Cholestyramine
   (C) Digoxin
   (D) Lithium
   (E) Theophylline

DIRECTIONS: 9–11. The following section consists of a list of lettered options followed by several numbered items. For each numbered item, select the ONE option that is most closely associated with it.
   (A) Allopurinol
   (B) Carbamazepine
   (C) Cholestyramine
   (D) Cimetidine
   (E) Clarithromycin
   (F) Cyclosporine
   (G) Digoxin
   (H) Erythromycin
   (I) Fluoxetine
   (J) Ibuprofen
   (K) Lovastatin
   (L) Phenelzine
   (M) Rifampin
   (N) Ritonavir
   (O) Theophylline

9. In AIDS patients the inhibitory action of this agent on drug metabolism has clinical value.

10. This drug enhances the toxicity of methotrexate by decreasing its renal clearance.

11. Concomitant use of St. John's wort is reported to increase the effectiveness of this drug.

ANSWERS

1. Quinidine and thiazide diuretics can both enhance the toxicity of digitalis. The action of quinidine is attributed to pharmacokinetic mechanisms, especially inhibition of its clearance. The plasma concentration of digoxin predictably increases when quinidine is added. The enhancement of digitalis toxicity by thiazides is due to a pharmacodynamic mechanism, namely, the action of these diuretics to reduce extracellular potassium. Sulfasalazine decreases plasma levels of digitalis by interfering with gut absorption of the drug. The answer is **D**.

2. Thiazides reduce the clearance of lithium by about 25%. They do not alter the clearance of the other agents listed. The answer is **D**.

3. Compounds in grapefruit juice can increase the rate and extent of bioavailability of several dihydropyridine calcium channel blockers, including felodipine and nifedipine. This interaction may be due to inhibition of the metabolism of the dihydropyridines by intestinal wall CYP3A4 or inhibition of the P-glycoprotein transporter in the same location. The answer is **C**.

4. This is a good example of an additive drug interaction resulting from 2 drugs acting on the same type of receptor. Most tricyclic antidepressants, phenothiazines, and older antihistaminic drugs (those available without prescription) are blockers of muscarinic receptors. Used concomitantly, any pair of these agents will demonstrate a predictable increase in atropine-like adverse effects. The answer is **A**.

5. The drug interaction between the inhibitors of monoamine oxidase used for depression and the drugs that selectively block serotonin reuptake (SSRIs) is called the serotonin syndrome. In the case of phenelzine and fluoxetine, the interaction has resulted in a fatal outcome. Key interventions include control of hyperthermia and seizures. The answer is **C**.

6. Rifampin is an effective inducer of hepatic P450 isozymes. Cyclosporine and tetracycline have no significant effects on drug metabolism. Ciprofloxacin and erythromycin are inhibitors of drug metabolism. The answer is **D**.

7. NSAIDs interfere with the antihypertensive action of angiotensin-converting enzyme inhibitors; the

other drugs listed enhance the blood pressure-lowering effects of captopril and other members of the "pril" drug family. The answer is **C**.

8. Azathioprine is converted to mercaptopurine, which is responsible for both its immunosuppressant action and its hematotoxicity. Allopurinol inhibits xanthine oxidase, the enzyme that metabolizes mercaptopurine. The answer is **A**.

9. Ritonavir inhibits the metabolism of other HIV protease inhibitors and is used in low-dose combinations with indinavir or lopinavir. The answer is **N**.

10. Several NSAIDs, including aspirin, ibuprofen, and piroxicam, increase serum levels of methotrexate by interfering with its renal clearance. The adverse effects of methotrexate, including its hematotoxicity, are predictably increased. The answer is **J**.

11. Concomitant use of St. John's wort enhances the effects of selective serotonin reuptake inhibitors. In contrast, use of the herbal decreases the effectiveness of other drugs (including cyclosporine, estrogens, and protease inhibitors) via its induction of drug-metabolizing enzymes. The answer is **I**.

SKILL KEEPER ANSWER: WARFARIN (SEE CHAPTER 34)

Warfarin inhibits coagulation by interfering with the vitamin K-dependent posttranslational modification of several clotting factors (prothrombin and factors VII, IX and X) and the anticoagulant proteins C and S. Without this posttranslational modification, these proteins are inactive. Because warfarin inhibits the synthesis of coagulation factors and not the function of preformed factors, it has a relatively slow onset and offset of activity. The anticoagulant effect of warfarin is monitored by the prothrombin time (PT) test. Excessive anticoagulation can be reversed by administration of vitamin K or by transfusion with fresh or frozen plasma, which contains functional clotting factors.

CHECKLIST

When you complete this chapter, you should be able to:

☐ Describe the primary pharmacokinetic mechanisms that underlie drug interactions.

☐ Describe how the pharmacodynamic characteristics of different drugs administered concomitantly may lead to additive, synergistic, or antagonistic effects.

☐ Identify specific drug interactions that involve (1) alcohol, (2) antacids, (3) cimetidine, (4) ketoconazole, (5) NSAIDs, (6) phenytoin, (7) rifampin, and (8) warfarin.

☐ List specific drug interactions that can occur in the management of HIV patients.

☐ Identify specific drug interactions that involve commonly used herbals.

Appendix I

Key Words for Key Drugs

The following list is a compilation of the drugs that are most likely to appear on examinations. Some of them are old, some are quite new. The brief descriptions should serve as a rapid review. The list can be used in 2 ways. First, cover the column of properties and test your ability to recall descriptive information about drugs picked at random from the left column; second, cover the left column and try to name a drug that fits the properties described. The numbers in parentheses at the end of each drug description denote relevant chapter(s).

Common abbreviations and acronyms: ANS, autonomic nervous system; AV, atrioventricular; BP, blood pressure; CNS, central nervous system; DMARD, disease-modifying antirheumatic drug; ENS, enteric nervous system; EPS, extrapyramidal system; GABA, γ-aminobutyric acid; GI, gastrointestinal; HF, heart failure; HR, heart rate; HTN, hypertension; LMW, low molecular weight; MI, myocardial infarct; NSAID, nonsteroidal anti-inflammatory drug; RA, rheumatoid arthritis; SANS, sympathetic nervous system; TCA, tricyclic antidepressant; TNF, tumor necrosis factor; *Tox,* toxicity; WBCs, white blood cells.

Drug	Properties
Abciximab	Monoclonal antibody that inhibits the binding of platelet glycoprotein IIb/IIIa (GPIIb/IIIa) to fibrinogen. Used to prevent clotting after coronary angioplasty and in acute coronary syndrome. Eptifibatide and tirofiban are also GPIIb/IIIa inhibitors. (34, 56)
Acetaminophen	Antipyretic analgesic: very weak cyclooxygenase inhibitor; not anti-inflammatory. Less GI distress than aspirin but dangerous in overdose. *Tox:* hepatic necrosis. *Antidote:* acetylcysteine. (36)
Acetazolamide	Carbonic anhydrase-inhibiting diuretic acting in the proximal convoluted tubule: produces a $NaHCO_3$ diuresis, results in bicarbonate depletion and metabolic acidosis. Has self-limited diuretic but persistent bicarbonate-depleting action. Used in glaucoma and mountain sickness. *Tox:* paresthesias, hepatic encephalopathy. Dorzolamide and brinzolamide are topical analogs for glaucoma. (15)
Acetylcholine	Cholinomimetic prototype: transmitter in CNS, ENS, all ANS ganglia, parasympathetic postganglionic synapses, sympathetic postganglionic fibers to sweat glands, and skeletal muscle endplate synapses. (6, 7)
Acyclovir	Antiviral: inhibits DNA synthesis in herpes simplex virus (HSV) and varicella-zoster virus (VZV). Requires activation by viral thymidine kinase (TK⁻ strains are resistant). *Tox:* behavioral effects and nephrotoxicity (crystalluria) but minimal myelosuppression. Famciclovir, penciclovir, and valacyclovir are similar but with longer half-lives. (49)
Adenosine	Antiarrhythmic: miscellaneous group; parenteral only. Hyperpolarizes AV nodal tissue, blocks conduction for 10–15 s. Used for nodal reentry arrhythmias. *Tox:* hypotension, flushing, chest pain. (14)
Albuterol	Typical rapid-acting β_2 agonist; important use in acute asthma. *Tox:* tachycardia, arrhythmias, tremor. Other drugs with similar action: metaproterenol, terbutaline. Slow-acting analogs: formoterol, salmeterol; used for prophylaxis. (9, 20)

Alendronate	Bisphosphonate: chronic treatment with low doses increases bone mineral density and reduces fractures. Higher doses lower serum calcium. Used in osteoporosis and for the hypercalcemia in Paget's disease and malignancies. *Tox:* gastric and esophageal irritation at low oral doses. Renal dysfunction and osteonecrosis of the jaw in high doses. Other bisphosphonates include etidronate, pamidronate, risedronate, etc. (42)
Allopurinol	Suicide inhibitor of xanthine oxidase; reduces production of uric acid. Used in gout and adjunctively in cancer chemotherapy. Inhibits metabolism of purine analogs (eg, mercaptopurine, azathioprine). (36)
Alprazolam	Benzodiazepine sedative-hypnotic: used in anxiety states including panic attacks and phobias. *Tox:* psychological and physiologic dependence, additive effects with other CNS depressants. (22)
Alteplase (t-PA)	Thrombolytic: human recombinant tissue plasminogen activator. Used to recanalize occluded blood vessels in acute MI, severe pulmonary embolism, stroke. *Tox:* bleeding. (34)
Amiloride	K^+-sparing diuretic: blocks epithelial Na^+ channels in cortical collecting tubules. *Tox:* hyperkalemia. (15)
Amiodarone	Class III (and other classes) antiarrhythmic: broad spectrum; blocks sodium, potassium, calcium channels, β receptors. High efficacy and very long half-life (weeks to months). *Tox:* deposits in tissues; skin coloration; hypo- or hyperthyroidism; pulmonary fibrosis. (14)
Amoxicillin	Penicillin: wider spectrum than penicillin G with activity similar to ampicillin but greater oral bioavailability; fewer adverse effects on GI tract than ampicillin. Susceptible to penicillinases unless used with clavulanic acid. *Tox:* penicillin allergy. (43)
Amphetamine	Indirect-acting sympathomimetic: displaces stored catecholamines in nerve endings. Marked CNS stimulant actions; high abuse liability. Used in attention deficit hyperactivity disorder, for short-term weight loss, and for narcolepsy. *Tox:* psychosis, HTN, MI, seizures. Other indirect-acting sympathomimetics that displace catecholamines: ephedrine, pseudoephedrine, methylphenidate. (9, 32)
Amphotericin B	Antifungal: polyene drug of choice for some systemic mycoses; binds to ergosterol to disrupt fungal cell membrane permeability. *Tox:* chills and fever, hypotension, nephrotoxicity (dose limiting; less with liposomal forms). (48)
Ampicillin	Penicillin: wider spectrum than penicillin G, susceptible to penicillinases unless used with sulbactam. Activity similar to that of penicillin G, plus *E coli, H influenzae, P mirabilis, Shigella.* Synergy with aminoglycosides versus *Enterococcus* and *Listeria. Tox:* penicillin allergy; more adverse effects on GI tract than other penicillins; maculopapular skin rash. (43)
Anastrozole	Aromatase inhibitor: prototype inhibitor of the enzyme that converts testosterone to estradiol. Used in estrogen-dependent breast cancer. Letrozole is similar. (40, 55)
Aspirin	NSAID prototype: inhibits cyclooxygenase (COX)-1 and -2 irreversibly. Antiplatelet agent as well as antipyretic, analgesic and anti-inflammatory drug. *Tox:* GI ulcers, allergy, bronchoconstriction, salicylism. Other NSAIDs: ibuprofen, indomethacin, ketorolac, and naproxen. (34, 36)
Atenolol	Beta$_1$-selective blocker: low lipid solubility, less CNS effect; used for HTN, angina. (**Mnemonic:** Generic names of $β_1$-selective blockers start with A through M except for carteolol, carvedilol, and labetalol.) *Tox:* asthma, bradycardia, AV block, heart failure. (10)
Atropine	Muscarinic cholinoceptor blocker prototype: lipid-soluble, CNS effects. *Tox:* "red as a beet, dry as a bone, blind as a bat, mad as a hatter," urinary retention, mydriasis. Cyclopentolate, tropicamide: antimuscarinics for ophthalmology; shorter duration than atropine (a few hours or less); cause cycloplegia and mydriasis. Glycopyrrolate: antimuscarinic with decreased CNS effects. (8)
Azithromycin	Macrolide antibiotic: similar to erythromycin but greater activity against *H influenzae,* chlamydiae, and streptococci; long half-life with renal elimination. *Tox:* GI distress but no

inhibition of drug metabolism. Clarithromycin is similar but has a shorter half-life, and inhibits drug metabolism. (44)

Baclofen	GABA analog, orally active: spasmolytic; activates $GABA_B$ receptors in the spinal cord. (27)
Benztropine	Muscarinic cholinoceptor blocker: centrally acting antimuscarinic prototype for parkinsonism. *Tox:* excess antimuscarinic effects. (8, 28)
Botulinum	Toxins produced by *Clostridium botulinum:* enzymes that cleave nerve terminal proteins (synaptobrevin, others) and block transmitter release from acetylcholine vesicles. Injected to treat muscle spasm, smooth wrinkles, and reduce excessive sweating. *Tox:* paralysis. (6, 27)
Bromocriptine	Ergot derivative: prototype dopamine agonist in CNS; inhibits prolactin release. Alternative drug in parkinsonism and hyperprolactinemia. *Tox:* CNS, dyskinesias, hypotension. Pergolide is similar. (16, 28, 37)
Bupivacaine	Long-acting amide local anesthetic prototype. *Tox:* greater cardiovascular toxicity than most local anesthetics. (26)
Buprenorphine	Opioid: long-acting partial agonist of mu receptors. Analgesic (not equivalent to morphine) and effective for detoxification and maintenance in opioid dependence. Other mixed agonist-antagonists: Nalbuphine activates kappa and weakly blocks mu receptors; pentazocine, kappa agonist and weak mu antagonist or partial agonist. (31)
Buspirone	Anxiolytic: partial agonist that interacts with $5-HT_{1A}$ receptors; slow onset (1–2 weeks). Minimal potentiation of CNS depressants, including ethanol; negligible abuse liability. (22)
Captopril	Angiotensin-converting enzyme (ACE) inhibitor prototype: used in HTN, diabetic nephropathy, and HF. *Tox:* hyperkalemia, fetal renal damage, cough ("sore throat"). Other "prils" include benazepril, enalapril, lisinopril, quinapril. (11, 13, 17)
Carbamazepine	Anticonvulsant: used for tonic-clonic and partial seizures; blocks Na^+ channels in neuronal membranes. Drug of choice for trigeminal neuralgia; backup drug in bipolar disorder. *Tox:* CNS depression, myelotoxic, induces liver drug-metabolizing enzymes, teratogenicity. (24, 29)
Carvedilol	Adrenoceptor blocker: racemic mixture, one isomer a nonselective β-blocker and the other an $α_1$-blocker. Used in HTN, prolongs survival in HF. *Tox:* cardiovascular depression, asthma. Labetalol is similar. (10, 13)
Cefazolin	First-generation cephalosporin prototype: bactericidal beta-lactam inhibitor of cell wall synthesis. Active against gram-positive cocci, *E coli, K pneumoniae*, but does not enter the CNS. *Tox:* potential allergy; partial cross-reactivity with penicillins. (43)
Cefoxitin	Second-generation cephalosporin: active against a wide spectrum of gram-negative bacteria, including anaerobes (*B fragilis*). Does not enter the CNS. Cefotetan is similar. (43)
Ceftriaxone	Third-generation cephalosporin: active against many bacteria, including pneumococci, gonococci (a drug of choice), and gram-negative rods. Enters the CNS and is used in bacterial meningitis. Cefotaxime and ceftazidime are other third-generation cephalosporins. (43)
Celecoxib	Selective COX-2 inhibitor. Less GI toxicity than nonselective NSAIDs. *Tox:* nephrotoxicity, increased risk of myocardial thrombosis and stroke. (36)
Chloramphenicol	Antibiotic: broad-spectrum agent; inhibits protein synthesis (50S); uses restricted to backup drug for bacterial meningitis, infections due to anaerobes, *Salmonella. Tox:* reversible myelosuppression, aplastic anemia, gray baby syndrome. (44)
Chloroquine	Antimalarial: blood schizonticide used for treatment and prophylaxis in areas in which *P falciparum* is susceptible. Binds to hemin, causing dysfunctional cell membranes; resistance resulting from efflux via P-glycoprotein pump. *Tox:* GI distress and skin rash at low doses; peripheral neuropathy, skin lesions, auditory and visual impairment, quinidine-like cardiotoxicity at high doses. (53)
Chlorpheniramine	Antihistamine first-generation H_1 blocker prototype. *Tox:* mild sedation, little antimuscarinic action. (16)
Chlorpromazine	Phenothiazine antipsychotic drug prototype: blocks most dopamine receptors in CNS. *Tox:* atropine-like, EPS dysfunction, hyperprolactinemia, postural hypotension, sedation,

seizures (in overdose), additive effects with other CNS depressants. Other phenothiazines: fluphenazine, trifluoperazine (antipsychotics), prochlorperazine (antiemetic), promethazine (preoperative sedation). (29)

Cholestyramine	Antihyperlipidemic: bile acid-binding resin prototype that sequesters bile acids in gut and diverts more cholesterol from the liver to bile acids instead of circulating lipoproteins. Used for hypercholesterolemia *Tox:* constipation, bloating; interferes with absorption of some drugs. Colestipol is similar. (35)
Cimetidine	H_2 blocker prototype: used in acid-peptic disease. *Tox:* inhibits hepatic drug metabolism; antiandrogen effects. Less toxic analogs: ranitidine, famotidine, nizatidine. (16, 60)
Ciprofloxacin	Second-generation fluoroquinolone antibiotic: bactericidal inhibitor of topoisomerases; active against *E coli, H influenzae, Campylobacter, Enterobacter, Pseudomonas, Shigella. Tox:* CNS dysfunction, GI distress, superinfection, collagen dysfunction (caution in children and pregnant women). *Interactions:* inhibits metabolism of caffeine, theophylline, warfarin. (46)
Cisplatin	Antineoplastic: platinum-containing alkylating anticancer drug. Used for solid tumors (eg, testes, lung). *Tox:* Neurotoxic and nephrotoxic. Carboplatin is similar. (55)
Clindamycin	Lincosamide antibiotic: bacteriostatic inhibitor of protein synthesis (50S); active against gram-positive cocci, *B fragilis. Tox:* GI distress, pseudomembranous colitis. (44)
Clomiphene	Selective estrogen receptor modulator (SERM): synthetic, used in infertility to induce ovulation by blocking pituitary estrogen receptors. May result in multiple births. (40)
Clonidine	Alpha$_2$ agonist: acts centrally to reduce SANS outflow, lowers BP. Used in HTN and in drug dependency states. *Tox:* mild sedation in normal doses, rebound HTN if stopped suddenly. (9, 11, 32)
Clopidogrel	Antiplatelet agent: irreversibly inhibits platelet ADP receptors and platelet aggregation. Used in transient ischemic attacks and to prevent strokes and restenosis after placement of coronary stents. *Tox:* bleeding, neutropenia. Ticlopidine is similar, but higher risk of neutropenia and thrombotic thrombocytopenic purpura (TTP). (34)
Clozapine	Atypical antipsychotic: low affinity for dopamine D_2 receptors, higher for D_4 and 5-HT$_{2A}$ receptors; fewer EPS adverse effects than other antipsychotic drugs. *Tox:* ANS effects, weight gain, agranulocytosis (infrequent but significant). (29)
Cocaine	Indirect-acting sympathomimetic that blocks amine reuptake into nerve endings: local anesthetic (ester type). Marked CNS stimulation, euphoria; high abuse and dependence liability. *Tox:* psychosis, HTN, cardiac arrhythmias, seizures. (9, 26, 32)
Colchicine	Microtubule assembly inhibitor: reduces mobility and phagocytosis by WBCs; used in chronic gout. *Tox:* GI (often severe), hepatic, renal damage. (36)
Cyclophosphamide	Antineoplastic, immunosuppressive: cell cycle-nonspecific alkylating agent. *Tox:* alopecia, GI distress, hemorrhagic cystitis (use mesna), myelosuppression. (55, 56)
Cyclosporine	Immunosuppressant: immunophilin ligand; inhibits synthesis of interleukins and interferon-γ, suppressing T-cell activation. *Tox:* nephrotoxicity (dose limiting), hypertension, peripheral neuropathy, seizures (in overdose). Tacrolimus and sirolimus are similar. (36, 56)
Cytokines, recombinant	DNA technology products: aldesleukin (IL-2, used in renal cancer); erythropoietin (epoetin alfa, used in anemias); filgrastim (G-CSF, used in neutropenia); interferon-α (used in hepatitis B and C and in cancer); interferon-β (used in multiple sclerosis); interferon-γ (used in chronic granulomatous disease); oprelvekin (IL-11, used in thrombocytopenia); thrombopoietin (used in thrombocytopenia); and sargramostim (GM-CSF, used in neutropenia). (33, 36, 49, 55, 56)
Dantrolene	Muscle relaxant: blocks Ca^{2+} release from sarcoplasmic reticulum of skeletal muscle. Used in muscle spasm (cerebral palsy, multiple sclerosis, cord injury) and in emergency treatment of malignant hyperthermia. (25, 27, 29)

Desmopressin	Vasopressin (ADH) analog, selective for V_2 receptors: used for pituitary diabetes insipidus and mild hemophilia A or von Willebrand disease. Vasopressin (ADH), an agonist for V_1 and V_2 receptors, is used in pituitary diabetes insipidus and bleeding esophageal varices. Conivaptan, an antagonist at V_{1a} and V_2 receptors, is used for hyponatremia. (15, 34, 37)
Diazepam	Benzodiazepine prototype: binds to BZ receptors of the $GABA_A$ receptor-chloride ion channel complex; facilitates the inhibitory actions of GABA by increasing the *frequency* of channel opening (compare phenobarbital). Uses: anxiety states, ethanol detoxification, muscle spasticity, status epilepticus. *Tox:* dependence, additive effects with other CNS depressants. (22, 24, 27, 32)
Digoxin	Cardiac glycoside prototype: positive inotropic drug for HF, half-life 40 h; inhibits Na^+/K^+ ATPase, also a cardiac parasympathomimetic. *Tox:* calcium overload arrhythmias, GI upset. (13, 14)
Diphenhydramine	Antihistamine (first-generation) H_1 blocker: used in hay fever, motion sickness, dystonias. *Tox:* antimuscarinic, α adrenoceptor blocker, strong sedative. Doxylamine is similar. (16, 60)
Dopamine	Neurotransmitter and agonist drug at dopamine receptors: used in shock to increase renal blood flow (low dose) and cardiac output (moderate dose). (6, 9, 13, 21, 28, 29, 37)
Doxorubicin	Antineoplastic: anthracycline drug (cell cycle-nonspecific); intercalates between base pairs to disrupt DNA functions, inhibits topoisomerases, and forms cytotoxic free radicals. *Tox:* cardiotoxicity (dexrazoxane is antidote), myelosuppression. Daunorubicin is similar. (55)
Doxycycline	Tetracycline antibiotic: protein synthesis inhibitor (30S), more effective than other tetracyclines against chlamydia and in Lyme disease; malaria prophylaxis. Unlike other tetracyclines, it is eliminated mainly in the feces. *Tox:* see tetracycline. (44, 53)
Edrophonium	Cholinesterase inhibitor: very short duration of action (15 min). Used in diagnosis of myasthenia gravis and to distinguish myasthenic crisis from cholinergic crisis. (7)
Efavirenz	Nonnucleoside reverse transcriptase inhibitor (NNRTI): used in combination regimens for HIV. *Tox:* skin rash, CNS effects, avoid in pregnancy. Other NNRTIs: delavirdine, nevirapine. (49)
Enfuvirtide	Antiviral: HIV fusion inhibitor used in combination regimens. *Tox:* injection site reactions and rare hypersensitivity. (49)
Enoxaparin	LMW heparin: used parenterally for anticoagulation. Primary effect is on factor Xa, less on thrombin. The aPTT test is unreliable. Other LMW heparins include dalteparin, tinzaparin. *Tox:* bleeding. (34)
Entacapone	COMT inhibitor: enhances levodopa access to CNS neurons; adjunctive use in Parkinson's disease. *Tox:* exacerbates levodopa effects. Tolcapone is similar in action and use but may be hepatotoxic. (28)
Ephedrine	Indirectly acting sympathomimetic: like amphetamine but less CNS stimulation, more smooth muscle effects. In botanicals (eg, ma huang) and products for weight loss that are banned in the United States. *Tox:* hypertension, stroke, MI. (9, 61)
Epinephrine	Adrenoceptor agonist prototype: product of adrenal medulla, some CNS neurons. Affinity for all α and all β receptors. Drug of choice in anaphylaxis; used as hemostatic and as adjunct with local anesthetics; cardiac stimulant; traditional use in asthma. *Tox:* tachycardia, hypertension, MI, pulmonary edema and hemorrhage. (6, 9)
Ergot alkaloids	Ergonovine, ergotamine: cause prolonged vasoconstriction and uterine contraction. Used in migraine and obstetrics. *Tox:* vasospasm (including coronaries). (16, 28, 37)
Erythromycin	Macrolide antibiotic: bacteriostatic inhibitor of protein synthesis (50S); activity includes gram-positive cocci and bacilli, *M pneumoniae, Legionella pneumophila, C trachomatis*. *Tox:* cholestatic jaundice (avoid estolate in pregnancy), inhibits liver drug-metabolizing enzymes, interactions with cisapride, theophylline, warfarin. Other macrolide antibiotics include azithromycin and clarithromycin. (44)
Etanercept	DMARD: recombinant protein that binds TNF. Infliximab has a similar mechanism of action. Effective (by injection) in RA and possibly other severe inflammatory diseases. *Tox:* injection site reactions include erythema, itching, and swelling; possible increased infection rate. (36, 56)

Ethanol	Sedative-hypnotic: acute actions include impaired judgment, ataxia, loss of consciousness, vasodilation, and cardiovascular and respiratory depression. Chronic use leads to dependence and dysfunction of multiple organ systems; fetal alcohol syndrome. *Note:* zero-order elimination kinetics. (23, 32)
Ethinyl estradiol	Synthetic estrogen: used in many hormonal contraceptives; mestranol is similar. (40)
Ethosuximide	Anticonvulsant: used in absence seizures; may block T-type Ca^{2+} channels in thalamic neurons. *Tox:* GI distress; safe in pregnancy. (24)
Ezetimibe	Antihyperlipidemic: cholesterol-lowering drug that inhibits GI transporter of dietary cholesterol and the cholesterol secreted in bile. Used for hypercholesterolemia, usually in combination with a statin. *Tox:* possible increased risk of hepatic damage when combined with statin. (35)
Fentanyl	Short-acting potent opioid agonist (see morphine) used commonly in anesthesia and for chronic pain (transdermal form). Remifentanil and sufentanil are similar. (25, 31,32)
Finasteride	Antiandrogen: steroid inhibitor of 5α-reductase that inhibits synthesis of dihydrotestosterone. Used in benign prostatic hyperplasia and male-pattern baldness. (40)
Flecainide	Class IC antiarrhythmic prototype: used in ventricular tachycardia and rapid atrial arrhythmias with Wolff-Parkinson-White syndrome. *Tox:* arrhythmogenic, CNS excitation. (14)
Fluconazole	Imidazole antifungal: inhibits ergosterol synthesis. CNS entry and renal elimination. Used in esophageal and vaginal candidiasis, in coccidioidomycosis, and in the prophylaxis and treatment of fungal meningitis. Adverse effects similar to those of ketoconazole but less severe. (48)
Fludrocortisone	Synthetic corticosteroid: high mineralocorticoid and moderate glucocorticoid activity; long duration of action. Used in Addison's disease. (39)
Flumazenil	Benzodiazepine receptor antagonist: used to reverse CNS depressant effects of benzodiazepines. (22, 59)
Fluorouracil	Antineoplastic: pyrimidine antimetabolite (cell cycle specific), irreversibly inhibits thymidylate synthase, resulting in dTMP deficiency and "thymine-less" cell death; used mainly for solid or superficial tumors. *Tox:* GI distress, myelosuppression. (55)
Fluoxetine	Antidepressant: selective serotonin reuptake inhibitor (SSRI) prototype. Less ANS adverse effects and cardiotoxic potential than tricyclics. *Tox:* CNS stimulation, sexual dysfunction, seizures in overdose, serotonin syndrome. Other SSRIs: citalopram, escitalopram, fluvoxamine, paroxetine, sertraline. (30)
Flutamide	Antiandrogen: prototype androgen receptor antagonist used in prostatic carcinoma. Others: bicalutamide, nilutamide. (40)
Furosemide	Loop diuretic prototype: blocks $Na^+/K^+/2Cl^-$ transporter in thick ascending limb; high efficacy; used in acute pulmonary edema, refractory edematous states, hypercalcemia, and HTN. *Tox:* ototoxicity, K^+ wasting, hypovolemia, increased serum uric acid. Ethacrynic acid is similar but causes less hyperuricemia and may even reduce uric acid levels. (13, 15)
Gabapentin	Anticonvulsant: structural analog of GABA that facilitates its inhibitory actions in the CNS; used for partial seizures, for neuropathic pain, and in bipolar disorder. *Tox:* sedation, movement disorders. (24, 27, 29)
Ganciclovir	Antiviral: effective against herpesviruses (cytomegalovirus [CMV] and herpes simplex virus [HSV]); for CMV requires bioactivation via viral phosphotransferase. *Tox:* myelosuppression, nephrotoxicity, neurotoxicity. (49)
Gemfibrozil	Antihyperlipidemic: fibrate prototype used for hypertriglyceridemia. Lowers serum VLDL and triglycerides and increases HDL by activating PPAR-α nuclear receptors. *Tox:* GI distress, cholelithiasis, skin rashes, increased risk of myopathy when combined with statins or niacin. (35)
Gentamicin	Aminoglycoside prototype: bactericidal inhibitor of protein synthesis (30S); active against many aerobic gram-negative bacteria. Narrow therapeutic window; dose reduction required in renal impairment. *Tox:* renal dysfunction, ototoxicity; once-daily dosing is effective (postantibiotic effect) and less toxic. Amikacin and tobramycin are similar. (45, 51)

Glipizide — Oral antidiabetic: second-generation, potent sulfonylurea secretagogue. Blocks K^+ channels in pancreatic B cells, causing depolarization and release of insulin. *Tox:* hypoglycemia, weight gain. Related drugs: glyburide and older sulfonylureas such chlorpropamide and tolbutamide; short-acting secretagogues include repaglinide and nateglinide. (41)

Glucagon — Hormone from pancreatic A cells. Increases blood sugar via increased cAMP. Used in hypoglycemia and as an antidote in β-blocker overdose. (41, 59)

Haloperidol — Antipsychotic butyrophenone: blocks brain dopamine D_2 receptors. *Tox:* marked EPS dysfunction, hyperprolactinemia; fewer ANS adverse effects than phenothiazines. (29)

Halothane — General anesthetic prototype: inhaled halogenated hydrocarbon. *Tox:* cardiovascular and respiratory depression and relaxation of skeletal and smooth muscle. Use is declining because of sensitization of heart to catecholamines and occurrence (rare) of hepatitis. Newer inhaled anesthetics include isoflurane and sevoflurane. (25)

Heparin — Anticoagulant: large polymeric molecule with activity against thrombin and factor X. Rapid onset, parenteral administration. *Tox:* bleeding. *Antidote:* protamine. See also enoxaparin. (34)

Hydralazine — Antihypertensive: arteriolar vasodilator, orally active; used in severe HTN, HF. Minoxidil, a similar but more powerful antihypertensive, is also used topically in baldness. *Tox:* tachycardia, salt and water retention, lupus-like syndrome (hydralazine). (11, 13)

Hydrochlorothiazide — Thiazide diuretic prototype: acts in distal convoluted tubule to block Na^+/Cl^- transporter; used in HTN, HF, nephrolithiasis. *Tox:* hypersensitivity reactions; increased serum lipids, uric acid, glucose; K^+ wasting. (11, 13, 15)

Hydroxychloroquine — DMARD: immunosuppressant used for rheumatoid arthritis. *Tox:* GI distress, ototoxicity, myopathy, neuropathy. Other older DMARDs: methotrexate, sulfasalazine, gold salts, penicillamine. (36)

Ibuprofen — NSAID: nonselective COX inhibitor with analgesic, antipyretic, and anti-inflammatory actions similar to aspirin, but no low-dose antiplatelet effect. *Tox:* GI, renal. (36)

Imipenem — Prototype carbapenem antibiotic: active against many aerobic and anaerobic bacteria, including penicillinase-producing organisms; a bactericidal inhibitor of cell wall synthesis. Used with cilastatin (which inhibits metabolism by renal dehydropeptidases). *Tox:* allergy (partial cross-reactivity with penicillins), seizures. Meropenem and ertapenem are similar but do not require cilastatin and are less likely to cause seizures. (43)

Imipramine — Tricyclic antidepressant (TCA): blocks reuptake of norepinephrine and serotonin. *Tox:* atropine-like, postural hypotension, sedation, cardiac arrhythmias in overdose, additive effects with other CNS depressants. Other TCAs: amitriptyline, clomipramine, doxepin. (30)

Indinavir — Antiviral: HIV protease inhibitor (PI) used as a component of combination regimens in AIDS. *Tox:* anemia, nephrolithiasis, metabolic disorders, inhibits P450 drug metabolism. Other PIs: amprenavir, nelfinavir, ritonavir (major P450 inhibitor, see below), and saquinavir. (49)

Indomethacin — NSAID: highly potent. Usually reserved for acute inflammation (eg, acute gout); neonatal patent ductus arteriosus. *Tox:* GI (bleeding), renal damage. (36)

Interferon alfa — Cytokine: treatment of hepatitis B and hepatitis C viral infections. *Tox:* "flu-like" syndrome, myelosuppression, neurotoxicity (49, 56)

Ipratropium — Antimuscarinic agent: aerosol for asthma, chronic obstructive pulmonary disease (COPD). Good bronchodilator in 30–60% of patients. Not as efficacious as β_2 agonists but less toxic in COPD. *Tox:* dry mouth. (8, 20)

Isoniazid — Antimycobacterial: primary drug in combination regimens for tuberculosis; used as sole agent in treatment of latent infection. Metabolic clearance via *N*-acetyltransferases (genetic variability). *Tox:* hepatotoxicity (age dependent), peripheral neuropathy (reversed by pyridoxine), hemolysis (in G6PD deficiency). (47)

Isoproterenol	Beta$_1$ and β$_2$ agonist catecholamine prototype: bronchodilator, cardiac stimulant. Always causes tachycardia because both direct and reflex actions increase HR. *Tox:* arrhythmias, tremor, angina. (9)
Ivermectin	Anthelmintic: drug of choice for onchocerciasis and threadworm infections. Intensifies GABA-mediated neurotransmission in nematodes, but no access to CNS in humans. *Tox:* in onchocerciasis causes headache, fever, hypotension, joint pain. (54)
Ketoconazole	Antifungal azole prototype: active systemically; inhibits the synthesis of ergosterol. Used for *C albicans,* dermatophytosis, and non-life-threatening systemic mycoses. Is sometimes used to suppress adrenocorticoid or gonadal hormone synthesis. *Tox:* hepatic dysfunction, inhibits steroid synthesis and P450-dependent drug metabolism. Others: fluconazole, itraconazole, and voriconazole have a wider spectrum and less inhibitory effects on hepatic cytochromes P450. (39, 40, 48)
Lamivudine	Nucleoside reverse transcriptase inhibitor (NRTI) also known as 3TC. Least toxic NRTI. Notable for use in chronic hepatitis B in addition to HIV infection. (49)
Lamotrigine	Newer antiepileptic drug for absence and partial seizures; also used in bipolar affective disorder. *Tox:* rash, possibly life threatening, especially in pediatric patients. (24, 29)
Leflunomide	DMARD: dihydroorotate dehydrogenase inhibitor that arrests T-cell proliferation. Used orally in RA. *Tox:* diarrhea, increased liver enzymes. (36, 56)
Leuprolide	GnRH analog: continuous therapy used to suppress gonadotropin and gonadal hormone synthesis, especially in concert with gonadotropins for ovulation induction and in prostatic carcinoma and endometriosis. Goserelin and nafarelin are similar. *Tox:* hot flushes, decreased bone density with prolonged use, gynecomastia (men). (37, 40, 55)
Levodopa	Dopamine precursor: used in parkinsonism, usually in combination with carbidopa (a peripheral inhibitor of dopamine metabolism). *Tox:* dyskinesias, hypotension, on–off phenomena, behavioral changes. (28)
Levonorgestrel	Progestin: used in many contraceptives including combined oral contraceptives, progestin-only oral contraceptives, the levonorgestrel IUD, subcutaneous implants, and the Plan B emergency contraceptive. (40)
Lidocaine	Amide local anesthetic, medium-duration amide prototype: highly selective use-dependent class IB antiarrhythmic; used for nerve block and acute post-MI ischemic ventricular arrhythmias. *Tox:* CNS excitation. Mexiletine: like lidocaine, but orally active. (14, 26)
Lithium	Antimanic prototype: a primary drug in mania and bipolar affective disorders; blocks recycling of the phosphatidylinositol second messenger system. *Tox:* tremor, diabetes insipidus, goiter, seizures (in overdose); teratogenic potential (Ebstein's malformations) now questionable. (29)
Loratadine	Second-generation H$_1$ antihistamine: used in hay fever. *Tox:* Much less sedation than first-generation antihistamines; no ANS effects. Others: desloratadine, cetirizine, fexofenadine. (16)
Losartan	Angiotensin AT$_1$ receptor blocker prototype: used in HTN. Effects and toxicity similar to those of ACE inhibitors but causes less cough. Other AT$_1$ blockers: candesartan, eprosartan, irbesartan, olmesartan, telmisartan, and valsartan. (11, 13, 17)
Lovastatin	Antihyperlipidemic: HMG-CoA reductase inhibitor prototype used for hypercholesterolemia. Acts in liver to reduce synthesis of cholesterol and indirectly increase LDL receptor synthesis. Other "statins": atorvastatin, fluvastatin, pravastatin, rosuvastatin, simvastatin. *Tox:* hepatotoxicity (elevated enzymes), muscle damage, teratogen. (35)
MAbs	Monoclonal antibodies include: abciximab (see above), daclizumab (blocks IL-2 receptors, used in renal transplants), infliximab (binds TNF, used in RA and Crohn's disease), palivizumab (used in RSV, respiratory syncytial virus), rituximab (used in non-Hodgkin's lymphoma), and trastuzumab (used in breast cancers with HER2/neu receptors). (56)
Malathion	Organophosphate insecticide cholinesterase inhibitor: prodrug converted to malaoxon. Less toxic in mammals and birds because metabolized to inactive products. Other organophosphates: parathion converted to paraoxon, and the nerve gases (eg, sarin, soman). (7, 57)

Mannitol	Osmotic diuretic: used short term for reduction of intracranial pressure or to promote excretion of renal toxins. *Tox:* initial expansion of extracellular fluid volume with resulting hyponatremia, headache, nausea. With excessive use, dehydration and hypernatremia. (15)
Mebendazole	Anthelmintic: important drug for common nematode infections. Inhibits microtubule synthesis and glucose uptake in nematodes. *Tox:* GI distress, caution in pregnancy. Albendazole (widely used) and thiabendazole (more toxic) are related anthelmintics. (54)
Medroxyprogesterone	Progestin: used in combination with an estrogen for treatment of menopausal symptoms and used as a long-acting injection (Depo-Provera) for contraception. (40)
Mefloquine	Antimalarial: unknown mechanism of action. Used for prophylaxis against and treatment of chloroquine-resistant malaria, but resistance emerging. *Tox:* GI distress, dizziness, seizures in overdose, arrhythmias. (53)
Meperidine	Opioid analgesic: synthetic, equivalent to morphine in efficacy but orally bioavailable. Strong agonist at mu opioid receptors; blocks muscarinic receptors; serotonergic activity. *Tox:* see morphine; normeperidine accumulation may cause seizures, serotonin syndrome with SSRIs. (31)
Metformin	Oral antidiabetic: prototype biguanide antidiabetic. Proposed mechanisms include decreased hepatic gluconeogenesis and stimulation of glycolysis. Minimal hypoglycemia or weight gain. *Tox:* GI distress, lactic acidosis possible but rare. (41)
Methadone	Opioid analgesic: synthetic mu agonist, equivalent to morphine in efficacy but orally bioavailable and with a longer half-life. Used as analgesic, to suppress withdrawal symptoms, and in maintenance programs. *Tox:* see morphine. (31, 32)
Methimazole	Antithyroid drug: inhibits tyrosine iodination and coupling reactions; orally active. *Tox:* rash, agranulocytosis (rare). Propylthiouracil is similar. (37)
Methotrexate	Antineoplastic, DMARD, immunosuppressant: cell cycle-specific drug that inhibits dihydrofolate reductase. Major dose reduction required in renal impairment. *Tox:* GI distress, myelosuppression, crystalluria. Leucovorin rescue used to reduce toxicity. (36, 55, 56)
Methyldopa	Antihypertensive: prodrug of methylnorepinephrine, a CNS-active α_2 agonist. Reduces SANS outflow from vasomotor center. *Tox:* sedation, positive Coombs test, hemolysis. (11)
Metoclopramide	Prokinetic agent: dopamine D_2 receptor agonist used to stimulate upper GI motility in patients with gastroparesis and as an antiemetic. *Tox:* Restlessness, insomnia, agitation, extrapyramidal effects, elevated prolactin. (60)
Metronidazole	Antiprotozoal antibiotic: drug of choice in extraluminal amebiasis and trichomoniasis (tinidazole is equivalent); effective against bacterial anaerobes, including *B fragilis* and in antibiotic-induced colitis resulting from *C difficile*. *Tox:* peripheral neuropathy, GI distress, ethanol intolerance, mutagenic potential. (50, 53)
Mifepristone	Progestin and glucocorticoid receptor antagonist: used in combination with prostaglandin analogs for medical abortion in early pregnancy. (39, 40)
Misoprostol	PGE_1 derivative: orally active prostaglandin used to prevent GI ulcers caused by NSAIDs. Also used with mifepristone as abortifacient. *Tox:* diarrhea. (18, 40, 60)
Morphine	Opioid analgesic prototype: strong mu receptor agonist. Poor oral bioavailability. *Tox:* constipation, emesis, sedation, respiratory depression, miosis, and urinary retention. Tolerance may be marked; high potential for psychological and physiologic dependence. Additive effects with other CNS depressants. (31, 32)
Nafcillin	Penicillinase-resistant penicillin: narrow spectrum, used for suspected or known staphylococcal infections; not active against methicillin-resistant *S aureus* (MRSA). *Tox:* penicillin allergy. Others in group include methicillin (the prototype, rarely used), oxacillin, cloxacillin, and dicloxacillin. (43, 51)
Naloxone	Opioid mu receptor antagonist: used to reverse CNS depressant effects of opioid analgesics (overdose or when used in anesthesia). Naltrexone (orally active), a related compound, is used in ethanol dependency states. (31, 59)

Neostigmine	Cholinesterase inhibitor: prototype synthetic quaternary nitrogen carbamate with little CNS effect. *Tox:* excess cholinomimetic effects. Pyridostigmine is similar but longer-acting. (7, 27)
Niacin	Antihyperlipidemic: inhibits release of VLDL from liver into circulation and release of fatty acids from adipose tissue. Lowers LDL cholesterol and triglycerides and raises HDL cholesterol. *Tox:* flushing, pruritus, liver dysfunction, increased risk of myopathy when combined with statins. (35)
Nifedipine	Dihydropyridine calcium channel blocker prototype: less cardiac depression than verapamil, diltiazem; used in angina, HTN. *Tox:* constipation, headache, tachycardia, arrhythmias (avoid rapid-onset forms). Others in the group include amlodipine, nimodipine (used in subarachnoid hemorrhage), and nicardipine. (11, 12)
Nitric oxide	Endogenous vasodilator released from vascular endothelium; neurotransmitter. Mediates vasodilating effect of acetylcholine, histamine, and hydralazine. Active metabolite of nitroprusside and of nitrates used in angina. Used as pulmonary dilator in neonatal hypoxia. *Tox:* excessive vasodilation, hypotension. (19)
Nitroglycerin	Antianginal vasodilator prototype: releases nitric oxide (NO) in smooth muscle of veins, less in arteries, and causes relaxation. Standard of therapy in angina (both atherosclerotic and variant). *Tox:* tachycardia, orthostatic hypotension, headache. Oral nitrates: isosorbide dinitrate, isosorbide mononitrate. (12, 13)
Norepinephrine	Adrenoceptor agonist prototype: acts at β_1 adrenoceptors and all α adrenoceptors; used as vasoconstrictor. Causes reflex bradycardia. *Tox:* ischemia, arrhythmias, HTN. (6, 9)
Olanzapine	Atypical antipsychotic: high-affinity antagonist at 5-HT$_2$ receptors with minimal extrapyramidal side effects; improves both positive and negative symptoms of schizophrenia. Other atypicals: quetiapine (short half-life), risperidone (possible EPS dysfunction), sertindole (QT prolongation), clozapine (agranulocytosis). (29)
Omeprazole	Proton pump inhibitor prototype: irreversible blocker of H^+/K^+ ATPase proton pump in parietal cells of stomach. Used in GI ulcers, Zollinger-Ellison syndrome, gastroesophageal reflux disease (GERD). Other "prazoles": lansoprazole, pantoprazole, rabeprazole. *Tox:* hypergastrinemia. (60)
Ondansetron	5-HT$_3$ receptor blocker prototype: very important antiemetic for cancer chemotherapy; also used postoperatively to reduce vomiting. *Tox:* extrapyramidal effects. Other "setrons": granisetron, dolasetron. (16, 60)
Oseltamivir	Antiviral: Neuraminidase inhibitor blocking release of mature virions of influenza A and B and decreasing their infectivity. Prophylactic and shortens duration of flu symptoms. Zanamivir is similar in action and use. (49)
Oxybutynin	Muscarinic cholinoceptor blocker: used to relieve bladder spasm and incontinence. Tolterodine, weaker but more selective for M$_3$ receptors, has similar uses. (8)
Paclitaxel	Antineoplastic plant alkaloid: cell cycle (M phase)-specific agent; inhibits mitotic spindle disassembly. *Tox:* hematotoxicity, peripheral neuropathy, hypersensitivity reactions. Docetaxel is similar. (55)
Penicillamine	Chelator, immunomodulator: treatment of copper, lead, mercury and arsenic poisoning. Also used in Wilson's disease and RA. (36, 58)
Penicillin G	Penicillin prototype: active against common streptococci, gram-positive bacilli, gram-negative cocci, spirochetes (drug of choice in syphilis), and enterococci (if used with an aminoglycoside); penicillinase susceptible. *Tox:* penicillin allergy. (43,51)
Phenelzine	Irreversible nonselective monoamine oxidase (MAO) inhibitor. Backup drug for atypical depression. *Tox:* Malignant hypertension with indirect-acting sympathomimetics and tyramine, serotonin syndrome with serotonergic drugs. (30)
Phenobarbital	Long-acting barbiturate: used as a sedative and for tonic-clonic seizures. Facilitates GABA-mediated neuronal inhibition (by increasing *duration* of channel opening) and may block excitatory neurotransmitters. Partial renal clearance that can be increased by urinary

alkalinization. Chronic use leads to induction of liver drug-metabolizing enzymes and ALA synthase. *Tox:* psychological and physiologic dependence; additive effects with other CNS depressants. (22, 24)

Phenoxybenzamine   Alpha-blocker prototype (nonselective): irreversible action. Phentolamine: similar with competitive action. Used in pheochromocytoma. *Tox:* excess hypotension; GI distress. (10)

Phenytoin   Anticonvulsant: used for tonic-clonic and partial seizures; blocks Na^+ channels in neuronal membranes. Serum levels variable because of first-pass metabolism and nonlinear elimination kinetics. *Tox:* sedation, diplopia, gingival hyperplasia, hirsutism, teratogenic potential (fetal hydantoin syndrome). Drug interactions via effects on plasma protein binding or induction of hepatic metabolism. (24)

Physostigmine   Acetylcholinesterase inhibitor prototype: alkaloid tertiary amine carbamate, enters eye and CNS readily. Used in glaucoma, atropine poisoning. *Tox:* convulsions, excess cholinomimetic effects. Others: neostigmine and pyridostigmine; echothiophate is a clinical organophosphate used rarely. (7, 59)

Pilocarpine   Muscarinic receptor partial agonist prototype: tertiary amine alkaloid. May cause paradoxic hypertension by activating muscarinic excitatory postsynaptic potential receptors in postganglionic sympathetic neurons. Used in Sjögren's syndrome, xerostomia, glaucoma. *Tox:* muscarinic excess. (7)

Pioglitazone   Oral antidiabetic: thiazolidinedione stimulator of peroxisome proliferator-activator receptors (PPAR) and enhances target tissue sensitivity to insulin. Less hypoglycemia and weight gain than secretagogue antidiabetics. *Tox:* fluid retention, heart failure, fractures in women. Rosiglitazone is similar. (41)

Piperacillin   Extended-spectrum penicillin active against selected gram-negative bacteria, including *Pseudomonas aeruginosa* (synergistic with aminoglycosides). Susceptible to penicillinases unless used with tazobactam. *Tox:* penicillin allergy. (43)

Pralidoxime   Acetylcholinesterase regenerator (antidote for organophosphate poisoning, used with atropine): chemical antagonist, very high affinity for phosphorus in organophosphates. *Tox:* neuromuscular weakness. (8, 57, 59)

Pramipexole   Dopamine D_3 receptor agonist in CNS (ropinirole similar): often a first-line drug in parkinsonism. *Tox:* postural hypotension, dyskinesias (less than bromocriptine) (28)

Praziquantel   Anthelmintic: important drug for trematode (fluke) and cestode (tapeworm) infections. Increases membrane permeability to Ca^{2+} causing muscle contraction followed by paralysis. *Tox:* headache, dizziness, GI distress, fever; potential abortifacient. (54)

Prazosin   Alpha$_1$-selective blocker prototype: used in HTN and benign prostatic hyperplasia. *Tox:* first-dose orthostatic hypotension but less reflex tachycardia than nonselective α-blockers. Other "osins": terazosin, doxazosin. Tamsulosin similar, used only in benign prostatic hyperplasia. (10, 11)

Prednisone   Glucocorticoid prototype: potent, short acting; much less mineralocorticoid activity than cortisol but more than dexamethasone, betamethasone, or triamcinolone. (20, 36, 39, 55, 56)

Probenecid   Uricosuric: inhibitor of renal weak acid secretion and reabsorption in proximal tubule; prolongs half-life of penicillin, accelerates clearance of uric acid. Used in gout. Sulfinpyrazone is similar. (36)

Procainamide   Class IA antiarrhythmic drug prototype: short half-life, metabolized by *N*-acetyltransferase. Similar to quinidine but more cardio-depressant and may cause a lupus-like syndrome. (14)

Propranolol   Nonselective β-blocker prototype: local anesthetic action but no partial agonist effect. Used in HTN, angina, arrhythmias, migraine, hyperthyroidism, tremor. *Tox:* asthma, AV block, HF. (8, 11, 14, 28, 38)

Prostacyclin PGI_2: endogenous prostaglandin vasodilator and inhibitor of platelet aggregation. An analog, epoprostenol, is used in primary pulmonary HTN. (18)

Pyrimethamine	Antiprotozoal: antifolate that inhibits DHF reductase and synergistic, via sequential block-ade, with sulfadiazine against *Toxoplasma gondii*. Folinic acid is needed to offset hemato-logic toxicity. (46, 52, 53)
Quinidine	Class IA antiarrhythmic: used (rarely) in atrial and ventricular arrhythmias. Used intra-venously in acute, severe malaria. *Tox:* cinchonism, GI upset, thrombocytopenic purpura, arrhythmogenic (torsade de pointes). (14)
Quinine	Antimalarial: blood schizonticide; no effect on liver stages. Interferes with nucleic acid metabolism in plasmodium. Isomer of quinidine, same toxicity. (53)
Raloxifene	Selective estrogen receptor modulator (SERM): partial agonist of estrogen receptors that regulate bone; estrogen antagonist in breast and endometrium; used for osteoporosis in women. (40, 42)
Ramelteon	Hypnotic: agonist at brain melatonin receptors; not a controlled substance. *Tox:* fatigue, increased prolactin and decreased testosterone. (22)
Reserpine	Antihypertensive (rarely used): selective inhibitor of vesicle catecholamine-H$^+$ antiporter; used in HTN, causes depletion of catecholamines and 5-HT from their stores. *Tox:* severe depression, suicide, ulcers, diarrhea. (6, 11)
Rifampin	Antimicrobial: inhibitor of DNA-dependent RNA polymerase used in drug regimens for tuberculosis and the meningococcal carrier state. *Tox:* hepatic dysfunction, induction of liver drug-metabolizing enzymes (drug interactions), flulike syndrome with intermittent dosing. Rifabutin similar but associated with fewer drug interactions. (47)
Ritonavir	Antiviral: HIV protease inhibitor (PI) used at low-dose as a component of combination regimens in AIDS to inhibit metabolism of other drugs (See indinavir). *Tox:* implicated in many drug interactions when used as sole PI.
Ropinirole	Dopamine receptor agonist: nonergot used in Parkinson's disease; more receptor selectivity and less toxicity than bromocriptine. *Tox:* dyskinesias, sedation. Pramipexole is similar. (28)
Selegiline	MAO-B inhibitor: selective inhibitor of the enzyme that metabolizes dopamine (no tyra-mine interactions). Used in Parkinson's disease. *Tox:* GI distress, CNS stimulation, dyski-nesias, serotonin syndrome if used with selective serotonin reuptake inhibitors. (28)
Sildenafil	Inhibits phosphodiesterase (PDE)-5, preventing breakdown of cGMP, which promotes vasodilation and smooth muscle relaxation. Used for erectile dysfunction. Tadalafil, varde-nafil are similar. *Tox:* severe hypotension when combined with nitrates, impaired blue-green color vision. (12)
Sotalol	Class III antiarrhythmic prototype: blocks I_K channels and β receptors. Used for atrial and ventricular arrhythmias. *Tox:* torsade de pointes arrhythmias. Others in group: ibutilide, dofetilide. (14)
Spironolactone	Aldosterone receptor antagonist: K$^+$-sparing diuretic action in the collecting tubules; used in aldosteronism, HTN, and female hirsutism (androgen receptor blocking action). *Tox:* hyperkalemia, gynecomastia. Eplerenone, used in HTN and HF, is a more selective aldos-terone antagonist. (13, 15, 39, 40)
Streptogramins	Antibiotics: Synercid is the combination of quinupristin and dalfopristin; bactericidal inhibitors of protein synthesis. Intravenous use for drug-resistant gram-positive cocci including MRSA (methicillin-resistant *S aureus*), VRE (vancomycin-resistant enterococci), and pneumococci. *Tox:* infusion-related pain, arthralgia, myalgia. Linezolid is another inhibitor of protein synthesis used for drug-resistant gram-positive cocci, including PRSP (penicillin-resistant *S pneumoniae*) strains. (44)
Streptokinase	Thrombolytic: protein from streptococci that accelerates plasminogen-to-plasmin conver-sion. *Tox:* bleeding, allergy. (34)
Succinylcholine	Depolarizing neuromuscular relaxant prototype: short duration (5 min) if patient has nor-mal plasma cholinesterase (genetically determined). No antidote (compare with tubocu-rarine). Implicated in malignant hyperthermia. (7, 27)

Sulfasalazine	Aminosalicylate anti-inflammatory drug: used for inflammatory bowel disease and rheumatoid arthritis. *Tox:* rash, GI disturbances, leukopenia. (36, 60)
Sumatriptan	5-HT$_{1D}$ receptor agonist: used to abort migraine attacks. *Tox:* coronary vasospasm, chest pain or pressure. Several other "triptans" are available. (16)
Tamoxifen	Selective estrogen receptor modulator (SERM): blocks estrogen receptors in breast tissue; activates endometrial receptors. Used in estrogen receptor-positive cancers, possibly prophylactic in high-risk patients. Toremifene is similar. Raloxifene, approved for osteoporosis, activates bone estrogen receptors but is an antagonist of breast and endometrial receptors. (40, 55)
Tetracycline	Antibiotic: tetracycline prototype; bacteriostatic inhibitor of protein synthesis (30S). Broad spectrum, but many resistant organisms. Used for mycoplasmal, chlamydial, rickettsial infections, chronic bronchitis, acne, cholera; a backup drug in syphilis. *Tox:* GI upset and superinfections, Fanconi's syndrome, photosensitivity, dental enamel dysplasia. (44)
Tetrodotoxin	Toxin: potent sodium channel blocker; blocks action potential propagation in nerve, heart, and skeletal muscle. From puffer fish, California newt. *Tox:* paresthesias, paralysis. Saxitoxin (paralytic shellfish poison) is similar. (6)
Trimethoprim-sulfamethoxazole (TMP-SMX)	Antimicrobial drug combination: causes synergistic sequential blockade of folic acid synthesis. Active against many gram-negative bacteria, including *Aeromonas, Enterobacter, H influenzae, Klebsiella, Moraxella, Salmonella, Serratia,* and *Shigella. Tox:* mainly due to sulfonamide; includes hypersensitivity, myelotoxicity, kernicterus, and drug interactions caused by competition for plasma protein binding. (46, 53)
Tubocurarine	Nondepolarizing neuromuscular blocking agent prototype: competitive nicotinic blocker. Analogs: pancuronium, atracurium, vecuronium, and other "-curiums" and "-oniums." *Tox:* respiratory paralysis. Releases histamine and may cause hypotension. *Antidote:* cholinesterase inhibitor, eg, neostigmine. (8, 26)
Tyramine	Indirect-acting sympathomimetic prototype: releases or displaces norepinephrine from stores in nerve endings. Presence in certain foods may cause potentially lethal hypertensive responses in patients taking MAO inhibitors. (27)
Valproic acid	Anticonvulsant: primary drug in absence, clonic-tonic, and myoclonic seizure states. Also used commonly for bipolar disorder. *Tox:* GI distress, hepatic necrosis (rare), teratogenic (spina bifida), inhibits drug metabolism. (24, 29)
Vancomycin	Glycopeptide bactericidal antibiotic: inhibits synthesis of cell wall precursor molecules. A drug of choice for methicillin-resistant staphylococci and effective in antibiotic-induced colitis. Dose reduction required in renal impairment (or hemodialysis). *Tox:* ototoxicity, hypersensitivity, renal dysfunction (rare). (43, 51)
Verapamil	Calcium channel blocker prototype: blocks L-type channels; cardiac depressant and vasodilator; used in HTN, angina, and arrhythmias. *Tox:* AV block, HF, constipation. Diltiazem, like verapamil, has more depressant effect on heart than dihydropyridines (eg, nifedipine). (11, 12, 14)
Vincristine	Antineoplastic: cell cycle (M phase)-specific plant alkaloid; inhibits mitotic spindle formation. *Tox:* peripheral neuropathy. Vinblastine, a congener, causes myelosuppression. (55)
Warfarin	Oral anticoagulant prototype: causes synthesis of nonfunctional versions of the vitamin K-dependent clotting factors (II, VII, IX, X). *Tox:* bleeding, teratogenic. *Antidote:* vitamin K, fresh plasma. (34)
Zidovudine (ZDV)	Antiviral: prototype NRTI used in combinations for HIV infections and in prophylaxis for needlesticks and vertical transmission. *Tox:* severe myelosuppression. Other NRTIs: abacavir, didanosine (ddI), amivudine (3TC), stavudine (d4T), and zalcitabine (ddC). (49)
Zolpidem	Nonbenzodiazepine hypnotic, acts via the BZ$_1$ receptor subtype and is reversed by flumazenil; less amnesia and muscle relaxation and lower dependence liability than benzodiazepines. Zaleplon and eszopiclone are similar. (22)

Appendix II

Examination 1

The following examination consists of 120 questions, mostly in the format ("single best answer") used in USMLE examinations. As in an actual examination, clinical descriptions, tables, or graphs are provided in many of the question stems.

It is suggested that you time yourself in taking this examination; in current USMLE examinations, the time allotted is approximately 1 min per question; thus, 2 h would be appropriate for this examination.

DIRECTIONS: Each numbered item or incomplete statement in this section is followed by answers or by completions of the statement. Select the ONE lettered answer or completion that is BEST in each case.

1. Phase 3 clinical trials typically involve
   (A) Measurement of the pharmacokinetics of the new drug in normal volunteers
   (B) Double-blind evaluation of the new drug in hundreds of patients with the target disease by specialists in academic centers
   (C) Postmarketing surveillance of drug toxicities
   (D) Evaluation of the new drug under conditions of actual use in several hundred to several thousand patients with the target disease
   (E) Collection of data regarding late-appearing toxicities from patients previously studied in phase 1 trials

2. A patient is admitted to the emergency department for treatment of a drug overdose. The identity of the drug is unknown, but it is observed that when the urine pH is acidic, the renal clearance of the drug is less than the glomerular filtration rate and that when the urine pH is alkaline, the clearance is greater than the glomerular filtration rate. The drug is probably a
   (A) Strong acid
   (B) Weak acid
   (C) Nonelectrolyte
   (D) Weak base
   (E) Strong base

3. A 45-year-old patient is to have reconstructive surgery on a hand that was recently injured in an accident. The anesthesiologist plans to use regional anesthesia of the arm for a fairly long procedure. The amide-type local anesthetic with the longest duration of action is
   (A) Bupivacaine
   (B) Cocaine
   (C) Lidocaine
   (D) Procaine
   (E) Tetracaine

4. A 60-year-old woman is in the coronary care unit after an acute myocardial infarction. She has developed signs of pulmonary edema of rapidly increasing severity. Aminophylline, dobutamine, and digoxin can each
   (A) Decrease conduction velocity in the atrioventricular node
   (B) Decrease venous return
   (C) Increase cardiac contractile force
   (D) Increase peripheral vascular resistance
   (E) Increase the amount of cAMP in cardiac muscle cells

5. An endogenous peptide that causes pain and edema in the area of release and is inactivated by angiotensin-converting enzyme is
   (A) Angiotensin II
   (B) Atrial natriuretic peptide
   (C) Bradykinin

(D) Endothelin-1

(E) Substance P

6. A patient has been receiving full doses of omeprazole for 7 weeks. A predictable clinical or laboratory finding after use of omeprazole is
(A) Agranulocytosis
(B) Antiestrogenic effects
(C) Hypergastrinemia
(D) Hypertension
(B) Systemic lupus erythematosus

7. A 67-year-old patient has recovered from the acute phase of a myocardial infarction but requires an antiarrhythmic drug for ventricular tachycardia. One property of quinidine that is NOT associated with procainamide is quinidine's
(A) Ability to control atrial as well as ventricular arrhythmias
(B) Activity by the oral route
(C) Prolongation of the PR interval
(D) Prolongation of the QRS interval
(E) Tendency to produce cinchonism

8. A patient discharged from the hospital after a myocardial infarction had been receiving small doses of procainamide to suppress a ventricular tachycardia. One month later, his local physician prescribed high-dose hydrochlorothiazide therapy for ankle edema, which was ascribed to congestive heart failure. Three weeks after beginning thiazide therapy, the patient was readmitted to the hospital with a rapid multifocal ventricular tachycardia. The most probable cause of this arrhythmia is
(A) Procainamide toxicity caused by inhibition of procainamide metabolism by the thiazide
(B) Direct effects of hydrochlorothiazide on the pacemaker of the heart
(C) Thiazide toxicity caused by the effects of procainamide on the kidneys
(D) Block of calcium current by the combination of procainamide plus thiazide
(E) Reduction of serum potassium caused by the diuretic action of hydrochlorothiazide

9. A 54-year-old woman presented with angina of effort. Laboratory assessment of her serum revealed elevated total and LDL cholesterol. The patient was placed on atorvastatin. This drug lowers serum cholesterol by
(A) Activating endothelial cell-associated lipoprotein lipase
(B) Increasing the shunting of hepatic cholesterol into the biochemical pathway of bile acid synthesis
(C) Indirectly increasing hepatic production of LDL receptors

(D) Inhibiting the uptake of cholesterol in epithelial cells that line the small intestine
(E) Stimulating hepatic fatty acid oxidation

10. The most appropriate drug for reversing myasthenic crisis in a patient who has missed several doses of his regular medication and is experiencing diplopia, dysarthria, and difficulty swallowing is
(A) Calcium
(B) Neostigmine
(C) Pralidoxime
(D) Succinylcholine
(E) Tubocurarine

11. A 4-year-old child was brought to an emergency department after ingesting a product found in the home. Her symptoms included an elevated temperature; hot, dry skin; moderate tachycardia; and mydriasis. The most likely cause of these symptoms is
(A) Acetaminophen overdose
(B) Amphetamine-containing diet pills
(C) Exposure to an organophosphate-containing insecticide
(D) Ingestion of a medication containing atropine
(E) Ingestion of phenylephrine-containing eye drops

12. A comatose patient is admitted to the emergency department 4 h after taking an overdose of phenobarbital. The plasma level of the drug at time of admission is 100 mg/L, and the apparent volume of distribution, half-life, and clearance of phenobarbital are 35 L, 4 days, and 6.1 L/day, respectively. The ingested dose was approximately
(A) 1 g
(B) 3.5 g
(C) 6.1 g
(D) 40 g
(E) 70 g

13. Most weak acid drugs as well as weak base drugs are absorbed primarily from the small intestine after oral administration because
(A) Both types are more ionized in the small intestine
(B) Both types are less ionized in the small intestine
(C) The blood flow is greater in the small intestine than that in other parts of the gut
(D) The small intestine has nonspecific carriers for most drugs
(E) The surface area of the small intestine is greater than other parts of the gut

14. Inhalation of carbon monoxide remains one of the leading causes of poisoning deaths in the United States. Death from carbon monoxide poisoning is due to

(A) Bronchial irritation resulting in bronchospasm and pulmonary edema

(B) CNS depression resulting in seizures, coma, and cardiorespiratory collapse

(C) Impaired oxygen delivery resulting in tissue hypoxia and multiorgan failure

(D) Interference with neurotransmission resulting in muscle weakness and respiratory failure

(E) Neuronal excitation resulting in rigidity, hyperthermia, and arrhythmia

15. A semiconscious patient in the intensive care unit is being artificially ventilated. Random spontaneous respiratory movements are rendering the mechanical ventilation ineffective. A useful drug to reduce the patient's ineffective spontaneous respiratory activity is
(A) Baclofen
(B) Dantrolene
(C) Pancuronium
(D) Pyridostigmine
(E) Succinylcholine

16. Which of the following drugs is used in ophthalmology, but causes mydriasis and cycloplegia lasting more than 24 h?
(A) Atropine
(B) Echothiophate
(C) Edrophonium
(D) Ephedrine
(E) Tropicamide

17. A 55-year-old surgeon has developed symmetric early morning stiffness in her hands. She wishes to take a nonsteroidal anti-inflammatory drug to relieve these symptoms. Which drug is an NSAID that is appropriate for chronic therapy of her arthritis?
(A) Colchicine
(B) Hydroxychloroquine
(C) Ibuprofen
(D) Indomethacin
(E) Sulfasalazine

18. A 59-year-old woman with a 60 pack-year smoking history was diagnosed with advanced lung cancer 2 mo ago. She now enters the hospital in a coma. Her serum calcium is 16 mg/dL (normal, 8.9–10.1 mg/dL). Which of the following (if given with IV fluids) would be most useful to reduce serum calcium in this patient?
(A) Acetazolamide
(B) Furosemide
(C) Hydrochlorothiazide
(D) Mannitol
(E) Spironolactone

19. A 50-year-old man has macrocytic anemia and early signs of neurologic abnormality. The drug that will probably be required in this case is
(A) Erythropoietin
(B) Filgrastim
(C) Folic acid
(D) Iron dextran
(E) Vitamin B_{12}

20. A patient in the coronary care unit has received warfarin for 2 weeks. As a result of this therapy, the patient will have
(A) Reduced plasma prothrombin (factor II) activity
(B) Reduced plasma factor VIII activity
(C) Reduced plasma plasminogen activity
(D) Increased tissue plasminogen activator activity
(E) Increased platelet adenosine stores

21–22. A 55-year-old man with a strong family history of cardiovascular disease has moderate hypertension and angina pectoris. Blood pressure is 160/109 mm Hg, and the ECG shows left ventricular hypertrophy. The rest of his physical examination and laboratory results are normal. His angina is precipitated by exercise. You have been asked to recommend a drug regimen for both conditions.

21. The antihypertensive drug most likely to aggravate angina pectoris is
(A) Captopril
(B) Clonidine
(C) Hydralazine
(D) Methyldopa
(E) Propranolol

22. A drug lacking vasodilator properties that is useful in angina is
(A) Isosorbide dinitrate
(B) Nimodipine
(C) Nitroglycerin
(D) Propranolol
(E) Verapamil

23. The eicosanoid that stimulates platelet aggregation most strongly is
(A) Leukotriene B_4
(B) Prostacyclin
(C) Prostaglandin E_2
(D) Prostaglandin F_2
(E) Thromboxane A_2

24. A drug that is used in the treatment of male impotence and inhibits a phosphodiesterase is
(A) Alprostadil
(B) Fluoxetine
(C) Mifepristone
(D) Sildenafil
(E) Zafirlukast

25. A drug useful in the prophylactic treatment of asthma but lacking bronchodilator action is
(A) Cromolyn
(B) Ephedrine
(C) Isoproterenol
(D) Metaproterenol
(E) Metoprolol

26. A physician was considering erythromycin for treatment of a 47-year-old man with an upper respiratory tract infection. However, the physician noted that the patient was taking simvastatin for treatment of hypercholesterolemia and realized that erythromycin, an inhibitor of cytochrome P340 3A enzymes, would inhibit the metabolism of simvastatin. The physician opted for a different class of antibiotic to avoid exposing the patient to higher concentrations of simvastatin and a risk of dose-dependent toxicity. The primary dose-dependent toxicity of simvastatin is
(A) Abdominal pain secondary to gallstone formation
(B) Blurred vision secondary to optic neuritis
(C) Elevated serum creatinine, possibly progressing to renal failure
(D) Increased serum uric acid concentration and increased risk of gout
(E) Muscle pain and weakness, possibly progressing to rhabdomyolysis

27. Although it does not act at any histamine receptor, epinephrine reverses many effects of histamine. Epinephrine is a
(A) Chemical antagonist of histamine
(B) Competitive inhibitor of histamine
(C) Metabolic inhibitor of histamine
(D) Noncompetitive antagonist of histamine
(E) Physiologic antagonist of histamine

28. Most drug receptors are
(A) Small molecules with a molecular weight between 100 and 1000
(B) Lipids arranged in a bilayer configuration
(C) Proteins located on cell membranes or in the cytosol
(D) DNA molecules
(E) RNA molecules

29. After an intravenous bolus injection of lidocaine, the major factors determining the initial plasma concentration are
(A) Dose and clearance
(B) Dose and apparent volume of distribution
(C) Apparent volume of distribution and clearance
(D) Clearance and half-life
(E) Half-life and dose

30. The graph shows the serum insulin level that results from a 2-injection regimen given to a child with type 1 diabetes. Assume that both injections (indicated by arrows along the time line) contain the same medication(s). The drug or drug combination that is most likely to generate the levels of insulin depicted in the figure is
(A) 100% Regular insulin
(B) 100% Lispro insulin
(C) 70% NPH insulin plus 30% regular insulin
(D) 100% NPH insulin
(E) 100% Insulin glargine

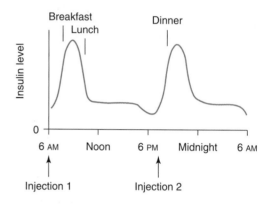

31. Intravenous administration of norepinephrine in a patient already taking an effective dose of atropine will often
(A) Decrease blood sugar
(B) Decrease total peripheral resistance
(C) Increase heart rate
(D) Increase skin temperature
(E) Reduce pupil size

32. A 26-year-old woman comes to the outpatient clinic with a complaint of rapid heart rate and easy fatigability. Laboratory work-up reveals low hemoglobin and microcytic red cell size. The most suitable therapy will be
(A) Ferrous sulfate
(B) Folic acid
(C) Iron dextran
(D) Pyridoxine
(E) Vitamin B$_{12}$

33. For a cumulative quantal dose–response graph, the variable that is plotted on the Y-axis (vertical axis) is the
(A) Cumulative efficacy of the experimental drug
(B) Log of the dose or concentration of the experimental drug
(C) Percent of a population with a specified response to the experimental drug

(D) Percent of receptors bound to the experimental drug

(E) Percent of the maximal response to the experimental drug or another drug that elicits the same response

34. The heart rate response to the infusion of a moderate dose of phenylephrine in conscious patients is not blocked by
(A) Atropine
(B) Hexamethonium
(C) Phenoxybenzamine
(D) Propranolol
(E) Scopolamine

35. An accepted clinical use of antimuscarinic drugs is for treatment of
(A) Alzheimer's disease
(B) Chronic obstructive pulmonary disease
(C) Constipation
(D) Hypertension
(E) Prostatic hyperplasia

36. An anticlotting drug that binds to and inhibits the platelet glycoprotein IIb/IIIa protein is
(A) Aspirin
(B) Clopidogrel
(C) Enoxaparin
(D) Fondaparinux
(E) Tirofiban

37. A 70-year-old man has severe urinary hesitancy associated with benign prostatic hyperplasia. He has tried α-blockers with little relief. His physician recommends a drug that blocks 5α-reductase in the prostate and writes a prescription for
(A) Finasteride
(B) Flutamide
(C) Ketoconazole
(D) Leuprolide
(E) Oxandrolone

38. The increase in heart rate and the force of cardiac contraction normally induced by electrical stimulation of sympathetic nerves can be blocked by
(A) Atropine
(B) Clonidine
(C) Hydralazine
(D) Neostigmine
(E) Propranolol

39. A treatment of angina that consistently decreases the heart rate and can prevent vasospastic angina attacks is
(A) Diltiazem
(B) Nifedipine
(C) Nitroglycerin

(D) Propranolol
(E) Timolol

40. Which of the following drugs can cause vasoconstriction in the absence of other drugs?
(A) Atenolol
(B) Ergotamine
(C) Phentolamine
(D) Propranolol
(E) Verapamil

41. In a study of new diuretics, an investigational drug was given twice daily for 8 days. The following data were obtained.

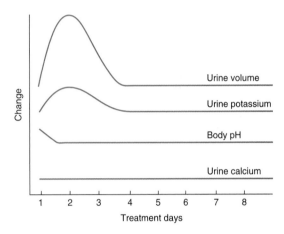

Which mechanism best explains the effects shown on the graph?
(A) Carbonic anhydrase inhibition
(B) Blockade of a $Na^+/K^+/2Cl^-$ transporter in the ascending limb of the loop of Henle
(C) Blockade of a NaCl transporter in the distal convoluted tubule
(D) Osmotic diuresis
(E) Block of aldosterone in the cortical collecting tubule

42. A diuretic that increases the delivery of poorly absorbed solute to the thick ascending limb of the nephron is
(A) Furosemide
(B) Indapamide
(C) Mannitol
(D) Spironolactone
(E) Vasopressin

43–44. A 65-year-old man with cardiomyopathy has recurrent congestive heart failure. Addition of digitalis to his regimen is being considered.

43. In a patient receiving digoxin for congestive heart failure, conditions that may facilitate the appearance of toxicity include
(A) Hyperkalemia
(B) Hypernatremia
(C) Hypocalcemia
(D) Hypomagnesemia
(E) Hypophosphatemia

44. The cellular cause of digitalis toxicity is
(A) Intracellular calcium overload
(B) Intracellular potassium overload
(C) Increased parasympathetic activity
(D) Increased adrenocorticosteroid levels
(E) Impaired sympathetic activity

45. Methylxanthine drugs such as theophylline cause
(A) Vasoconstriction in many vascular beds
(B) Decrease in the amount of cAMP in mast cells
(C) Bronchodilation
(D) Activation of the enzyme phosphodiesterase
(E) Sedation

46. A drug used in asthma that often causes tachycardia and tremor is
(A) Albuterol
(B) Cromolyn sodium
(C) Ipratropium
(D) Montelukast
(E) Prednisone

47. The drug with the most useful effects in the treatment of inoperable metastatic pheochromocytoma secreting mostly norepinephrine is
(A) Clonidine
(B) Minoxidil
(C) Phenoxybenzamine
(D) Propranolol
(E) Reserpine

48. An agent that can readily cause edema if released or injected near capillaries is
(A) Angiotensin II
(B) Epinephrine
(C) Histamine
(D) Norepinephrine
(E) Serotonin

49. Typical responses to β receptor activation include
(A) Hypoglycemia
(B) Lipolysis
(C) Glycogen synthesis
(D) Decreased skeletal muscle tremor
(E) Decreased renin secretion

50. A patient has been taking aspirin for rheumatoid arthritis for 8 years. Exacerbations are becoming worse, and she asks the physician about drugs that might stop the progression of the disease. Which of the following is a disease-modifying antirheumatic drug (DMARD)?
(A) Colchicine
(B) Epoprostenol
(C) Methotrexate
(D) Naproxen
(E) Zafirlukast

51. A neuronal cell body located in the raphe nuclei has fine axonal projections to most brain levels. The neurotransmitter that it releases, which can be either excitatory or inhibitory, is most likely to be
(A) Acetylcholine
(B) Dopamine
(C) Glutamic acid
(D) Glycine
(E) Serotonin

52–53. A 40-year-old man had been consuming alcoholic beverages at lunch and in the evenings all his adult life. During the last 2 years, his alcohol consumption had steadily increased, continuing throughout the day. In response to family pressures, he abruptly stopped drinking alcohol, and within a few hours he became increasingly anxious and agitated and showed symptoms of autonomic hyperexcitability. At this point, he was brought to the hospital.

52. In the emergency department, the symptoms increased in severity, with hyperreflexia progressing to seizures. He was given an intravenous injection of a drug that controlled the seizure activity and was then hospitalized. During the recovery period, the same agent was used in oral form with gradual dose tapering. The drug he received as an injection and then as an oral pill was
(A) Clonidine
(B) Diazepam
(C) Haloperidol
(D) Naltrexone
(E) Phenytoin

53. In the first week of this patient's recovery, he is at increased risk of a syndrome that is characterized by
(A) Ascites, mental confusion, and elevated serum transaminases
(B) Headache, hypotension, and widespread petechiae
(C) Hyperglycemia, acidosis, and stupor
(D) Respiratory depression, miosis, and mental confusion
(E) Tremor, delusions, and visual hallucinations

54. The pharmacokinetic characteristics of several hydantoin derivatives, each with anticonvulsant

Drug	Oral Bioavailability(%)	Plasma Protein Binding (%)	Elimination Kinetics	Cytochrome P450 Induction
ABC	10	90	First order	++
DEF	90	50	First order	++
GHI	50	98	Zero order	None
JKL	85	10	First order	None
MNO	95	10	First order	++

activity equivalent to that of phenytoin, were examined in phase 1 clinical trials. The rationale was to identify a drug with more desirable kinetic properties than those of phenytoin.

Based on the data shown in the table above, which drug has the optimum pharmacokinetic properties for oral use in the management of patients with seizure disorders?
(A) ABC
(B) DEF
(C) GHI
(D) JKL
(E) MNO

55. Which statement concerning anesthetic agents is accurate?
(A) Anesthetic potency is quantitated by the minimum alveolar concentration (MAC) that causes 50% of subjects to fail to respond to a standardized painful stimulus
(B) General anesthesia is associated with increased blood pressure and total peripheral resistance
(C) If an anesthetic agent is very soluble in the blood, it will have a relatively fast onset of action
(D) Inhalational agents are used for long procedures because intravenous anesthetics are too toxic to use for more than a few minutes
(E) Surgical anesthesia is associated with complete muscle paralysis

56. A patient is to undergo day surgery and a short-acting intravenous agent with a fast onset will be used. Recovery, unhampered by postoperative nausea, will be rapid because the clearance of the drug is greater than hepatic blood flow. The drug to be used is
(A) Fentanyl
(B) Ketamine
(C) Propofol
(D) Thiopental
(E) Zolpidem

57. A patient with an incurable cancer is suffering from pain that is gradually increasing in intensity. In the management of pain in such a patient
(A) Meperidine is more effective than morphine in cancer pain states
(B) Nonsteroidal anti-inflammatory drugs may control symptoms during a significant portion of the course of the disease
(C) Physical dependency always occurs in the later stages of the disease
(D) The placebo effect is absent
(E) To delay the development of dependency, opioid analgesics should never be given for initial management of chronic pain

58. Which effect of morphine is established to be mediated via activation of mu receptors?
(A) Cough suppression
(B) Elevation of arterial P_{CO_2}
(C) Mydriasis
(D) Relaxation of vascular smooth muscle
(E) Tachycardia

59. There is a wide range of receptor types and receptor mechanisms that mediate the effects of endogenous signaling molecules and the drugs that mimic or block their effects. Which drug mediates its effects by binding to and activating an intracellular receptor that, when activated, acts as a transcription factor?
(A) Albuterol
(B) Captopril
(C) Erythropoietin
(D) Morphine
(E) Prednisone

60. A drug that is currently a first-choice drug in the management of absence seizures as well as partial, primary generalized, and tonic-clonic seizures is
(A) Carbamazepine
(B) Ethosuximide
(C) Gabapentin
(D) Phenytoin
(E) Valproic acid

61. If one patient is taking amitriptyline and another patient is taking chlorpromazine, they are both likely to experience
(A) Excessive salivation
(B) Extrapyramidal dysfunction
(C) Gynecomastia
(D) Increased gastrointestinal motility
(E) Postural hypotension

62. The following data concern the relative activities of hypothetical investigational drugs as blockers of the membrane transporters (reuptake systems) for 3 CNS neurotransmitters.

	Blocking Actions on CNS Transporters for		
Drug	Dopamine	Serotonin	Norepinephrine
UCSF 1	+++	None	None
UCSF 2	+++	++++	++
UCSF 3	None	++	++
UCSF 4	None	+++	++
UCSF 5	+	+	None

Key: Number of + signs denotes intensity of blocking actions.

Which drug is likely to be effective in the treatment of major depressive disorders but may also cause marked adverse effects, including thought disorders, delusions, hallucinations, and paranoia?
(A) UCSF 1
(B) UCSF 2
(C) UCSF 3
(D) UCSF 4
(E) UCSF 5

63. A 38-year-old woman who lived alone visited a psychiatrist because she was depressed. Her symptoms included low self-esteem, with frequent ruminations on her worthlessness, and hypersomnia. She was hyperphagic and overweight and complained that her limbs felt heavy. An initial diagnosis was made of a depressive disorder. Treatment was initiated with imipramine, but after 2 mo the patient had not improved significantly. Which drug is most likely to have therapeutic value in this depressed patient?
(A) Baclofen
(B) Citalopram
(C) Clonazepam
(D) Nortriptyline
(E) Risperidone

64. Psychiatric evaluation of a patient after 6 weeks of treatment with a monoamine oxidase inhibitor (MAOI) shows no improvement. The psychiatrist now writes a prescription for fluoxetine, which the patient starts 2 days after her final dose of the MAOI. Because the MAOIs used as antidepressants continue to exert effects for 2 or more weeks after discontinuance, the most likely result of the administration of fluoxetine now will be to cause
(A) A rapid amelioration of her depressive symptoms
(B) Electrocardiographic abnormalities
(C) Extrapyramidal dysfunction
(D) The serotonin syndrome
(E) Weight gain

65. A 45-year-old woman was suspected of having Cushing's syndrome. To confirm the diagnosis, the patient was given an oral medication late in the evening and had blood drawn the following morning for laboratory testing. The oral medication was
(A) Dexamethasone
(B) Fludrocortisone
(C) Glucose
(D) Ketoconazole
(E) Propylthiouracil

66. An atypical antipsychotic drug that is quite sedating and associated with significant weight gain, hyperlipidemia, and increased risk of type II diabetes is
(A) Bupropion
(B) Clonazepam
(C) Haloperidol
(D) Olanzapine
(E) Trifluoperazine

67. A psychiatric patient taking medications develops a tremor, thyroid enlargement, and leukocytosis. The drug he is taking is most likely to be
(A) Clomipramine
(B) Haloperidol
(C) Imipramine
(D) Lithium
(E) Sertraline

68. The mechanism of action of benzodiazepines is
(A) Activation of $GABA_B$ receptors
(B) Antagonism of glycine receptors in the spinal cord
(C) Blockade of the action of glutamic acid
(D) Increased GABA-mediated chloride ion conductance
(E) Inhibition of GABA aminotransferase

69. A drug that is used in the treatment of parkinsonism and will also attenuate reversible extrapyramidal side effects of neuroleptics is

(A) Amantadine
(B) Levodopa
(C) Pergolide
(D) Selegiline
(E) Trihexyphenidyl

70. After a very large overdose of a benzodiazepine, a patient is admitted to the hospital. Administration of which of the following will reverse the action of the benzodiazepine?
(A) Atropine
(B) Etomidate
(C) Flumazenil
(D) Naloxone
(E) Zolpidem

71. A 65-year-old man with bacteremia is to be treated with a combination of antibiotics. The inclusion of the aminoglycoside amikacin in the therapy will provide coverage against
(A) *Bacteroides fragilis*
(B) *Klebsiella pneumoniae*
(C) *Legionella* species
(D) Methicillin-resistant *Staphylococcus aureus*
(E) *Neisseria meningitidis*

72. If an aerobic gram-negative rod causing bacteremia proves to be resistant to aminoglycosides, the mechanism of resistance is most likely due to
(A) Changed pathway of bacterial folate synthesis
(B) Decreased intracellular accumulation of the drug
(C) Drug inactivation by bacterial group transferases
(D) Induced synthesis of beta-lactamases
(E) Production of drug-trapping thiol compounds

73. A 54-year-old woman with a recent history of deep vein thrombosis had been stable on warfarin therapy for the past 2 mo. However, her most recent prothrombin time (PT) test revealed a markedly reduced INR. When asked about changes in diet or medication during the last several weeks, the woman said that she had recently begun taking an over-the-counter supplement recommended by a friend. Based on this information, the supplement is most likely to contain
(A) Ginkgo
(B) Ginseng
(C) Kava
(D) Ma-huang
(E) St. John's wort

74. Beta-lactamase production by strains of *Haemophilus influenzae, Moraxella catarrhalis,* and *Neisseria gonorrhoeae* confers resistance against penicillin G. Which of the following antibiotics is most likely to be effective against all strains of each of these organisms?
(A) Ampicillin
(B) Ceftriaxone
(C) Clindamycin
(D) Gentamicin
(E) Piperacillin

75–76. A 36-year-old patient is hospitalized for injuries sustained in an automobile accident. After several days, he develops a urinary tract infection resulting from *Pseudomonas aeruginosa.* Current drug treatment of the patient is limited to opioid analgesics and ibuprofen for pain. The patient's drug history includes a severe skin rash after treatment of otitis media with cefaclor. The following data show the antimicrobial sensitivity of aerobic isolates from urine sources in the hospital during the past year.

75. If a single drug is to be administered to this patient, the most appropriate choice in terms of efficacy and safety is
(A) Ampicillin
(B) Cefepime

| | Percentage of Isolates from Urine Sources Susceptible to | | | | |
Organism	Ampicillin	Ciprofloxacin	Tobramycin	Cefepime	Ticarcillin-Clavulanate
E coli	50	99	98	100	50
K pneumoniae	5	100	99	100	50
P mirabilis	90	98	98	100	90
P aeruginosa	0	86	90	94	90
S marcescens	8	70	80	85	82
S aureus	13	67	0	0	13
S epidermidis	14	67	0	0	12

(C) Ciprofloxacin
(D) Ticarcillin-clavulanate
(E) Tobramycin

76. Because the mortality rate approaches 50% in patients who develop sepsis caused by *Pseudomonas aeruginosa*, it is usually advisable to use a combination of antibiotics known to have synergistic activity against this microorganism. Which pair of antibiotics is established to be synergistic against *Pseudomonas aeruginosa*?
    (A) Ampicillin and tobramycin
    (B) Cefepime and vancomycin
    (C) Ciprofloxacin and ampicillin
    (D) Tobramycin and ticarcillin/clavulanate
    (E) Trimethoprim and sulfamethoxazole

77. A 24-year-old woman is to be treated with ciprofloxacin for a urinary tract infection. A contraindication to the use of ciprofloxacin in this patient is a history of
    (A) Deep vein thrombosis
    (B) Glucose-6-phosphate dehydrogenase (G6PD) deficiency
    (C) Gout
    (D) Joint-related medical problems
    (E) Use at the present time of a combined hormonal contraceptive

78. A 19-year-old woman with recurrent sinusitis has been treated with different antibiotics on several occasions. During the course of one such treatment, she developed a severe diarrhea and was hospitalized. Sigmoidoscopy revealed colitis, and pseudomembranes were confirmed histologically. Which of the following drugs, administered orally, is most likely to be effective in the treatment of colitis caused by *C difficile*?
    (A) Ampicillin
    (B) Cefazolin
    (C) Clindamycin
    (D) Doxycycline
    (E) Metronidazole

79. In the management of patients with AIDS, the sulfonamides are often used in combination with inhibitors of dihydrofolate reductase to prevent infection resulting from
    (A) *Campylobacter jejuni*
    (B) *Mycobacterium avium-intracellulare*
    (C) *Neisseria gonorrhea*
    (D) *Pneumocystis jiroveci*
    (E) *Treponema pallidum*

80. In a cancer cell, decreased ability to phosphorylate pyrimidines could result in resistance to the anticancer action of

(A) Cisplatin
(B) Etoposide
(C) Fluorouracil
(D) Mercaptopurine
(E) Methotrexate

81. A 65-year-old woman with endometrial cancer came to an outpatient cancer treatment center for her first cycle of platinum-based chemotherapy. To prevent chemotherapy-induced nausea and vomiting, this patient is likely to be given
    (A) Cisapride
    (B) Famotidine
    (C) Mesalamine
    (D) Ondansetron
    (E) Sumatriptan

82. A 20-year-old foreign exchange student attending college in California is to be treated for pulmonary tuberculosis acquired while he was living in Southeast Asia. Because drug resistance is anticipated, the proposed antibiotic regimen includes ethambutol, isoniazid (with supplementary vitamin B_6), pyrazinamide, and rifampin. Provided that his disease responds well to the drug regimen and that the microbiology laboratory results show sensitivity to the drugs, it would be appropriate after 2 mo to
    (A) Change his drug regimen to prophylaxis with isoniazid
    (B) Discontinue pyrazinamide
    (C) Establish baseline ocular function
    (D) Monitor amylase activity
    (E) Stop the supplementary vitamin B_6

83. An antifungal drug that binds to ergosterol and disrupts fungal membrane integrity is
    (A) Amphotericin B
    (B) Flucytosine
    (C) Griseofulvin
    (D) Ketoconazole
    (E) Terbinafine

84–85. A 20-year-old college student is brought to the emergency department after taking an overdose of a nonprescription drug. The patient is comatose. He has been hyperventilating and is now dehydrated with an elevated temperature. Serum analyses demonstrate that the patient has an anion gap metabolic acidosis.

84. The most likely cause of these signs and symptoms is overdosage of
    (A) Aspirin
    (B) Acetaminophen
    (C) Dextromethorphan
    (D) Diphenhydramine
    (E) Ethanol

85. In the management of this patient, it would be MOST appropriate to
    (A) Administer acetylcysteine
    (B) Administer fomepizole
    (C) Administer glucagon
    (D) Alkalinize the urine
    (E) Induce vomiting with syrup of ipecac

86. The drug or drug combination that has efficacy against methicillin-resistant *Staphylococcus aureus* and most strains of *Enterococcus faecalis* is
    (A) Ceftriaxone
    (B) Gentamicin
    (C) Imipenem/cilastatin
    (D) Piperacillin/tazobactam
    (E) Vancomycin plus gentamicin

87. Chemoprophylaxis for travelers to geographic regions where chloroquine-resistant *P falciparum* is endemic is effectively provided by
    (A) Doxycycline
    (B) Malarone (atavaquone-proguanil)
    (C) Mefloquine
    (D) Quinine
    (E) Any of the drugs listed above

88. A cardiac Purkinje fiber was isolated from an animal heart and placed in a recording chamber. One of the Purkinje cells was impaled with a microelectrode, and action potentials were recorded while the preparation was stimulated at 1 stimulus per second. A representative control action potential is shown in black in the graph. After equilibration, oxygenation was reduced and a drug was added to the perfusate while recording continued. A representative action potential obtained at the peak of drug action is shown as the superimposed action potential (color). Identify the drug from the following list.

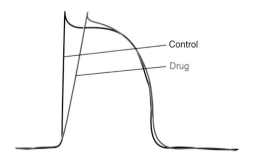

(A) Amiodarone
(B) Bretylium
(C) Diltiazem
(D) Flecainide
(E) Fluoxetine

(F) Lidocaine
(G) Nitroglycerin
(H) Propranolol
(I) Sotalol
(J) Verapamil

89. In patients with chronic granulomatous disease, a drug that increases the synthesis of tumor necrosis factor and thereby stimulates phagocytosis is
    (A) Aldesleukin
    (B) Cyclosporine
    (C) Filgrastim
    (D) Infliximab
    (E) Interferon-γ

90. A 43-year-old woman was brought to a hospital emergency department by her brother. Visiting the halfway house in which she lived, he had found her to be lethargic, with slurred speech. The patient had a long history of treatment for psychiatric problems, and the brother feared that she might have overdosed on 1 or more of the several drugs that had been prescribed for her. Physical examination revealed tachycardia with irregular heart rate, shallow respiration, decreased bowel sounds, dilated pupils, and hyperthermia. An ECG revealed a widened QRS complex with diffuse T-wave changes. If this patient had taken a drug overdose, the most likely causative agent was
    (A) Clozapine
    (B) Fluoxetine
    (C) Lithium
    (D) Thioridazine
    (E) Zolpidem

91. Cocaine intoxication commonly leads to treatment in hospital emergency departments. Severe intoxication with cocaine can result in
    (A) Bradycardia, hypotension, and coma
    (B) Coma, miosis, and respiratory depression
    (C) Cough, wheezing, and pneumonia
    (D) Hyperthermia, seizures, and cardiac arrhythmia
    (E) Hypokalemia, nausea, and paralysis

92–93. A 30-year-old hospitalized patient with AIDS has a CD4 cell count of 50/μL. He is being treated with a highly active antiretroviral therapy (HAART) regimen consisting of zidovudine (ZDV), lamivudine (3TC), and indinavir. Other drugs being administered to this patient include acyclovir, clarithromycin, rifabutin, and trimethoprim-sulfamethoxazole.

92. The drug in this patient's regimen that inhibits posttranslational modification of viral proteins is
    (A) Acyclovir
    (B) Indinavir

(C) Lamivudine
(D) Rifabutin
(E) Zidovudine

93. None of the drugs being administered to this patient are useful for prevention or treatment of opportunistic infections caused by
(A) *Candida albicans*
(B) Cytomegalovirus
(C) *M avium-intracellulare*
(D) *Pneumocystis jiroveci*
(E) *Toxoplasma gondii*

94. A 62-year-old woman who presented with pain in her hips, knees, and several vertebrae was diagnosed with Paget's disease. She had been mostly immobile lately due to bone pain and presented with lethargy, fatigue, muscle weakness, anorexia, and constipation. Her serum calcium concentration was found to be 14 mg/dL (normal 9–10 mg/dL). In addition to the bisphosphonates, another drug that has proved useful in reducing bone pain and lowering serum calcium in female patients with Paget's disease is
(A) Calcitonin
(B) Fluoride
(C) Hydrochlorothiazide
(D) Raloxifene
(E) Teriparatide (recombinant form of PTH)

95. Chronic lead poisoning is likely to cause
(A) Erythema and urticaria
(B) Glomerulonephritis
(C) Hair loss
(D) Jaundice
(E) Radial nerve palsy

96. Reserpine provides an antihypertensive effect by
(A) Accelerating the rate of enzymatic inactivation of amine neurotransmitters in the CNS
(B) Activating α_2 adrenoceptors located in the presynaptic membranes of CNS neurons that regulate peripheral SANS activity
(C) Blocking the transport of amine neurotransmitters from the cytoplasm to the inside of synaptic transmitter storage vesicles
(D) Inhibiting the uptake of amine neurotransmitters from the extracellular fluid into the cytoplasm in the presynaptic nerve terminus
(E) Interfering with the fusion of the membranes of synaptic vesicles with the plasma membrane

97. Which agent used in hypertension is a prodrug that is converted to its active form in the brain?
(A) Clonidine
(B) Doxazosin

(C) Methyldopa
(D) Nitroprusside
(E) Verapamil

98. A drug that blocks the uptake of dopamine and norepinephrine into presynaptic nerve terminals and also blocks sodium channels in axonal membranes is
(A) Cocaine
(B) Dextroamphetamine
(C) Ephedrine
(D) Fluoxetine
(E) Phenelzine

99. The consumption of shellfish harvested during a "red tide" (resulting from a large population of a dinoflagellate species) is not recommended. This is because the shellfish are likely to contain
(A) Arsenic
(B) Botulinum toxins
(C) Cyanide
(D) Saxitoxin
(E) Tetrodotoxin

100. A nonselective β-blocker that is also an α_1 selective antagonist is
(A) Atenolol
(B) Carvedilol
(C) Nadolol
(D) Pindolol
(E) Timolol

101. A 35-year-old woman who has never been pregnant suffers each month from pain, discomfort, and mood depression at the time of menses. She may benefit from the use of this selective inhibitor of the reuptake of serotonin.
(A) Amitriptyline
(B) Bupropion
(C) Mirtazapine
(D) Paroxetine
(E) Trazodone

102. A 23-year-old man was brought to a hospital suffering from marked bradykinesia, muscle rigidity, and tremor at rest. Unfortunately, the extrapyramidal dysfunction was permanent in this patient, as a result of self-administration of MPTP, a drug that is cytotoxic to nigrostriatal dopaminergic neurons. The drug known to protect against the neuronal toxicity of MPTP is
(A) Benztropine
(B) Bromocriptine
(C) Entacapone
(D) Levodopa
(E) Selegiline

103. Which drug is an opioid derivative that lacks analgesic activity but is useful as a cough suppressant?
    (A) Codeine
    (B) Dextromethorphan
    (C) Hydrocodone
    (D) Meperidine
    (E) Pentazocine

104. Drugs that selectively inhibit D_2 dopamine receptors in the CNS have efficacy in the treatment of schizophrenia. Efficacy in the treatment of schizophrenia is also seen with drugs that block
    (A) α adrenoceptors or D_1 dopamine receptors
    (B) D_4 dopamine receptors or 5-HT_2 serotonin receptors
    (C) $GABA_A$ receptors or 5-HT_3 serotonin receptors
    (D) H_1 histamine receptors or β adrenoceptors
    (E) β adrenoceptors or NMDA receptors

105. A 44-year-old patient suffering from alcoholism enters a residential treatment program that emphasizes group therapy and also uses pharmacologic agents adjunctively. The patient is given a drug that decreases the craving for alcohol. Because the drug will not cause adverse effects if the patient consumes alcoholic beverages, it can be identified as
    (A) Bupropion
    (B) Disulfiram
    (C) Olanzapine
    (D) Naltrexone
    (E) Sertraline

106. A 22-year-old woman presents with left lower quadrant abdominal pain and a purulent vaginal discharge that, on Gram stain, revealed gram-negative rods. A diagnosis is made of pelvic inflammatory disease possibly involving both *N gonorrhoeae* and *C trachomatis*. A drug or drug combination that provides adequate empiric coverage of the organisms involved in this infection is
    (A) Azithromycin
    (B) Ceftriaxone plus doxycycline
    (C) Metronidazole
    (D) Norfloxacin plus ampicillin
    (E) Trimethoprim-sulfamethoxazole

107. This agent, which is used in the chemotherapy of Hodgkin's lymphoma, is an agonist of a hormone receptor.
    (A) Dacarbazine
    (B) Doxorubicin
    (C) Prednisone
    (D) Procarbazine
    (E) Vinblastine

108. A tyrosine kinase enzyme inhibitor that is used to treat chronic myelogenous leukemia is
    (A) Anastrozole
    (B) Imatinib
    (C) Mitomycin
    (D) Rituximab
    (E) Teniposide

109. A 17-year-old high school student presents with headache, fever, and cough of 2 days' duration. Sputum is scant and nonpurulent, and a Gram stain reveals many white cells but no organisms. Because this otherwise healthy patient appears to have a community-acquired pneumonia (CAP), you should initiate treatment with
    (A) Azithromycin
    (B) Chloramphenicol
    (C) Clindamycin
    (D) Gentamicin
    (E) Quinupristin-dalfopristin

110. Relative to ciprofloxacin, levofloxacin has improved activity against
    (A) *Bacteroides fragilis*
    (B) *Escherichia coli*
    (C) *Haemophilus influenzae*
    (D) *Mycoplasma pneumoniae*
    (E) *Streptococcus pneumoniae*

111. The drug of choice for the management of osteoporosis caused by high-dose use of glucocorticoids is
    (A) Alendronate
    (B) Anastrozole
    (C) Mestranol
    (D) Omeprazole
    (E) Oxandrolone

112. The mechanism of action of cyclosporine involves
    (A) Activation of phospholipase A_2
    (B) Block of interleukin-2 receptors
    (C) Competitive inhibition of inosine monophosphate dehydrogenase
    (D) Inhibition of enzymes involved in purine metabolism
    (E) Inhibition of the cytoplasmic phosphatase calcineurin

113. A drug that is appropriate for treating a patient with moderate to severe rheumatoid arthritis but is not appropriate for treating a patient with moderate to severe osteoarthritis is
    (A) Acetaminophen
    (B) Etanercept
    (C) Ibuprofen
    (D) Ketorolac
    (E) Oxycodone

114–115. An anesthetized subject was given an intravenous bolus dose of a drug (**Drug 1**) while the systolic and diastolic blood pressures (color) and the heart rate were recorded, as shown on the left side of the graph below. While the recorder was stopped, **Drug 2** was given (center). **Drug 1** was then administered again, as shown on the right side of the graph.

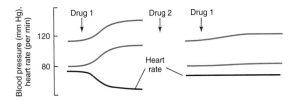

114. Identify Drug 1 from the following list
  (A) Atropine
  (B) Diphenhydramine
  (C) Echothiophate
  (D) Endothelin
  (E) Epinephrine
  (F) Histamine
  (G) Isoproterenol
  (H) Norepinephrine
  (I) Phentolamine
  (J) Phenylephrine
  (K) Terbutaline

115. Identify Drug 2 from the following list
  (A) Angiotensin II
  (B) Atropine
  (C) Bethanechol
  (D) Diphenhydramine
  (E) Endothelin
  (F) Epinephrine
  (G) Isoproterenol
  (H) Norepinephrine
  (I) Phentolamine
  (J) Phenylephrine
  (K) Terbutaline

116. An anthelmintic drug with a wide spectrum of activity that includes *Schistosoma* species (blood flukes), *Clonorchis sinensis* (liver fluke), and *Paragonimus westermani* (lung fluke) is
  (A) Ivermectin
  (B) Mefloquine
  (C) Metronidazole

  (D) Praziquantel
  (E) Thiabendazole

117. In the treatment of hypothyroidism, thyroxine is preferred over liothyronine because thyroxine
  (A) Can be made more easily by recombinant DNA technology
  (B) Has a longer half-life
  (C) Has higher affinity for thyroid hormone receptors
  (D) Is faster acting
  (E) Is more likely to improve a patient's mood

118. A 29-year-old G1P1 woman presents with infertility of 12 months' duration. Questioning reveals that the patient has had only 4 menstrual periods in the past year and that she sometimes notices breast nipple discharge. She has not been taking any prescription medications during the past year. A serum prolactin measurement reveals a concentration of 90 ng/mL (normal for a nonpregnant woman is <25 ng/mL). Based on these findings, which of the following drugs is most likely to help make this woman's ovulation more regular and restore her fertility?
  (A) Bromocriptine
  (B) Desmopressin
  (C) Leuprolide
  (D) Prochlorperazine
  (E) Spironolactone

119. A young woman seeks advice because she had unprotected sexual intercourse 12 h earlier. Based on her menstrual cycle, she believes that conception is possible. Which drug should she use as a postcoital contraceptive?
  (A) Clomiphene
  (B) Diethylstilbestrol plus raloxifene
  (C) Flutamide
  (D) Letrozole plus finasteride
  (E) L-Norgestrel

120. A 55-year-old woman with type 2 diabetes was going to be started on metformin. Before initiating therapy, it is important to confirm that the patient has normal renal function because patients with unrecognized renal insufficiency who take normal doses of metformin are at increased risk of
  (A) Hypoglycemia
  (B) Interstitial nephritis
  (C) Lactic acidosis
  (D) Liver failure
  (E) Torsade de pointes cardiac arrhythmia

ANSWER KEY FOR EXAMINATION 1*

1. D (5)	**31.** C (6, 8, 9)	**61.** E (29, 30)	**91.** D (59)
2. B (1)	**32.** A (33)	**62.** B (29, 30)	**92.** B (49)
3. A (26)	**33.** C (2)	**63.** B (30)	**93.** A (48, 49)
4. C (9, 13, 20)	**34.** D (6, 9, 10)	**64.** D (30)	**94.** A (42)
5. C (17)	**35.** B (8, 20)	**65.** A (37, 39)	**95.** E (58, 59)
6. C (16, 60)	**36.** E (34)	**66.** D (29)	**96.** C (6, 11)
7. E (14)	**37.** A (40)	**67.** D (29)	**97.** C (11)
8. E (14, 15)	**38.** E (6, 10)	**68.** D (21, 22)	**98.** A (6, 9, 30)
9. C (35)	**39.** A (12)	**69.** E (28, 29)	**99.** D (6)
10. B (7)	**40.** B (16)	**70.** C (22, 59)	**100.** B (10)
11. D (8, 59)	**41.** A (15)	**71.** B (45, 51)	**101.** D (30)
12. B (3)	**42.** C (15)	**72.** C (45)	**102.** E (28)
13. E (1)	**43.** D (13)	**73.** E (3, 61, 63)	**103.** B (31)
14. C (57, 59)	**44.** A (13)	**74.** B (43, 51)	**104.** B (29)
15. C (27)	**45.** C (20)	**75.** E (43, 45, 51)	**105.** D (23, 31, 32)
16. A (8)	**46.** A (20)	**76.** D (43, 45)	**106.** B (43, 44, 51)
17. C (36)	**47.** C (10, 11)	**77.** D (46)	**107.** C (39, 55)
18. B (15, 42)	**48.** C (16)	**78.** E (43, 50, 51)	**108.** B (55)
19. E (33)	**49.** B (9)	**79.** D (46, 53)	**109.** A (44, 51)
20. A (34)	**50.** C (18, 36)	**80.** C (55)	**110.** E (46)
21. C (11, 12)	**51.** E (21)	**81.** D (60)	**111.** A (42)
22. D (12)	**52.** B (22, 23, 59)	**82.** B (47)	**112.** E (56)
23. E (18, 34)	**53.** E (23, 32)	**83.** A (48)	**113.** B (36)
24. D (12, 18, 19)	**54.** D (3)	**84.** A (36, 59)	**114.** J (9)
25. A (20)	**55.** A (25)	**85.** D (59)	**115.** I (10)
26. E (35)	**56.** C (25)	**86.** E (43, 45)	**116.** D (54)
27. E (2)	**57.** B (31, 36)	**87.** E (53)	**117.** B (38)
28. C (2)	**58.** B (31)	**88.** D (14)	**118.** A (37)
29. B (3)	**59.** E (2, 39)	**89.** E (56)	**119.** E (40)
30. C (41)	**60.** E (24)	**90.** D (29, 30, 59)	**120.** C (41)

---

*Numbers in parentheses are chapters in which answers are found.

Appendix III

Examination 2

DIRECTIONS: Each numbered item or incomplete statement in this section is followed by answers or by completions of the statement. Select the ONE lettered answer or completion that is BEST in each case.

1. Which of the following is a common effect of both muscarinic stimulant drugs and opioids?
   (A) Decreased peristalsis
   (B) Decreased secretion by salivary glands
   (C) Hypertension
   (D) Inhibition of sweat glands
   (E) Miosis

2. Which statement about nitric oxide is false?
   (A) Nitric oxide is synthesized in vascular endothelium and the brain
   (B) Nitric oxide is released from storage vesicles by acetylcholine
   (C) Nitric oxide is released from exogenous molecules (eg, nitrates and nitroprusside)
   (D) Nitric oxide synthase is stimulated by histamine
   (E) Nitric oxide synthase exists in both inducible and constitutive forms

3. Regarding pharmacokinetics, the bioavailability of a drug is
   (A) Greater for women than men
   (B) Greater for drugs with large volumes of distribution
   (C) Determined by the AUC (area under the curve) for the route of administration divided by the AUC for IV administration
   (D) Determined by renal blood flow divided by hepatic blood flow
   (E) Determined by the oral dose divided by the IV dose

4. Receptors that communicate their activation by turning on an integral intracellular tyrosine kinase include
   (A) Acetylcholine nicotinic receptors
   (B) G protein-coupled receptors

   (C) Insulin receptors
   (D) Steroid receptors
   (E) Vitamin D receptors

5. A patient with an arrhythmia is to receive lidocaine by constant IV infusion. The target plasma concentration is 3 mg/L. The pharmacokinetic parameters for lidocaine in the general population are V_d 70 L, CL 35 L/h, and $t_{1/2}$ 1.4 h. An infusion is begun. The plasma concentration of lidocaine is measured 2.8 h later and reported to be 1.5 mg/L. This indicates that the final steady state plasma concentration in this patient will be
   (A) 1.5 mg/L
   (B) 2.0 mg/L
   (C) 3.0 mg/L
   (D) 6.0 mg/L
   (E) Insufficient data to answer

6. A new drug is to be evaluated. Before human trials are begun, FDA regulations require that
   (A) The drug be studied in 3 mammalian species
   (B) All acute and chronic animal toxicity data be submitted to the FDA
   (C) The drug must be shown to be safe in animals with the target disease
   (D) The drug must be shown to be free of carcinogenic effects
   (E) The effect of the drug on reproduction must be studied in at least 2 animal species

7. A drug that blocks the heart rate effect of a slow intravenous infusion of phenylephrine is
   (A) Atropine
   (B) Haloperidol
   (C) Physostigmine
   (D) Pilocarpine
   (E) Propranolol

8. A patient is admitted to the emergency department while vomiting blood. Her supine blood pressure is

100/60 mm Hg; sitting up, her BP is 50/0. Which of the following most accurately describes the probable autonomic response to the bleeding?
(**A**) Slow heart rate, dilated pupils, damp skin
(**B**) Rapid heart rate, dilated pupils, damp skin
(**C**) Slow heart rate, dry skin, increased bowel sounds
(**D**) Rapid heart rate, dry skin, constricted pupils, increased bowel sounds
(**E**) Rapid heart rate, constricted pupils, warm skin

9. A 65-year-old man has chronic open-angle glaucoma. The drug that is LEAST likely to have therapeutic value for this condition is
(**A**) Acetazolamide
(**B**) Isoproterenol
(**C**) Latanoprost
(**D**) Pilocarpine
(**E**) Timolol

10. A new drug was administered to a group of normal volunteers. Intravenous bolus doses produced the changes in blood pressure and heart rate shown in the graph below. The most probable receptor affinities of this new drug are
(**A**) α_1, α_2, and β_1
(**B**) α_1 and α_2 only
(**C**) β_1 and β_2 only
(**D**) Muscarinic M_3 only
(**E**) Nicotinic N_N only

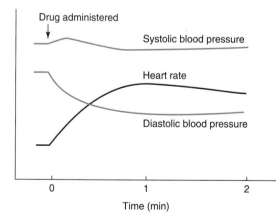

Drug administered

Systolic blood pressure

Heart rate

Diastolic blood pressure

| 0 | 1 | 2 |

Time (min)

11. Persons who ingest three or more alcoholic drinks daily can develop severe hepatotoxicity after doses of acetaminophen that are not toxic to individuals with normal liver function. This increased sensitivity to acetaminophen's toxicity is due to
(**A**) Decreased availability of acetaldehyde dehydrogenase

(**B**) Decreased hepatocellular stores of NADPH
(**C**) Increased extraction of acetaminophen by the cirrhotic liver
(**D**) Increased activity of cytochrome P450 mixed function oxidase isozymes
(**E**) Increased liver blood flow

12. An example of a phase I drug-metabolizing reaction is
(**A**) Acetylation
(**B**) Glucuronidation
(**C**) Hydroxylation
(**D**) Methylation
(**E**) Sulfation

13–14. A 52-year-old plumber comes to the office with a complaint of periodic onset of chest pain, described as a sensation of heavy pressure over the sternum that comes on when he exercises and disappears within 15 min when he stops. After a full physical examination and further evaluation, you make the diagnosis of angina of effort.

13. In considering medical therapy for this patient, which of the following correctly describes the beneficial action of nitroglycerin in this condition?
(**A**) Dilation of coronary arterioles reduces resistance and increases coronary flow through ischemic tissue
(**B**) Dilation of peripheral arterioles increases cardiac work
(**C**) Dilation of systemic veins results in decreased diastolic cardiac size
(**D**) Increased sympathetic outflow increases coronary flow
(**E**) Tachycardia increases diastolic coronary flow

14. A drug that is useful in angina but causes constipation, edema, and increased cardiac size is
(**A**) Atenolol
(**B**) Hydralazine
(**C**) Isosorbide dinitrate
(**D**) Nitroglycerin
(**E**) Verapamil

15. A drug suitable for producing a brief (5- to 15-min) increase in cardiac vagal effects is
(**A**) Digoxin
(**B**) Edrophonium
(**C**) Ergotamine
(**D**) Pralidoxime
(**E**) Pyridostigmine

16. A patient with a 30-year history of type 1 diabetes comes to you with a complaint of bloating and sour belching after meals. On several occasions,

vomiting has occurred after a meal. Evaluation reveals delayed emptying of the stomach, and you diagnose diabetic gastroparesis. Which drug would be most useful in this patient?
(A) Famotidine
(B) Metoclopramide
(C) Misoprostol
(D) Omeprazole
(E) Ondansetron

17. An important difference between nonselective α receptor antagonists and α_1-selective antagonists is that α_1-selective antagonists
(A) Are more likely to cause hypoglycemia
(B) Are more likely to precipitate bronchoconstriction in patients with asthma
(C) Have greater efficacy in relaxing smooth muscle in the urinary tract
(D) Produce less reflex tachycardia
(E) Reduce mean arterial blood pressure to a greater extent

18–19. A 47-year-old sales associate has developed severe congestive heart failure and digoxin is prescribed for his condition. In addition to the signs and symptoms of heart failure, he has become very depressed about his poor prognosis.

18. The most accurate description of the mechanism of action of digitalis in congestive heart failure is that
(A) Increased cytoplasmic sodium concentration results in increased calcium stores in sarcoplasmic reticulum
(B) Blockade of the sodium pump results in increased calcium entry through calcium channels
(C) Blockade of potassium transport results in increased intracellular potassium
(D) Actin-myosin filaments are sensitized to calcium
(E) Increased inward trigger calcium influx causes increased release of calcium from the sarcoplasmic reticulum

19. Six months after starting digoxin therapy, the patient attempts suicide by swallowing 75 digoxin tablets (0.25 mg each). He is discovered by his wife and brought to the emergency department by paramedics. His blood pressure is 100/50 mm Hg, heart rate 40/min, and respirations 15/min. Toxicity caused by suicidal digoxin overdose should be treated by
(A) Administration of digoxin antibodies
(B) Administration of phenytoin intravenously
(C) Administration of sodium bicarbonate

(D) Lowering the serum magnesium
(E) Raising the serum potassium to 7 mEq/L

20–21. A 70-year-old woman fell 2 years ago during a spell of dizziness and broke her hip. Now she is to be treated for a blood pressure of 170/100 mm Hg.

20. When treating hypertension chronically, orthostatic hypotension is greatest with
(A) Clonidine
(B) Guanethidine
(C) Hydralazine
(D) Prazosin
(E) Propranolol

21. Which of the following is usually associated with orthostatic hypotension for the first few doses only?
(A) Clonidine
(B) Guanethidine
(C) Hydralazine
(D) Prazosin
(E) Propranolol

22. A drug that promotes the healing of gastric and duodenal ulcers primarily by adhering to the damaged tissue and forming a protective cover is
(A) Cholestyramine
(B) Cimetidine
(C) Metoclopramide
(D) Misoprostol
(E) Sucralfate

23–24. A 52-year-old woman is admitted to the emergency department with a history of drug treatment for several conditions. Her serum electrolytes are found to be as follows (normal values in parentheses):

Na^+: 140 mEq/L (135–145) K^+: 6.5 mEq/L (3.5–5)
Cl^-: 100 mEq/L (98–107)   pH: 7.3 (7.31–7.41)

23. This patient has probably been taking
(A) Acetazolamide
(B) Atenolol
(C) Digoxin
(D) Furosemide
(E) Spironolactone

24. In view of the electrolyte panel shown (and regardless of its cause), the patient will be less sensitive to the toxic actions of
(A) Cimetidine
(B) Digoxin
(C) Dobutamine
(D) Fexofenadine
(E) Omeprazole

25. A drug that decreases blood pressure when given orally and may be followed by rebound hypertension if stopped suddenly is
(A) Atenolol
(B) Clonidine
(C) Morphine
(D) Nitroprusside
(E) Prazosin

26. Ventricular muscle from a cardiac biopsy was prepared for transmembrane potential recording in an isolated muscle chamber. Action potentials were recorded before and after application of drug X. Identify drug X from the following list.

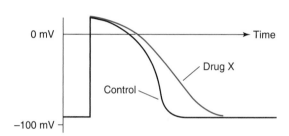

(A) Adenosine
(B) Dofetilide
(C) Esmolol
(D) Procainamide
(E) Verapamil

27. Propranolol and hydralazine have which of the following effects in common?
(A) Decreased cardiac force
(B) Decreased cardiac output
(C) Decreased mean arterial blood pressure
(D) Increased systemic vascular resistance
(E) Tachycardia

28. A 54-year-old male farmer has a 5-year history of frequent, recurrent, and very painful calcium-containing kidney stones. The patient has hypercalciuria caused by a primary defect in renal calcium reabsorption. Appropriate chronic therapy for this man is a(n)
(A) Aldosterone antagonist
(B) Loop diuretic
(C) NSAID
(D) Strong opioid
(E) Thiazide diuretic

29. A 55-year-old executive has cardiomyopathy and congestive heart failure. He is being treated with diuretics. The mechanism of action of furosemide is best described as
(A) Interference with H^+/HCO_3^- exchange
(B) Blockade of a $Na^+/K^+/2Cl^-$ transporter
(C) Blockade of a Na^+/Cl^- cotransporter
(D) Blockade of carbonic anhydrase
(E) Inhibition of genetic expression of DNA in the kidney

30. A peptide that causes arteriolar vasoconstriction is
(A) Brain natriuretic peptide (BNP)
(B) Calcitonin gene-related peptide
(C) Endothelin
(D) Substance P
(E) Vasoactive intestinal peptide

31. Cyclooxygenase-1 and -2 are responsible for the
(A) Conversion of GTP to cyclic GMP (cGMP)
(B) Conversion of ATP to cyclic AMP (cAMP)
(C) Metabolic degradation of cAMP
(D) Synthesis of leukotrienes from arachidonate
(E) Synthesis of prostaglandins from arachidonate

32–33. A 16-year-old student has had asthma for 8 years. The number of episodes of severe bronchospasm has increased recently, and you have been asked to review the therapeutic plan.

32. Which of the following agents is LEAST likely to be of therapeutic value in an ordinary acute bronchospastic attack?
(A) Albuterol
(B) Beclomethasone
(C) Ipratropium
(D) Metaproterenol
(E) Theophylline

33. A long-acting β_2-selective antagonist that is used as an inhaled therapy for moderate or severe asthma is
(A) Formoterol
(B) Ipratopium
(C) Terbutaline
(D) Theophylline
(E) Zafirlukast

34. Lidocaine is commonly used as a local anesthetic. If a patient mistakenly receives a toxic dose of lidocaine intravenously, the patient is likely to exhibit
(A) Excessive salivation, mydriasis, and diarrhea
(B) Generalized paralysis resulting in respiratory failure
(C) Hyperthermia and hypertension
(D) No effects immediately but then delayed, massive hepatocellular damage
(E) Seizures and coma

35. Early in an anesthesia procedure, which includes the use of succinylcholine and halothane, a surgical patient develops severe muscle rigidity, hypertension, and hyperthermia. Management of this patient will almost certainly include the administration of
(A) Baclofen
(B) Cyclobenzaprine
(C) Dantrolene
(D) Naloxone
(E) Tubocurarine

36. A 34-year-old woman in her second trimester of pregnancy presented with a tender, red, swollen calf that was diagnosed as a deep vein thrombosis (DVT) and was treated successfully. However, because of the high risk of recurrence of the DVT, she was treated with an anticoagulant for the remainder of her pregnancy. The drug used was most likely
(A) Aspirin
(B) Clopidogrel
(C) Enoxaparin
(D) Lepirudin
(E) Warfarin

37. Which drug is correctly associated with its clinical application?
(A) Erythropoietin: macrocytic anemia
(B) Filgrastim (G-CSF): thrombocytopenia resulting from myelocytic leukemia
(C) Ferrous sulfate: microcytic anemia of pregnancy
(D) Folic acid: hemochromatosis
(E) Oprelvekin (IL-11): rheumatoid arthritis

38. A 23-year-old woman with signs and symptoms of a lower urinary tract infection was treated effectively with an oral antibiotic. The drug achieves effective concentrations in the urine, but systemic levels are inadequate for treatment of blood or respiratory tract infections. The drug used was
(A) Aztreonam
(B) Cephalexin
(C) Gentamicin
(D) Linezolid
(E) Norfloxacin

39. Which match of an antifungal drug to a characteristic feature of the agent is accurate?
(A) Amphotericin B: dose-limiting hepatotoxicity
(B) Caspofungin: inhibition of $\beta(1-3)$ glucan synthesis
(C) Flucytosine: effective in the treatment of onychomycosis
(D) Itraconazole: binds to ergosterol to form artificial membrane "pores"
(E) Ketoconazole: induction of hepatic cytochrome P-450 drug-metabolizing enzymes

40. Which match of an antiviral drug to a characteristic feature of the agent is accurate?
(A) Acyclovir: inhibits viral thymidine kinase
(B) Enfuvirtide: antisense oligonucleotide active versus CMV
(C) Lamivudine: least toxic of the NRTIs and also useful in HBV
(D) Ritonavir: potent inhibitor of viral neuraminidase
(E) Zanamivir: inhibitor of hepatic cytochrome P450 drug-metabolizing enzymes

41. A 5-year-old boy was diagnosed as having an intestinal infection with *Enterobius vermicularis* (pinworm). He should be treated with
(A) Ivermectin
(B) Mebendazole
(C) Nitrofurantoin
(D) Praziquantel
(E) Quinine

42. Which agent is the drug of choice in severe amebic disease and for hepatic abscess?
(A) Diloxanide furoate
(B) Doxycycline
(C) Iodoquinol
(D) Pentamidine
(E) Tinidazole

43. An oral antidiabetic drug that inhibits an enzyme in the gastrointestinal tract that converts polysaccharides to monosaccharides and thereby reduces postprandial hyperglycemia is
(A) Acarbose
(B) Glipizide
(C) Metformin
(D) Rosiglitazone
(E) Sitagliptin

44. A young patient with end-stage kidney disease receives a transplant from a living related donor who is HLA-identical and red blood cell ABO matched. To prevent rejection, the transplant recipient is treated with cyclosporine. Two years after initiating cyclosporine therapy, the patient developed evidence of cyclosporine-induced nephrotoxicity and hypertension. He was switched to an immunosuppressant that lacks renal toxicity and produces its immunosuppressant effect by inhibiting the de novo pathway of purine synthesis. The new immunosuppressant is
(A) Azathioprine
(B) Etanercept
(C) Mycophenolate mofetil
(D) Tacrolimus
(E) Thalidomide

45. Blizzard weather conditions have forced a family living on welfare to stay in their poorly ventilated apartment for several days. During this time, all family members have developed slight nausea, headache, and dizziness. When the youngest member of the family becomes confused, starts breathing rapidly, and then faints, she is brought to the emergency department of the local hospital. The condition of this patient is most likely due to
(A) Glue sniffing
(B) Ingestion of lead-based paints (pica)
(C) Inhalation of carbon monoxide
(D) Malnutrition
(E) Sulfur dioxide poisoning

46. A young female patient using an oral contraceptive is to be treated for pulmonary tuberculosis. She is advised to use an additional method of contraception since the efficacy of the oral agents is commonly decreased if her drug regimen includes
(A) Amikacin
(B) Ethambutol
(C) Isoniazid
(D) Pyrazinamide
(E) Rifampin

47. A 2-year-old girl was brought to the emergency department because of vomiting, bloody diarrhea, and hypotension. An abdominal x-ray film showed multiple radiopaque pills, and a relative at the child's home reported the discovery of an open bottle of iron pills behind a large piece of furniture. In addition to supportive care, treatment of the child is most likely to include
(A) Intravenous administration of acetylcysteine
(B) Intravenous administration of deferoxamine
(C) Intravenous administration of pralidoxime

(D) Oral administration of activated charcoal
(E) Oral administration of edetate (EDTA)

48. The primary site of action of tyramine is
(A) Ganglionic receptors
(B) Gut and liver catechol-*O*-methyltransferase
(C) Postganglionic sympathetic nerve terminals
(D) Preganglionic sympathetic nerve terminals
(E) Vascular smooth muscle cell receptors

49. In the treatment of hypertension, the combination of enalapril and spironolactone is ill-advised because of the risk of
(A) Bone loss and osteoporosis
(B) Calcium-containing kidney stones
(C) Hyperkalemia
(D) Metabolic acidosis
(E) Postural hypotension

50. Baclofen activates specific spinal cord receptors for this inhibitory neurotransmitter.
(A) Acetylcholine
(B) GABA
(C) Glycine
(D) Serotonin
(E) Substance P

51–52. The research division of a pharmaceutical corporation has characterized the receptor blocking actions of 5 new drugs, each of which may have potential therapeutic value. The relative intensities of their blocking actions are shown in the following table. Because each of these drugs is lipophilic and can cross the blood-brain barrier, they are expected to have CNS effects.

51. Based on the data shown in the table below, which drug is most likely to exacerbate the symptoms of Parkinson's disease?

	Blocking Action on CNS Receptors			
Drug	Adrenergic (Beta)	Cholinergic (M)	Dopaminergic (D₂)	GABAergic (A)
A	++	+++	+++	None
B	None	None	None	++++
C	None	++++	+	None
D	+	None	+++	+
E	None	+	+	+

Key: Number of + signs denotes intensity of blocking actions.

(A) Drug A
(B) Drug B
(C) Drug C
(D) Drug D
(E) Drug E

52. Based on the data shown in the table above, which drug is most likely to lower the threshold to seizures?
(A) Drug A
(B) Drug B
(C) Drug C
(D) Drug D
(E) Drug E

53. A 20-year-old man who had become physiologically dependent after illicit use of secobarbital ("reds") is undergoing severe withdrawal symptoms, including nausea, vomiting, delirium, and periodic seizures. These symptoms would be alleviated by the administration of
(A) Buprenorphine
(B) Bupropion
(C) Fluoxetine
(D) Lorazepam
(E) Meperidine

54. In attempted suicides involving a drug overdose, flumazenil is likely to reverse the CNS depressant effects of
(A) Chloral hydrate
(B) Eszopiclone
(C) Ethanol
(D) Meperidine
(E) Secobarbital

55. An individual who ingested an antifreeze solution containing ethylene glycol was brought to a hospital emergency department. In an attempt to prevent severe acidosis and renal damage, the patient was given fomepizole. Fomepizole is useful in ethylene glycol poisoning because it inhibits
(A) Alcohol dehydrogenase
(B) Aldehyde dehydrogenase
(C) Enzymes in the microsomal ethanol-oxidizing system (MEOS)
(D) Enzymes that require thiamin as a cofactor
(E) Glutathione transferase

56. A drug that exerts its anticonvulsant effects by blocking voltage-gated sodium channels in neuronal membranes is
(A) Diazepam
(B) Ethosuximide
(C) Gabapentin
(D) Phenytoin
(E) Vigabatrin

57. A young woman suffering from myoclonic seizures was receiving effective single-drug therapy with valproic acid. Because she was planning a pregnancy, her physician switched her to an alternative medication with less potential for teratogenicity. Which one of the following drugs is effective in myoclonic seizures but often makes the patient extremely drowsy at the dose level required for effective seizure control?
(A) Carbamazepine
(B) Clonazepam
(C) Ethosuximide
(D) Lamotrigine
(E) Topiramate

58. The mechanism of local anesthetic action of cocaine is
(A) Activation of G protein-linked membrane receptors
(B) Block of the reuptake of norepinephrine at sympathetic nerve endings
(C) Competitive pharmacologic antagonism of nicotinic receptors
(D) Inhibition of blood and tissue enzymes that hydrolyze acetylcholine
(E) Use-dependent blockade of voltage-gated sodium channels

59. A patient is brought to the emergency department suffering from an overdose of an illicit drug. She is agitated, has disordered thought processes, suffers from paranoia, and "hears voices." The drug most likely to be responsible for her condition is
(A) Gamma-hydroxybutyrate (GHB)
(B) Hashish
(C) Heroin
(D) Marijuana
(E) Methamphetamine

60. A patient undergoing surgery is given a drug for skeletal muscle relaxation. The anesthesiologist notes a marked drop in blood pressure and an increase in airway resistance immediately after the injection. Intravenous administration of diphenhydramine quickly restores the patient's blood pressure and airway diameter. The muscle relaxant used was probably
(A) Baclofen
(B) Dantrolene
(C) Diazepam
(D) Tubocurarine
(E) Zolpidem

61. The following table contains data on 2 properties of different compounds under study for use as inhalational anesthetics.

Properties of Inhalational Anesthetics		
Anesthetic	Blood: Gas Partition Coefficient	Minimal Alveolar Anesthetic Concentration (%)
A	0.8	9.7
B	1.4	1.46
C	9.8	0.66
D	2.3	0.86
E	1.8	1.76

The agent most likely to have the slowest rate of recovery from its anesthetic action is
(A) Anesthetic A
(B) Anesthetic B
(C) Anesthetic C
(D) Anesthetic D
(E) Anesthetic E

62. Although fentanyl or one of its congeners is usually administered in the early stages of a general anesthesia procedure, it is likely that the patient will receive an injection of morphine during the last phase. The rationale for switching from fentanyl to morphine is that
(A) Morphine has a longer duration of action
(B) Morphine has greater analgesic efficacy
(C) Morphine has more of a "ceiling effect" and is less likely to cause respiratory failure
(D) Morphine is a nonselective opioid receptor agonist, whereas fentanyl is a selective kappa receptor agonist
(E) The effects of morphine are more completely reversed by naloxone

63. Mental retardation, microcephaly, and underdevelopment of the midface region in an infant is associated with chronic heavy maternal use during pregnancy of
(A) Cocaine
(B) Diazepam
(C) Ethanol
(D) Heroin
(E) Methylenedioxymethamphetamine (MDMA)

64. After ingestion of a meal that included sardines, cheese, and red wine, a patient taking phenelzine experienced a hypertensive crisis. The most likely explanation for this untoward effect is that phenelzine

(A) Acts to release tyramine from these foods
(B) Inhibits MAO type B
(C) Inhibits the metabolism of catecholamines
(D) Is an activator of tyrosine hydroxylase
(E) Promotes the release of norepinephrine from sympathetic nerve endings

65. Which one of the following is characteristic of succinylcholine?
(A) Actions in phase I block are reversed by neostigmine
(B) Is an antagonist at muscarinic receptors
(C) Blocks the release of histamine
(D) May cause hyperkalemia
(E) Is metabolized by acetylcholinesterase

66. A 48-year-old surgical patient was anesthetized with an intravenous bolus dose of propofol, then maintained on isoflurane with vecuronium as the skeletal muscle relaxant. At the end of the surgical procedure, she was given pyridostigmine and glycopyrrolate. Postoperative pain was managed by parenteral morphine. Which statement about the drugs used in this case is accurate?
(A) Continuous infusion of propofol is contraindicated because of its emetic effects
(B) Glycopyrrolate protects against potential cardiovascular effects due to pyridostigmine
(C) Muscle fasciculation resulting from vecuronium causes postoperative pain
(D) Pyridostigmine is likely to cause CNS effects
(E) Skeletal muscle-relaxing effects are less with isoflurane than other inhalation anesthetics

67. A woman taking haloperidol develops a spectrum of adverse effects that include the amenorrhea-galactorrhea syndrome and extrapyramidal dysfunction. Another antipsychotic drug is prescribed and since weekly blood tests are necessary, the drug is
(A) Bupropion
(B) Clozapine
(C) Nefazodone
(D) Olanzapine
(E) Sertraline

68. Naloxone will not antagonize or reverse
(A) Analgesic effects of morphine in a cancer patient
(B) Drug actions resulting from activation of mu opioid receptors
(C) Opioid-analgesic overdose in a patient on methadone maintenance
(D) Pupillary constriction caused by levorphanol
(E) Respiratory depression caused by overdose of nefazodone

69. Several drugs used in patients with advanced Parkinson's disease allow patients to lower their

dose of L-dopa/carbidopa, and thus reduce the incidence of L-dopa-induced dyskinesias. These drugs also decrease the amount of "off" time for the patient. Which drug is used in this way but does not, if used alone, ameliorate the symptoms of early Parkinson's disease or enhance CNS dopaminergic activity?

(A) Amantadine
(B) Bromocriptine
(C) Entacapone
(D) Pramipexole
(E) Selegiline

70. Ramelteon, a drug prescribed for insomnia, is thought to act in the CNS via

(A) Activation of benzodiazepine receptors
(B) Activation of melatonin receptors
(C) Block of the GABA transporter
(D) Inhibition of GABA metabolism
(E) Stimulation of glutamate receptors

71–72. A young man comes to a community clinic with a urogenital infection that, based on the Gram stain, appears to be due to *Neisseria gonorrhoeae.* Questioning suggests that the patient acquired the infection while vacationing abroad. The physician is concerned about drug resistance of the gonococcus. He notes that the patient has a history of an anaphylactic reaction to penicillin G.

71. Which drug is both most likely to be effective in the treatment of gonorrhea in this patient and safe to use?

(A) Amoxicillin-clavulanate
(B) Ceftriaxone
(C) Clarithromycin
(D) Ofloxacin
(E) Tetracycline

72. The physician is also concerned about the possibility of a nongonococcal urethritis in this patient. Although several antibiotics in the list below are active in such infections, these infections can usually be eradicated by the administration of a single dose of

(A) Azithromycin
(B) Doxycycline
(C) Erythromycin
(D) Tetracycline
(E) Trimethoprim-sulfamethoxazole

73. The antibacterial action of aminoglycosides is due to their ability to

(A) Activate autolytic enzymes
(B) Bind to the 30S ribosomal subunit and block initiation of bacterial protein synthesis

(C) Inhibit bacterial topoisomerases II and IV
(D) Inhibit the synthesis of precursors of the linear peptidoglycan chains of the bacterial cell wall
(E) Interfere with the synthesis of tetrahydrofolate

74. A 26-year-old woman with chronic bronchitis lives in a region of the country where winter conditions are harsh. Her physician recommends prophylactic use of oral tetracycline during the winter season. Which statement about the tetracycline antibiotics is accurate?

(A) Absorption from the gastrointestinal tract is enhanced by yogurt
(B) Elimination is predominantly via cytochrome P450 mediated hepatic metabolism
(C) Formation of drug-metabolizing enzymes is a primary mechanism of resistance to tetracyclines
(D) The patient should discontinue the tetracycline if she becomes pregnant
(E) The tetracylines suppress vaginal candidiasis

75. The long-term daily oral administration of therapeutic doses of prednisone results in

(A) Anemia
(B) Decreased bone density
(C) Elevated serum calcium concentration
(D) Hyperplasia of cells in the zona fasciculata and zona reticularis of the adrenal cortex
(E) Increased male-pattern hair growth in women

76. A 67-year-old man with osteoporosis was being treated with once-weekly alendronate. This medication has the unusual toxicity of

(A) A bluish hue to skin color
(B) Esophageal irritation
(C) Impairment of blue-green color vision
(D) Priapism
(E) Tendinitis

77. Clarithromycin has good activity against

(A) *Bacteroides fragilis*
(B) *Enterococcus faecalis*
(C) *Mycobacterium avium-intracellulare*
(D) *Pseudomonas aeruginosa*
(E) *Treponema pallidum*

78. A 30-year-old male patient who is HIV positive has a CD4 T-lymphocyte count of 450 cells/μL (normal, 600–1500 cells/μL) and a viral RNA load of 11,000 copies/mL. His treatment involves a 3-drug antiviral regimen (HAART) consisting of zidovudine, didanosine, and efavirenz. Efavirenz limits HIV infection by

(A) Binding to the active site of HIV reverse transcriptase

(B) Blocking the binding of HIV virions to the CD4 receptor on T cells

(C) Inhibiting the HIV enzyme that cleaves sialic acid residues from the surface of HIV virions

(D) Inhibiting the HIV protease

(E) Serving as an allosteric inhibitor of HIV reverse transcriptase

79–80. A 73-year-old patient has chronic pulmonary dysfunction requiring daily hospital visits for respiratory therapy. She is hospitalized with pneumonia, and it is not clear whether the infection is community or hospital acquired.

79. If she has a community-acquired pneumonia (CAP), coverage must be provided for pneumococci and atypical pathogens. In such a case, the most appropriate drug treatment in this patient is

(A) Ampicillin plus tobramycin

(B) Ceftriaxone plus erythromycin

(C) Penicillin G plus norfloxacin

(D) Ticarcillin-clavulanic acid

(E) Trimethoprim-sulfamethoxazole

80. If she has a hospital-acquired pneumonia (HAP), coverage must be provided for gram-negative bacteria (especially *Pseudomonas aeruginosa*) and for *S aureus,* many of which can be multiple drug resistant (MDR) organisms. In such a case, empiric treatment is likely to involve

(A) Amoxicillin-clavulanic acid

(B) Cefazolin plus metronidazole

(C) Linezolid

(D) Quinupristin-dalfopristin

(E) Vancomycin plus piperacillin/tazobactam

81. Resistance to acyclovir is most commonly due to mutations in a viral gene that encodes a protein that

(A) Converts viral single-stranded RNA into double-stranded DNA

(B) Phosphorylates acyclovir

(C) Synthesizes glutathione

(D) Transports acyclovir into the cell

(E) Transports acyclovir out of the cell

82. A male patient with AIDS has a CD4 T-lymphocyte count of 50 cells/μL (normal, 600–1500 cells/μL). He is being maintained on a multidrug regimen consisting of acyclovir, clarithromycin, dronabinol, fluconazole, lamivudine, indinavir, trimethoprim-sulfamethoxazole, and zidovudine. The drug that provides prophylaxis against cryptococcal infections of the meninges is

(A) Acyclovir

(B) Clarithromycin

(C) Fluconazole

(D) Lamivudine

(E) Trimethoprim-sulfamethoxazole

83–84. A patient with diffuse non-Hodgkin's lymphoma is treated with a combination drug regimen that includes bleomycin, cyclophosphamide, vincristine, doxorubicin, and prednisone.

83. The patient's cumulative dose of bleomycin will be carefully monitored because high cumulative doses are associated with

(A) Cardiotoxicity

(B) Hemorrhagic cystitis

(C) Hypoglycemia

(D) Peripheral neuropathy

(E) Pulmonary fibrosis

84. Dexrazoxane is thought to protect against the distinctive toxicity of which drug in this patient's regimen?

(A) Bleomycin

(B) Cyclophosphamide

(C) Doxorubicin

(D) Prednisone

(E) Vincristine

85. After delivery of a healthy infant, a young woman begins to bleed extensively because her uterus has failed to contract. Which drug should be administered to this woman?

(A) Betamethasone

(B) Desmopressin

(C) Leuprolide

(D) Oxytocin

(E) Prolactin

86. Adding a progestin to the estrogenic component of hormone replacement therapy for postmenopausal women

(A) Prevents thromboembolic events

(B) Provides better control of problematic hot flushes

(C) Reduces the risk of endometrial cancer

(D) Restores regular vaginal bleeding

(E) Slows bone loss

87. Based on the data in the table below concerning the antimicrobial drug sensitivity of bacterial isolates, which of the drugs listed appears to be the best choice for treatment of acute otitis media?

(A) Amoxicillin

(B) Ceftriaxone

(C) Ciprofloxacin

(D) Erythromycin

(E) TMP-SMX

Antimicrobial Sensitivity of Aerobic Isolates from Non-Urine Sources					
	% of Isolates Susceptible to				
Organism	Amoxicillin	Ceftriaxone	Ciprofloxacin	Erythromycin	TMP-SMX
E coli	50	99	98	20	70
H influenzae	5	95	97	23	87
K pneumoniae	90	98	98	98	90
M catarrhalis	20	86	76	91	96
L pneumophila	8	20	48	100	88
S pneumoniae	13	97	85	90	39
S aureus	14	87	65	50	50

88. Relative to fexofenadine, diphenhydramine is more likely to
(A) Be used for treatment of asthma
(B) Be used for treatment of gastroesophageal reflux disease
(C) Cause cardiac arrhythmias in overdose
(D) Have efficacy in the prevention of motion sickness
(E) Increase the serum concentration of warfarin

89. Chronic heart failure is commonly treated with a combination of drugs that both improve symptoms and provide long-term benefits. Three drugs or drug groups that have been shown in clinical trials to provide benefits in patients with chronic heart failure are
(A) ACE inhibitors, carvedilol, and spironolactone
(B) Alpha$_1$-selective antagonists, hydrochlorothiazide, and amrinone
(C) Digoxin, β agonists, and nitroglycerin
(D) Dobutamine, propranolol, and furosemide
(E) Verapamil, isosorbide dinitrate, and furosemide

90. A drug that inhibits the synthesis of thyroid hormone by preventing coupling of iodotyrosine molecules is
(A) Dexamethasone
(B) Ipodate
(C) Lithium
(D) Methimazole
(E) Propranolol

91. Long-term use of meperidine for analgesia is avoided because the accumulation of normeperidine, a metabolite of meperidine, is associated with risk of
(A) Constipation
(B) Dependence

(C) Neutropenia
(D) Renal impairment
(E) Seizures

92. A 60-year-old man with a history of a mild myocardial infarction was discovered to have low serum HDL cholesterol and moderately high serum triglyceride level. His serum total and LDL cholesterol concentrations were well below the upper limit of normal. The drug that is likely to result in the greatest lowering of this patient's serum triglyceride concentration and elevation of his serum LDL cholesterol concentration is
(A) Cholestyramine
(B) Ezetimibe
(C) Gemfibrozil
(D) Lovastatin
(E) Rosiglitazone

93. Protamine can be used to reverse the anticoagulant effect of
(A) Abciximab
(B) Clopidogrel
(C) Fondaparinux
(D) Unfractionated heparin
(E) Warfarin

94. A drug that reduces the need for platelet transfusions in patients undergoing cancer chemotherapy is
(A) Cyanocobalamin
(B) Erythropoietin
(C) Iron dextran
(D) Oprelvekin (interleukin-11)
(E) Tranexamic acid

95. In a patient with familial combined hyperlipidemia that is associated with increased VLDL and LDL, the drug that is most likely to *increase* plasma triglycerides while also decreasing plasma LDL is

(A) Cholestyramine
(B) Ezetimibe
(C) Gemfibrozil
(D) Niacin
(E) Rosuvastatin

96. A drug was given as an intravenous bolus to an anesthetized subject while the blood pressure was recorded. The results are shown in the figure below. Systolic and diastolic blood pressures in response to Drug X are shown. Drug X behaves most like which one of the following?

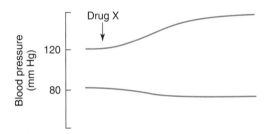

(A) Angiotensin
(B) Epinephrine
(C) Isoproterenol
(D) Norepinephrine
(E) Phenylephrine
(F) Terbutaline
(G) Tyramine

97. One of the health benefits of the use of combined oral contraceptives in premenopausal women is that these contraceptives reduce the risk of
(A) Deep vein thrombosis
(B) Episodes of migraine headache
(C) Ischemic stroke
(D) Ovarian cancer
(E) Pituitary adenoma

98. Hypercoagulability and dermal vascular necrosis resulting from protein C deficiency is known to be an early-appearing adverse effect of treatment with
(A) Aspirin
(B) Clopidogrel
(C) Heparin
(D) Streptokinase
(E) Warfarin

99. A 45-year-old woman suffers from abdominal pain and bloody diarrhea that has been diagnosed as Crohn's disease. A first-line drug for treatment of Crohn's disease that acts locally in the gastrointestinal tract to provide an anti-inflammatory effect is
(A) Aluminum hydroxide
(B) Metoclopramide

(C) Misoprostol
(D) Mesalamine
(E) Ranitidine

100. A 24-year-old man with a history of partial seizures has been treated with standard anticonvulsants for several years. He is currently taking valproic acid, which is not fully effective, and his neurologist prescribes a new drug approved for adjunctive use in partial seizures. Unfortunately, the patient develops toxic epidermal necrolysis. The new drug prescribed was
(A) Felbamate
(B) Gabapentin
(C) Lamotrigine
(D) Tiagabine
(E) Vigabatrin

101. The introduction of this drug may represent a novel approach to the treatment of major depressive disorders because it appears to act as an antagonist at α_2 adrenoceptors in the CNS.
(A) Amoxapine
(B) Bupropion
(C) Citalopram
(D) Mirtazapine
(E) Paroxetine

102. A drug that is commonly given as an intravenous bolus for the purpose of converting AV nodal arrhythmias to normal sinus rhythm is
(A) Adenosine
(B) Amiodarone
(C) Lidocaine
(D) Quinidine
(E) Sotalol

103. Which one of the following pairs of drug and indication is accurate?
(A) Amphetamine: Alzheimer's dementia
(B) Bupropion: acute anxiety
(C) Fluoxetine: insomnia
(D) Ropinirole: Parkinson's disease
(E) Trazodone: attention deficit disorder

104. Which one of the following toxic compounds is correctly paired with an antidote that is used in the treatment of a patient poisoned with the toxic compound?
(A) Acetaminophen: vitamin K
(B) Beta-blocker: dobutamine
(C) Ethanol: methanol
(D) Cyanide: sodium nitrite
(E) Tricyclic antidepressants: physostigmine

105. This cell cycle-nonspecific agent is commonly used as a component of cancer chemotherapy

regimens, including those for non-Hodgkin's lymphoma and for breast cancers; administration of mercaptoethanesulfonate (mesna) decreases the risk of hematuria.
(A) Cyclophosphamide
(B) Cytarabine
(C) Fluorouracil
(D) Methotrexate
(E) Vinblastine

106. Ganciclovir has much greater activity than acyclovir against
(A) Cytomegalovirus
(B) Hepatitis B virus
(C) Herpes simplex virus
(D) HIV
(E) Influenza A virus

107. Standard chemoprophylaxis of vivax and ovale malaria does not eradicate liver hypnozoite forms. To reduce the likelihood of a relapse after completion of travel to an endemic area, most authorities recommend the use of
(A) Atovaquone
(B) Chloroquine
(C) Mefloquine
(D) Primaquine
(E) Quinine

108. A cell cycle-specific anticancer drug that acts in the M-phase of the cell cycle to prevent disassembly of the mitotic spindle is
(A) Dactinomycin
(B) Etoposide
(C) Paclitaxel
(D) Procarbazine
(E) Vinblastine

109. The dose of this immunosuppressive prodrug must be significantly reduced in patients who are also taking the xanthine oxidase inhibitor allopurinol.
(A) Azathioprine
(B) Cyclosporine
(C) Hydroxychloroquine
(D) Methotrexate
(E) Tacrolimus

110. A 57-year-old man presented with signs and symptoms of acute gout that included intense pain in the first metatarsophalangeal joint of his right big toe of 1 day's duration and a joint that was swollen, tender, and red. Examination of synovial fluid removed from the joint revealed crystals of uric acid. The patient had a serum uric acid concentration of 10 mg/dL (normal 3.0–8.2 mg/dL). This was the patient's first episode of gout. He did not have any other medical illnesses and was not taking any medications. The drug that is most

appropriate for immediate treatment of this acute attack of gout is
(A) Allopurinol
(B) Indomethacin
(C) Methotrexate
(D) Morphine
(E) Probenicid

111. A cytokine that appears to play a central role in the pathogenesis of rheumatoid arthritis and is a target of drugs like etanercept is
(A) Cyclophilin
(B) Granulocyte colony-stimulating factor (G-CSF)
(C) Interferon-α
(D) Interleukin-11 (IL-11)
(E) Tumor necrosis factor-α (TNF-α)

112. A newborn was diagnosed as having a congenital abnormality that resulted in transposition of her great arteries. While preparing the infant for surgery, the medical team needed to keep the ductus arteriosus open. They did this by infusing
(A) Cortisol
(B) Indomethacin
(C) Ketorolac
(D) Misoprostol
(E) Tacrolimus

113. A 42-year-old woman developed a syndrome of polyuria, thirst, and hypernatremia after surgical removal of part of her pituitary gland. These signs and symptoms will be treated with
(A) Bromocriptine
(B) Desmopressin
(C) Octreotide
(D) Prednisone
(E) Somatropin

114. Relative to Lugol's solution, propylthiouracil has
(A) A faster onset of antithyroid action
(B) A greater inhibitory effect on the proteolytic release of hormones from the thyroid gland
(C) Increased likelihood of causing exophthalmos during the first week of treatment
(D) Increased risk of fetal toxicity
(E) More sustained antithyroid activity when used continuously for several months

115. Regarding verapamil, which one of the following statements is most accurate?
(A) Chronic heart failure is an important indication for the use of verapamil
(B) Contraindicated in the asthmatic patient
(C) Contracts intestinal smooth muscle
(D) Prolongs the repolarization phase of the action potential in AV nodal cells
(E) Used in management of supraventricular tachycardias

116. A 54-year-old woman was found to have node-positive breast cancer. Following her surgery, she was treated with a drug that prevents the conversion of testosterone to estradiol. The drug was

(A) Anastrozole
(B) Ethinyl estradiol
(C) Finasteride
(D) Spironolactone
(E) Tamoxifen

117. The drug that is most likely to cause hypoglycemia when used as monotherapy in the treatment of a patient with type 2 diabetes is

(A) Acarbose
(B) Glipizide
(C) Metformin
(D) Miglitol
(E) Rosiglitazone

118. Anticoagulation is needed immediately in a patient with deep vein thrombosis. The patient has a history of heparin-induced thrombocytopenia. The most appropriate drug for parenteral administration in this patient is

(A) Clopidogrel
(B) Lepirudin
(C) Ticlopidine
(D) Unfractionated heparin
(E) Warfarin

119–120. A drug (Drug 1) was given as an IV bolus to a subject while blood pressure and heart rate were recorded as shown on the left side of the graph below. After recovery from the effects of Drug 1, a long-acting dose of Drug 2 was given. After the recorder was turned back on, Drug 1 was repeated with the results shown on the right side of the graph.

119. Identify Drug 1 from the following list.

(A) Angiotensin
(B) Endothelin
(C) Epinephrine
(D) Guanethidine
(E) Hexamethonium
(F) Isoproterenol
(G) Norepinephrine
(H) Phenylephrine
(I) Prazosin
(J) Propranolol

120. Identify Drug 2 from the following list.

(A) Angiotensin
(B) Endothelin
(C) Epinephrine
(D) Guanethidine
(E) Hexamethonium
(F) Isoproterenol
(G) Norepinephrine
(H) Phenylephrine
(I) Prazosin
(J) Propranolol

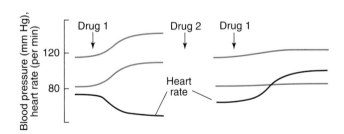

ANSWER KEY FOR EXAMINATION 2*

1. E (7, 31)	**31.** E (18)	**61.** C (25)	**91.** E (31)
2. B (19)	**32.** B (20)	**62.** A (31)	**92.** C (35)
3. C (1, 3)	**33.** A (20)	**63.** C (23)	**93.** D (34)
4. C (2)	**34.** E (26)	**64.** C (9, 30, 62)	**94.** D (33)
5. B (3)	**35.** C (25, 27)	**65.** D (27)	**95.** A (35)
6. E (5)	**36.** C (34)	**66.** B (7, 8, 27)	**96.** B (9, 10)
7. A (6, 8, 9)	**37.** C (33)	**67.** B (29)	**97.** D (40)
8. B (6)	**38.** E (50)	**68.** E (30, 31)	**98.** E (34)
9. B (10)	**39.** B (48)	**69.** C (28)	**99.** D (60)
10. C (9)	**40.** C (49)	**70.** B (22)	**100.** C (24)
11. D (4, 23, 36)	**41.** B (54)	**71.** D (43, 46)	**101.** D (30)
12. C (4)	**42.** E (53)	**72.** A (44)	**102.** A (14)
13. C (12)	**43.** A (41)	**73.** B (45)	**103.** D (28)
14. E (12)	**44.** C (56)	**74.** D (44)	**104.** D (59)
15. B (7)	**45.** C (57)	**75.** B (39)	**105.** A (55)
16. B (60)	**46.** E (47, 62)	**76.** B (42)	**106.** A (49)
17. D (10)	**47.** B (58, 59)	**77.** C (44, 47)	**107.** D (53)
18. A (13)	**48.** C (6, 9)	**78.** E (49)	**108.** C (55)
19. A (13, 59)	**49.** C (11, 15)	**79.** B (43, 44, 46)	**109.** A (55, 56)
20. B (11)	**50.** B (27)	**80.** E (43, 44, 46)	**110.** B (36)
21. D (11)	**51.** D (21, 28)	**81.** B (49)	**111.** E (33, 36, 56)
22. E (60)	**52.** B (21, 24)	**82.** C (48)	**112.** D (18)
23. E (15)	**53.** D (22, 32)	**83.** E (55)	**113.** B (37)
24. B (9, 14, 16)	**54.** B (22, 30)	**84.** C (55)	**114.** E (38)
25. B (11)	**55.** A (23)	**85.** D (37)	**115.** E (12, 14)
26. B (14)	**56.** D (24)	**86.** C (40)	**116.** A (40, 55)
27. C (10, 11)	**57.** B (24)	**87.** B (43, 51)	**117.** B (41)
28. E (15, 42)	**58.** E (26)	**88.** D (16)	**118.** B (34)
29. B (15)	**59.** E (32)	**89.** A (13)	**119.** G (9, 10)
30. C (17)	**60.** D (27)	**90.** D (38)	**120.** I (10)

*Numbers in parentheses are chapters in which answers are found.

Appendix IV

Strategies for Improving Test Performance

There are many strategies for studying and exam taking, and decisions about which ones to use are partly a function of individual habit and preference. However, basic study rules may be applied to any learning exercise; test-taking strategies depend on the type of examination. For those interested in test-*writing* strategies, the Case and Swanson reference is strongly recommended (see References).

FIVE BASIC STUDY RULES

1. When studying dense textual material, stop after a few pages to write out the gist of it from memory. If necessary, refer to the material just read. After finishing a chapter, construct your own tables of the major drugs, receptor types, mechanisms, and so on, and fill in as many of the blanks as you can. Refer to tables and figures in the book as needed to complete your notes. Create your own mnemonics if possible. Look up other mnemonics in books if you can't think of one yourself. These are all active learning techniques; mere reading is passive and far less effective unless you happen to have a photographic memory. Your notes should be legible or typed on a computer, and saved for ready access when reviewing for exams.

2. Experiment with other study methods until you find out what works for you. This may involve solo study or group study, flash cards, or text reading. You won't know how effective these techniques are until you have tried them.

3. Don't scorn "cramming," but don't rely on it either. Some steady, day-by-day reading and digestion of conceptual material is usually needed to avoid last-minute indigestion. Similarly, don't substitute memorization of lists (eg, the Key Words list, Appendix I) for more substantive understanding.

4. If you are preparing for a course examination, make every effort to attend all the lectures. The lecturer's view of what is important may be quite different from that of the author of a course textbook, and chances are good that exam questions will be based on the instructor's own lecture notes.

5. If old test questions are legitimately available (as they are for the USMLE and courses in most medical schools), make use of these guides to study. By definition, they are a strong indicator of what the examination writers have considered core information in the recent past (also see Point 4).

STRATEGIES APPLICABLE TO ALL EXAMINATIONS

Three general rules apply to all examinations.

1. When starting the examination, scan the entire question set before answering any. If the examination has several parts, allot time to each part in proportion to its length. Within each part, answer the easy questions first, placing a mark in the margin by the questions to which you will return. Practice saving enough time for the more difficult questions by scheduling 1 minute or less for each question on practice examinations such as those in Appendices II and III in this book. (The time available in the USMLE examination is approximately 55–60 seconds per question.)

2. Students are often advised to avoid changing their first guess on multiple-choice questions. However, research has shown that students who are unsure of the answer to a question make a change from the incorrect answer to the correct answer about 55% of the time. So if you are unsure of your first choice for a particular question and on further reflection

see an answer that looks better, research supports your making one—but only one—change.

3. Understand the method for scoring wrong answers. The USMLE does not penalize for wrong answers; it scores you only on the total number of correct answers. Therefore, even if you have no idea as to the correct answer, make a guess anyway; there is no penalty for an incorrect answer. In other words, *do not leave any blanks on a USMLE answer sheet or computer screen.* Note that this may not be true for some local examinations; some scoring algorithms do penalize for incorrect answers. Make sure you understand the rules for such local examinations.

STRATEGIES FOR SPECIFIC QUESTION FORMATS

A certain group of students—often characterized as "good test-takers"—may not know every detail about the subject matter being tested but seem to perform extremely well most of the time. The strategy used by these people is not a secret, although few instructors seem to realize how easy it is to break down their questions into much simpler ones. Lists of these strategies are widely available (eg, in the descriptive material distributed by the National Board of Medical Examiners to its candidates). A paraphrased compendium of this advice is presented next.

A. Strategies for the "Choose the One Best Answer" (of 5 Choices) Type Question

1. Many of the newer "clinical correlation" questions on the Board exam have an extremely long stem that provides a great deal of clinical data. Much of the data presented may be irrelevant. The challenge becomes one of *finding out what is being asked*. One method for rapidly narrowing the search is to scan the answer list *first* when confronted with a very long stem. The nature of the answers will provide a clue to the parts of the stem that are relevant and those that are not.

2. If 2 statements are contradictory (ie, only 1 can be correct), chances are good that 1 of the 2 is the correct answer (ie, the other 3 choices may be distracters). For example, consider the following:

1. In treating quinidine overdose, the best strategy would be to
   (A) Acidify the urine
   (B) Administer a calcium chelator such as EDTA
   (C) Alkalinize the urine
   (D) Give potassium chloride
   (E) Give procainamide

The correct answer is **A**: acidify the urine. In the pair of contradictory statements (choices A and C), the

instructor revealed what was being tested and then used the other three as "filler." Therefore, if you don't know the answer, you are better off guessing **A** or **C** (a 50% success probability) than **A** or **B** or **C** or **D** or **E** (a 20% success probability). Note that this strategy is only valid if you **must** guess; many instructors now introduce contradictory pairs as distracters. Another "rule" that should only be used if you must guess is the "longest choice" rule. When all the answers in a multiple-choice question are relatively long, the correct answer is often the longest one. Note again that sophisticated question writers may introduce especially long **incorrect** choices to foil this strategy.

3. Statements that contain the words "always," "never," "must," and so on are usually false. For example,

Acetylcholine always increases the heart rate when given intravenously because it lowers blood pressure and evokes a strong baroreceptor-mediated reflex tachycardia.

The statement is false because, although acetylcholine often increases the heart rate, it can also cause bradycardia. (When given as a bolus, it may reach the sinus node in high enough concentration to cause initial bradycardia.) The use of trigger words such as "always" and "must" suggests that the instructor had some exception in mind. However, be aware that there are a few situations in which the statement with a trigger word is correct.

4. Choices that do not fit the stem grammatically are usually wrong. For example,

1. *A drug that acts on a β receptor and produces a maximal effect that is equal to one half the effect of a large dose of isoproterenol is called a*
   (A) Agonist
   (B) Analog of isoproterenol
   (C) Antagonist
   (D) Partial agonist

The use of the article *a* at the end of the stem rather than *an* implies that the answer must start with a consonant (ie, choice **D**). Similar use may be made of disagreements in number. Note that careful question writers will avoid this problem by placing the articles in the choice list, not in the stem.

5. A statement is not false just because changing a few words will make it somewhat more true than you think it is now. "Choose the one best answer" does not mean "Choose the only correct statement."

B. Strategies for "All of the Following Are Accurate Except" Questions

1. This type of question is largely avoided now on the USMLE because of problems with ambiguity;

however, this type still is used in many local examinations because question-writers perceive them to be relatively easier to construct. When faced with this type of question, approach it as a nested set of true/false questions in which (hopefully) only one is true. It may help to mark each choice as either "T" or "F" as you read through them.

2. If 2 statements are contradictory, then 1 of them is certain to be the correct (false) answer because they cannot both be accurate statements, and yet this type of question cannot have 2 false answers. For example, consider the following:

1. All of the following may result from the use of thiazide diuretics EXCEPT
   (A) Hyperglycemia
   (B) Hypernatremia
   (C) Hyponatremia
   (D) Hyperuricemia
   (E) Metabolic alkalosis

The correct answer is **B:** hypernatremia. The possibility that thiazide diuretics do not affect serum sodium concentrations is not tenable because that would produce 2 false choices. It is also highly unlikely that a drug could cause 2 opposite effects; therefore, the probability that 1 of the opposites is the correct (false) answer is extremely high.

3. If the choices contain 2 drugs that are highly similar, then neither is likely to be the correct (false) answer. For example, consider the following:

1. *A young man who had become physiologically dependent after illicit use of secobarbital is undergoing severe withdrawal symptoms, including nausea, vomiting, delirium, and periodic seizures. Which one of the following drugs will NOT alleviate these symptoms?*
   (A) Buspirone
   (B) Chlordiazepoxide
   (C) Diazepam
   (D) Midazolam
   (E) Phenobarbital

The correct answer is **A:** buspirone. If you recognize that chlordiazepoxide, diazepam, and midazolam are all benzodiazepine drugs with virtually identical pharmacologic effects, then you can quite safely rule out all three of them.

C. STRATEGIES FOR MATCHING TYPE QUESTIONS

Matching questions usually test name recognition, and the most efficient approach consists of reading each stem item and then scanning the list of choices from the start and picking the first clear "hit." This is especially important on extended matching questions in which just reading the list can be time consuming. (It should

be noted, however, that the strategy suggested by the National Board of Medical Examiners for the USMLE differs from the above; see their *General Instructions* publication.) Occasionally, the strategies described above for the single best answer type question can be applied to the matching and extended matching type.

D. STRATEGIES FOR THE "ANSWER A IF 1, 2, AND 3 ARE CORRECT" TYPE QUESTION

This type of question, known as the "K type," has been dropped from the USMLE and, therefore, is no longer represented among the practice questions provided in this review book. However, it is still used in some local examinations.

For this type of question, one rarely must know the truth about all 4 statements to arrive at the correct answer. The instructions are to select
   (A) if only (1), (2), and (3) are correct;
   (B) if only (1) and (3) are correct;
   (C) if only (2) and (4) are correct;
   (D) if only (4) is correct;
   (E) if all are correct.

Useful strategies include the following:

1. If statement 1 is correct and 2 is wrong, the answer must be **B** (ie, 1 and 3 are correct). You don't need to know anything about 3 or 4.

2. If statement 1 is wrong, then answers **A, B,** and **E** are automatically excluded. Concentrate on statements 2 and 4.

3. The converse of 1 above: If choice 1 is wrong and 2 is correct, the answer must be **C** (ie, 2 and 4 are correct).

4. If statement 2 is correct and 4 is wrong, the answer is **A** (ie, 1 and 3 must be correct and you need not even look at them). (See example below.)

5. If statements 1, 2, and 4 are correct, the answer must be **E.** You need not know anything about 3.

6. Similarly, if statements 2 and 3 are correct and 4 is wrong, the answer must be **A,** and statement 1 must be correct.

7. If statements 2, 3, and 4 are correct, then the answer must be **E,** and statement 1 must be correct.

No doubt more of these rules exist. In general, if you know whether 2 or 3 of the 4 statements in each question are right or wrong (ie, 50–75% the material), you should achieve a perfect score on this kind of question. The best way to learn these rules is to apply them to practice questions until the principles are firmly ingrained.

Consider the following question. Using the above rules, you should be able to answer it correctly even though there is no reason why you should know anything about the information contained in 2 of the 4 statements. The answer follows.

Which of the following statements is (are) correct?

1. The "struck bushel" is equal to 2150.42 cubic inches.

2. Medicine is one of the health sciences.

3. The fresh meat of the Atlantic salmon contains 220 IU of vitamin A per 100 g edible portion.

4. Hippocrates was the founder of modern psychoanalysis.

The answer is **A.** Because statement 2 is clearly correct and 4 is just as patently incorrect (let's give Freud the credit), the answer can only be **A,** and statements 1 and 3 must be correct. (The data are from Lentner C, editor: *Geigy Scientific Tables,* 8th ed. Vol. 1. Ciba-Geigy, 1981.)

REFERENCES

Bhushan V, Le T: *First Aid for the USMLE STEP 1 2007.* McGraw-Hill, 2006.

Case SM, Swanson DB: *Constructing Written Test Questions for the Basic and Clinical Sciences,* 2nd ed. National Board of Medical Examiners, 1998. Available only from the World Wide Web (www.nbme.org; Guide for Writing Test Items).

Fischer MR, Herrmann S, Kopp V: Answering multiple-choice questions in high-stakes medical examinations. Medical Education 2005;39:890.

Step 1 content description and sample test materials. National Board of Medical Examiners, 2007. Available from the USMLE World Wide Web page at www.usmle.org.

Subject Index

NOTE: Page numbers in **boldface** indicate a major discussion. Page numbers followed by *f* and *t* indicate figures and tables, respectively. A *b* following a page number indicates a boxed feature.